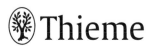

Herbal Medicine

Third Edition

Volker Fintelmann, MD
Professor
Specialist for Internal Medicine
Formerly Member and Chairman of the Commission E
Hamburg, Germany

Rudolf Fritz Weiss†, MD
Formerly Professor of Phytotherapy
University of Tübingen
Professor h.c.
Member of the Commission E
Tübingen, Germany

Kenny Kuchta, PhD, FLS
Professor h.c.
Zhejiang Institute of TCM and Natural Medicine,
Hangzhou, China;
Forschungsstelle für Fernöstliche Medizin（漢方医学研究拠点）
Department of Vegetation Analysis and Phytodiversity
Albrecht von Haller Institute of Plant Sciences
Georg August University
Göttingen, Germany

117 illustrations

Thieme
Stuttgart • New York • Delhi • Rio de Janeiro

Library of Congress Cataloging-in-Publication Data is available from the publisher.

This book is an authorized and revised translation of the 13th German edition published and copyrighted 2016 by Karl F. Haug Verlag in Georg Thieme Verlag KG, Stuttgart, Germany. Title of the German edition: Lehrbuch Phytotherapie.

Translator: Johanna Cummings-Pertl
Hopland, California, USA

Photographer: © Dr. Roland Spohn, Engen

Important note: Medicine is an ever-changing science undergoing continual development. Research and clinical experience are continually expanding our knowledge, in particular our knowledge of proper treatment and drug therapy. Insofar as this book mentions any dosage or application, readersmay rest assured that the authors, editors, and publishers have made every effort to ensure that such references are in accordance with **the state of knowledge at the time of production of the book.**

Nevertheless, this does not involve, imply, or express any guarantee or responsibility on the part of the publishers in respect to any dosage instructions and forms of applications stated in the book. **Every user is requested to examine carefully** the manufacturers' leaflets accompanying each drug and to check, if necessary in consultation with a physician or specialist, whether the dosage schedules mentioned therein or the contraindications stated by the manufacturers differ from the statements made in the present book. Such examination is particularly important with drugs that are either rarely used or have been newly released on the market. Every dosage schedule or every form of application used is entirely at the user's own risk and responsibility. The authors and publishers request every user to report to the publishers any discrepancies or inaccuracies noticed. If errors in this work are found after publication, errata will be posted at www.thieme.com on the product description page.

Some of the product names, patents, and registered designs referred to in this book are in fact registered trademarks or proprietary names even though specific reference to this fact is not always made in the text. Therefore, the appearance of a name without designation as proprietary is not to be construed as a representation by the publisher that it is in the public domain. Thieme addresses people of all gender identities equally. We encourage our authors to use gender-neutral or gender-equal expressions wherever the context allows.

Thieme Publishers Stuttgart
Rüdigerstrasse 14, 70469 Stuttgart, Germany
+49 [0]711 8931 421, customerservice@thieme.de

Cover design: © Thieme Publishing Group
Cover photo: Dr. Roland Spohn, Engen
Typesetting by TNQ Technologies, India

Printed in Germany by Westermann Druck Zwickau GmbH

5 4 3 2 1

DOI: 10.1055/b000000219

ISBN: 978-3-13-241423-5

Also available as an e-book:
eISBN (PDF): 978-3-13-241424-2
eISBN (epub): 978-3-13-258233-0

In Memoriam

Rudolf Fritz Weiss (1895–1991)

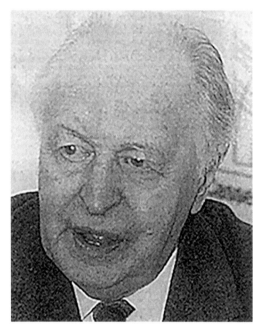

Prof. Dr. med. Rudolf Fritz Weiss

Rudolf Fritz Weiss was born on 28 July 1895 in Berlin-Charlottenburg, Germany. In his own words, he felt drawn to "botany, floristics, and plant biography" from an early age. Even as a youth, he was an eager collector of the local flora and created his own comprehensive herbarium. This enabled him early on to develop a firm understanding of plants based on his immediate experience in nature. After he graduated from high school, he studied human medicine and botany at the University of Berlin. After receiving his medical license in 1922, he began specialty training to become an internist at the famous Berlin Charité hospital. As of 1931, Weiss taught plant medicine at the Akademie für Ärztliche Fortbildung (Academy for Continuing Medical Education) in Berlin. From 1939–1945, Weiss was head physician of the internal medicine department at the Berlin-Britz hospital, and as a medical officer of the reserve, he was responsible for the military rehabilitation branch at that hospital. For seven years, from 1945–1952, Weiss was a prisoner of war in the Soviet Union. During this period, he provided intensive medical care for his fellow prisoners. His profound knowledge of plants was very helpful during this time. It enabled him to collect the medicinal plants he was able to find in the prisoner compounds and to use them as medicine in their simplest form. In 1987, he was awarded the 1st Class Order of Merit of the Federal Republic of Germany (Bundesverdienstkreuz 1. Klasse) for his tireless and immense medical service by Richard von Weizsäcker, the then president of the Federal Republic of Germany.

In 1952, Weiss established his internal medicine practice in Hannover, where he practiced until 1961. He then moved to Aitrach in the Bavarian Allgäu region to dedicate himself entirely to his scientific work. From 1978–1990, he was a permanent member of the commission responsible for the authorization and processing of herbal drugs for human use, commonly known as Commission E, at the German Federal Ministry of Health. In 1984, at the age of 88, he took on a teaching assignment at the pharmaceutical faculty of the University of Tübingen and lectured in "modern phytotherapy in practice."

Weiss's mission was to provide a scientific rationale for plant medicine, for which he later used the term "phytotherapy," in reference to the term coined by the French physician Henry Leclerc. Weiss considered it essential that this scientific development of modern phytotherapy was carried out by practicing and clinical physicians. At the same time, he also valued the more theoretical work of pharmacists and medical historians. His life goal was the recognition of phytotherapy as an indispensable component of medicine. He tirelessly devoted his almost 100-year-long life to this goal.

At the urging of his students, his many years of lectures at the Akademie für Ärztliche Fortbildung (Academy for Continuing Medical Education) in Berlin were collected in the book *Pflanzenheilkunde in der ärztlichen Praxis* (Herbal Medicine in Medical Practice), which was published in 1944 by the Hippokrates-Verlag Marquardt & Cie, Stuttgart. In the ensuing years, he developed it into his textbook on herbal medicine, *Lehrbuch der Phytotherapie*, which is considered a classic in phytotherapy literature. He guided the textbook's publication through its sixth edition in 1985, which formed the basis for the textbook's first English edition, published in 1988.

In his foreword to the 1944 edition, Weiss states that the book is based on a purely medical viewpoint, and that the content is determined by practical medical experience in treating patients in accordance with scientific knowledge. In 1980, Weiss founded the magazine *Zeitschrift für Phytotherapie* (Journal of Phytotherapy), which he published for an extended period. He published more than 100 original articles and various monographs, including *Das neue große Kneippbuch* (The New and Comprehensive Kneipp Book) and the follow-on publication *Das große Kräuterheilbuch des Pfarrers Künzle* (A Comprehensive Guide to the Herbal Medicine of Pastor Künzle).

Rudolf Fritz Weiss, together with the thorough scientific work of some university pharmacists, can be credited with enabling phytotherapy to take its place within modern medicine. He was by far the most profound expert in this line of therapy. His lectures and writings were always based on extensive practical experience and in consensus with scientifically oriented medicine ("Western medicine") of which he viewed phytotherapy a part. In 1985, he was awarded the title "Professor" for his groundbreaking work, his tireless battles on behalf of phytotherapy, and his diligence in medical training and further education by Lothar Späth, the then governor of the German state of Baden-Württemberg. Weiss was exceptionally physically fit and mentally and spiritually active well into advanced age, and until shortly before his death. Even after he was partially blind, he was able to guide me through his garden in "Vogelherd" and show me all his plant treasures, which were growing wild, without specific botanical order, but extremely healthy. Rudolf Fritz Weiss died on 27 November 1991 in Memmingen, Germany.

In the history of medicine, he will be honored as one of the most distinguished physicians of the 20th century.

Volker Fintelmann

Contents

Contents

Contents

Preface

The 3rd English edition of *Herbal Medicine* is based on the content of the 13th German edition of *Lehrbuch Phytotherapie* that was published in 2016. This edition is the first to be published together with my coauthor, Kenny Kuchta, with whom I entrusted the main responsibility for its pharmaceutical content. He was already very familiar with the entire content of the book due to his work on its recent Japanese edition. In this current edition, he initiated the decisions to include several new plants and the reinstatement of some plants that had been withdrawn from previous editions based on the findings of contemporary scientific research. Furthermore, he reworked and updated both the content and the corresponding references of the chapter on drug interactions, which now represents the state of the art on this topic in our book. He also critically proofread the English translation in close coordination with the publisher. Over the past years, we have developed a very trusting collaboration.

The development of medicine in the 21st century, an essential topic already described in the 2nd edition by Mark Blumenthal in the Foreword and by me in the Preface, remains the scope of this edition. Phytotherapy concedes its therapeutic effect to the consequence of the pharmacological effects of the chemical constituents of medicinal plant extracts; its guiding principle is, therefore, the same scientific method as that of the natural sciences. Just as in chemical pharmacotherapy, phytotherapy is based not on speculation but on observed and empirically documentable effects. However, phytotherapy methodically makes the observable—the observation—the starting point of further cognition. In doing so, it lays claim to a holism that has, unfortunately, been largely lost in the past half century through the objectification of standard therapy.

Herbal medicinal products, based on a sound footing in pharmaceutical science, should guide prescribing therapists, especially medical doctors, back to an understanding of their patients as whole human beings. In this context, the medicinal plant should not be seen reductively as an interesting supplier of various substances, but as a complex entity that starts to correspond with the human body and primarily interacts with the body's autoregulatory mechanisms. Beyond an interest in pure scientific knowledge, contemplating the therapeutic properties pertaining to any specific medicinal plant will give the therapist empathy toward its innate, creative, and healing principles. This empathy should then be directed toward the human being and contribute in a major way to therapeutic effectiveness.

Going forward, the view that limits herbal drugs to the purely objective criterion of efficacy and restricts the view of the human body to its states of health and sickness, will not suffice. One's subjective state of health, mood, and presence of mind are also part of human nature. Future medical strategies, even those with a pronounced scientific approach like phytotherapy, need to address these issues in order for them to be humane, i.e., fit for humans. It stands to reason that such an integrative and individualized holistic practice of medicine will be able to restore the bond between doctor and patient that we are in danger of losing in the increasing objectification of standard therapy.

Further, the importance of prevention should be rediscovered and implemented in therapy. It is characteristic of medicinal plant extracts to act, by and large, in synergy with the physiological self-regenerative processes of the human body, not to counteract them as is typical for many synthetic chemical compounds. This characteristic also accounts for the comparatively low occurrence of side effects associated with medicinal plant extracts. It is my deep conviction that the medical sciences will need to shift their attention from the treatment of diseases to the preservation of health (i.e., prevention) in order to remain of continuous benefit.

Please note that in order to enhance readability, the binomial nomenclature in this edition has not been presented in italics as per standard style. I wish to thank the publisher, and especially Angelika-Marie Findgott, the editor responsible for this 3rd edition, and my coauthor Kenny Kuchta, for their good work.

I hope that our book will find an interested and engaged readership and one that actively participates in establishing medicinal plant therapy in the future as an accepted component of a humane and individualized medicine.

Volker Fintelmann

Part 1

Introduction

1

1 What Is Phytotherapy?

Phytotherapy encompasses the application of botanical medicine for the prevention, treatment, and healing of disease. Its basic principles are often difficult to extrapolate due to the manifold effects of phytotherapeutics. This is compounded by the fact that the combined effects of its constituents cannot yet be sufficiently assessed through scientific studies. In the words of Johann Wolfgang von Goethe: "To know and note the living, you'll find it best to first dispense with the spirit: Then with the pieces in your hand, Ah! You've only lost the spiritual bond" (Faust, act 1, scene 4).

This chapter describes the basic requirements for "modern" phytotherapy. Based on contemporary research, it seeks to overcome the impossibility postulated by Goethe of connecting the spirit with its individual constituents, which is what makes phytotherapy such an important therapeutic modality.

1.1 Definition

The term phytotherapy describes the use of plants and parts of plants, such as leaves, flowers, roots, fruits, or seeds and their preparations for the prevention and treatment of diseases and health issues. Plants suited to this application have traditionally been referred to as **medicinal plants**. Of key importance is the fact that the medicinal plant or its parts are used as a holistic substance. Plant medicines therefore always represent **multicomponent mixtures.** In numerous countries, the quality, effectiveness, and safety of plant medicines must meet the requirements of national drug legislation—for example, in Germany, the Medicininal Products Act (Arzneimittelgesetz—AMG).

The application of isolated, chemically defined constituents derived from plants falls outside of the definition of phytotherapy according to the current AMG. Such products are instead aptly labeled as "natural products as medicines." Weiss accepted this approach as a part of phytotherapy and classified isolated active constituents as *Forte-Phytotherapeutics* (powerful phytotherapy). However, according to the definition of the Commission E of the German Federal Ministry of Health, which has jurisdiction over phytotherapy, the application of isolated plant constituents no longer represents phytotherapy. For example, digitalis glycosides such as digoxin or digitoxin extracted from foxglove

(Digitalis purpurea, Digitalis lanata) were categorized as phytotherapy in several of the initial German editions of this book. Chemically or synthetically altered derivatives such as acetyl or methyl digoxin, however, are not classified as phytotherapy under any definition because they do not occur "in nature" in this form. In addition, constituents formerly isolated from plants are today primarily chemically synthesized and the source material frequently no longer has any connection with the original medicinal plant.

1.1.1 Constituents and Structural Composition

Understanding phytotherapy seems to require viewing the specific combination of constituents of a whole plant as a **compositional secret**. What von Goethe recognized as an "open secret" also applies to understanding medicinal plants. Today's physiochemical processes enable us to analyze a plant or its constituents down to the finest detail. However, this analysis does explain the often incredible diversity of constituents of a single plant or how the plant continuously maintains its characteristic wholeness even though its composition constantly changes with the seasons, growth environment, geological conditions, and other factors. The structural composition of a medicinal plant, can be quantitatively verified, but plants also exhibit a qualitative nature that eludes absolute proof and can only be described.

Nowadays, the natural sciences frequently reduce the spiritual foundational principle referred to in the von Goethe quote above to genetics. No doubt genes are an important physical prerequisite for the survival of a species. It is important to remember, though, that genes are "composed" or created according to their specificity and type of articulation. Musicians also compose symphonies according to the rules of intervals, keys, and rhythms. Even though these are identical for each composer, each finished composition is unique and carries an individual "signature." A musical expert can listen to a composition and recognize its creator, the composer. In the same way, plant experts can employ pharmacognosy to identify a plant from the whole plant down to its specific composition.

The goal of phytotherapy is not only to discover the plant, its growing conditions, and its constituents, but also its composition and thereby its **singularity**, the property that differentiates it from all others. Detailed knowledge of the composition of a plant must be in tune with the discovery of its compositional secret, the "spiritual bond."

1.1.2 Phytotherapy and Herbal Medicine

Phytotherapy is only one part of the comprehensive field of herbal medicine, which includes phytochemistry, phytopharmacy, and phytopharmacology, and phytotherapy.

Phytochemistry exclusively studies the constituents (chemicals) in plants. Its mission is to identify the chemical composition of plants, verify, or control its fingerprint, and to describe potential constituents that can be examined pharmacologically for its effects. The atomistic view of phytochemistry is focused solely on the parts and not the whole. Phytochemistry provides the impulse to examine active constituents for their potential to be synthesized in order to become independent from harvesting in nature.

Phytopharmacy focuses on the drug that provides the basis for an herbal medicinal, and how it is used directly, for example, in teas or in various forms of pharmaceutically prepared extracts. Descriptions of plants in this book name the associated pharmaceutical drug. Pharmacognosy, or the identification of a drug through visual inspection, is an important part of phytopharmacy. In the past, pharmacognosists identified plants by looking at, touching, tasting, and smelling the plant. This approach to identifying and determining the quality of a medicinal plant can still be important. However, in the meantime, highly specialized physiochemical analysis methods are the preferred method of identifying drugs. It is not unusual for a pharmacist to know and be able to differentiate the entire fingerprint of a medicinal herb, but to no longer be able to recognize the plant in nature. There are now many pharmacologists in pharmaceutical university faculties who examine the pharmacokinetics and pharmacodynamics of medicinal plants under a primary pharmaceutical point of view.

Medical schools are still in the beginning stages of recognizing **phytopharmacology** as a specific field of study. An increasing number of pharmacologists study plant constituents, but they rarely practice the specific task of analyzing the pharmacokinetics and pharmacodynamics of multichemical and polychemical compositions. This monocausal approach to medicine seems to impede a shift in thinking. Clinical pharmacology, the stepchild of pharmacology, could certainly play a significant role in assessing the efficacy of phytotherapeutics. Phytotherapeutics are known more for their comprehensive efficacy than for their specialized effects. Therefore, they should be studied directly in human trials because transferring the results of animal trials of these multicomponent substances to humans is much more problematic than for defined isolated synthetic constituents. The same applies to manifold questions of toxicology. Frequently, risks of medicinal plants are cited in an entirely unscientific manner based on a purely theoretical background or self-selected paradigm even though these results have not been observed in humans.

Phytotherapy is the fourth component of the comprehensive field of herbal medicine. It describes the possibilities and limitations of using medicinal plants to treat indications in human medicine. It belongs primarily in the hands of physicians or other therapists such as chiropractors, physical therapists, nursing professionals, or—especially in the legal framework of the United States—certified herbalists and naturopaths, using herbal medicine. Many phytopharmaceuticals are also suited for self-medication, especially in a preventive sense.

Practicing pharmacists play an important advisory role in this context. For this reason, the possibilities and limitations of phytotherapy should be covered even more comprehensively in the education of pharmacists. Prof. Weiss frequently observed in his day that pharmacists recommended synthetic-chemical drugs for minor illnesses when a phytopharmaceutical with similar efficacy, but more favorable tolerability, could have been the drug of first choice. Most pharmacists at German universities learn at least the basics of pharmacognosy. In contrast, the present curriculum for medical doctors does not include any training in herbal medicine. In contrast to the time of Prof. Weiss, contemporary medical doctors in Germany are therefore not sufficiently exposed to phytotherapy during their training.

1.2 History

Medicinal plant therapy is found **worldwide** in medical systems that are often thousands of years old.

Examples include East Asian (Chinese, Japanese, Korean), Tibetan, and Indian Ayurvedic medicine. Shamans of the Indigenous peoples of Africa and North America, South America, and Oceania always also used plants. Many of these plants are now standard phytotherapy drugs, for example, the purple coneflower (Echinacea purpurea) or devil's claw (Harpagophytum procumbens). The priests of ancient Egypt and Greece; Galen, the personal physician of the Roman emperor Marcus Aurelius; the healer and abbess Hildegard von Bingen; and Paracelsus (b. Theophrastus von Hohenheim, 1493–1541), all understood the healing power of certain plants and incorporated them into their therapy systems.

More recently, famous German physicians such as **Christoph Wilhelm Friedrich Hufeland** (1762–1836), **Carl Gustav Carus** (1789–1869) and **Sebastian Kneipp** (1821–1897) valued and utilized medicinal plants, often also referred to as medicinal herbs. Of interest in this context are the indications referred to especially during the Middle Ages or even earlier periods. Our understanding of medical science makes the indications listed during those periods seem imprecise, unscientific or even incomprehensible because we can no longer decipher or translate the medical thinking of the time. This is especially true for the great medical pioneer, Paracelsus. At the same time, we are often surprised to discover that medicinal plants whose action and efficacy we are very familiar with have been successfully used in the past for similar indications. Dismissing this abundance of often very broad indications for medicinal plants as medical lore or "indicational lyricism" indicates a profound lack of understanding: The connections between illness, humans, nature and cosmos were experienced very differently in the past than in the increasingly abstractive medical science of the 20th century. However, this is not to propagate a "back to nature" (Rousseau, 1712–1778) approach or a return to older and ostensibly better days.

Phytotherapy was introduced as a scientific term by the French physician **Henri Leclerc** (1870–1955), who lived and practiced in Paris. He wrote numerous papers about the application of medicinal plants, most of which were published in the leading French medical periodical *La Presse médicale*. Leclerc summarized his experience in his handbook *Précis de Phytothérapie*.

Phytotherapy owes its renaissance in Germany to the revision of the Medicinal Products Act (Arzneimittelgesetz—AMG), which took effect on 1 January 1978 and has since been amended and supplemented several times. This law incorporated a plurality of therapeutic modalities into socially accepted modern medicine and assigned phytotherapy the role of a "particular therapeutic system." Phytotherapy also owes its transition to a modern, contemporary form to the Nestor of phytotherapy in Germany, **Rudolf Fritz Weiss** (1895–1991). Already in 1944, his first presentations and writings had been published in a book on phytotherapy - the 1st German edition of the work at hand - and he actively wrote, presented, and promoted the medical applications of medicinal plants well into his old age.

This modernization of phytotherapy is also a result of the efforts of numerous pharmacists at German universities who intensively studied medicinal plants from modern pharmaceutical, pharmacological, and clinical perspectives despite the risk of discrimination. Although not authorized to directly treat patients, they frequently crossed the limits of their profession as pharmacists by passing on many therapeutic suggestions and prescriptions. Close cooperation between pharmaceutical and clinical research is therefore essential in order to further the scientific understanding of phytotherapy in the future.

The history of phytotherapy is also a history of our modern medicine. Since its inception during the mid-19th century, it has defined itself as oriented toward natural science. It is not the task of this book to praise its accomplishments or to condemn it where it went astray. The style of this book, however, will illustrate that phytotherapy demands modern medicine broaden its very tight boundaries of scientificity and seek new opportunities for discovery and understanding. Using science to test modern phytotherapy as it has been passed on to us by age-old traditions of plant-based therapy to assess its efficacy and safety is appropriate.

1.3 Phytotherapy: A Particular Therapeutic System?

In Germany, according to the Medicinal Products Act (Arzneimittelgesetz—AMG), phytotherapy—in addition to homeopathy and anthroposophical medicine —is considered a "particular therapeutic system," and therefore plays a special role within the health care system. The following presents and discusses the background for this classification in more detail.

1.3.1 Phytotherapy and Mainstream Medicine

Most representatives of modern phytotherapy view it as part of science-based (mainstream) medicine. Their aspiration to apply the same scientific methods to phytotherapeutics as to synthetic drugs and to view phytotherapy as an **integral component** of modern pharmacotherapy deserves to be supported. In this context, it should be mentioned that phytotherapy, unlike homeopathy and anthroposophical medicine, does not rely on its own epistemology or scientific method. It has been and continues to be a natural science in the truest sense of the word, although, in the past, it was viewed in a more comprehensive context than today. Understanding phytotherapy required the physician to pass "nature's exam" (Paracelsus). The application areas for phytotherapy were continuously adapted to its time without being redefined in principle. The majority of its applications is derived from centuries or even millennia of experience with medicinal herbs. We do not understand how this knowledge was developed. However, the process of "cultural evolution" may offer a general understanding of the overall processes (see section 1.3.1.1 Cultural Evolution below).

One example for the delineation of phytotherapy from homeopathy is the question of application areas. Hahnemann's uses of medicinal plants as he described them often exhibit entirely different indications than in phytotherapy.

One possible discovery method suggested and practiced by Goethe is based on "observant judgment." Goethe suggests that this ability develops in observers of plants, if they encounter a plant without preconceptions and discover the plants very own nature. In discussions with the Kantian Schiller, who argued along the lines of today's scientific thinking, Goethe posited the thesis that Schiller's method led to a sensory perception of the underlying idea.

1.3.1.1 Cultural Evolution

Recent anthropological research data has led to the astounding conclusion that traditional herbal medicine most probably has a longer history than humankind: Apes have been observed using medicinal plants for the treatment of diseases (Huffman). Moreover, human populations that settled in the same region of Africa use the same plants for very similar indications (Huffman). One example for this transfer of medicinal knowledge from animals to humans is Vernonia amygdalina Del. Chimpanzees (Pan troglodytes) have been observed on numerous occasions to chew on the bitter pith of this plant as self-medication in cases of parasitic nematode infections (Huffmann). Traditional healers of the WaTongwe people of the Mahale Mountains in Tanzania, where the use of V. amygdalina by chimpanzees has also been observed, use this plant to treat intestinal parasites, diarrhea, and stomach upset. Phytochemical research has demonstrated that sesquiterpene lactones in V. amygdalina possess anthelmintic, antiamoebic, antitumor, and antibiotic properties (Huffman).

We can thus propose a long-term coevolution between man and his food and medicinal plants, resulting in the adaptation of human pharmacology to bioactive plant metabolites. The fact that as early as 50,000 years ago Neanderthals used yarrow (Achillea millefolium) and chamomile (Matricaria chamomilla)–two plants still registered as medicinal plants in the European Pharmacopoeia– as well as poplar buds (Populus spec.) as medicine (Hardy, Weyrich), demonstrates that contemporary phytotherapeutic practice goes back to the dawn of man. The accumulated body of knowledge (referred to as "tradition" or "culture") is transferable in humans from person-to-person, which enables close relatives to learn successful behaviors. The process of the improvement and distribution of this knowledge can be referred to as "cultural evolution." The evolutionary pressure that drives this cultural evolution is the survival benefit held by those with knowledge of effective treatments.

Weiss maintained that the knowledge derived from developing an intimate, trusting relationship with a plant was an essential prerequisite for its successful therapeutic application. This position, no doubt, explodes the narrow boundaries imposed upon itself by science-based medicine in which all nonphysical components of therapy are to be eliminated for the sake of science (double-blind studies). Alphons Martini (1829–1880) referred to the millennia of practical therapeutic experience as real experience and considered it scientifically equal to pharmacologic-experimental experience. Even major representatives of science-based medicine of the 20th century do not accept this separation of science and experience. The Heidelberg physiologist Hans Schäfer (1979) commented on this issue as follows: "Intuition and science are not opposites. The part of medical diagnosis and therapy that requires empathy and compassion (sympathy with the sick person) is intuitive. Our current medical system is adversarial towards intuition, to the detriment of all. Physicians should know that – and change it."

Evidence-based medicine (EBM), which was originally referred to by Sackett as evidence-based practice (EBP), is proclaimed as the current definitive standard of natural science-based medicine. According to Sackett, it "represents the conscientious, explicit and judicious use of current best evidence in making decisions about the care of the individual patient. It means integrating individual clinical expertise with the best available external clinical evidence from systematic research." He formulated the levels of evidence shown in ▶ Table 1.1.

In his critical overview of EBM, Loew contrasted it with **experience-based medicine**. He accepted EBM for phytotherapy provided it encompasses the translation of current scientific findings from experimental data, clinical-pharmacologic research, and clinical studies into decision guidelines for rational diagnostic and therapeutic medicine. EBM is a decision guide for practical medicine, but because of its self-imposed limitations, it must be viewed as an aid in finding diagnostics and therapy, and not as the only viable path. Too many aspects of practical medical reality, and especially the influence of individual differences, are only partially, or not at all, addressed by EBM. Appointing EBM as the "new paradigm," or the only permissible path of discovery in medicine, threatens to produce, according to Keil, an historian of medicine, a "progressive absolutism that does not represent progress, but instead regression into the period of mindless enlightenment." With a view toward the uniqueness of phytotherapy, Loew therefore suggests a different weighting of evidence-producing criteria (▶ Table 1.2).

The key question in the context of discussing the scientific nature of medicine is whether it allows itself to be guided by reality and the needs of patients and of people seeking good health or whether it determines the nature of these components from within an ivory tower. In the context of this discussion, Thure von Uexküll, a prominent representative of psychosomatic medicine in the 20th century, referred to "patient-oriented medicine" as a means of supplementing EBM. In addition, Meyer referred to the significant differences in mentalities and cultural influences on medical practice and demanded a **culture-based medicine**. Finally, Kiene coined the term **cognition-based medicine** in 2001. It is based on evidence-supported individual epistemology assessment and documentation in polarity to systemic collective analysis.

This brief discussion about the significance and relevance of EBM shows that it describes an essential aspect of medical science without encompassing the reality of medicine as a whole. This means that the characteristics of EBM apply to phytotherapy, but phytotherapy, with a view to Schäfer's statements, pushes its overly tight boundaries. Kraft and März provide a good overview of the scientific nature of phytotherapy. They emphasize the synergistic effects of phytopharmaceuticals as polychemical (multicomponent) mixtures that have demonstrated their therapeutic superiority

Table 1.1 Evidence-Based Practice (EBP): Levels of evidence according to Sackett (Perlett).

	Study Documentation
Level 1	Systematic review, foundation: randomized, controlled trials
Level 2	At least one sufficiently large randomized, controlled trial, orintervention trial
Level 3	Nonrandomized or nonprospective trials, for example, cohort trials, or case-control trials
Level 4	At least one nonexperimental observational trial
Level 5	Expert opinions; consensus process

Table 1.2 Experience-Based Medicine: Levels of Evidence according to Loew.

	Study Documentation
Level 1	Systematic and current overviews based on prospective cohort or case-control trials
Level 2	Prospective cohort or case-control trials without study-induced intervention into physician–patient interaction
Level 3	Retrospective, prospective cohort, or case-control trials
Level 4	Pooled, structured expert interviews
Level 5	Expert opinion, consensus process

compared to isolated single constituents also experimentally. They conclude that evidence is an important factor in assessing efficacy, but not the only one: "The lack of evidence of efficacy is not the evidence of the lack of efficacy."

Regaining the intuitive component in addition to the analytical science-based component of the discovery method used is vital for the humane development of modern medicine. Medicinal plants, or phytotherapeutics, can play an important mediating role. Asclepius, the god of healing and medicine in Greek and Roman mythology, referred to this role about 3,000 years ago in his proclamation to his student Hippocrates: "First the word—then the plant—last the knife!" Weiss updated this aspiration as follows: "First the word—then the plant—then the large store of synthetic chemotherapeutics—and last, the knife."

This emphasis on the word as the first order of therapy refers to other important aspects. Today, the distinction is made between silent, scientific medicine and talking, alternative medicine. This animates demands for raising reimbursement rates for talking medicine compared to those of the predominant technical medicine. What a declaration of bankruptcy for modern medicine! The word is also at the center of Christianity and to be viewed as the ethical, interdenominational foundation of therapy, described by Weiss as follows: "Especially today, there appears to be cause for emphasizing that the 'word' needs to be the beginning of all medical efforts. This was true in the past, and today we are again becoming more conscious of this fact. The 'word' is spiritual medicine and therefore initially addresses the psyche, but from there can profoundly impact the physical sphere. This has been confirmed by the teachings of psychosomatics. The 'word,' spoken in the right manner, is a force greater in its effect and range than we have been inclined to assume in a materialistic world. Combining an intensive doctor–patient conversation in the simplest of manners with the simultaneous administration of a medicinal herb provides an ideal form of medicine that should be sufficient in the great majority of diseases. This is especially true for many cases physicians see in their daily practice. Clinicians, however, should also be more mindful of this basic fact of all healing, especially with a view toward the discoveries in psychosomatics. They will not regret it."

From this perspective, the special role of phytotherapy as a therapy method could point the way

toward the necessary supplementation of the scientific method by **embracing the whole** and thereby clarifying and hopefully overcoming the one-sidedness of exclusively physiochemical processes. This is yet another example of the spiritual law of "one and the other" overcoming the strictly analytical "either-or." The pharmacologically defined, always repeatable, mostly monocausal effect is complemented by therapeutic effects that, based on the author's experience, act on a mental level as well as on overall health. They individually encompass the entire human being in their mental state or overall state of health, with their different levels of being: body, soul, and spirit.

1.3.2 Effect and Efficacy

One special aspect of phytotherapy is its breadth of indication areas. The medical use of the whole plant or "whole" parts of the plant, special mixtures derived through extraction or isolated single components, all involve specialization that ranges from comprehensive therapeutic efficacy to a pharmacologically definable effect. The more constituents contained in a phytotherapeutic, the broader its indication area. The therapeutic effect of polychemical (multicomponent) mixtures is broader than that of certain constituents in a standardized extract or of a defined monosubstance, usually in the form of a synthetic derivative. For the treating physician, this gradation creates a multitude of indication possibilities especially for phytopharmaceuticals.

Milk thistle (Silybum marianum) is a good example. Milk thistle has been in use for centuries for an extraordinarily large number of indications that go well beyond the currently known special reference to the liver. Rademacher discovered its effect on liver disorders, commonly summed up as hepatopathies in the 19th century, and named this indication for the tincture of the milk thistle fruit he used, Tinctura Rademacheri. Around 1930, Hörhammer described silymarin, an extract of the milk thistle fruit. Today we know it to be a flavone mixture with three components: silicristin, silidianin, and silibinin. Modern pharmacologic and clinical studies have shown silymarin to be protective and curative for toxic liver disorders (hepatosis). A semisynthetic derivative of water-soluble silibinin (silibinin-C-2',3-dihydrogensuccinate, disodium salt) became the antidote for specific, acute, life-threatening liver intoxication resulting from

Amanita phalloides (death cap) poisoning. This shows the entire range of phytotherapy: from broad, nonspecific applications to still general, but organ-specific applications to specialization for a narrower indication of toxic liver disorders. At the same time, the more limited efficacy represents a crossing over the border to synthetics, which provide a specific antidote for a single, specific disorder.

Any type of ideology that says that only holistic models provide healing is just as one-sided and questionable as the dominant view today that verifiable therapeutic results can only be achieved with chemically defined single substances. The situation of the patient defines which of the methods introduced here is most likely to result in healing.

1.3.3 Phytotherapy and Prevention

According to a study of natural medicine conducted by the Allensbach Institute in 2002, 38% of all German adults taking preventive medications took natural medicines exclusively and 41% took natural medicines among other medications (IfD). This acceptance of, and even preference for, natural medicines has increased since 2002. In a representative survey conducted by the opinion research institute Emnid in 2004 (Pascoe Study), 81% of those adults surveyed were convinced by the medicinal properties of natural medicines and 80% would choose natural medicines over chemically synthesized medicines if they had a choice (Pascoe). A follow-up study in 2007 (Pascoe Study) confirmed these results.

This data is also precisely confirmed by a 2015 study by the market research institute TNS Infratest led by Professor Wasem. More than 90% of the German adults surveyed were familiar with the term "natural medicines." Herbal medicines were named most frequently (87%), about half of the respondents named homeopathy, and 38% named anthroposophical medicine. A high percentage of the natural remedies mentioned (86%) were home remedies such as poultices, baths, and teas. The study showed that, in Germany, pharmacies continue to be the main source of natural medicines. When asked why they preferred natural medicine, 89% of those Germans surveyed responded "because they are well tolerated, efficacious and useful" and 84% of respondents reported positive personal experience with natural medicine. The study also documents the high economic impact of natural medicine.

Health care policy makers are increasingly demanding a shift in emphasis from treatment of manifest diseases to prevention. This is not so much due to a resurrection of the old medical theorem that "prevention is better than cure," but rather to the increasing cost of health care. Diagnosing diseases in their development or latency stages and seeking treatment is indeed consistent with medical–ethical responsibilities. However, most often, treatment is delayed until a disease has manifested and can in many cases be objectively and demonstrably diagnosed. Until now, medical science has not addressed the question whether disease expresses as functional disorders in its early stage or whether, even earlier, and more succinctly, a disposition toward disease expresses as changes in mood or presence of mind. Appropriate assessment of phytopharmaceuticals within the framework of modern holistic pharmacotherapy, however, requires consideration of treatment in its early or latency stages, especially for diseases that tend toward becoming chronic.

Even medical dictionaries do not usually differentiate between prophylaxis and prevention. In the following, **prophylaxis** means the prevention of possible diseases, for example, as manifested in immunizations. **Prevention** means preventing manifest and chronic courses of disease by treating them in their latent prestages or early stages. Familial and constitutional dispositions may also require preventive measures. The author is convinced that the hypothesis that effective prevention represents large potential cost reductions is correct.

The author's decade-long practical medical experience indicates that phytopharmaceuticals are especially well suited as preventive medicine. The following chapters will provide many examples. The fact that phytopharmaceuticals are **well tolerated** plays a significant role here because of their often long-term use. In the past, the term "transposition therapy" was used to describe that the goal of treatment was not to block individual functions or intermediary metabolism steps and thereby achieve purely symptomatic effects. Rather, prevention means to teach the body's own organization and regulation systems to perform their healthy functions. This can be achieved through substitution, stimulation, or soothing. The medicinal plant can provide a kind of model for the disturbed function and "educate," correspond with and create encounters with the organism. It is up to the healing art of the physician to determine, in each case, when this "educational process" is complete and to terminate therapy at the right time. Unnecessarily prolonging treatment can begin to increase the risk of undesirable effects. Experience has shown a correlation between the extent of side effects and whether the organism positively responds to or rejects the therapy. This presupposes that the organism can access a perception potential (immune system) that can determine the positive or negative effects of the administered components (remedy).

Physiologists, pathologists, and even pharmacologists, who view all organism processes as self-regulated automatisms, reject these ideas, or at least view them skeptically. Some readers of this book may also find them to be unfamiliar. Medicine in the 21st century, however, will increasingly encounter these regularities as well as the functional and regulation systems described here, and will assess them scientifically. Practical experience with phytopharmaceuticals and their efficacy will convince physicians of their existence (Fintelmann).

1.4 Importance of Proof of Efficacy

The question of evidence of drug efficacy has been discussed with much intensity and controversy, but without definitive results. The dogma of conclusive proof provided by double-blind, randomized, controlled trials began to be eroded by Kienle, but was by no means abandoned. Kiene revisited this question again and researched its dimension. The objective was twofold: on the one hand, to attempt to evaluate the effect of an isolated remedy within a given therapy and, on the other hand, to objectify the results gained in the process. The scientifically verified **placebo problem** is that the development of placebo effects is not understood. Kienle published a detailed description and scientific discussion of the placebo effect.

What must be termed outside the realm of scientific discussion is the attempt to discriminate against **therapeutic experience**. No patient wants to be treated by physicians without any experience who derive their knowledge strictly from results of double-blind studies. A well-known US adage describes the importance of experience: "You can fool all the people some of the time, and some of the people all the time, but you can't fool all the

people all the time." Transposed to the field of pharmacotherapy, this means: Long-term use of a drug that is repeatedly requested by patients and prescribed by physicians proves its efficacy—even without a double-blind trial.

1.4.1 Legal Foundation in Germany

During the drafting of the new Medicinal Products Act (Arzneimittelgesetz – AMG) enacted on 1 January 1978, and revised and amended multiple times since then, the Youth, Family, and Health Committee developing the act issued the following statement on 28 April 1976: "The committee has unanimously concluded that it cannot and must not be the task of law makers to one-sidedly define methods of proving drug efficacy that elevate one of many competing therapy directions into the position of generally binding 'state-of-the-art knowledge' and thereby making it the only yardstick for the approval of a drug. Rather, the decision process of the committee regarding approval legislation, and especially in developing approval requirements, was guided by the political goal that the approval process must clearly reflect the scientific plurality present in drug therapy."

This statement was emphatically confirmed in the Medicinal Products Act (Arzneimittelgesetz—AMG). According to Section 26, subsection 2, sentence 2 of the act, scientific evidence includes experiential (empirical) results that are documented using scientific methods. Section 25, subsections 6 and 7 call for the creation of specific commissions to evaluate documentation submitted for approval of drugs that were on the market and approved at the time the Medicinal Products Act (Arzneimittelgesetz – AMG) was enacted and to process the scientific data in accordance with Section 22, subsection. 3 and Section 23, subsection 3, sentence 2. The so-called Commission E (Zulassungs- und Aufbereitungskommission für den humanmedizinischen Bereich, phytotherapeutische Therapierichtung und Stoffgruppe) was especially established for herbal medicinal products and is "in charge of the scientific evaluation of efficacy, safety and pharmaceutical quality of medicinal products appertaining to the 'particular therapeutic systems' and of traditional medicinal products." The Commission E first met in the spring of 1978 and has since operated with a varying membership (members serve 3-year terms).

The available scientific data was compiled by external experts and evaluated by Commission E working groups in preparation for plenary deliberation and adoption following extensive discussion. Following a draft phase, the commission resumed deliberation, with each member invited to propose amendments for subsequent evaluation and approval in the plenary. At the conclusion of this process, a monograph for each medicinal plant was approved and published by the German Federal Ministry of Health and published in the German Federal Gazette (*Bundesanzeiger*).

Since then, ca. 380 such monographs have been developed. Some of these have been revised to reflect new discoveries and have been supplemented by monographs for typical drug combinations and standard monographs. In addition to **positive (approved) monographs** documenting positive evaluations for many medicinal plants, the Commission E also created **negative (unapproved) monographs** when proof of efficacy was not provided by the available scientific data or when its use was outweighed by too great a risk. Risk assessment, especially for questions of toxicology, was extremely difficult because even a relatively small risk resulted in a negative assessment. The usefulness of the plant in question tended to be easily understated.

The Commission E was aware of the fact that proof of efficacy for phytotherapeutics cannot be one-sidedly judged by criteria that have been established for controlled trials and statistical evaluation of synthetic drugs. It had to meet its legal requirement of allowing for medical experience as scientific data for the evaluation of medicinal plants.

The Medicinal Products Act (Arzneimittelgesetz—AMG) represented a turning point for phytotherapy, especially as a modern therapy evaluated by applying scientific criteria. In 1978, phytotherapy was relatively unknown and was practiced by only a few physicians. Today, its remedies are public knowledge. They are viewed as indispensable components of modern medicine and are receiving increasing approval from practicing physicians. The fact that herbal medicine is especially well tolerated—and that the risks of modern synthetic drugs and their limited possibilities within the context of chronic disease management have become increasingly obvious—contributed significantly to this development.

Definition

The efficacy of phytotherapeutics is judged to be certain or sufficiently likely if at least one of the following **conditions** is met:
1. Effect and efficacy are documented in reputable overview papers, manuals, or textbooks.
2. Results of controlled trials in comparison with placebo or reference substances are available.
3. Clinical studies are documented but are insufficient for a recommendation for approval; however, experimental study results are known and point in the same direction.
4. Scientifically documented evidence is available.
5. Experiential data is available that is not sufficient for a recommendation for approval; however, conclusive experimental study results or further evaluable observations or evidence are available.

1.4.2 International Standards

Today, drug laws in Europe are no longer exclusively a national domain, as the European Union is unifying the evaluation of drugs and related legislation. To achieve common standards for phytopharmaceuticals, the **European Scientific Cooperative on Phytotherapy** (ESCOP) has created its own monographs, which are referenced in the appendix of this book (p. 403). They are based on the Commission E monographs, but have been amended with special considerations for other countries and are much more comprehensive.

In preparation for harmonizing the approval of drugs in the EU, the Directive 2001/83/EG summarizes all previous regulations in one document. This document also contains definitions for herbal medicines. The term "well-established use" was created. Since the individual member countries had very different applications for plant-based (and other complimentary) drugs, another directive, 2004/24/EG, was created to harmonize the related questions. This connects the standard that previously existed in Germany for traditional drugs and their traditional applications with a simplified registration (Stolte and Knöss). The Herbal Medicinal Products Committee (HMPC) created by the European Medicines Agency (EMA) in 2004 also developed transnational monographs. By early 2014, 125 such HMPC monographs had been published. The scientific data described in these documents (Commission E, ESCOP, HMPC), including plausibility criteria, now forms the basis for approval of herbal medicines in the European Union. Helmstädter and Staiger have created a pharmaco–historical overview of this topic.

We will need to seek new paths to provide appropriate answers to the question of proof of efficacy. The **Delphi method** derives its name from processes practiced by the wise priestesses of Delphi in ancient Greece. The method involves providing all available documentation, including biographical information, initially to three experts who are not known to each other and also not known to any other participants except to one central agency. This agency receives all "verdicts," collates them anonymously, and forwards them to three other experts who also remain anonymous. If they return their deliberations, and if there is consensus or a clear dominance of one opinion, the assessment can be considered complete. If not, the process continues. In the United States, 12 such exchanges are considered the rule and 14 are desirable. This process creates a recognized positive or negative result and resembles the work of the Commission E in developing its monographs.

Application observation has been established as a defined and practiced method, especially since the publication of the recommendations for implementing application observations by the German Society for Medical Informatics, Biometry and Epidemiology (GMDS). It collects, reviews, and evaluates data about the application of already approved, registered, or fictitiously approved drugs in an open study.

It is characteristic for this method that the individual doctor–patient relationship in terms of indication, choice, and implementation of therapy is hardly influenced.

Outcomes research, which were first developed in the United States, are based on the criterion that therapy never consists of only one remedy or one process but instead demands comprehensive concepts. Outcome research trials review and evaluate therapy concepts in comparison to each other. This method is also increasingly being viewed favorably in Germany.

Whether new ways toward determining efficacy are adopted, and which ones, remains open.

Certainly, there will continue to be a need for controlled trials. Well-documented individual case studies, which have been shown to be reliable for determining undesirable drug side effects, deserve more recognition (Kienle and Kiene). For rare disorders, large controlled case studies are not even possible. In those cases, a demonstrable standard therapy needs to serve as the basis for comparison. Therapeutic concepts can also be compared with each other, provided target criteria and statistical evaluation are identical.

All ethical questions related to controlled trials are receiving renewed recognition lately and have led to the establishment of institutionalized ethics commissions. However, there is a need to recognize that efficacy evaluations solely at the diagnostic level do not do justice to the possibilities and realities of phytotherapeutics and the holistic entity "human being." Appropriate proof of efficacy must consider all aspects of human existence.

1.4.3 Findings and Feeling

Opponents of herbal medicine often maintain that these medicines are only suitable for improving a state of disorder or discomfort. The denigration implied here shows the inability of these scientists to understand the reality of a person who is ill. Against a backdrop of ideological one-sidedness, the increasingly dogmatic field of medical science has constructed abstract assessments of therapies oriented solely toward objectively provable findings. In their daily practice, however, physicians continuously observe that people who are ill, experience and suffer discomfort much more directly than their pathological findings or diagnosis indicate. However, modern medicine has managed to get more and more patients to fixate on their findings or pathologies. Patients judge the value of therapy by these findings and then seek out a different physician or alternative practitioner for alleviation of their discomfort or lack of well-being.

However, there is no doubt that everyone who is ill seeks to regain their health in both areas: findings as well as feeling. Strangely, scientific medicine has long criticized "cosmetic diagnostics." For example, it has been shown that treatment of chronic hepatitis with glucocorticosteroids produced dramatic improvements in transaminase levels. However, histological assessments have shown that actual disease progression and chronic destructive inflammation of the liver not only did not improve, but often worsened dramatically during therapy. This was referred to as the "**whitewash effect.**" It led to cortisone therapy for chronic hepatitis becoming obsolete.

One representative of anthropology who appropriately valued the topic of feeling or discomfort without ignoring pathological findings or diagnostics is the Heidelberg clinician Plügge, who wrote in 1962: "Even though each consultation starts with the patient telling the physician about their feeling of discomfort, thereby making the appearance of how patients experience their discomfort a vital element in this meeting of the physician and the patient, medicine still completely lacks a theory of well-being and discomfort. A patient's level of discomfort is a diagnostic guidepost and is the target of the therapy we provide. It takes on the role of a mediator between the physician and the objective diagnosis, as a path toward the patient and often as a troublemaker in their relationship. In spite of the interesting and, it seems to me, dominant role played by a person's well-being, everything we commonly refer to as discomfort, feeling, well-being, and states of health has remained a stepchild of medicine. Interestingly, we as physicians are not interested in a theory of types of well-being, which naturally would need to be a theory of the types of mind-body experiences. This is rooted in the character of today's medicine: We tend not to spend too much time on how the patient feels because our focus quickly shifts toward diagnosing the underlying pathology. To state this in an extreme manner: We view the objective diagnosis as the principle task, the most important, that which we feel responsible for. The objective diagnosis becomes the purported 'truth.' We tend to assume that discomfort can be misleading but diagnostics cannot, that objective diagnosis makes up our scientific substrate. The subjective side is not of significant importance and ideally, is dispensable. "

This statement continues to be true, although even scientifically oriented physicians are increasingly recognizing that the subjective view of discomfort can no longer be disregarded, especially in the context of diagnostics and therapy. For example, the question of **quality of life** is receiving more attention in conjunction with therapy in oncology.

As was mentioned in the context of the uniqueness of phytotherapy, the author's practical experience leads to the hypothesis that plant medicines seem to primarily work in areas where the human organism experiences well-being that changes into discomfort as a result of disease. **Well-being** is an expression of an overall holistic sense of health, ideally a sense of wellness. **Feelings of comfort or discomfort**, on the other hand, are an expression of individual symptoms, for example, localized pain, sense of bloating in the upper abdomen, discomfort in the extremities or dysuria. The objectifiable level of findings or diagnostics is created by analytical thinking that starts with the whole and breaks it down into parts. It seeks to derive its knowledge from ever greater differentiation. Assessing feelings of discomfort requires synthesizing thinking that directs the focus from symptoms as an expression of holistic beings to the whole being. The world of feelings of comfort or discomfort is an expression of the subjectiveness of the individual and is generally not provable. It can only be described and understood (▶ Fig. 1.1). Some disorders are entirely dominated by findings and show no symptoms or feelings of discomfort, such as hypertonicity, or hypercholesteremia. Other disorders are entirely within the realm of feelings of discomfort, without the possibility of objectifiable diagnosis, for example, migraines. Both nosological units of a disease process cannot be differentiated according to which is more "correct," worthy of recognition or exists in a scientific sense. Disorders

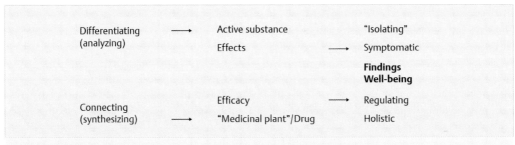

Fig. 1.1 Holistic view of human beings from objective and subjective perspectives.

that combine discomfort and pathological findings are even more frequent.

We would like to introduce the working hypothesis that phytotherapeutics primarily influence the sense of well-being because they communicate with the body's endogenous regulation and organization systems by substituting, calming, or stimulating them. Phytotherapy works (heals) primarily **with** the body. Therapy that acts on an objectifiable level works primarily **against** the body. For this reason, many modern drugs have names like antidiabetic, antihypertensive, or antidepressant. One should not conclude from this choice of words, however, that it reflects a valuation of desirable or unsatisfactory but necessary therapy methods. Modern physicians must move beyond the "either-or" they have become used to and move toward "both" because both options encompass the reality of holistic human beings in medicine: In many areas, for example in emergency medicine or in intensive care, a drug is intended to work immediately and absolutely. Many disorders, however, especially chronic disorders and minor ailments with a high proportion of an impaired sense of well-being, require a normalization of organic dysfunction and restoration of a sense of well-being.

Physicians practicing phytotherapy are often excited to observe that improvements on a diagnostic level do not coincide with primary improvements in well-being, but do tend toward normalization after a significant delay. The hypothetical concepts discussed in this book contribute toward understanding this process.

The worlds of finding and feeling exist in parallel and require different therapeutics, depending on which side of the disorder is dominant. Some disorders require treatment exclusively with synthetics.

Some are only treatable with phytotherapeutics. Other disorders require both types of therapy and these therapies are complementary. This results in the following four categories, illustrated in ▶ Table 1.3.

The **holistic human being** is characterized by the levels of finding and feeling as well as the criteria mood and presence of mind.

Findings indicate pathologies in the physiochemical dimension of the body. Feeling is an expression of the body's functionality, its life force. **Mood** describes the psychosomatic level, the unity of body and soul. Today, the words "psyche" and "psychogenic" tend to be used rather loosely. Much of what is labeled with these terms is derived from the level of functionality or life, not directly from the connections between body and soul. These are holistically expressed in a wide range of moods. The fact that modern medicine is, or at least was, conscious of this fact can be deduced from the pathologically oriented use of the term "mood disorders."

Objectifiably accessible areas of this psychosomatic dimension can primarily be found in endocrinology and immunology. Psychoneuroimmunology is a scientifically accepted specialty and no physician, no matter how scientifically oriented, will be able to deny the high percentage of psychologic symptoms associated with endocrine disorders. If the reader would indulge us, we would like to mention that the concept of tuning or attunement also has its place in music. In order for an orchestra or a chamber music ensemble to play together harmoniously, all musical instruments have to be in tune with each other. Would such attunement between organs, organ systems, and their manifold functions in the entire organism not also result in better health?

Table 1.3 Therapeutic categories for phytotherapeutics (according to Fintelmann et al.)

	Characteristics
Category 1	Indications for which phytotherapeutics are the drug of first choice and that have no synthetic alternatives, for example, toxic liver diseases.
Category 2	Indications for which phytotherapeutics may be used as an alternative to synthetics, for example, anxiety, mild to moderate depression, functional dyspepsia, and nonspecific urinary tract infections.
Category 3	Indications for which phytotherapeutics are used as an adjuvant to basic therapy, for example, adjuvant therapy for heart, liver, and respiratory disorders.
Category 4	Indications for which the use of phytotherapeutics is not appropriate or viewed as malpractice because it prevents or delays rational therapy using synthetics.

Presence of mind describes the dimension of the mind in the human body. It is the instrument used to express human individuality to the world and for human beings to experience themselves as "I." This is where we enter the mental/spiritual dimension of medicine. Carl Gustav Carus considered this to be self-evident in the 19th century and Rudolf Steiner newly described it in the 20th century.

Proof of efficacy that truly serves human medicine will need to expand its scope from a strict focus on findings to the levels of feeling, mood and presence of mind (Fintelmann). However, there is still a great need for basic scientific foundations.

1.5 Side Effects

A statement heard frequently is that phytotherapeutics "can't do harm." Such nonsensical statements also imply the opinion of opponents of phytotherapy that it cannot do harm "because it doesn't work"! At the same time, many proponents of phytotherapy also frequently emphasize the supposed inability of herbal medicine to do harm.

According to modern pharmacology and its associated toxicology, all drugs have side effects, that is, they have **desirable** and **undesirable** effects. This almost paradigmatic statement is justified if drugs have been studied in large collective trials with average findings without making a connection to individual patients. It contradicts, however, the age-old medical–ethical precept of "first, do no harm" (*primum non nocere*) and provokes a basic question: Can ethical human medicine continue to tolerate the potential harm inflicted on individual humans by not basing therapy on individuals, but rather on statistically developed collective data?

One of the goals of this books is to restore the ability of physicians to more effectively address the needs of each patient's personality and to freely prescribe the individual therapy that is appropriate for each patient's constitution and disorder. Truly modern phytotherapy will primarily be **individual therapy** that rejects any type of therapy schematics.

At the same time, we can, and must, accept that even with individualized therapy approaches, the response of the individual to the chosen therapy cannot be predicted with absolute certainty. For this reason, it is impossible to refer to a therapy of any kind as a priori harmless. One proof of this statement is the potential for allergic reactions, which cannot be underestimated especially for phytotherapeutics. The four dimensions illustrated above—finding, feeling, mood, and presence of mind—must be considered. Physicians need to learn how to appropriately assess the effects of therapy on these different levels of being. In so doing, they will arrive at the conclusion that undesirable effects occur more frequently than previously thought.

Phytotherapeutics and synthetics differ in frequency and intensity of side effects, but both have side effects. Without a doubt, phytotherapeutics are more well tolerated than synthetics, which have substantial potential side effects. The reason for this seems simple: Plants and humans have **evolved together** and have therefore evolved adaptive processes in their metabolism for much longer and more successfully than for synthetics, which, in part, were not discovered and used until the 20th century. The metabolic processes used by the human body to break down foreign substances, primarily in the liver, displays virtually archaic features.

This is why the organism chooses metabolic steps to process synthetic foreign substances (xenobiotics) that, for example, create radicals. This turns an initially indifferent substance into an aggressive noxious substance. One of the most well-known examples is carbon tetrachloride, which develops liver toxicity when broken down into carbon trichloride.

1.5.1 Risks and Undesirable Effects

Definition

In his 1990 article about **risks and undesirable effects of herbal medicine**, Frohne differentiates between:

- Plants with highly active constituents and correspondingly high-risk potential. These plants have mostly disappeared from modern medicine or are used only as isolated, pure substances.
- Plant medicines with active constituents that may cause undesirable effects if overdosed or used chronically (misuse).
- Plant medicines for which therapeutic efficacy has not been demonstrated or has been judged controversially, but which certainly may have undesirable effects.
- Plant medicines that may have dangerous side effects due to unidentified additional constituents.

For a long time, the discussion about the pros and cons of phytotherapeutics focused primarily on their efficacy. Meanwhile, the focus has shifted primarily to risk assessment, with an emphasis on proven **mutagenic** or **carcinogenic** and, much more rarely, teratogenic effects. One of the first plants in this category was **birthwort** (Aristolochia clematitis), when long-term use of isolated aristolochic acid was shown to cause malignant tumors. Since then, such mutagenic or carcinogenic potential has been deduced for various medicinal herbs based on experiments. The most intense discussion revolved around pyrrolizidine alkaloids, anthraquinones, and quercetin. The data on which such assessments are based needs to be seriously questioned. The issues associated with transferability of animal studies or certain cell lines to the holistic human organism have already been discussed. It leaves out a multitude of repair mechanisms available to the human immune system and individual responses. Animals respond much more appropriately to their species, but they also develop a uniform response by inbreeding (Wistar rat).

Vogel (1984; 1985) refers to the problems of mutagenicity and carcinogenicity, which is discussed in detail for medicinal plants containing pyrrolizidine alkaloids, such as comfrey (symphytum), coltsfoot (tussilago farfara), butterbur (petasites), and others. The potentially mutagenic or carcinogenic pyrrolizidine alkaloid content of such plant medicines meanwhile has been limited by establishing a maximum administrable dose.

Allergic reactions are also a topic of discussion for the undesirable effects of plant medicines. Hausen and Vieluf have conducted essential scientific research in this area, which has been published in the second edition of their book *Allergiepflanzen–Pflanzenallergene* (Allergy-inducing Plants–Plant Allergens).

1.5.2 Relationship between Dosage and Effect

Another extremely problematic area is ignorance about the relationship between dosage and effect. The therapeutic dosage used in almost all animal experiments that gave rise to suspicions about the carcinogenicity of phytotherapeutics was extremely different from similar experiments centered on human beings. This is compounded by the completely abnormal feeding situation to which these experimental animals are subjected. They are (force) fed the drug to be tested via a gavage for months or years, which places them in an unnatural situation that by itself can cause pathologic changes in organs. One of the paradigms of toxicology states that even a single molecule of a potentially mutagenic or carcinogenic substance can cause cell mutations and, therefore, no dose-dependent prescription should be allowed. The most serious argument here is that no human toxicology exists for this problem, and that it was also not replaced by applicable epidemiological studies. In the case of pyrrolizidine alkaloids, it was shown that when comfrey (Symphytum officinale (p. 294)) was eaten by humans or fed to animals in extremely high daily or long-term doses and compared to the therapeutic application of Symphytum officinale (p. 294), no increase in carcinomas occurred in humans or animals. Despite this finding, the theoretically formulated risk was maintained.

An article in the *Frankfurter Allgemeine Zeitung* (2000) illustrates the tendency to malign phytopharmaceuticals, especially those that are successful in the marketplace. The headline "Treacherous St.-John's-Wort" (Tückisches Johanniskraut) refers to publications at the time about the interactions between St.-John's-wort and, for example, the HIV/AIDS drug indinavir. St.-John's-wort reduced the effect of this drug and of cyclosporine. This interaction was shown in two patients who had received heart transplants and who had taken a St.-John's-wort preparation for depressive mood disorder. In keeping with the frequently postulated statement "No effect without side effect (or interaction)," such observations should be viewed as more proof of the effects of St.-John's-wort. Instead, this plant medicine is maligned as "treacherous," a term that, based on our experience with synthetic drugs and their predominantly obligatory interactions, is completely uncommon. At the same time, such observations are highly significant and should be seriously considered when prescriptions are issued.

Plant medicines no doubt possess a documentable potential for undesirable effects, but toxicology is not yet able to make reliable statements regarding the issues raised here. Toxicology's predominantly hypothetical and paradigmatic approach is not restricted to phytopharmaceuticals. It also impacts synthetics and other substances in our environment.

1.6 Interactions

The basic characteristics of a drug include a description of its potential or proven interactions with other drugs. One central problem in this context is the fact that insufficient data is available for most drugs. This is because when an interaction is suspected, the criteria of evidence-based medicine call for randomized, double-blind, and placebo-controlled studies that provide conclusive results about the observed question of interaction. However, this is not the current state of scientific knowledge. Instead, *in vitro* studies are conducted and based on the results, and conclusions are drawn for *in vivo* conditions. This establishes clinical relevance using a very questionable mode of transmission.

For a long time, the topic of interactions did not seem to be relevant in reference to plant medicines. Nearly all Commission E monographs contain the laconic statement "none known." This began to change more recently following the observation of interactions between St.-John's-wort and cyclosporine, which is used in organ transplant patients to prevent organ rejections. Since then, there has been a lively public discussion about the dangers resulting from not yet studied or not yet known possible interactions for plant medicines. Critics of complementary medicine are using this discussion for their own purposes. For example, in 2012, a highly controversial publication about this topic (Tsai et al.) referred to the "tip of the iceberg." Since then, the discussion has tended toward more rationality because numerous studies on this topic have mostly provided the "all clear" signal about this topic in reference to plant medicines.

Basically, the discussion about interaction needs to differentiate between desirable and undesirable, in the same way as is done for effects. This is because the combination drugs that are so typical for phytotherapy rest on the assumption of "desired" interactions between various partners. Of course, medicine as a bioscience seeks to emphasize treatments using primarily chemically defined single constituents. However, in reality, pathology, or especially cases of comorbidity, will almost never be treated with only one drug constituent. Quite the contrary: The number of concurrently prescribed drugs for typical disorders of our time such as high blood pressure, coronary heart disease, rheumatoid arthritis, etc. are legion. And is it really possible to document the appropriateness of each of those individual physician's prescriptions through evidence-based studies?

Two basic mechanisms regulate the bioavailability of medications absorbed by the metabolism: First, metabolic changes performed by enzymes, and second, transport processes performed by influx and efflux pumps. Metabolic changes are primarily caused by cytochrome P450 (CYP) enzymes (phase I metabolism) and glucuronosyltransferase (phase II metabolism). P-glycoproteins are responsible for efflux transport and OATPs (Organic Anion Transporting Polypeptides) are responsible for influx transport.

Research into chemosynthetic drugs has shown that the most important and most frequent drug interactions occur when the bioavailability of an active substance is increased or decreased by inhibition or induction of one of the metabolic changes or transport processes described above. This is referred to as pharmacokinetic interaction (Saller et al.).

Clinically relevant interactions of phytomedicines based on this mechanism are well documented for extracts of St.-John's-wort (Hypericum perforatum) that contain hyperforin. After a few days, these can cause increased expression of CYP enzymes and P-glycoproteins, especially in the liver and small intestine. This leads to a clinically relevant reduction in the bioavailability of many substances that are metabolized by these two systems (Sugimoto et al.).

These reports about the interaction potential of St.-John's-wort extracts containing hyperforin have raised serious concerns among patients and with regulatory agencies about similar risks for other medicinal plants. Despite that, intensive research has, so far, only produced *in vivo* results of doubtful clinical relevance in many cases, which have frequently already been disproven experimentally.

For example, a clinical study of the effects of hawthorn (Crataegus oxyacantha) leaves and flowers on the metabolization of the p-glycoprotein substrate digoxin showed that the extract used did not cause clinically relevant changes in the maximum plasma concentration or in the elimination half-life of digoxin. This indicates that concurrent use of hawthorn preparations and drugs whose bioavailability is dominated by p-glycoprotein is highly unlikely to lead to drug interactions (Tankanow et al.).

In the case of valerian (Valeriana officinalis), a clinical study of the CYP system showed that even 28 days of therapy using a daily dose of 375 mg of valerian extract showed no clinically significant changes in the activity of the enzyme systems involved. This supports the conclusion that clinically relevant interactions with substrates of this metabolic pathway are not to be expected (Gurley et al.).

In the case of milk thistle (Silybum marianum), in vitro experiments showed irreversible inactivation of CYP enzymes caused by silymarin. Initially, this made interactions of such extracts with other pharmaceutical substances seem plausible (Unger 2010). In a clinical study using irinotecan as a model substance, the pharmacokinetic parameters of the starting substance as well as its most important metabolites remained unchanged even after up to 12 days of administration of a milk thistle product (Baker et al.). Sometimes, a clinical study is cited as proof of the possible interaction potential of milk thistle extracts, which documented a doubling of the bioavailability of losartan on average for study participants (Han et al.). However, these results have not been replicated to date and the data from this study is based on a very small population of six patients.

In the case of ginkgo extracts, despite multiple in vivo studies that pointed to strong interaction potential (Unger 2013), clinical use did not show relevant impacts on the bioavailability of other pharmaceutical substances (Unger 2013). In a systematic review and meta-analysis of 18 controlled clinical studies involving 1,985 patients, Kellermann and Kloft showed no verifiable increased risk of bleeding.

In this context, it should be mentioned that even in the case of St.-John's-wort (Hypericum perforatum)—the only common medicinal plant for which clinically relevant drug interactions have been unequivocally documented—the data refers only to a subgroup of preparations: extracts that contain a high concentration of hyperforin, which is being discussed by some as one of the active constituents. These findings are contrasted by other studies of St.-John's-wort extracts without hyperforin, which, surprisingly, have been shown in clinical trials to be just as effective as extracts containing hyperforin. These studies show no indication for the high interaction potential that was shown for the above mentioned high-concentration hyperforin extracts (Butterweck et al., Madabushi et al.).

It seems that this is not a typical characteristic of the Hypericum perforatum drug, but rather a specific problem in the extraction process. This problem is amplified by the fact that currently, a number of St.-John's-wort preparation marketed in Germany have been manufactured in a way that knowingly enriches their hyperforin content.

The HMPC monographs include interactions, but they only appear in about one out of five monographs and the validity of this information varies widely (Pittner). Current scientific knowledge indicates that clinically relevant interactions for medicinal plants are rarely to be expected, with the exception of high-concentration hyperforin St.-John's-wort extracts. This demonstrates again the special tolerability of phytopharmaceuticals as compared to modern, chemically defined synthetics.

Medicinal Plants

Medicinal plants for which the German Federal Ministry of Health has postulated **interaction suspicion** and ordered studies regarding their interaction potential. Nevertheless, the clinical relevance of herbal drug interactions is minimal provided phytotherapeutics are used at commonly recommended doses.

- Artichoke, Cynara cardunculus
- Stinging nettle, Urtica dioica/urens
- Eucalyptus, Eucalyptus globulus
- Turmeric, Curcuma longa
- Ginkgo, Ginkgo biloba
- Autumn crocus, Colchicum autumnale
- St.-John's-wort, Hypericum perforatum
- German chamomile, Matricaria recutita
- Onion, Allium cepa
- Milk thistle, Silybum marianum
- Peppermint, Mentha piperita
- Licorice, Glycyrrhiza glabra

Bibliography

Definition

Dingermann T, Loew D. Phytopharmakologie. Experimentelle und klinische Pharmakologie pflanzlicher Arzneimittel. Stuttgart: Wissenschaftliche Verlagsgesellschaft; 2003

Eberwein E, Vogel G. Arzneipflanzen in der Phytotherapie. Bonn: Kooperation Phytopharmaka; 1990

Fintelmann V, Menßen HG, Siegers CP. Phytotherapie Manual. 2nd ed. Stuttgart: Hippokrates (Helsinki): 1993

Frohne D. Heilpflanzenlexikon. 8th ed. Stuttgart: Wissen-schaftliche Verlagsgesellschaft; 2002

Frohne D, Jensen U. Systematik des Pflanzenreichs. Unter besonderer Berücksichtigung chemischer Merkmale und pflanzlicher Drogen. 5th ed. Stuttgart: Wissenschaftliche Verlagsgesellschaft; 1998

Hänsel R. Phytopharmaka. 2. ed Berlin: Springer; 1991

Hänsel R, Sticher O, Steinegger E. Pharmakognosie – Phytopharmazie. 8. ed Berlin: Springer; 2007

Hausen BM, Vieluf IK. Allergiepflanzen, Pflanzenallergene. Kontakallergene. 2nd ed. Munich: ecomed; 2001

Nowak R. Notfallhandbuch Giftpflanzen. Berlin: Springer; 1998

Saller R, Reichling J, Hellenbrecht D. Phytotherapie. Heidelberg: Haug; 1995

Schilcher H. Kammerer p. Leitfaden Phytotherapie. 3. ed Munich: Elsevier; 2007

Schulz V, Hänsel R. Rationale Phytotherapie. 5. ed Berlin: Springer; 2004

Vogel G, Gaisbauer M, Winkler W. Phytotherapie in der Praxis. Cologne: Deutscher Ärzte–Verlag; 1990

Wagner H, Wiesenauer M. Phytotherapie: Phytopharmaka und pflanzliche Homöopathika. 2nd ed. Stuttgart: Wissen-schaftliche Verlagsgesellschaft; 2003

Wichtl M, Ed. Teedrogen und Phytopharmaka. 5. ed Stuttgart: Wissenschaftliche Verlagsgesellschaft; 2008

Phytotherapy: A Particular Therapeutic System?

Bosse A. Vertrauen in die Naturheilkunde wächst und wächst. Z Phytother. 2007; 28:195–196

Fintelmann V. Die Phytotherapie als Wissenschaftsfrage. Gibt es eine Erfahrungsmedizin? Z Phytother. 1985; 6:169–171

Fintelmann V. Zukunftsaspekte der Phytotherapie. Z Phytother. 1987; 8:97–101

Fintelmann V. Erkenntnistheoretische Erwägungen. In: Intuitive Medizin. 5. ed Stuttgart: Hippokrates 2007: 19–26

Fintelmann V, Menßen HG. Gegenwart und Zukunft einer modernen Phytotherapie. Natur- und Ganzheitsmedizin. 1992; 5:111–119

Franz G. Phytotherapie: Alte Probleme – neue Tendenzen. ÄrzteZ. Naturheilverfahren 1989;30:113–118

Goethe von JW. Die Metamorphose der Pflanzen. In: Steiner R, ed Naturwissenschaftliche Schriften. Dornach: Steiner; 1975: 17–59

Hänsel R. Möglichkeiten und Grenzen pflanzlicher Arzneimittel (Phytotherapie). Dtsch Apoth Ztg. 1987; 127:2–6

Hardy K, Buckley S, Collins MJ, et al. Neanderthal medics? Evidence for food, cooking, and medicinal plants entrapped in dental calculus. Naturwissenschaften. 2012; 99(8):617–626

Huffman MA. Self-Medicative Behavior in the African Great Apes: An Evolutionary Perspective into the Origins of Human Traditional Medicine. 2001; 51(8):651–661

IfD. (Institut für Demoskopie Allensbach; Hrsg.). Naturheilmittel 2002. Wichtigste Erkenntnisse aus Allensbacher Trendstudien. Allensbach: IfD; 2002

Keil TU. Kontroverse um Silikonimplantate in der plastischen Chirurgie. Prüfung der Argumente unter den Kriterien der Evidence-Based Medicine. Fortschr Med. 1998; 116(7):1

Kiene H. Komplementäre Methodenlehre der klinischen Forschung. Cognition-based Medicine. Berlin: Springer; 2001

Koch V. Phytotherapie—(k)eine besondere Therapierichtung? Hufeland-Journal: HJ. 1994; 9:90–94

Kraft K, März R. Die wissenschaftliche Basis der Phytotherapie. Z Phytother. 2006; 27:279–283

Loew D. EBM: Evidence-based (phyto) medicine versus Experience-based (phyto) medicine. Z Phytother. 2000; 21(2):71–77

Ludewig R. Schulmedizin und Naturmedizin im Meinungsstreit um Arzneimittel. Plädoyer für eine Modus vivendi. Natur- und Ganzheitsmedizin. 1989; 2:40–47

Meyer R. "Culture-based medicine." Landessitten und Thera-pierichtlinien. Dtsch Aerztebl. 1999; 96:C2084

Pascoe ED. Pascoe-Studie 2004. Gießen: Pascoe GmbH; 2004:1–7

Pascoe ED. Pascoe-Studie 2007. Gießen: Pascoe GmbH; 2007: 1–15

Perlett M. Gegenwärtiger Stand der evidenzbasierten Medizin. Z Allg Med. 1998; 74:450–454

Rademacher JG. Erfahrungsheillehre (1. Bd.). Berlin: Reimer; 1851: 140

Sackett DL, Richardson WS, Rosenberg W, Haynes RB. Evidence-based Medicine. How to practice and teach EBM. New York, USA: Churchill Livingstone; 1997

Schäfer H. Die Zukunft der Medizin. Dtsch Aerztebl. 1975; 72(8): 520–523

Schäfer H. Plädoyer für eine neue Medizin. Munich: Piper; 1979

Schilcher H. Naturheilmittel aus wissenschaftlicher und praktischer Sicht. Therapeutikon. 1990; 4:247–254

Uexküll T, Herrmann JM. Evidenz-basierte und Patienten-orientierte Medizin. Munch Med Wochenschr. 1999; 141:23–25

Vogel G. Besonderheiten pflanzlicher Arzneimittel – Mythos oder Wirklichkeit? Dtsch Apoth Ztg. 1979; 119:2029–2003

Wagner H, Hörhammer L, Münster R. Zur Chemie des Silymarins (Silybin), des Wirkprinzips der Früchte von Silybum marianum (L.) Gaertn. (Carduus marianus L.) [On the chemistry of silymarin (silybin), the active principle of the fruits from Silybum marianum (L.) Gaertn. (Carduus marianus L.]. Arzneimittelforschung. 1968; 18(6):688–696

Wasem J. Studie des Marktforschungsinstituts TNS Infratest. Zit. n. Phytokompass—Aktuelles aus Forschung und Praxis,. 2015; 2: 6–7

Weyrich LS, Duchene S, Soubrier J, et al. Neanderthal behaviour, diet, and disease inferred from ancient DNA in dental calculus. Nature. 2017; 544(7650):357–361

Winterhoff H, Gumbinger HG. Pharmakologische Unter-suchungen mit Pflanzenextrakten. Probleme und Lösungsmö-glichkeiten. Dtsch Apoth Ztg. 1990; 130:2667–2670

Importance of Proof of Efficacy

Bleuler E. Das autistisch-undisziplinierte Denken in der Medizin und seine Überwindung. 5. ed Berlin: Springer; 1962

Carus CG. Erfahrungsresultate aus ärztlichen Studien und ärztlichem Wirken. Leipzig: Brockhaus; 1859

Der Placebo-Effekt NP. MMW Munch Med Wochenschr. 1977; 119: 203–208

Dorn M. Zur Problematik klinischer Prüfungen mit Phytopharmaka. Ärztez Naturheilverfahren 1993;34:848–855

Eberwein B. Zur Bewertung von Kombinationsarzneimitteln im Rahmen der Arzneimittel-Zulassung. Ärztez Naturheilverfahren 1990;31:117–123

Fahrländer H, Truog P. Placebowirkung und Alternativmedi-zin.Placebo action and alternative medicine]. Schweiz Med Wochenschr. 1990; 120(16):581–588

Fintelmann V. Befund und Befindlichkeit. Z Phytother. 1990; 11: 10–13

Fintelmann V. Intuitive Medizin. 6. ed Stuttgart: Hippokrates; 2016

Fintelmann V. Kombinationsarzneimittel aus medizinischer Sicht. Z Phytother. 1988; 9:58–62

Fintelmann V. Quo vadis? Medizin am Scheideweg. Stuttgart: Mayer; 2000

Fülgraff G. Der kontrollierte Versuch–Eine kritische Würdigung. Pharmazeut Ztg. 1985; 130:3309–3313

GMDS. (Deutsche Gesellschaft für Medizinische Informatik, Biometrie und Epidemiologie; Hrsg.). Empfehlungen zur Durchführung von Anwendungsbeobachtungen (Recommen-dations concerning the conduct of "Anwendungsbeo-bachtungen") der Deutschen Gesellschaft für Medizinische Informatik, Biometrie und Epidemiologie (GMDS). Informatik, Biometrie und Epidemiologie in Medizin und Biologie 1997; 4: 247–252

Helmstädter A, Staiger C. Traditionelle Anwendung: Eine Betrachtung zu pflanzlichen Arzneimitteln aus pharmaziehis-torischer Sicht. Forsch Komplementmed [Forschende Komplementarmedizin]. 2012; 19:93–98

Hornung J. Was ist ein Placebo? Die Bedeutung einer korrekten Definition für die klinische Forschung. Forsch Komplementmed. 1994; 1(4):160–165

Kiene H. Kritik der klinischen Doppelblindstudie. Munich: MMV Medizin; 1993

Kienle G. Arzneimittelsicherheit und Gesellschaft. Stuttgart: Schattauer; 1974

Kienle GS. Der sogenannte Placeboeffekt. Stuttgart: Schattauer; 1995

Kienle GS, Kiene H. Zur Bedeutung von Fallberichten. In: Kienle GS, Fintelmann V, Treichler M. Onkologie auf anthroposophischer Grundlage. Frankfurt: Info3 Verlag. 2016

Loew D. Wirksamkeit und Sicherheit praxisrelevanter Phytopharmaka. Z Phytother. 2005; 26(3):119–125

Medicinal Products Act (Arzneimittelgesetz–AMG) http://www.gesetze-im-internet.de/englisch_amg/index.html (Accessed 28 October 2021)

Plügge H. Wohlbefinden und Missbefinden. Tübingen: Niemeyer; 1962

Steiner R, ed Naturwissenschaftliche Schriften. Dornach: Steiner; 1975

Stolte F, Knöss W. „Tradition" und traditionelle pflanzliche Arzneimittel. Z Phytother. 2014; 35(02):63–67

Victor N, Windeler J, Hasford J, et al. Empfehlungen zur Durchführung von Anwendungsbeobachtungen. Informatik. Biometrie und Epidemiologie in Medizin und Biologie. 1997; 28 (4):247–252

Vogel G. Wirksamkeitsnachweis bei Phytopharmaka. Dtsch Apoth Ztg. 1985; 125:485–489

Side Effects

Anonymus. Tückisches Johanniskraut. Lebensgefährliche Wechselwirkung mit anderen Arzneimitteln. Frankfurter Allgemeine Zeitung. 2000; 45:1

Frohne D. Sind pflanzliche Arzneimittel unschädlich? Dtsch Apothek Z. 1990; 130:1861–1871

Hausen BM, Vieluf IK. Allergiepflanzen, Pflanzenallergene. Kontaktallergene. 2nd ed. Munich: Ecomed; 2001

Schulz V. Arzneimittelinteraktionen: Relevanz für Phytopharmaka? Z Phytother. 2004; 25(6):283–288

Thesen R. Phytotherapeutika–nicht immer harmlos. Pharm Ztg. 1988; 133:38–43

Vogel G. Phytopharmaka–Arzneimittel ohne Risiko? Dtsch Apoth Ztg. 1984; 124:639–642

Vogel G. Wissenschaftliche Erkenntnisse zu Wirksamkeit und Unbedenklichkeit pflanzlicher Arzneimittel. Therapiewoche. 1984:4078–4086

Interactions

Baker SD, Zhao M, Rudek MA, Guchelaar HJ, et al. Effect of milk thistle (Silybum marianum) on the pharmacokinetics of irinotecan. Clin Cancer Res. 2005; 11(21):7800–7806

Butterweck V, Christoffel V, Nahrstedt A, Petereit F, Spengler B, Winterhoff H. Step by step removal of hyperforin and hypericin: activity profile of different Hypericum preparations in behavioral models. Life Sci. 2003; 73(5):627–639

Gaus W, Westendorf J, Diebow R, Kieser M. Identification of adverse drug reactions by evaluation of a prescription database, demonstrated for "risk of bleeding.". Methods Inf Med. 2005; 44 (5):697–703

Gurley BJ, Gardner SF, Hubbard MA, et al. In vivo effects of goldenseal, kava kava, black cohosh, and valerian on human cytochrome P450 1A2, 2D6, 2E1, and 3A4/5 phenotypes. Clin Pharmacol Ther. 2005; 77(5):415–426

Han Y, Guo D, Chen Y, Chen Y, Tan ZR, Zhou HH. Effect of silymarin on the pharmacokinetics of losartan and its active metabolite E-3174 in healthy Chinese volunteers. Eur J Clin Pharmacol. 2009; 65(6):585–591

Kellermann AJ, Kloft C. Is there a risk of bleeding associated with standardized Ginkgo biloba extract therapy? A systematic review and meta-analysis. Pharmacotherapy. 2011; 31(5):490–502

Madabushi R, Frank B, Drewelow B, Derendorf H, Butterweck V. Hyperforin in St. John's wort drug interactions. Eur J Clin Pharmacol. 2006; 62(3):225–233

Madeira S, Melo M, Porto J, et al. The diseases we cause: Iatrogenic illness in a department of internal medicine. Eur J Intern Med. 2007; 18(5):391–399

Pittner H. Wechselwirkungen mit pflanzlichen Arzneimitteln: Was steht in den HMPC-Monographien? Phytotherapie Austria 2014; 8(1): 4–7

Saller R, Kasper S, Dimpfel W, et al. Phytotherapie in der Geriatrie und Gerontologie. Forsch Komplement Med. 2014; 21 Suppl 1: 2–18

Seden K, Dickinson L, Khoo S, Back D. Grapefruit-drug interactions. Drugs. 2010; 70(18):2373–2407

Sugimoto K, Ohmori M, Tsuruoka S, et al. Different effects of St. John's wort on the pharmacokinetics of simvastatin and pravastatin. Clin Pharmacol Ther. 2001; 70(6):518–524

Tankanow R, Tamer HR, Streetman DS, et al. Interaction study between digoxin and a preparation of hawthorn (Crataegus oxyacantha). J Clin Pharmacol. 2003; 43(6):637–642

Tsai HH, Lin HW, Simon Pickard A, Tsai HY, Mahady GB. Evaluation of documented drug interactions and contrain-dications associated with herbs and dietary supplements: a systematic literature review. Int J Clin Pract. 2012; 66(11):1056–1078

Unger M. Pharmakokinetische Arzneimittelinteraktionen durch pflanzliche Arzneimittel: Kritische Bewertung und klinische Relevanz. Wien Med Wochenschr. 2010; 160(21–22):571–577

Unger M. Pharmacokinetic drug interactions involving Ginkgo biloba. Drug Metab Rev. 2013; 45(3):353–385

2 Specific Aspects

This chapter discusses the basic requirements for phytotherapeutics and introduces the "old" art of prescribing, which is particularly well suited to phytotherapeutics. Special consideration is given to the use of medicinal plants for medicinal teas and herbal baths. These therapies have been established for centuries. They allow the excellent healing effects of medicinal plants to unfold in a very specific way that is finely tuned to a patient's state of health.

2.1 Quality Assurance

The three main requirements of the Medicinal Products Act (Arzneimittelgesetz—AMG) for medical products in Germany are pharmaceutical quality, efficacy, and safety. For phytopharmaceuticals, this means that the type of preparation is of key importance because medicinal plants are rarely used in their "natural" state, except perhaps the application of cabbage leaves or onion slices. Creating medicine from a medicinal plant always involves drugs and their pharmaceutic preparations. In modern phytotherapy, this usually involves **extracts**. The substance and structural composition of extracts should represent the substantive and structural composition of the medicinal plant and its special characteristics.

Against this backdrop, Gaedcke refers to plant extracts in their natural, unadulterated, substantive wholeness as the actual active substance, which he divides into active substances, constituent and substance groups that determine efficacy, pharmaceutically relevant constituents or groups of constituents that co-determine efficacy, lead substances, coeffectors, adjuvants, and fillers. He further differentiates **adjuvants** into undesirable substances—for example, those possessing allergenic or toxic potential—and ubiquitous substances, such as carbohydrates, proteins, fatty oils, chlorophyll, etc. Standardization encompasses all measures leading to reproducible quality for the drug and for the extracts derived from the drug. If additional constituents that determine efficacy are known to exist for the standardized extract, the potency of those constituents can be standardized as well. Hefendehl and Lander refer to standardization as the "formulation of a drug powder or extract according to a fixed standard value, listing the minimum and maximum potency of a substance or substance group that is considered a determinant of efficacy."

One essential consideration is the **quality of the source (parent) drug**. Many important native medicinal plants are no longer collected in the wild, as was the case in the past, but are farmed in a standardized manner. This mean that the growing conditions of the plant need to be suitable for producing a drug that is equal to or exceeds the quality of the original, wild harvested plant. Controlled farming certainly guarantees a more balanced composition of the pharmaceutical drug but will never achieve the precision of synthetic monosubstances. Conditions such as climate, soil quality, harvest and drying conditions substantially influence the drug. Wild harvesting continues to make sense for personal use, but it is important to look for plants in areas likely to have low levels of contamination with pollutants.

Wild harvesting of protected plants (for example, **Arnica montana**) or of exotic plants such as the South African devil's claw, is a different matter. For these plant populations, destructive wild-harvesting poses a real threat. For this reason, the German Federal Agency for Environmental Protection (Bundesamt für Naturschutz, BfN) initiated an international standard for sustainable wild harvesting of medicinal plants in cooperation with the World Wide Fund for Nature (WWF) and the International Union for Conservation of Nature (IUCN), within the framework of the international Trade Records Analysis of Flora and Fauna in Commerce (TRAFFIC) (Pätzold and Honnef).

2.1.1 Finished Pharmaceutical Products

Finished pharmaceutical products used in phytotherapy should meet certain labeling guidelines that the prescriber can verify at any time.

Optionally, substances that co-determine efficacy and/or **lead substances** may be listed. These represent chemically defined constituents of plant medicines that are important for verification and quality assurance. The drug extract ratio (DER) allows practitioners to calculate whether therapeutically effective or rational dosing is possible. Listing the extraction agent is essential. For example, water is an insufficient extraction agent for lipophilic constituents.

Understanding the preparation methods with their possibilities and limitations as well as meeting clear labeling guidelines are indispensable components of modern phytotherapy. These criteria have been adopted by the manufacturers of phytopharmaceuticals who joined together in the Committee for Research into Natural Medicines (Komitee Forschung Naturmedizin, KFN). Their goal is to guarantee phytopharmaceuticals to prescribers that go beyond meeting precise criteria and that can demonstrate results of original experimental and clinical research. These criteria no longer refer to drug monographs and their seeming universality, but to individual, scientifically tested and approved medicinal products. Results are published and revised regularly in the *Kompendium Phytopharmaka*.

One problem, which is not to be underestimated, is how to compare defined extracts with extracts from the same plant, but without comparable criteria regarding location of growth, extraction process, and other manufacturing processes. This phytoequivalence of different medicinal products from the same medicinal plant is a question that has not yet been addressed by science. It creates, for example, the need to exclude generic plant medicines (Ullmann).

> **Definition**
>
> Dingermann considers the following **criteria** of significance for phytopharmaceuticals:
> - Type of active constituent, for example, drug, tincture, extract, fluid extract, dry extract, or other extracts
> - Amount of active constituent per single dose (for solid medicinal products) or per package (for fluid medicinal products), for example, 200 mg dry extract per pill or 100 mL fluid extract
> - Ratio of drug to active constituent (the drug extract ratio, DER)
> - Type and concentration of extraction agent
> - Indication
> - Daily dose

2.1.2 Preparation Methods

▶ Table 2.1 provides an overview of the preparation methods for plant medicines.

Table 2.1 Drug preparation methods

Preparation Method	Description
Medicinal teas (Species)	Tea blend (most often more than one plant drug)
Infusion (Infusum)	Infusion (of tender plant parts: flowers, leaves, seeds)
Decoction (Decoctum)	Simmering (of very hard drugs: wood, bark, roots)
Maceration (Maceratio)	Soaking in cold water (primarily for mucilaginous drugs)
Succus	Sap or juice expressed from a fresh plant
Extraction (Extractum)	Extract (dry, thick fluid)
Hydrosol (Aqua aromatic)	Aromatic water (produced by distilling fresh leaves, fruits, flowers, and other plant materials)
Syrup (Sirupus)	Liquid preparation in a concentrated solution (as a corrigent for infusions and mixtures)
Spirit (Spiritus)	Tincture (alcohol-based solution) (primarily for external application, for example, calamus spirit; less frequently for internal use, for example, peppermint spirit, peppermint drops)
Suppositories (Suppositorium)	Suppository (containing powdered drugs, for example, chamomile flos, or made from extracts)
Ointment (Unguentum)	Topical salve (from tinctures or extracts using a hydrophilic base, for example, unguentum molle, unguentum cereum, etc.)
Finished pharmaceutical products	Tablet, pill, capsule, drops, vial, syrup, etc.

2.2 Guidelines for Prescribing Medicinal Plants

Today's pharmacotherapy is so heavily dominated by finished pharmaceutical products that younger physicians are rarely still familiar with the art of prescribing. Phytotherapy provides the impetus for physicians to relearn how to compose their own **prescriptions**, especially because, as mentioned above, medicinal plant therapy helps physicians to understand the individuality of disease. Moving from schematic to individualized therapy provides increased professional satisfaction for physicians. Patients notice that the physician is addressing their individual needs. This is certainly one of the factors that has led to increased recognition of natural medicine. In a representative survey of 2,111 Germans over the age of 16 published on 18 May 2001 by the *Deutsches Ärzteblatt*, a German publication for physicians, respondents responded as follows: 83% expressed spontaneous support for natural remedies, 45% believed physicians underutilized the possibilities of alternative medicine, 50% believed without reservation in the efficacy of natural medicines, 67% with prior experience with natural medicine and alternative remedies wished for more physicians with experience in this area. These wishes did not represent a rejection of conventional medicine: 81% of respondents were convinced that the approaches are complementary (Bühring). More recent survey results are discussed in section 1.3.3 Phytotherapy and Prevention (p. 9).

Teas are the simplest prescription and the one most well suited to individualized prescriptions, although they are not necessarily the primary type of prescription. Among other preparations, **tinctures** are also especially well suited to individualized prescriptions. And in modern phytotherapy, like in so many other areas, finished pharmaceutical products dominate. Their advantages include standardized manufacturing processes using high-quality source drugs, which generally assures a stable share of the essential constituents.

Individualized prescriptions offer economic advantages because individually prescribed tea or tincture blends are often substantially less expensive than finished pharmaceutical products. This also offers economic benefits to the prescription budgets allocated to physicians working within managed care or national health systems, for example, the German public health insurance system.

The following section introduces brief guidelines for prescribing phytotherapeutics. The practical application section of this book contains numerous prescription suggestions and especially suitable drugs for these application areas.

2.2.1 Basic Principles

Prescriptions for phytotherapeutics should be rational in the same way as is common for synthetic drugs. They should also be subject to all criteria used for pharmacological assessment of synthetics. This includes known undesirable effects, specific contraindications, and especially interactions with other drugs or remedies.

There is still little precise information about interactions between phytotherapeutics (caveat: not in reference to chemically defined individual components). For this reason, physicians starting to prescribe phytotherapeutics and desiring to compose their own individual prescriptions should give preference to **monotherapy**. This path allows physicians to become familiar more quickly with the actions of individual medicinal plants. These actions are often more difficult to differentiate in combination remedies.

Previously, many **combination medicinal products** used in phytotherapy consisted of numerous medicinal plants. They were referred to as "desk combinations," because their compositions were frequently not rationally comprehensible. Since that time, the EU guideline 5/318 (Part 3, Chapter II, C2) or, in Germany, the Medicinal Products Act require the composition of combination drugs to be substantiated much more precisely. At the same time, the Medicinal Products Act, Section 22, subsection 3a in its 12 December 2005 revision requires that each component of combination drugs is described and justified: "If the medicinal product contains more than one active substance, evidence shall be provided to prove that every active substance contributes to the positive assessment of the medicinal product."

EU guidelines go a step further: The 2017 edition of the *Guideline on Clinical Development of Fixed Combination Medicinal Products* of the European Medicines Agency (EMA) states: "Particular attention should be given to the doses of each active substance in the fixed combination medicinal product, with each dose combination being scientifically justified and clinically relevant. The use of all active substances in the indication applied for should be justified." The guideline goes on to say: "For any fixed combination medicinal product, it is necessary to assess the potential clinical advantages of combination therapy against the use of monotherapies, in order to determine whether the product meets the requirements with respect to efficacy and safety." It states further: "The evidence base for establishing the contribution to an overall effect and favorable benefit-risk balance of the fixed combination is expected to ...[d] demonstrate that each active substance contributes to efficacy and/or benefit-risk balance. Active substances may have additive effects or synergistic effects.

The general assumption is that combination drugs should not contain more than **three combination partners**. This rule may be disregarded for some individual applications—for example, in cases of well-documented traditional use of historically fixed combinations of several herbal raw drugs.

To demonstrate the practical application of these guidelines, the Commission E compiled and published a number of approved fixed combinations.

The main positive criteria for fixed combinations are to simplify therapy and to enhance drug efficacy. **Simplification of therapy** is a motivation that applies to all aspects of medicine and is especially relevant in clinical practice. Fixed combination drugs may also improve patient compliance because patients may experience several mechanisms of action at the same time while taking a single preparation. The predominant reason for fixed combinations is likely to be the **enhancement of drug efficacy** according to the simple formula: "Divided we are weak, together we are strong!" It is not really possible to apply the yardstick of the scientific pharmacologic method to the additive, superadditive, concordance, and equivalency effects of fixed combinations. Fixed combinations imitate the creative principles of nature in a positive sense to invent new therapeutic "wholes" or holistic combinations. Such combination drugs therefore can only be judged using the criteria of therapeutic efficacy.

Combination preparations to be rejected are those for which ideological justification is sought or that were created for clearly recognizable personal gain. Market success of combination drugs seems to be enhanced by the addition of more combination partners. In phytotherapy, single component prescriptions are preferable to combination drugs. Only physicians who are very familiar with the efficacy of drugs derived from single medicinal plants can freely combine them or judge the efficacy of combination drugs.

Definition

The German Commission E rates **fixed combinations as positive** if they meet at least one of the following criteria:
- Additive synergistic effects of the components with equal or various targets exist, and/or
- A more than additive effect of the fixed combination occurs compared to the single components, and/or
- Side effects of a single component are lessened or negated (e.g., dosage reduction of components acting in the same direction), and/or
- The combination instigates a therapy simplification or improvement in therapy safety. This can be the case if an improvement of compliance (by reduction of the medication frequency and/or simplification of dosage administration), and/or an improvement in absorption, and/or an avoidance of galenic incompatibilities is obtained, and/or
- One of the medicinally active components lessens or negates one or more of the side effects of another component, if the side effect normally occurs.

Safety concerns regarding fixed combinations are characterized by the following parameters:
- Considerable pharmacokinetic and/or pharmacodynamic interactions exist that do not improve the benefit/risk ratio, or even worsen it.
- The half-life and/or the duration of the actions of the medicinally active components differ widely.

The second criteria can be disregarded if the combination is proven to be clinically valuable and/or if it contains a component that is intended to affect an unpleasant reaction, in order to prevent abuse.

However, **fixed combinations** are a useful and indispensable component of a physician's therapeutic repertoire.

2.2.2 Important Terms and Prescription-Writing Guidelines

See ▶ Table 2.2, ▶ Table 2.3, and ▶ Table 2.4.

2.3 Medicinal Teas

As a basic rule, the physician needs to carefully assess which of the prescription methods listed in in ▶ Table 2.1 is the most suitable for a specific condition. Tinctures, for example, are very well suited for combination remedies. Teas are a very important therapy type in phytotherapy.

Table 2.2 Naming conventions and abbreviations for plant medicines

Abbreviation	Latin Name	English Name
bacc.	Bacca	Berry
bulb.	Bulbus	Bulb
cort.	Cortex	Bark
Flos	Flos	Flower
fol.	Folium	Leaf
gland.	Glandula	Gland
gem.	Gemma	Bud
herb.	Herba	Herb (above-ground parts)
lich.	Lichen	Lichen
lign.	Lignum	Wood
pericarp.	Pericarpium	Peel (pericarp)
rad.	Radix	Root
rhiz.	Rhizoma	Rootstock (rhizome)
sem.	Semen	Seed
stip.	Stipes	Stem
sum.	Summitas	Branch tip
tub.	Tuber	Tuber
tur.	Turio	Sprout

2.3.1 Composition

Prescriptions for combination remedies contain a main or **basic constituent** (*remedium cardinale*), an **adjuvant** that amplifies or complements the effect of the basic constituent in a certain direction, possibly a **filler** (constituent), and often a **corrigent** for improving flavor or tolerability.

Fillers are drugs that lend a pleasing or noticeable appearance to the tea mixture due to their striking color and/or their peculiar shape. Ready-made tea mixtures often contain such fillers. Medicinal teas composed according to a physician's individual prescription do not require them. Of course, thin parts of herbs or twigs that are a drab gray-green in color are less impressive than mixtures containing bright yellow or blue components. Yellow components are usually sandy everlasting (Helichrysum arenarium), which in prescriptions may still be referred to by their previous name, Stoechados citrinae flos. Blue flowers may be cornflower (Centaurea cyanus) or lavender (Lavandula angustifolia). Roman chamomile (Anthemis nobilis) flowers are strikingly white and calendula flowers (Calendula officinalis) are large and orange in color. The common tea variety of the tree mallow (Malva arborea) flowers are even larger and peculiarly dark purple or blackish in color.

2.3.2 Naming

Every prescription requires the precise names of the drugs, which are noted as abbreviations (▶ Table 2.2).

Table 2.3 Terms used in plant medicine preparation

Abbreviation	Latin Name	English Name
conc., concis.	concisus/-a/-um	Chopped
cont.	contusus/-a/-um	Crushed
dep.	depuratus/-a/-um	Purified
pulv.	pulveratus/-a/-um, pulvis	Powdered, powder, pulverized, ground
pulv. subt.	pulveratus/-a/-um subtile	Finely powdered (finely ground)
expulp.	expulpatus/-a/-um	Pulp removed

Table 2.4 General Prescription Guidelines

Abbreviation	Latin Name	Meaning
Rx	Recipe	Prescription (introductory designation for every prescription)
āā or aa	ana partes aequales	Equal parts of each (for multiple constituents)
M. f. or M. Ft. or M. et ft. spec. pulv. pil. ungt. supp.	Misce fiat species pulvis pillulae unguentum suppositorium	Mix and make (the prescription), for example: Tea Powder Pills Ointment, unguent Suppositories
D.S. or Sig:	Da Signa	Give (the patient) Label as follows (dosage instructions)
D. ad scat.	Da ad scatulam	Place (for example, powder) into a container
D. tal. dos. Nr....	Da tales doses Nr....	Divide into individual doses of...

2.3.3 Instructions for Use

At the beginning of treatment, patients should be advised that teas are only effective if they are used regularly and over a long period of time. Weiss uses the term regimen because it signals use over a certain period of time. However, teas should not be taken for an unlimited time because the summation of small effects can lead to intolerability, habituation, or even harm.

Every tea prescription must contain detailed instructions for its use. These instructions need to state whether the tea needs to be prepared by pouring hot water over it, or whether it needs to be simmered and for how long. All drugs containing volatile oils should be prepared by pouring hot water over them, covering them, and letting them steep for 5–10 minutes. Boiling such teas would cause most of the volatile oils to evaporate and the tea would lose its efficacy.

Instructions for dosage of teas generally can be a little more relaxed than for fixed drug combinations containing specific constituents. The usual dosage for teas is 1–2 teaspoons of the tea mixture in 1 glass or 150 mL of water. The Commission E monographs always indicate an average daily dosage for tea preparations.

Timing of use is also a consideration. One cup of tea should be taken in the morning and another in the evening at bedtime. Frequently, a third cup is added at noon or, better yet, in the afternoon, a few hours after the midday meal. Teas should be consumed on an empty stomach unless there are special reasons not to.

Teas should be enjoyed while still very warm and, as Kneipp said, in a "dietetic manner." This means that teas should be treated like a good meal and consumed slowly, in small sips. The term "dietetic" describes a comprehensive aspiration expressed by Hufeland and also by von Feuchtersleben in his book *Die Diätetik der Seele* (The Dietetics of the Soul), which is well worth reading. It refers to measures that influence the body and soul with the goal of harmonizing and thereby increasing general vitality. Teas should be consumed in an atmosphere of utmost physical and mental quietude. Sitting comfortably in a chair and maintaining a mental attitude that is supportive to healing of the disorder are helpful.

> **Caution**
>
> Within the context of all prescriptions in this book, the terms "hot water" and "boiling water" always refer to water that has been heated to the boiling point in an electric or stovetop tea kettle. Never use hot tap water because using it for preparation will lead to the swift growth of bacteria in the liquid!
>
> Furthermore, teas should always be covered during steeping, if not specifically mentioned in the prescription instructions to prepare otherwise.

The taste of medicinal teas can sometimes be improved by sweetening them with sugar. However, this is not advisable for bitter teas. Teas containing volatile oils are more suited to being sweetened using sugar. Honey is even better than sugar. With teas for soothing coughs, honey can even enhance the tea's healing effect. Glucose is not preferable to plain sugar (sucrose) or honey. The use of synthetic sweetening agents is not advisable. Sweetening is not necessary. Many patients prefer to drink their medicinal teas entirely without sweeteners. It increases the "medicinal' aspect." Even such seemingly minor details should be taken into consideration by practitioners.

2.3.4 Instant Teas and Ready-Made Tea Blends

Instant teas, which are prepared by adding hot water, represent technical progress. These products go beyond tea in its original sense. They are extracts produced using high-end technical processes. One established process is spray drying using drying times of only a few seconds. This creates a completely dry and long-lasting powder that dissolves into water without changes or residue. Experiments using paper chromatograms showed that spray drying maintains the spectrum of constituents very well, even for vitamin C, which is very sensitive. The same applies to freeze-drying.

Instant teas have proven to be practical and effective. In our hectic times, they contribute toward making tea therapy more accessible to a larger group of people with illnesses. For example, instant teas can be freshly prepared during a lunch break at the workplace or at anytime away from home.

Tea bags have also been shown to be useful. Their active constituents quickly and thoroughly infuse into liquid. In Germany, preparations available at pharmacies guarantee higher quality than teas offered in supermarkets, as the latter are required by law to contain a much smaller dose of the active material according to the Medicinal Products Act (Arzneimittelgesetz—AMG).

Sample Prescriptions

Prescriptions

Mild Laxative Tea for Chronic Gallbladder Disorders

Rx
Absinthii herb. 30.0 (wormwood herb)
(= base constituent)
Frangulae cort. 10.0 (buckthorn bark)
(= adjuvant)
Menth. pip. fol. 10.0 (peppermint leaves)
(= corrigent)
Stoechados flos 10.0 (sandy everlasting flowers, Helichrysum arenarium)
(= constituent)
M. f. spec. (tea)
Add 1 cup of boiling water to 1 teaspoon of tea. Cover and steep for 15 minutes; then strain.
D.S.
Drink one cup of warm tea in the morning on an empty stomach and one in the evening before bedtime for 3 weeks.

Definition

Six Rules for a Tea Prescription
1. Prescribe only **one base constituent**, if possible, or a maximum of two to three.
2. Only one **adjuvant**, at the most two, to better assess the effect.
3. **Corrigents**, if used, should be comparable to the base constituent in their effect and should improve taste (drugs containing volatile oils).
4. The effect of drugs chosen as **constituents** should be similar to those of the base constituent.
5. **Instructions for preparation** must be very precise:
   - Leaves, flowers, and seeds should be prepared by pouring hot water over them.
   - Roots, bark, and wood should be simmered in hot water for 10–15 minutes or should be placed in cold water and then be brought to a brief boil. In tea blends, the base constituent determines the preparation method.
6. Always include precise instructions for use. As a rule, these are as follows:
   - 1–3 teaspoons in 1 cup or 1 glass of water.
   - 2–3 cups per day; the first cup on an empty stomach in the morning, the second cup in the evening at bedtime and, if needed, a third cup in the afternoon.
   Duration of treatment: 3–4 weeks.

Tincture Combination Amplified by Essential Oil

Rx

Tinct. Absinthii 10.0 (wormwood tincture)
(= base)
Tinct. Belladonnae 5.0 (belladonna tincture)
(= adjuvant)
Ol. Carvi 2.0 (caraway essential oil)
(= corrigent)
Tinct. Valerian. aeth. ad 30.0 (ethereal valerian tincture)
(= constituent)
D.S.
Take 30 drops 3 × a day after meals in a shot glass of water. Use for 2 weeks.

Prescription

Suppositories Using a Powdered Herb

Rx

Chamomill. flos pulv. 0.5 (powdered German chamomile flower)
(= base)
Extr. Belladonnae 0.02 (belladonna extract)
(= adjuvant)
Ol. Cacao 1.5 (cocoa butter)
(= constituent)
M. f. spec.
D. tal. dos. Nr. IV (divide into 4 doses)
D.S.
Use one suppository each in the morning and the evening.

2.4 Phytobalneology

Bathing in water that contains medicinal plants is an age-old tradition. We need to differentiate between cosmetic and therapeutic baths. For cosmetic baths, the most important aspects are pleasing scents and a nice bath water color. Herbal medicinal baths, on the other hand, have to meet very different, medical requirements. Phytobalneology experienced a significant increase in popularity through the work of Sebastian Kneipp. He resurrected the ancient practice of adding plant components to bath water. He combined this with his warm water treatments, which unfortunately are not yet as well known as his much more famous cold water treatments. Kneipp has been quoted as saying: "I very rarely or never use only water for all my warm water treatments. I always add components of various medicinal herbs to the water."

Medicinal Plants

Herbs Used in Therapeutic Baths

- Common horsetail, Equisetum arvense
- Valerian, Valeriana officinalis
- Oak bark, Quercus cortex
- Norway spruce needles, Picea abies folium
- Oat straw, Avenae stramentum
- Hay flower, Graminis flos
- Calamus, Acorus calamus
- German chamomile, Matricaria recutita
- Lavender, Lavandula angustifolia
- Lemon balm, Melissa officinalis
- Rosemary, Rosmarinus officinalis
- Yarrow, Achillea millefolium
- Thyme, Thymus vulgaris
- Wheat bran, Furfur tritici

There has been much discussion about the efficacy of herbal baths and their mechanism of action. The assertions that the therapeutic effects of herbal baths result only from the purely physical effects of water and that herbs do not add specific effects has been disproven. Many studies have shown the skin to be a good and reliable **absorption organ**. This is evidenced by transdermal applications of pharmaceutical drugs, such as in nitroglycerin and estrogen patches. According to galenics, the constituents of medicinal herbs in bath additives are equally well absorbed. This has been shown by Römmelt et al. Volatile oils have been measured in blood levels and in exhaled air. One very interesting aspect in this context is that these plasma concentrations occur with some delay and reach their maximum after the end of the bath. Concentrations measured in exhaled air reach their maximum even later.

Aromatherapy is often cited as a possible mechanism because it causes changes in well-being by stimulating the central nervous system via the olfactory organ. No doubt, scents can cause stimulation or repulsion. However, their therapeutic effects seem to be derived primarily via the absorption of volatile oil components through the mucous membranes of the nose and—in the case of balneology—via the entire surface of the skin into the blood stream.

2.4.1 Types of Applications

The degree of absorption of volatile oils also depends on water temperature, and rises as the temperature increases. **Bath oils** are a primary method. Their efficacy depends very much on sufficient distribution of the oils into the full or partial bath. **Emulsions** of medicinal plants containing volatile oils are also well suited as additions to baths. Both application methods are simple and also make it easier to clean the bathtub.

Whole plant extracts are also very effective, but their syrupy consistency and murky appearance makes them less popular. They have their place for applications where other components, in addition to the absorption of volatile oils are important, for example with common horsetail (Equisetum arvense). **Chopped or ground herbs** may also be added to baths. This is the original and, certainly still, valid method. According to Kneipp, the herbs used, for example, oak bark or horsetail, are cooked into a thick slurry which is then added to the bath water. Another method is to tie the herbs used into a small linen bag and to agitate the bag in the bath water. This method is useful for partial baths and wet compresses.

2.4.2 Instructions for Use

When prescribing therapeutic baths, **water temperature** is important. In general, it should be moderate, between 36–38 °C (96.5–100 °F), depending on personal sensitivity. Bath duration for full or partial baths should not exceed 10–15 minutes unless specifically prescribed otherwise. A 30-minute period of rest should follow baths unless the bath is designed to be "energizing." Calming baths are best taken in the evening.

Baths, especially full baths, are strenuous. They frequently tax the circulatory system and should only be prescribed for patients whose circulatory system can be presumed to be stable. Congestive heart failure and heart arrhythmia, for example, are absolute contraindications for a full bath. **Partial baths**, for example, hand, foot, lower arm or sitz baths, can certainly be useful in such cases, but always with close medical or caregiver supervision.

Oil dispersion baths, in accordance with Junge, are useful for distributing bath oils in full or partial baths. They require a small apparatus that can be attached to every faucet or handheld shower head. The apparatus contains the bath oil and distributes it very finely into the bath water instead of creating a film of oil on the surface of the water.

Medicinal Plants for Balneology

Norway Spruce (Picea abies)

Norway spruce baths are the most prevalent and most thoroughly studied type of herbal bath. Norway spruce has been shown to develop a specific stimulating effect that can be fairly well dosed. In addition to Norway spruce (Picea abies), fir (Abies alba) or pine (Pinus sylvestris) may also be used. Norway spruce baths have many therapeutic uses, for example, for nerve disorders and rheumatic and neuralgic conditions.

Norway spruce extracts involve four manufacturing steps: (1) distillation to obtain the essential oil from spruce needles, (2) extraction to obtain the water-soluble components, (3) thickening into a syrupy state in a vacuum concentrator and (4) adding back the essential oil derived from the spruce needles in the first step of the process. The best and most potent source is whole Norway spruce needle extract derived from needles and small twigs of younger branches of trees that are between 60 and 80 years old.

Common Oak (Quercus robur), Sessile Oak (Quercus patraea)

Oaks are a common leaf tree in our landscape. In Europe, the common oak (Quercus robur; ▶ Fig. 9.1) and sessile oak (Quercus petraea) are the most common.

Oak bark differs in two significant ways from spruce needles in its therapeutic application: It does not contain volatile oils, only tannins, and its tannin content is substantially higher, about 26–30% on average. The tannin in oak bark exerts substantial localized, but very intense effects. This makes oak bark well suited for special applications, such as chronic and localized skin disorders, especially plantar hyperhidrosis. Other important applications include exudative eczemas and inflammatory eye disorders, which should be treated using compresses.

For application, a small handful of oak bark is simmered in 1 L of water until the liquid is reduced to about 0.5 L. This amount of liquid can now be used for hand or foot baths. For compresses, the bark should be boiled for a shorter time into a decoction, about 10–15 minutes. It is important to completely remove all pieces of oak bark and splinters from the decoction before use. Compresses should be applied loosely and air- and watertight to prevent skin damage.

Ready-made oak bark extracts are also available. One teaspoon to one tablespoon of this extract can be added to partial baths.

Wheat (Triticum aestivum)

Wheat bran is calming for the skin and is used for acute skin disorders and for sensitive skin that does not tolerate soap well.

Valerian (Valeriana officinalis)

Valerian baths are calming and promote sleep. They should be used in the evening. Sometimes the patient needs to be prevented from falling asleep in the bath! One full bath requires 100 g valerian root (Radix Valerianae) or 250 g valerian tincture. Ready-made whole plant valerian extracts are available.

Lemon Balm (Melissa officinalis)

Lemon balm baths are also calming and relaxing and indicated especially for nervous heart disorders, general anxiety, and difficulty falling asleep. Ready-made whole plant extracts are available for this application. Alternatively, 1–2 tablespoons of pure lemon balm oil may be added to the bath water.

Calamus (Acorus calamus)

Calamus has general tonifying effects. This makes calamus leaves a good remedy for general exhaustion during convalescence and low blood pressure with circulatory system disorders, anemia, metabolic disorders, diabetes, etc. Since calamus baths are stimulating, they are best taken in the morning. With dysautonomia and similar conditions, calamus baths on (a weekend) morning, followed by 1 hour of bedrest can be helpful. In Japan, calamus baths (shobu-yu) for little boys are a fixed feature of Children's Day on May 5th.

Rosemary (Rosmarinus officinalis)

The main applications for rosemary baths are constitutional hypertension, circulatory disorders, and varicose veins as well as rheumatic pain, bruises, sprains, and similar disorders. An infusion of 50 g of rosemary leaves in 0.5 L of water is added to a full bath. Ready-made preparations of good quality are also available. Rosemary baths, like calamus baths, have a tonifying effect. They should be taken in the morning, followed by a sufficient period of rest.

Thyme (Thymus vulgaris)

Thyme volatile oil is absorbed in sufficient quantities and mostly excreted via the lungs. Combined with the indications for thyme volatile oil itself, thyme baths can have positive effects on all disorders where thyme is indicated, such as an antispasmodic and broncholytic for chronic coughs, emphysema, whooping cough in children, etc.

German Chamomile (Matricaria recutita)

Applied externally, chamomile primarily promotes healing of slow-healing wounds, acts as an antispasmodic with hemorrhoids and relieves itching in chronic eczema. An infusion of 100 g of chamomile flowers or a ready-made extract is added to a full bath. German chamomile is used more frequently for partial baths and compresses. One well-known and popular application is steam baths for inflamed hemorrhoids. Their application is simple: pour a handful of chamomile flowers into the bottom of a bucket and add 2–3 L of boiling water. Patients then sit on the bucket opening, thereby covering the top of the bucket, and cover themselves with a blanket.

Yarrow (Achillea millefolium)

The effects of yarrow are comparable to those of chamomile, primarily anti-inflammatory and antispasmodic. In addition, yarrow contains a tonifying bitter substance and tannins. This gives yarrow a special note and application area, primarily for gynecological disorders. Yarrow is primarily used for sitz baths, but also in full baths. Ready-made bath extracts are the simplest to use.

Lavender (Lavandula angustifolia, Lavandula officinalis)

Lavender, due to its lavender volatile oil, acts as a general stimulant and tonic for the nervous system. This makes lavender flowers (along with its upper stalk and leaves) a good remedy for women during states of dysautonomia related to menopause.

Lavender is also considered a mild sedative when applied externally in oil dispersion baths. The Commission E therefore issued a positive monograph with indications for external use during states of exhaustion. In clinical practice, these are most likely to be stress related and frequently present as general anxiety.

Lavender baths are also strongly recommended for another indication, based on the latest research results for lavender: In a published clinical study (Kaspar and Dienel), a lavender oil preparation taken internally showed significant efficacy compared to a placebo and was as effective as the reference substance lorazepam with anxiety of different causes, especially generalized anxiety disorder. The study also demonstrated effective improvements for symptoms of depression that often accompany anxiety disorders. The most important components of the preparation used in the study included linalool, linalyl acetate, 1,8-cineol, ß-ocimene, terpinen-4-ol, and camphor. Since lavender baths involve the purely external application of lavender oil, significantly weaker effects can be expected, but the basic effect should still be present based on absorption of the lavender oil components via the skin and the olfactory epithelium.

Common Horsetail (Equisetum arvense)

Common horsetail contains silicic acid, which is primarily locally stimulating, but in a different way than calamus. It appears to have special efficacy that has not yet been verified by detailed clinical studies on the metabolism of the skin and subcutaneous tissue as well as tendons and ligaments (for example, the damage that is associated with skiing accidents) and for all types of complaints related to fallen arches and pes planus. Other indications for horsetail include rheumatic and neuralgic conditions, eczema, neurodermatitis, local circulation problems, frost bite, postthrombosis swelling, pain caused by fallen arches, and similar complaints.

Hay Flower (Graminis flos)

The characteristic scent of hay flower stems from sweet vernal grass (Anthoxanthum odoratum), one of the most common grasses. It contains coumarin glycoside—and similar to sweet woodruff (Asperula odorata)—gives off the scent of coumarin

as it wilts. Applied externally, hay flower increases hyperemia and skin stimulation. Hay flower baths are used primarily to treat rheumatism and metabolic disorders. For a full bath, a decoction of 500 g hay flowers in 4–5 L of water is added to the bath water. For partial baths, which are also very popular, proportionally less of the herb is used.

Bibliography

Quality Assurance

Dingermann T, Ed. Transparenzkriterien für pflanzliche, homöopathische und anthroposophische Arzneimittel. Basel: Karger; 2000

Dingermann T, Loew D. Phytopharmakologie. Experimentelle und klinische Pharmakologie pflanzlicher Arzneimittel. Stuttgart: Wissenschaftliche Verlagsgesellschaft; 2003

Dingermann T, Ed. Kompendium Phytopharmaka. Qualität-skriterien und Verordnungsbeispiele. Stuttgart: Deutscher Apotheker Verlag; 2015

Fintelmann V, Ed. Kompendium Phytopharmaka. Neu-Isenburg: MMI; 2008

Gaedcke F. Ist die Qualität pflanzlicher Extrakte angemessen gesichert? Z Phytother. 1999; 20:254–263

Hefendehl FW, Lander C. Qualitätssicherung pflanzlicher Arzneimittel—Anforderungen bei der Zulassung. In: Hanke G, ed Qualität pflanzlicher Arzneimittel. Paperback APV; 1982

Pätzold B, Honnef S. Internationaler Standard zur nachhaltigen Wildsammlung von Heilpflanzen. Z Phytother. 2005; 26:245–246

Ullmann M. Phytoäquivalenz: Kriterium für generische Zulassung? Phytokompass. 2015; 2:19–21

Weimer F, Stumpf H. Qualität quantifizierter Pflanzenex-trakte. Dtsch Apoth Ztg. 2006; 147(17):50–57

Guidelines for Prescribing Medicinal Plants

American Botanical Council. The Complete German Commission E Monographs. http://cms.herbalgram.org/commissione/index.html (Accessed 28 October 2021)

Bühring P. Meinungsforschung: Ganzheitliche Therapie gewünscht. Dtsch Aerztebl. 2001; 98(20):1307

European Medicines Agency. Guideline on clinical development of fixed combination medicinal products. http://www.ema.europa.eu/docs/en_GB/document_library/Scientific_guideline/2017/03/WC500224836.pdf (Accessed 28 October 2021)

Medicinal Products Act (Arzneimittelgesetz – AMG), version 4.4. 2016 (BGBl. I p. 569), https://www.gesetze-im-internet.de/englisch_amg/englisch_amg.html (Accessed 28 October 2021)

Medicinal Teas

von Feuchtersleben E. Zur Diätetik der Seele. Leipzig: Reclam; 1848

Fintelmann V. Praktische Tee-Therapie. Stuttgart: Wissenschaftliche Verlagsgesellschaft; 2005

Phytobalneology

Brüggemann W. Moderne Phyto-Balneotherapie. Phys Med Rehab. 1973; 13:262–267

Kaspar S, Dienel A. Silexan (WS 1265) vermindert begleitende depressive Symptome bei Patienten mit Angsterkrankungen. Z Phytother. 2013; 34 Suppl. 1:58

Oil dispersion bath. https://www.jungebad.de/das-jungebad.html. (Accessed 9 March 2022)

Pratzel A. Haut und Wasser—biochemische und bio-physikalische Phänomene. Z Angew Bader Klimaheilkd. 1977; 24:123–126

Pratzel HG, Schnizzer W. Handbuch der Medizinischen Bäder. Heidelberg: Haug; 1992

Römmelt H, Drexel H, Dirnagl K. Wirkstoffaufnahme aus pflanzlichen Badezusätzen. Heilkunst. 1978; 91:240–256

Römmelt H, Zuber A, Dirnayl K, Drexel H. Zur Resorption von Terpenen aus Badezusätzen. Munch Med Wochenschr. 1974; 116:537–540

Uehleke B. Phytobalneologie. Z Phytother. 2011; 32:54–59

Wagner H, Wiesenauer M. Phytotherapie: Phytopharmaka und pflanzliche Homöopathika. 2nd ed. Stuttgart: Wissenschaftliche Verlagsgesellschaft; 2003

Wieck WP. Balneotherapie gynäkologischer Erkrankungen. Therapeutikon. 1987; 2:124–127

Part 2

Practical Applications

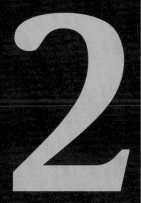

3 Gastrointestinal and Metabolic Disorders

This chapter illustrates the broad spectrum of therapeutic applications for medicinal plants with gastroenterological and metabolic disorders. The special efficacy and wide-ranging indications of phytotherapy once again emphasize the outstanding role phytotherapeutics have played for centuries in disorders of the gastrointestinal system. Phytotherapeutics are especially well tolerated and offer a genuine therapeutic alternative to many synthetic drugs.

The comprehensive spectrum of indications for phytotherapy and its remedies in conjunction with gastroenterological disorders make this the largest chapter of this book. Many of these gastroenterological indications correspond well to categories 1 and 2 of the therapeutic categories for phytotherapeutics as described in **Table 1.3**. These are either remedies of first choice or ones that offer the prescribing practitioner genuine well-tolerated alternatives to synthetics for the same indications, especially for conditions requiring long-term treatment.

This chapter is also a good example for illustrating the essential differences between synthetics and phytopharmaceuticals. The indications for phytotherapeutics are rarely as clear and well defined as they are for synthetics. They are also rarely focused on clear and undisputable findings but rather target functional disorders, i.e., when the patient is not feeling well (see Section 1.4.3 "Findings and Feeling" (p. 12)). In this context we also have to discuss latent diseases that exhibit measurable imbalances of important functions, but where a serious morphological diagnosis cannot (yet!) be made. One example in this context is the sufficient production of gastric acid with atrophic gastritis. Science-based medicine is beginning to share this view, as is illustrated, for example, by the definition of "functional dyspepsia" (see Chapter 3.5 "Functional Dyspepsia" (p. 121)). Gastroenterological and metabolic disorders present with predominantly functional symptoms that each patient experiences very individually. These conditions are very unlikely to be treated successfully by a single constituent finished pharmaceutical product. This illustrates the advantages of phytotherapeutic multicomponent remedies, the ability of the practitioner to formulate individualized prescriptions, or the use of combination remedies recommended frequently in this chapter. Many of the remedies discussed in this chapter derive from R.F. Weiss's treasure trove of experience and are presented as exemplary treatment options to encourage practitioners to formulate their own individualized prescriptions.

Unfortunately, this field offers few newer, innovative remedies. The research potential for this field is extremely limited by two factors: The almost complete lack of manufacturer-independent funding and the fact that this indication framework is viewed as an imbalanced state of health, which is largely excluded from insurance reimbursement and consequently largely self-medicated.

Some of the medicinal plants presented in this chapter have additional indications that are discussed in other chapters. Chamomile is one such example. Its role as the best antiphlogistic "surface remedy" for the skin and mucous membranes makes it comprehensively efficacious in many areas and this is why it is cited repeatedly. There are also many overlapping indication areas, for example, between the chapters on chronic gastric disorders and peptic ulcer disorder or between the plants presented in the liver and gallbladder sections. Phytotherapeutics cannot be as easily categorized and delineated as we have become accustomed to for synthetic, symptom-oriented drugs.

Medicinal Plants

Acute Stomatitis, Acute Pharyngitis, Nonpyogenic Tonsillitis
Mallow, Malva sylvestris
Sage, Salvia officinalis
Marshmallow, Althaea officinalis
German Chamomile, Matricaria recutita, Matricaria chamomilla
Arnica, Arnica montana

Chronic Stomatitis, Chronic Pharyngitis
Tormentil, Potentilla tormentilla
Bilberry (European Blueberry), Vaccinium myrtillus
Centaury, Centaurium minus
Bogbean, Menyanthes trifoliata
Yellow Gentian, Gentiana lutea

Cold Sores, Herpes Simplex (Herpes Labialis)
Lemon Balm, Melissa officinalis

Acute Gastritis
German Chamomile, Matricaria recutita, Matricaria chamomilla
Pineapple Weed, Matricaria matricarioides
Roman Chamomile, Anthemis nobilis
Peppermint, Mentha piperita
Spearmint, Mentha spicata, syn. Mentha crispa
Horsemint, Wild Mint, Mentha sylvestris/longifolia
Lemon Balm, Melissa officinalis

Irritable Stomach
German Chamomile, Matricaria recutita, Matricaria chamomilla

Chronic Gastritis, Lack of Appetite
Centaury, Centaurium minus
Yellow Gentian, Gentiana lutea
Cinchona Bark, Cinchona pubescens
Bogbean Leaves, Menyanthes trifoliata
Condurango Bark, Marsdenia condurango
Bitter Orange, Citrus aurantium ssp. amara
Angelica Root, Angelica archangelica
Blessed Thistle, Cnicus benedictus, syn. Carduus benedictus, syn. Centaurea benedicta
Calamus, Acorus calamus
Wormwood, Artemisia absinthium
Ginger, Zingiber officinalis
Galangal, Alpinia officinarum
Iceland Moss, Cetraria islandica
Usnea, Usnea barbata
Flaxseed, Linum usitatissimum

Gastric and Duodenal Ulcers
Licorice, Glycyrrhiza glabra
German Chamomile, Matricaria recutita, Matricaria chamomilla
Belladonna, Atropa belladonna

Irritable Bowel Syndrome
German Chamomile, Matricaria recutita, Matricaria chamomilla
Fennel, Foeniculum vulgare
Caraway, Carum carvi
Peppermint, Mentha piperita

Meteorism, Roemheld Syndrome
Caraway, Carum carvi
Fennel, Foeniculum vulgare
Anise, Pimpinella anisum

Star Anise, Illicum verum
Coriander, Coriandrum sativum

Crohn's Disease
Frankincense, Boswellia serrata
Wormwood, Artemisia absinthium

Diarrhea
Tormentil, Potentilla tormentilla
Bilberry (European Blueberry), Vaccinium myrtillus
Blackberry, Rubus fruticosus
Oak, Quercus
Uzara, Xysmalobium undulatum
Poppy, Papaver somniferum

Chronic Slow Transit Constipation
Senna, Senna alexandrina, syn. Cassia acutifolia, syn. Cassia angustifolia
Rhubarb, Rheum palmatum/officinale
Aloe Vera, Aloe vera
Alder Buckthorn, Rhamnus frangula
Cascara Sagrada, Frangula purshiana, Rhamnus purshiana
Flaxseed, Linum usitatissimum
Psyllium Seed, black, Plantago psyllium
Psyllium Seed, blond, Plantago ovata
Castor Bean, Ricinus communis

Proctitis
German Chamomile, Matricaria recutita, Matricaria chamomilla
Calamus, Acorus calamus
St.-John's-wort, Hypericum perforatum

Hemorrhoids
Butcher's-broom, Ruscus aculeatus
Witch Hazel, Hamamelis Virginiana
Aspen (quaking), Populus tremula
Tormentil, Potentilla tormentilla
German Chamomile, Matricaria recutita, Matricaria chamomilla
Arnica, Arnica montana
Oak, Quercus

Hepatic Disorders
Milk Thistle, Silybum marianum
Artichoke, Cynara cardunculus
Beet, Beta vulgaris
Yarrow, Achillea millefolium

Biliary Dyskinesia
Wormwood, Artemisia absinthium
Celandine, Chelidonium majus
Fumitory, Fumaria officinalis
Boldo, Peumus boldus
Radish, Raphanus sativus

Postcholecystectomy Syndrome
Wormwood, Artemisia absinthium
Celandine, Chelidonium majus
Fumitory, Fumaria officinalis
Boldo Leaf, Peumus boldus
Radish, Raphanus sativus

Functional Dyspepsia
Turmeric, Curcuma longa
Artichoke, Cynara cardunculus
Dandelion, Taraxacum officinale
Wormwood, Artemisia absinthium
Milk Thistle, Silybum marianum
Peppermint, Mentha piperita
Bitter Candytuft, Iberis amara
Haronga, Harungana madagascariensis
Papaya, Carica papaya
Bromelain (pineapple), Ananas comosus

Diabetes Mellitus
White Kidney Bean, Phaseolus vulgaris

Lipometabolic Disorders
Artichoke, Cynara cardunculus
Garlic, Allium sativum

Hyperthyroidism
Bugleweed, Lycopus virginicus/europaeus
Motherwort, Leonurus cardiaca

3.1 Mucous Membrane Disorders of the Mouth and Throat

Oral rinses and gargling are time-tested and reliable treatments for many different mucous membrane disorders of the mouth and throat. They should be considered especially for tonsillitis, stomatitis, and gingivitis as well as acute and chronic pharyngitis. Severe pyogenic tonsillitis caused by *Streptococcus*, for example, requires antibiotics. The antibacterial action of the antibiotic can, however, be supported by phytotherapeutic remedies that speed up and optimize recovery.

The medicinal plants listed here are primarily demulcent, topical antiphlogistic, astringent, and tonic remedies. They cleanse and effect hyperemia of the oral mucosa. They also contain mucilage, glycosides, volatile oils, bitters, and tannins, among other substances, and can provide localized tissue healing. Repeated and thorough rinsing of the mouth helps to reduce pain and positively impacts the healing process as it causes acute symptoms to subside more quickly and shortens illness duration.

▶ **Note.** Studies also show that the virostatic action of lemon balm leaves significantly reduces the symptoms of **herpes simplex** (cold sores).

3.1.1 Acute Stomatitis, Acute Pharyngitis, Nonpyogenic Tonsillitis

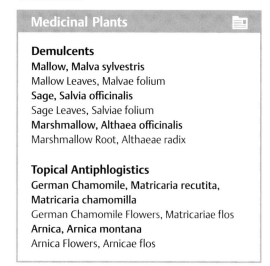

Medicinal Plants

Demulcents
Mallow, Malva sylvestris
Mallow Leaves, Malvae folium
Sage, Salvia officinalis
Sage Leaves, Salviae folium
Marshmallow, Althaea officinalis
Marshmallow Root, Althaeae radix

Topical Antiphlogistics
German Chamomile, Matricaria recutita, Matricaria chamomilla
German Chamomile Flowers, Matricariae flos
Arnica, Arnica montana
Arnica Flowers, Arnicae flos

Stomatitis, pharyngitis, and nonpyogenic tonsillitis are primarily treated with demulcents and topical antiphlogistics. They alleviate subjective symptoms and support the self-healing powers of mucous membranes. They do not replace antibiotics if their use is indicated.

Plants for Treatment

Mallow (Malva sylvestris)

For more information about this plant, see Mallow (p. 185).

> **Preparation**
>
> - **Tea**
>   Add 2 cups of boiling water to 2–3 teaspoons of the drug. Steep covered for 5 minutes, then strain.
>   Gargle and rinse mouth while tea is lukewarm.

Sage (Salvia officinalis)

This shrub grows to a height of 0.5–1 m and is found primarily on sunny hillsides in limestone soil. Its elongated leaves are gray-green on the surface and white/feltlike on the bottom. Its flowers are light blue to purple. Sage is native to the Mediterranean region.

Parts of plant used: Sage leaves (**Salviae folium**).

▶ **Pharmacology.** Sage contains volatile oil, lamiaceae tannins, diterpene bitter principles, triterpenes, steroids, and flavones.

> **Preparation**
>
> - **Tea**
>   See preparation for mallow (Malva sylvestris)

Marshmallow (Althaea officinalis)

For more information about this plant, see Marshmallow (p. 183).

> **Preparation**
>
> - **Tea**
>   See preparation for mallow (Malva sylvestris)

German Chamomile (Matricaria recutita, Matricaria chamomilla)

For more information about this plant, see German Chamomile (p. 42).

▶ **Indications.** German chamomile is especially well suited for the treatment of **acute, painful infections**, and **nonpyogenic tonsillitis**.

> **Preparations**
>
> - **Tea**
>   Add 1 cup of hot water to 2–3 teaspoons of the drug. Steep covered for 5–10 minutes. Gargle hourly using freshly prepared, warm tea.
> - **Fluid Extract**
>   Add 10 drops to 1 glass of water, gargle, or rinse several times a day.
>   Fluid extract is helpful for painful stomatitis.
> - **Chamomile Flower—Sage Leaf Gargle Combination (Gargarisma Chamomillae compositum)**
>   Mix equal amounts of each herb and make a decoction in the ratio of 1 cup of water per 3 teaspoons of the drug mixture. Let the decoction steep covered for 15 minutes. Add about 1 tablespoon of the decoction to 1 cup of warm milk and use this liquid to rinse.

> **Prescriptions**
>
> Rx
> Extract. Salviae fluid. (sage fluid extract)
> Extract. Chamomilla fluid. āā 20.0 (German chamomile fluid extract)
> D.S.
> Add 20–30 drops to 1 glass of water and use to gargle.

Arnica (Arnica montana)

For a description of this plant, see Arnica (p. 144).

▶ **Indications.** Primarily used for **acute pharyngitis**. It increases peripheral circulation and local immune response of mucous membranes.

> **Preparation**
>
> - **Tincture**
>   Add 1 teaspoon to 1 glass of water and use for rinsing the mouth and gargling. Use several times a day.

▸ **Therapy Recommendations.** It is often helpful to alternate the application of arnica and chamomile. With peritonsillar abscesses, this method frequently causes a spontaneous opening and draining of pus with immediate improvement of symptoms. Patients should gargle deep in the pharynx every 30 minutes using plenty of the liquid, as hot as can be tolerated.

3.1.2 Chronic Stomatitis, Chronic Pharyngitis

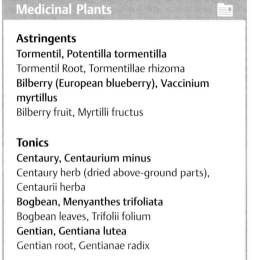

Medicinal Plants

Astringents
Tormentil, Potentilla tormentilla
Tormentil Root, Tormentillae rhizoma
Bilberry (European blueberry), Vaccinium myrtillus
Bilberry fruit, Myrtilli fructus

Tonics
Centaury, Centaurium minus
Centaury herb (dried above-ground parts), Centaurii herba
Bogbean, Menyanthes trifoliata
Bogbean leaves, Trifolii folium
Gentian, Gentiana lutea
Gentian root, Gentianae radix

Subacute or chronic stomatitis and gingivitis, chronic pharyngitis, and persistent smoker's catarrh are treated using primarily plants referred to as **astringents** due to their tannin content. These plants are also often helpful in cases of globus sensation without organic causes.

Indications for astringents can also be successfully treated using plants that contain certain bitters, called **tonics**. A special indication for tonics is dry mouth (xerostomia), also resulting from sicca syndrome or radiation treatment.

Plants for Treatment

Tormentil (Potentilla tormentilla, Potentilla erecta)

For more information about this plant, see Tormentil (p. 84).

Preparations

- **Decoction**
  Add 2–3 tablespoons of tormentil roots to 1 L of water, cover, and bring to a boil. Use this decoction to rinse several times a day.
- **Tincture**
  The tincture is suitable for rinses and can be used together with sage.

Prescription

Rx
Tincture. Tormentillae 20.0 (tormentil tincture)
D.S.
Add 1 teaspoon to 1 glass of water and use for rinsing the mouth.

Prescription

Rx
Tincture Tormentillae (tormentil tincture)
Tincture Salviae āā 10.0 (sage tincture)
D.S.
Add 1 teaspoon to 1 glass of water and use for rinsing the mouth.

- **Combination of Tormentil and Arnica Tinctures**

Prescription

Rx
Tincture Tormentillae (tormentil tincture)
Tincture Arnicae āā 20.0 (arnica tincture)
D.S.
Add 1 teaspoon to 1 glass of water and use for rinsing the mouth.

- Both tormentil tincture and arnica tincture are used to treat **periodontitis** by painting the gums with the undiluted tincture. This treatment has no drawbacks compared to Rhatany root tincture

(Tinctura Ratanhiae) or Areca catechu tincture and should be the primary treatment of choice.

- **Combination of Tormentil and Myrrh Tinctures**
- Myrrh tincture (Tinctura Myrrhae) is an aromatic medicine that contains a volatile oil, resin, and oleo-gum. The composition of myrrh is very different from tormentil, and it is a good complement to tormentil.
- The prescription should specify both tinctures in equal parts.

Prescription	

Rx
Tincture. Tormentillae (tormentil tincture)
Tincture. Myrrhae āā 20.0 (myrrh tincture)
D.S.
Brush the undiluted tincture on the gums (topical).

- **Tormentil Tincture** (Tinctura Tormentillae, according to the German Prescription Formulas, DRF)
- This composition is identical to the above prescription combining tormentil and myrrh.

Bilberry (European Blueberry) (Vaccinium myrtillus)

For more information about this plant, see Bilberry (p. 86).

Medicinal applications use the **bilberry fruit** (berries, Myrtilli fructus).

Preparation	

- **Tea**
  Boil 1–3 tablespoons of dried bilberries in 1 L of water for about 15 minutes. Use this blackish-blue tea to "bathe" the mouth for an extended period several times a day. This simple treatment is every effective with acute glossitis and aphthous stomatitis (canker sore).

Centaury (Centaurium minus, Centaurium erythraea)

For more information about this plant, see Centaury (p. 53).

Preparation	

- **Tea**
  Add 1 cup of boiling water to 1–2 teaspoons of the chopped herb. Steep covered for 2 minutes and strain. Use as a rinse several times a day.

Bogbean (Menyanthes trifoliate)

For more information about this plant, see Bogbean (p. 56).

Preparation	

- **Tea**
  Add 1 cup of boiling water to 1–2 teaspoons of the chopped herb. Steep covered for 2 minutes and strain. Use as a rinse several times a day.

Gentian (Gentiana lutea)

For more information about this plant, see Gentian (p. 54).

Preparations	

- **Tea**
  Add 1 cup of boiling water to 1–2 teaspoons of the chopped herb. Steep covered for 2 minutes and strain. Use as a rinse several times a day.
- **Tincture**
  Add 20–40 drops to 1 glass of lukewarm water. Gargle or rinse several times a day.

▶ **Therapy Recommendations.** Astringents should be alternated with demulcents. Demulcents form a protective layer on the pharyngeal mucosa. This replaces the substance that can no longer be produced by the atrophic mucous glands.

3.1.3 Herpes Simplex, Herpes Labialis (Cold Sores)

Medicinal Plants	

Lemon Balm, Melissa officinalis
Lemon Balm Leaves, Melissae folium

Plants for Treatment

Lemon Balm (Melissa officinalis)

For more information about this plant, see Lemon Balm (p. 48).

▶ **Indications.** Research documents specific virostatic actions of **lemon balm leaves** (Melissae folium), against the herpes virus.

▶ **Research.** Research by May and Willuhn showed inhibition of the herpes simplex virus by lemon balm extract using a plaque inhibition test and Fintner color test. Lemon balm was also found to have antiphlogistic and astringent actions, which are attributed to the tannin content of lemon balm leaves. Subsequent studies showed excellent results for a proprietary lemon balm leaf extract with respect to speed of healing, recurrence-free interval and tolerability (Wölbling and Milbradt; Wölbling and Rapprich). Vogt et al. confirmed these results in a subsequent, placebo-controlled, double-blind study.

Bibliography

May G, Willuhn G. Antivirale Wirkung wässriger Pflanzenextrakte in Gewebekulturen [Antiviral effect of aqueous plant extracts in tissue culture]. Arzneimittelforschung. 1978; 28(1):1–7

Vogt HJ, Tausch I, Wölbling RH, Kaiser PM. Melissenextrakt bei Herpes simplex (eine Placebo-kontrollierte Doppelblind-Studie). Allgemeinarzt. 1991; 13:832–841

Wölbling RH, Milbradt R. Klinik und Therapie des Herpes simplex. Vorstellung eines neuen phytotherapeutischen Wirkstoffes. Therapiewoche. 1984; 34:1193–1200

Wölbling RH, Rapprich K. Herpes simplex. Zur Verträglichkeit von Lomaherpan®-Creme bei der Behandlung des Herpes simplex. Therapiewoche. 1985; 35:4057–4058

Questions

1. Which shared characteristic of certain medicinal plants is especially well suited for treatment of stomatitis, pharyngitis, and nonpyogenic tonsillitis?
2. Which symptoms call for treatment with German Chamomile?
3. Which constituents characterize plant-based astringents?
4. Which plant is effective against herpes labialis (cold sores)?

Answers (p. 421) for Chapter 3.1

3.2 Gastric Disorders

Phytotherapy plays an especially important role in the treatment of gastroenterological disorders (Barton; Fintelmann). Frequently, disorders in this area can be treated using only plant medicines, along with the dietary and physical measures that are almost always indispensable. In many other cases, plant medicines can provide very valuable adjuvant therapy. Tea therapy has been used and proven to be very helpful for centuries to treat gastrointestinal disorders. Simple tincture combinations and/or essential oils also provide valuable treatment options.

Acute gastric disorders encompass conditions of varying genesis, including simple overloading of the stomach, all types of nausea and vomiting, acute gastritis, and irritable stomach, a functional disorder. Stomach spasticity is one of the main symptoms in this area. Without question, the underlying causes of gastric complaints need to be investigated. At the same time, the patient needs to be immediately provided with symptomatic relief.

Chronic gastric disorders are characterized primarily by chronic (atrophic) gastritis and many functional digestive disorders referred to as functional dyspepsia. The latter are discussed in Chapter 3.5 (p. 121) "Functional Dyspepsia" (p. 121) because they involve several upper abdominal organs. Lack of appetite represents a multilayered symptom complex with causes that go beyond stomach disorders. Since its typical treatment involves bitters (amara), it is discussed in this context as well. The goals of phytotherapy for this condition are to stimulate secretions and gastric acid production, protect mucous membranes, and provide mild spasmolytic as well as carminative effects.

Peptic ulcer disease is also discussed in section 3.2.4 Gastric and Duodenal (Peptic) Ulcers (p. 66).

For references corresponding to the preceding section, see Bibliography following 3.2.1 (p. 49).

3.2.1 Acute Gastritis

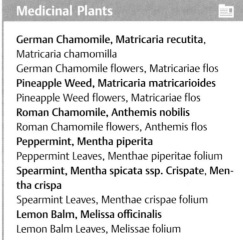

Medicinal Plants

German Chamomile, Matricaria recutita, Matricaria chamomilla
German Chamomile flowers, Matricariae flos
Pineapple Weed, Matricaria matricarioides
Pineapple Weed flowers, Matricariae flos
Roman Chamomile, Anthemis nobilis
Roman Chamomile flowers, Anthemis flos
Peppermint, Mentha piperita
Peppermint Leaves, Menthae piperitae folium
Spearmint, Mentha spicata ssp. Crispate, Mentha crispa
Spearmint Leaves, Menthae crispae folium
Lemon Balm, Melissa officinalis
Lemon Balm Leaves, Melissae folium

True acute gastritis is rare. It is usually caused by diet or, for example, excessive alcohol consumption, and, less frequently, by viral infections. Its symptoms include nausea, usually burning upper abdominal pain, and lack of appetite. Short-term phytotherapy almost always provides immediate improvement.

The most important medicinal plants used to treat acute, noninfectious gastric disorders are **chamomile, peppermint**, and **lemon balm**.

Plants for Treatment

German Chamomile (Matricaria recutita, Matricaria chamomilla)

German chamomile (▶ Fig. 3.1) (also referred to as "true" or "blue chamomile") is a member of the Compositae (Asteraceae) family of plants. This plant is ubiquitous in Germany, where it grows wild along country roads, as a weed in agricultural fields, and even in gardens. In North America, the plant has been introduced and has naturalized in many areas. Chamomile used medicinally is almost always cultivated. The quality of chamomile grown

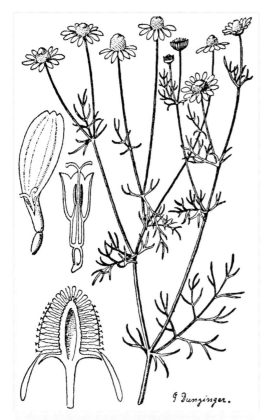

Fig. 3.1 German Chamomile, Matricaria recutita (Matricaria chamomilla).

in Germany is very high and often superior to that of imports. The volatile oil content of chamomile grown in Germany, for example, is 0.6–1.0% compared to 0.3–0.56% of that grown in Hungary.

The annual consumption of chamomile in Germany is 3,000 tons—an astonishingly high amount. About 500 tons are used for medicinal purposes and 2,500 tons for foodstuffs; the cost per kilo is about 1.50–5.00 €/kg, depending on quality. To supplement its own domestic supply and to meet the demands of the market, Germany imports from the countries of Argentina, Egypt, Poland, and Croatia.

Medicinal applications use the **German chamomile flower heads** (Matricariae flos).

One additional type of chamomile is **Matricaria inodora**, or scentless chamomile (also known as scentless mayweed). This is a relative of German chamomile and true to its name; it is completely scentless, unlike German chamomile. The plant is also much larger, taller, and firmer. Matricaria

inodora is a common garden weed and often grows alongside true chamomile. Paying attention to the plants' scents (or lack of) will avoid confusing these two types of chamomile. Matricaria inodora is not used medicinally.

▶ **Pharmacology.** German chamomile is **antiphlogistic, spasmolytic**, and **carminative**. In addition to these actions, which have been well demonstrated pharmacologically, this plant also has been proven to have bacteriostatic and fungistatic effects. Its active principles include volatile oil, flavonoids, and mucilages.

The various components of German chamomile's volatile oil are primarily antiphlogistic, but also spasmolytic. Obtaining sufficient amounts of this volatile oil requires alcoholic extraction. Aqueous extractions such as teas only contain about 15% of the volatile oil contained in German chamomile flowers.

Distillates of German chamomile volatile oil contain the terpenoids chamazulene (up to 15%), (-)-α-bisabolol (up to 25%), (-)-bisabolol oxides A, B, C, and one cis-/trans-en-yn-dicycloether (up to 30%). The bisabolol terpenoids and chamazulene are classified as sesquiterpenes.

German chamomile's antiseptic action and its efficacy in protecting against and healing ulcers were demonstrated in 1975 by Isaac and Thiemer and confirmed by subsequent researchers.

Flavonoids are found in alcoholic extracts as well as in tea infusions. Their action is primarily spasmolytic and is equivalent to about 30–50% of the spasmolytic efficacy of papaverine. Specific chamomile flavones include apigenin, luteolin, and quercetin.

Wurm et al. showed that the antiphlogistic action of chamomile is based on its inhibitory effects on prostaglandin synthesis and lipoxygenases.

German chamomile contains about 10% mucilages which consist of uronic acid containing acidic heteroxylanes. These substances are not present in purely alcoholic extractions. Topical use of these mucilages is **anti-inflammatory** and **anti-irritant**. Some *in vitro* test models have also shown immune-stimulating effects. The mucilaginous components of chamomile flowers complement the primary action of its volatile oil and flavonoids.

Acute or chronic toxicity is practically nonexistent.

▶ **Research.** Typical pharmacologic studies involve the carrageenan- and dextran-induced rat paw edema models, the adjuvant arthritis model of the rat and the UV erythema model of the guinea pig. These models produced many animal study results that are described in detail by Schilcher as well as by Wagner and Wiesenauer.

Isaac and Thiemer along with Szelenyi et al. showed that ulcers caused by indomethacin, stress or alcohol were inhibited by α-bisabolol. These studies also showed an increase in the rate of healing for peptic ulcers. It is safe to assume that chamomile's **protective effects against ulcers or its ability to heal ulcers** is not only derived from α-bisabolol. More likely, other constituents also promote local endogenous prostaglandin synthesis, which strengthens the mucosal protective barrier. This treats the cause of ulcers, similar to the action of licorice root because it stimulates the protection provided by mucus against the negative, aggressive impact of acid. Other studies show that some components of the chamomile flower, especially (-)-α-bisabolol and chamazulene, inhibit cyclooxygenase and lipoxygenase in the arachidonic acid cascade (Schilcher).

Since Aggag and Yousef reported bacteriostatic and **bactericidal** effects for chamomile essential oils, other extensive experimental studies have confirmed these effects along with fungicidal and **fungistatic** effects. Schilcher provides a detailed overview of these study results. These effects are weaker than those of synthetic antibiotics, chemotherapeutics or antifungals, but they are significant given the manifold indications for chamomile.

Kraul and Schmidt along with Barton conducted experimental animal studies that seem to indicate the influence of azulen and its derivatives on cancer genesis and the inhibition of metastasis. However, these results were not studied further. Revisiting these early studies may present new questions for further study.

Frequently cited allergic reactions to chamomile, especially contact dermatitis, have been studied by Hausen whose critical examination did not show a connection between such reactions and the prescription of chamomile.

▶ **Indications.** German chamomile is primarily used to treat **acute gastritis** of varying etiology.

Chamomile preparations are extremely well tolerated. Contact or inhalation allergies are very rare. The fact that chamomile pollen contributes to general pollen allergies, or pollinosis, is not relevant for the assessment of medical prescriptions for chamomile.

The Commission E monograph for chamomile lists the following indications: skin and mucous membrane inflammations, bacterial skin diseases, including those of the oral cavity and gums, inflammations and irritations of the respiratory tract, anal or genital inflammation as well as spastic gastrointestinal disorders and inflammatory diseases of the gastrointestinal tract.

Acute gastritis is frequently associated with acute mucous membrane inflammation of the upper gastrointestinal tract. Esophagitis or enteritis in conjunction with mostly viral infections also respond well to chamomile preparations.

Chamomile is also increasingly used in cosmetics because of its antiphlogistic effects. Biochemical studies have shown that chamomile extract influences skin metabolism and can increase oxidative phosphorylation and improve skin tissue regeneration (Isaac and Thiemer).

Preparations

- **Tea**
  Add 1 cup of hot water to 2–3 teaspoons of chamomile flowers, but do not boil. Steep covered for 5–10 minutes, then strain. Drink 1 cup 3–4 × day, slowly, in small sips (dietary consumption).
- **Tincture**
  Add 20 drops to 1 glass of lukewarm water and drink slowly in small sips.
- **Fluid Extract**
  Take 10–20 drops several times a day.

▶ **Chamomile Tea Therapies**
- When using **prepackaged chamomile tea bags**, it is best to use 2 teabags per cup.
- **Chamomile regimen**: Drink 1 cup of chamomile tea 3–4 × day, ideally on an empty stomach in the morning before breakfast, twice during the day between meals, and 1 cup in the evening at bedtime.
- **Chamomile tea "rolling regimen"**: Drink 2 cups of chamomile tea (best if freshly prepared) in the early morning on an empty stomach. Then lie down for 5 minutes in each of these positions, respectively: first on the back, then on the left side, then on the stomach, and finally on the right side. In addition to its pharmacologically defined action, this treatment also provides a calming psychogenic effect.

- For **acute gastrointestinal colic**: Drink 2–3 cups of freshly prepared chamomile tea every 20–30 minutes. Defined chamomile extract products may be used. The chamomile "rolling regimen" is also indicated for this condition.

▶ **Therapy Recommendations.** Even though many ready-made chamomile preparations are available commercially, prescriptions should focus on chamomile **tea**. When chamomile treatment is indicated, practitioners should write a prescription for this otherwise over-the-counter medicine to underscore the gravity of the prescription.

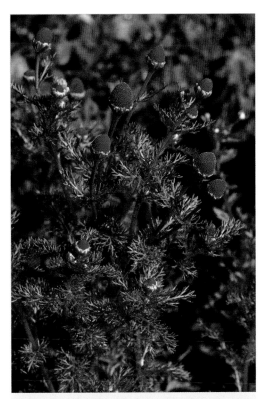

Prescriptions

Rx
Matricariae flos 100.0 (German chamomile flowers)
M. f. spec.
Add 1 cup of hot water to 2 teaspoons. Steep covered for 5–10 minutes, then strain.
D. S.
Drink, slowly, in small sips, while still comfortably warm.

Fig. 3.2 Pineapple Weed, Matricaria matricarioides (Matricaria discoidea). Photo: Dr. Roland Spohn, Engen.

Pineapple Weed (Matricaria matricarioides, Matricaria discoidea, Matricaria suaveolens)

Pineapple weed (also known as rayless chamomile, wild chamomile, or disc mayweed) lacks the white flower petals (ray florets) surrounding the yellow flower cone in German chamomile. Pineapple weed is a low-lying weed that always grows in large clumps close to the ground (▶ Fig. 3.2). Its chamomile-like scent is noticeable even from a distance. However, closer inspection quickly reveals that pineapple weed does not have the pleasant aromatic chamomile scent. Its scent is rather pungent, almost unpleasant.

Pineapple weed grows throughout Germany along garden fences, country roads, and even alongside garbage dump sites. As a ruderal species, it prefers proximity to human settlements.

Pineapple weed is used medicinally.

▶ **Note.** Pineapple weed is native to East Asia and western North America. During the middle of the 19th century, specimens of it "escaped" from the old Botanical Garden in Berlin. It spread astoundingly quickly first in the area around Berlin, and then along roads and especially along railroad tracks throughout Germany, and beyond. During World War II, people hoped to find a substitute for German chamomile in this easy-to-collect and abundant type of chamomile. However, its status as a substitute for German chamomile was not confirmed.

Preparation	

- **Tea**
  For preparation instructions, see German Chamomile.

Roman Chamomile (Anthemis nobilis, Chamemaelum nobile L.) Stinking Chamomile (Mayweed, Dog Fennel) (Anthemis cotula L.)

The anthemis varietals are commonly viewed as chamomile. Botanists also refer to them as chamomile, even though they are a separate species that is not related to German chamomile.

The constituents and action of Roman chamomile are similar to those of German chamomile, but weaker overall. Roman chamomile's dried, full flower heads are larger and better looking, which is why they are frequently used to "beautify" chamomile tea blends.

The European Pharmacopoeia lists Roman chamomile flowers as Chamomillae romanae flos.

Stinking chamomile (Anthemis cotula) is even more abundant than German chamomile in Germany and is often mistaken for it. Although it grows in similar sites, stinking chamomile prefers abandoned roads and squares and is also found as a weed in gardens. In fields, it is much less common than German chamomile. Stinking chamomile smells like a doghouse, which also explains one of its common names, dog fennel. It does, however, have a slight chamomile scent. Stinking chamomile (Anthemis cotula) has naturalized in the Americas.

Definition

Stinking chamomile and German chamomile flowers **differ** in two simple ways:

- With German chamomile, the receptacle of older flowers curves upward in a cone shape and its center is hollow. With stinking chamomile, the receptacle, even in more mature flowers, shows no or very little curvature and its center is solid.
- The quickest way to differentiate German chamomile from stinking chamomile is to cut the flower in half lengthwise using scissors or a knife, or even a thumb nail. Close inspection reveals that stinking chamomile flowers have a small, scale shaped chaff next to each small individual flower in the receptacle. Its peripheral white flower petals are horizontal, similar to those of daisies. In German chamomile, the peripheral white flower petals, at least in older flowers, are often folded down and the chaff is missing.

Stinking chamomile has no medicinal use. Adding it to German chamomile can result in **allergic reactions** because stinking chamomile contains a higher level of the sesquiterpene lactone anthecotulid, which has strong antigenic effects.

Peppermint (Mentha × piperita)

Peppermint (▶ Fig. 3.3) is a cross between Mentha aquatica and Mentha spicata (Mentha spicata is a cross between Mentha rotundifolia and Mentha longifolia). This cross seems to have been coincidental and first appeared in England at the end of the 17th century. It was first described scientifically in 1696 by the British naturalist and theologian John Ray. These plants were further cultivated and soon found a wide spectrum of use in phytotherapy. As is the rule with hybrids, it can only be propagated asexually by rootstock division. Peppermint is a relatively new hybrid, but its parent plants (especially Mentha longifolia) are some of the oldest known medicinal plants. They were mentioned by Greek and Roman authors in antiquity and even in the Bible. The present-day indications for peppermint are based on these traditional uses of its ancestors.

Peppermint is part of the Labiatae family of plants. It has decussated, wide lanceolate leaves that exhibit several punctiform, translucent glands on the underside of the leaf when the leaf is held up to light.

Centuries of cultivation have refined the peppermint plant but have also made it more vulnerable. If it grows in the same location for a longer period of time, it begins to regress and becomes more like curly mint (Mentha spicata, see below), and its leaves become more crispate, and its scent and flavor weaken.

Peppermint is cultivated commercially in high volume in some areas of southern and central Germany. However, it is also suitable for small scale cultivation and home gardens. An area the size of

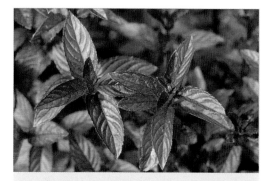

Fig. 3.3 Peppermint, Mentha piperita. Photo: Dr. Roland Spohn, Engen.

one-half to one square meter is enough to supply sufficient peppermint to last a long time. Peppermint plants need to be transplanted every 2 years.

Peppermint is much less expensive than chamomile. Its cultivation and trade are well organized and high-quality peppermint is available from many sources, including health food stores and farmers' markets.

Medicinal applications use the **peppermint leaves** (Menthae piperitae folium).

▶ **Pharmacology.** The active constituents of peppermint include volatile oil (minimum of 1.2%), tannins (6–12%), and bitters.

Peppermint essential oil (Menthae piperitae aetheroleum) contains a minimum of 4.5% up to a maximum of 10% ester (calculated as menthyl acetate), a minimum of 44% free alcohols (calculated as menthol), and a minimum of 15% up to a maximum of 32% ketones (calculated as menthones). Peppermint oil is **antispasmodic** for the smooth muscles of the gastrointestinal system. It is also **cholagogic** and **carminative**. Peppermint oil has also been shown to have antibacterial properties.

Peppermint is well tolerated and there are no known side effects or interactions with other drugs to date.

▶ **Indications.** Peppermint is a natural combination medicine, primarily for **functional spastic epigastric symptoms**. It combines spasmolytic, cholagogic, carminative and antibacterial actions. This makes peppermint a reliable plant medicine, whether used alone or combined with other gastrointestinal remedies. It is especially suitable for conditions dominated by nausea, the urge to vomit, and spastic pain.

The Commission E monograph for peppermint leaves lists the following indications: spastic complaints of the gastrointestinal tract as well as gall bladder and bile ducts, irritable bowel syndrome (IBS), inflammation of the oral mucosa, upper respiratory catarrh, myalgia, and neuralgiform symptoms. For more information, see the separate chapters about these conditions.

Treatments may make use of the whole plant, plant leaves, or isolated essential oils. Pure peppermint essential oil concentrates the medicinal action of the plant, with a primary focus on its spasmolytic action on the stomach, intestines, and bile duct. Successful treatment requires using a sufficient amount of peppermint.

> ### Caution
>
> Caution is advised in case of severe gastric acid dyspepsia, which can be worsened by peppermint tea.

> ### Preparations
>
> Peppermint tea is the most well-known application of peppermint, either used on its own or combined with other medicinal plants.
> - **Tea**
>   Add 1 cup of hot water to 1–2 teaspoons of the drug. Do not boil. Steep covered for 10–15 minutes, then strain.
>   Drink warm, in small sips, best after or between meals.
> - **Tincture**
>   Take 10–20 drops in one glass of water. Preferable for acute symptoms.
> - **Peppermint Hydrosol (Aqua Menthae piperitae)**
>   Take by the tablespoonful. May be substituted for the tea, but the effect is less potent.
> - **Syrup**
>   Syrup is used as a flavor corrigent in blends.

Other Types of Mint

Other mints are sometimes used for menthol production, but they are not substitutes for peppermint's medicinal quality. They are listed here for information purposes.

Spearmint (Mentha crispa, Mentha spicata ssp. crispate)

Spearmint (Mentha crispa) is very similar to peppermint. It represents a curly leafed variety of true peppermint. Its leaves are almost round.

The volatile oil content of spearmint fluctuates; the chemical composition of the oil is inconsistent.

Spearmint is used in the same manner as peppermint. There does not seem to be an advantage or difference compared to peppermint. Medicinal applications use the **spearmint leaves** (Menthae crispae folium).

Preparation

Largely the same as peppermint preparations.

Horse Mint (Mentha sylvestris, Mentha longifolia)

Horsemint's main characteristic is its gray pubescent stems. Crushing its leaves releases a pronounced peppermint scent.

Preparations

Horsemint is primarily suited to external applications.
- **Herbal Baths**
- **Herb Pillows**

Pennyroyal (Mentha pulegium)

European pennyroyal (Mentha pulegium) grows wild and is also cultivated in the Mediterranean countries. It supplies an essential oil that is used in menthol production. Pennyroyal is not directly used as a medicinal plant in Germany.

Caution ⚠

Pulegone, the main constituent in pennyroyal volatile oil, is very toxic, and can induce abortion.

Lemon Balm (Melissa officinalis)

Lemon balm is one of our oldest medicinal plants (► Fig. 3.4). It originates from southern Europe and is widely planted in gardens. It has become naturalized in many regions of North and South America. Its name derives from the lemonlike scent released when its leaves are crushed.

Like peppermint, lemon balm is a member of the Labiatae family. Its flowers are inconspicuously small, whitish, and form verticillate whorls of three to five flowers at the leaf axils. Its leaves are wide and ovate except for the bottom leaves, which are almost heart shaped.

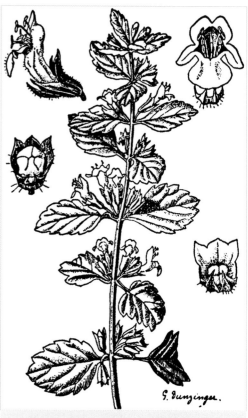

Fig. 3.4 Lemon Balm, Melissa officinalis.

Medicinal applications use the **lemon balm leaves** (Melissae folium).

► **Note.** Lemon balm is sometimes confused with beebalm or Oswego tea (Monarda didyma), which is also known as "bergamot" because of its aromatic scent that is very similar to that of the bergamot orange (Citrus bergamia). For tea preparations, **beebalm herb** (dried above-ground parts, Monardae herba) is used. Beebalm is native to North America–where it is traditionally used by some Indigenous peoples for the treatment of excessive flatulence—and is also cultivated in Germany. It contains a volatile oil, bitters, and the anthocyanin monardaein. The plant is an aromatic and primarily used as a flavor corrigent in tea blends.

► **Pharmacology.** Lemon balm leaves contain a minimum of 0.05% volatile oil (Oleum Melissae), consisting primarily of citronellal, citral A and B, and linalool as well as other monoterpenes and sesquiterpenes. Other constituents include tannins, flavonoids, and bitters.

Lemon balm is mainly used as a **mild sedative**. Its sedative effects are primarily attributed to its volatile oil content. However, lemon balm's minuscule volatile oil content does not seem to explain its entire therapeutic effect. Lemon balm is also a carminative based on its spasmolytic and antibacterial actions.

▶ **Research.** Wagner and Sprinkmeyer showed that 3–10 mg/kg of lemon balm essential oil induces sedation in spontaneous motility tests in mice. They also showed spasmolytic actions for the lemon balm constituents of citral and linalool. Wagner and Wiesenauer posit that the effect of lemon balm likely derives from the additive and potentiating actions of all lemon balm constituents.

▶ **Indications.** The main indications for lemon balm are **functional gastrointestinal disorders** with a tendency toward meteorism.

The Commission E monograph for lemon balm lists the following indications: nervous sleeping disorders (problems falling asleep) and functional gastrointestinal complaints.

Lemon balm is well tolerated, with no known side effects or interactions with other drugs.

▶ **Note.** Lemon balm is also discussed in the chapter about nervous system and psychological disorders (see Chapter 8.1 "Nervous Unrest and Sleep Disorders" (p. 252)). This plant is also indicated for nervous restlessness, especially in conjunction with functional heart disorders, and problems falling asleep. Lemon balm's special action with herpes simplex infections (cold sores) is discussed in Section 3.1.3 Lemon Balm (Melissa officinalis) (p. 41).

Preparations

- **Tea**
  Add 1 cup of hot water to 2 teaspoons of the drug. Steep covered for 10–15 minutes, then strain. Drink several times a day in small sips, preferably warm, and optionally sweetened with honey.
- **Combination with Peppermint**
  Combine 2 teaspoons of peppermint leaves (Menthae piperitae folium) and 2 teaspoons of lemon balm leaves. Prepare tea as described above. Drink 1 cup in the evening.
- **Lemon Balm Hydrosol (Aqua Melissae)**
  Take 1–2 tablespoons several times a day. This inexpensive preparation may be substituted for tea, but its action is less potent.

▶ **Therapy Recommendations.** It frequently makes sense to combine lemon balm and peppermint. Lemon balm supports peppermint's action with its sedative component and frequently improves the flavor of peppermint. This is especially advantageous when peppermint needs to be taken long term, when a change in flavor is often welcomed.

Bibliography

Aggag ME, Yousef RT. Study of antimicrobial activity of chamomile oil. Planta Med. 1972; 22(2):140–144

Barton H. Zum Wirkungsmechanismus des 1,4-Dimethyl-7-isopropylazulens auf die Tumorzelle. Acta Biol Med Ger. 1959; 2:555–567

Fintelmann V. Modern phytotherapy and its uses in gastrointestinal conditions. Planta Med. 1991; 57 Suppl 1:48–52

Fintelmann V. Phytopharmaka in der Gastroenterologie. Z Phytother. 1994; 15:137–141

Hausen BM, Busker E, Carle R. Über das Sensibilisierungsvermögen von Compositenar. VII. Experimentelle Untersuchungen mit Auszügen und Inhaltsstoffen von Chamomilla recutita und Anthemis cotula. Planta Med. 1984; 42:205–284

Isaac D. Die Kamillentherapie—Erfolg und Bestätigung. Dtsch Apoth Ztg. 1980; 120:567–570

Isaac O, Thiemer R. Biochemische Untersuchungen von Kamilleninhaltsstoffen. III. In vitro-Versuche über die antipeptische Wirkung des (-)-α-Bisabolols. Arzneimittel Forschung. 1975; 25:1086–1087

Kraul MA, Schmidt F. Über die wachstumshemmende Wirkung bestimmter Extrakte aus Flores Chamomillae und eines synthetischen Azulenpräparates auf experimentelle Mäusetumoren. Arch der Pharm. 1957; 290:66–74

Schilcher H. Die Kamille. Stuttgart: Wissenschaftliche Verlagsgesellschaft; 1987

Szelenyi I, Isaac O, Thiemer K. Pharmakologische Untersuchungen von Kamillen-Inhaltsstoffen. III. Tierexperimentelle Untersuchungen über die ulkusprotektive Wirkung der Kamille. Planta Med. 1979; 35(3):218–227

Wagner H, Sprinkmeyer L. Über die pharmakologische Wirkung von Melissengeist. Dtsch Apoth Ztg. 1973; 113:1159–1166

Wagner H, Wiesenauer M. Phytotherapie: Phytopharmaka und pflanzliche Homöopathika. 2nd ed. Stuttgart: Wissenschaftliche Verlgesellschaft; 2003

Wurm G, Baumann K, Geves U. Beeinflussung des Arachidonsäurestoffwechsels durch Flavonoide. Dtsch Apoth Ztg. 1982; 122: 2062–2068

Questions

1. Which medicinal plants are especially suited to treating acute gastritis?
2. What are the important pharmacologic effects of German chamomile?
3. What is a "rolling regimen"?
4. Which plant family does peppermint belong to?
5. What is peppermint's main effect on the stomach?
6. What caution needs to be taken when prescribing peppermint for acute gastritis?

Answers (p. 421) for Chapter 3.2.1

3.2.2 Irritable Stomach

For references corresponding to the preceding section, see Bibliography following 3.2.3 (p. 71).

Medicinal Plants

German Chamomile, Matricaria recutita
German Chamomile leaves, Matricariae flos

Irritable stomach is a **classic psychosomatic disorder** or imbalance. Diagnostics focused on findings are not able to identify organic morphologic changes. However, patients suffer from symptoms characterized by pain, pressure, and possibly heartburn that significantly impact their quality of life. Patients also frequently develop cancer phobia and search for "hidden" causes because they do not understand the discrepancy between their symptoms and the practitioner's statement that no disease processes related to the stomach can be found.

Irritable stomach is not a minor ailment and is always a primary indication for the use of phytopharmaceuticals. The primary remedy of choice is German chamomile because of its antispasmodic action. In case of severe spastic symptoms, chamomile may be combined with belladonna (Atropa belladonna).

Plants for Treatment

German Chamomile (Matricaria recutita)

For more information about this plant, see German Chamomile (p. 42).

Preparations

- **Tea**
  Add 1 cup of hot water to 2–3 teaspoons of the drug. Steep covered for 5–10 minutes, then strain.
  Drink slowly between meals.
  The daily intake should be divided into several doses, including the morning "rolling regimen." (p. 45)
- **Tea with Belladonna Tincture**
  Add 5–10 drops of belladonna tincture (p. 70) to 1 cup of chamomile tea.
  This tea is used for very severe spastic symptoms.

3.2.3 Chronic Gastritis, Lack of Appetite

Medicinal Plants

Tonic Bitters (Amara tonica)
Centaury, Centaurium minus
Centaury herb, Centaurii herba
Gentian, Gentiana lutea
Gentian root, Gentianae radix
Cinchona, Cinchona pubescens
Cinchona bark, Cinchonae cortex
Bogbean, Menyanthes trifoliate
Bogbean leaf, Menyanthis folium
Condurango, Marsdenia condurango
Condurango bark, Condurango cortex
Bitter Orange, Citrus aurantium ssp. amara
Bitter Orange peel, Aurantii pericarpium

Aromatic Bitters (bitters containing volatile oils, Amara aromatica)
Angelica, Angelica archangelica
Angelica root, Angelicae radix
Blessed Thistle, Cnicus benedictus, syn. Carduus benedictus; syn. Centaurea benedicta
Blessed Thistle herb, Cnici benedicti herba
Calamus, Acorus calamus
Calamus root, Calami rhizome
Wormwood, Artemisia absinthium
Wormwood herb, Absinthii herba

Acrid Bitters (Amara acria)
Ginger, Zingiber officinalis
Ginger root, Zingiberis rhizome
Galangal, Alpinia officinarum
Galangal root, Galangae rhizome

Demulcents
Iceland Moss, Cetraria islandica
Icelandic Moss lichen, Lichen islandicus
Usnea, Usnea barbata
Usnea, Usnea
Flax, Linum usitatissimum
Flaxseed, Lini semen

Chronic gastritis that has been diagnosed histologically exhibits all degrees of changes in gastric mucosa. In its final stage, it presents as chronic atrophic gastritis.

The primary cause of chronic gastritis is bacterial infection with **Helicobacter pylori.** Stomach cancer often occurs in conjunction with *Helicobacter pylori* infections of the gastric mucosa. The goal, therefore, is to eradicate this pathogen as completely as possible using antibiotic combination therapy to prevent the development of carcinomas. Research also points to the action of plant medicines specifically against *Helicobacter pylori*, for example, licorice (p. 66). Treatments using such phytopharmaceuticals during or after antibiotic treatment to eradicate this pathogen make sense.

Another type of gastric mucosa disorder is drug-induced, often erosive gastritis. Many different drugs, especially salicylates and nonsteroidal anti-inflammatory drugs (NSAID), can lead to drug-induced damage of the gastric mucosa. The first step in treating this type of gastritis is to stop the medication causing damage. The gastric mucosa can be healed with chamomile tea, peppermint tea, flaxseed gruel (mucilage), and a short-term bland diet. These treatments will usually cause symptoms to subside and disappear quickly.

Phytopharmaceuticals cannot reverse morphological changes of the gastric mucosa associated with chronic gastritis. However, in its early stages, phytopharmaceuticals can support gastric mucosa in its role as a protector against aggressive factors by stimulating and maintaining the secretion and production of mucus. Prevention is a key aspect of therapy in this context. Functional dyspepsia is an expression of reduced function not only of the stomach, but also of other upper abdominal organs. That is why this topic is discussed in a separate chapter. One of the key symptoms of diminished gastric mucosa function is lack of appetite. Treatments for lack of appetite are discussed in conjunction with chronic gastritis.

There are two large groups of medicinal plants available for the treatment of chronic gastric disorders: **bitters** (amara) and **demulcents that contain mucilage.** Demulcents create a protective layer of mucus on the gastric mucosa, which can reduce inflammation. In some cases and for some combinations, spasmolytics (see Sections 3.2.1 "Acute Gastritis (p. 42)" and 3.2.2 "Irritable Stomach (p. 51)") and carminatives (see Chapter 3.3 "Gastroenterological Disorders" (p. 72)) may be added.

Plants for Treatment: Bitters (Amara)

A very large number of plants contain bitters. Of those, a very high number contain other active constituents beside bitters. The term "bitters" refers to plants with a predominantly **bitter action** and where this action determines its effects and medical indication.

For clinical and practical application, bitters (amara) are divided into three categories: tonic bitters (Amara tonica), aromatic bitters (Amara aromatica), and acrid bitters (Amara acria). The pharmacologic actions and clinical effects of these plants are largely identical. This is why these aspects are discussed before presenting the descriptions of the individual plants.

▶ **Pharmacology.** Most bitters are monoterpenes and sesquiterpenes. The iridoid ester glycoside amarogentin contained in gentian is the most bitter natural compound known. Its bittering power is 1:58 million. Absinth contained in wormwood also has a high bittering power of 1:13 million. Other bitters include alkaloids (quinine), flavanone glycosides, and substances exhibiting steroid structures.

Bitters **increase secretions,** primarily by stimulating the bitter receptors in the taste buds at the base of the tongue and secondarily, by stimulating gastrin release when the bitters reach the stomach together with food. Gastrin stimulates motility in the upper gastrointestinal tract and the production of gastric acid, bile, and pancreatic secretions.

▶ **Research.** Amann and Maiwald showed the release of gastrin and pepsinogen for several bitters.

▶ **Indications.** Important indications for bitters include **motility disorders of the upper digestive tract**, especially of the stomach. Bitters can frequently provide sustained improvement for conditions presenting with a large, atonic stomach with very little motility or as tonic gallbladder and pancreas disorders.

The most well-known application for bitters is **lack of appetite** caused by general exhaustion, recent infection, anorexia, or constitutional factors. Lack of appetite as a symptom of serious organic disorders such as cancer does not usually respond as well to bitters.

The Commission E lists the indications lack of appetite and dyspeptic symptoms.

Bitter plant medicines are most effective if they are taken 15–30 minutes before meals. They also need to be taken in sufficient amounts to be effective. However, excessive amounts can cause the opposite effects (Wagner and Wiesenauer).

> ### Caution ⚠
>
> All bitters (amara), but especially acrid bitters (Amara acria), are contraindicated for gastric and duodenal ulcers. Stimulation of acid secretion is not desirable with these conditions. Experience has shown that bitters can also intensify subjective symptoms in patients with these conditions.

▶ **Note.** Observant clinicians and practitioners will note that bitters demonstrate more generalized actions that go beyond the upper digestive tract. They can stimulate and strengthen in cases of exhaustion and vegetative functional disorders. Hyperventilation tetany can be stopped immediately by quick administration of a few drops of gentian tincture on the tongue. In children, bitters can provide sustained improvement for mild anorexia that has not yet progressed to serious anorexia nervosa. Bitter medicinals do not produce additional effects for patients who have a normal appetite and normal reflex secretion.

Tonic Bitters

Tonic bitters are also referred to as Tonica amara, stomachics, or aperitifs.

Of the large number of tonic bitters, two to three common plants can usually cover most therapeutic requirements in practice. These plants all belong to the Gentianaceae family.

Centaury (European) (Centaurium minus, Centaurium erythraea)

Centaury (also known as feverwort) is an inconspicuous plant that usually grows in large patches in boggy meadows. The plant is easy to identify by its peculiar, stiff stem. The lower leaves form a rosette that is often wilted by the time the plant goes into bloom. Centaury's square stem starts to branch toward the upper part of the plant, which causes the flowers to crowd. The flowers are small and pale pink to blood red and, occasionally, white. The leaves are decussate. They grow in sets of two opposite leaves, and the next-higher pair of leaves grows at a right angle to the lower pair (▶ Fig. 3.5).

All parts of the plant taste bitter. The stem is the most bitter. The flowers and leaves are slightly less bitter; however, the flowers taste more bitter than the leaves.

Medicinal applications use the **centaury herb** (dried above-ground parts, Centaurii herba). Dried centaury is easily identified. The flowers prominently appear as reddish dots in a mass of nondescript, greenish leaves. Centaury does not have a distinct scent.

▶ **Note.** Two other types of centaury should be mentioned in this context: branched or dwarf centaury (Centaurium pulchellum) and seaside centaury (Centaurium vulgare). Centaurium

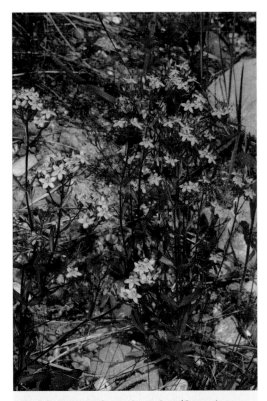

Fig. 3.5 Centaury, Centaurium minus (Centaurium erythraea). Photo: Dr. Roland Spohn, Engen.

pulchellum is small and delicate. It grows in the same locations as Centaurium minus but is less common. Centaurium vulgare grows in salt marshes inland or along the coast. Both of these types of century have effects similar to Centaurium minus, but are not much used for medicinal purposes because they cannot be harvested in large amounts. However, combining them with centaury herb is not considered an adulteration.

▶ **Pharmacology.** The bitter taste of the centaury herb can be detected in aqueous extractions of up to a dilution of 1:3500. In addition to a bitter glycoside (erythaurin), the plant contains 0.1% oleanolic acid and resins. Bitters, however, dominate centaury's action, with significant local and general tonifying effects.

▶ **Indications.** Centaury is especially effective for the treatment of **postinfectious achylous conditions**.

▶ **Note.** Centaury was formerly used as a fever remedy based on its tonifying effects, but this indication is no longer relevant.

Preparations

- **Tea**
  Add 1 cup of boiling water to 1–2 teaspoons of the drug. Steep covered for 5–10 minutes, then strain.
  Drink 1 cup at room temperature at least 15 minutes before meals.
- **Extract**
  Take single doses of 1–2 g of centaury extract several times a day.
  Centaury extract is frequently added to bitter tinctures or combination remedies.

▶ **Therapy Recommendation.** Centaury should be taken long term because its tonifying effects on the stomach and the human organism generally take some time to fully manifest.

Gentian (Gentiana lutea)

The medicinal herb gentian should not be confused with the beautiful, blue-blossomed gentian that grows in the European Alps. Gentiana lutea is a much larger and more robust plant that looks completely different. As its name indicates (Latin *luteus* = yellow), its blossoms are yellow instead of blue (▶ Fig. 3.6).

Gentian is considered a pure bitter. Its bittering power is 1:20,000, which means that its bitter flavor can still be detected in a solution of 1 part in 20,000 parts of water. This makes gentian the most bitter native herb in Germany.

Gentian roots do not contain tannins. This means that gentian does not have any astringent effects and does not irritate the stomach. Its bitter action can be applied in isolation, justifying its classification as a pure bitter.

Gentian in all its preparations—including gentian liqueur—is very popular in European Alpine regions and known worldwide. By stimulating stomach secretions, motility, and tone, gentian promotes the digestion of many foods that are difficult to digest.

Medicinal applications use the **gentian root** (Gentianae radix).

▶ **Pharmacology.** Gentian contains 2–3% bitters such as amarogentin and gentiopicroside and has a minimum bittering power of 10,000.

▶ **Indications.** The main indications for gentian are achylic and atonic conditions referred to as **sensitive stomach**. Gentian, like centaury, begins its action on the oral mucosa, which is why gentian should be retained in the mouth for a brief period before being swallowed. However, research shows, without a doubt, that gentian acts directly on the gastric mucosa by stimulating the release of gastrin.

Caution

Use with caution in cases of sensitive irritable stomach with hyperacidity. Gentian can increase hyperacidity symptoms.

▶ **Research.** An observational study of 205 patients tested the efficacy and tolerability of a dry gentian extract (Enziagil capsules). The study showed good therapeutic efficacy and good tolerability of the extract even though, due to its galenic preparation, the bitter action of the extract was not activated until it reached the stomach and could not be tasted (Wegener).

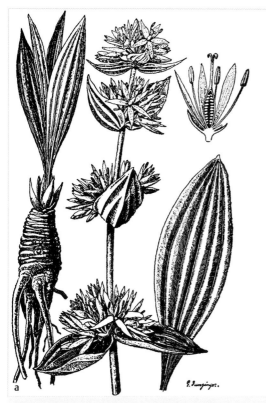
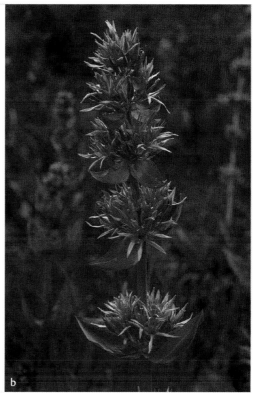

Fig. 3.6 a and b Gentian, Gentiana lutea. Photo: Dr. Roland Spohn, Engen.

- **Tea**
  Add 1 cup of cold water to 1 teaspoon of the drug. Bring to a boil and steep covered for 5 hours.
  Alternatively, add 1 cup of boiling water to 1 teaspoon of the finely chopped drug, steep covered for 5 minutes, then strain.
  Drink tea 30 minutes before meals, if possible.
- **Extract**
  Take as gentian capsules several times a day.

Star Gentian (Felwort, Star Swertia) Swertia perennis)

Swertia perennis is part of the Gentianaceae family and is the only Swertia species native to Germany. It also grows in western North America and in parts of Eurasia. Its habitat is moist soil around springs at high elevations. Several other Swertia species are very common in Japan, where swertia bitters are used more widely than gentian bitters.

Cinchona (Cinchona pubescens, Cinchona succirubra)

Cinchona trees reach a height of 25 m and are native to western South America. They are evergreen and mostly solitary, with blunt-edged, hair-covered branches. The outer layer of their bark is reddish brown, with deep fissures. Its leaves are about 20 cm long and 12 cm wide, egg-shaped, and thin.

Medicinal applications use the **cinchona bark** (Cinchonae cortex).

▶ **Pharmacology.** Of the alkaloids contained in cinchona bark, a minimum of 30% and a maximum of 60% are quinines. Cinchona bark also contains bitters and tannins.

Cinchona bark bitters stimulate gastric secretions and are also tonifying.

▶ **Indications.** Cinchona bark is recommended for **lack of appetite** and **dyspeptic symptoms**.

Preparations

- **Fluid Extract**
  Take 20 drops in plenty of water before meals.
  Cinchona bark fluid extract is intensely bitter. It contains sufficient diluted quinine to cause a tonic bitter effect.
- **Cinchona Composite Tincture** (Tinctura Chinae composita, according to the German Pharmacopoeia, DAB)
  This combination contains 10 parts cinchona bark, 4 parts bitter orange peel, 4 parts gentian root, and 2 parts "true"cinnamon bark (Cinnamomum zeylanicum, syn. Cinnamomum verum).
  Take 15–20 drops diluted in ½ glass of water before meals.

Prescriptions

Cinchona Bark–Rhubarb Combination
Rx
Tinct. Chinae comp. (cinchona composite tincture)
Tinct. Rhei vinosae āā 25.0 (rhubarb tincture, wine extraction)
D. S.
Take 1 teaspoon 3 × a day before meals.

This combination is used as a tonic or aperitif for fatigue and exhaustion, for example, following infection or surgery.

Other Tonic Bitters

Bogbean (Menyanthes trifoliate)

True to its name, bogbean is a characteristic inhabitant of boggy parts of meadows and moors (fens), and seems to prefer this habitat. Its peculiar, whitish-reddish flowers occur in clusters, with the tips of their crowns covered by beard-like hair (▶ Fig. 3.7). In somewhat more dry peat meadows, bogbean leaves are recognizable by their single leaves above the peat moss surface. Its large leaves and long stems are arranged in clusters of three

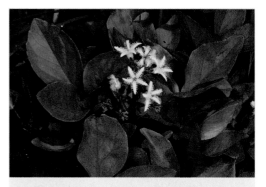

Fig. 3.7 Bogbean, Menyanthes trifoliata. Photo: Dr. Roland Spohn, Engen.

(trifoliate), the same as clover, which is how the plant derives part of its Latin name.

Medicinal applications use the **bogbean leaves** (Menyanthis folium). Its bittering power is 1:1500, which is weaker than gentian or centaury. In addition to bitter glycosides, bogbean also contains tannins and flavonoids. Unlike gentian, bogbean is not considered a "pure" tonic bitter.

Bogbean is used much less frequently than centaury or gentian.

Caution

Caution is advised when using bogbean due to its irritating effects on the stomach. For this reason, bogbean is mostly used only in combination with other medicinal plants.

Preparations

- **Tea**
  Add 1 cup of boiling water to 1 teaspoon of the finely chopped drug. Steep covered for 10 minutes, then strain.
  Drink 1 cup unsweetened 15–30 minutes before meals.
- **Decoction**
  Add 1 cup of cold water to 1 teaspoon of the finely chopped drug and bring to a brief boil. Steep covered for 10 minutes, then strain.
  Drink 1 cup before meals.
- **Tincture**
  Add 20–40 drops to ½ glass of water and drink slowly.

Condurango (Marsdenia condurango)

Condurango is a climbing shrub native to South America and belongs to the Asclepiadaceae family. Its bark, **Condurango cortex**, is used as a bitter drug that tastes bitter and harsh, and is almost exclusively used in combination remedies due to its fairly weak effect.

▶ **Note.** In the past, condurango bark was used to make condurango wine.

Bitter Orange (Citrus aurantium ssp. amara)

For more information about this plant, see Bitter Orange (p. 334).

Bitter orange has a pleasant taste and is a **mild sedative**. It is not a strong bitter and is used primarily in special circumstances that require a weaker effect. It is also indicated for young children.

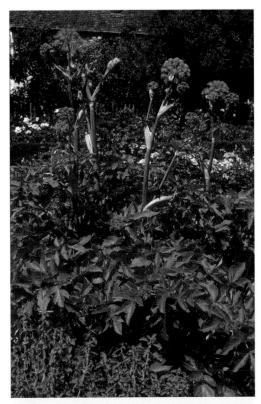

Fig. 3.8 Angelica, Angelica archangelica. Photo: Dr. Roland Spohn, Engen.

Preparation
• Tincture Add 20–40 drops to 1 glass of lukewarm water and drink in small sips about 30 minutes before meals.

Aromatic Bitters

The most commonly used aromatic bitters to treat chronic gastric disorders are angelica, blessed thistle, yarrow and, in some instances, calamus. These bitter medicinal plants are referred to as "aromatic" because they contain volatile oils in addition to bitters. Their action is based on a combination of bitters and spasmolytic, carminative, or cholagogic/choleretic principles. Their indication areas differ from those of "pure" bitters. Their general tonic effect is weaker and their local effect on the stomach is stronger.

Angelica (Angelica archangelica)

This rare, tall, and very striking plant belongs to the Apiaceae family. It can grow up to 2 m tall, and its leaves are large and pinnately divided twice to about halfway (bipinnatipartite). It has farinose pubescent umbels with many small, greenish flowers (▶ Fig. 3.8). In Europe, it is native to higher elevation regions such as the Giant Mountains (Czech Republic and Poland) or the Iser Mountains (Czech Republic) but also grows in lowland areas. Angelica archangelica is cultivated and has naturalized in many regions of North America.

Medicinal applications use **angelica rootstock and roots** (Angelicae radix). Frequently, the roots form braids that look as if they were artificially braided. These braids are considered to be an especially high-quality drug. Angelica used in plant medicine is almost always cultivated.

▶ **Pharmacology.** Angelica root contains 0.35–1.3% volatile oil as well as coumarins and furanocoumarins. Angelica is carminative, cholagocic, and mildly spasmolytic. It is used as an constituent in several well-known herbal digestive liqueurs such as Benedictine and Chartreuse because of its spicy and bitter flavor.

▶ **Note.** Angelica's appearance is very similar to several wild plants frequently found in Germany and other areas of the world. In Germany, it bears a close resemblance to wild angelica, Angelica sylvestris, which grows in ditches, along the edges of meadows and in moist forest areas. Wild angelica does not have the imbuing, aromatic scent of Angelica archangelica. Wild angelica is also easily differentiated from Angelica archangelica by its round leaf stalks (petioles) that feature slight grooves on the upper surface. The leaf stalks of Angelica archangelica are broadly tubular and not grooved on the upper surface.

In North America, Angelica archangelica may be confused with several similar plants. Some of these plants are highly toxic, such as poison hemlock (Conium maculatum), water hemlock (Cicuta maculate, Cicuta douglasii, Cicuta bolanderi), and some, such as giant hogweed (Heracleum mantegazzianum or maximum), may cause severe contact dermatitis.

Czygan provides a detailed description of the medical and cultural historical significance of angelica.

▶ **Indications.** Pharmaceutical biologists usually classify Angelica archangelica as belonging to the category of medicinal plants containing volatile oils. From a clinical practice point of view, classification as an aromatic bitter is more appropriate because this describes angelica's main application.

The Commission E monograph for angelica root lists the following indications: **loss of appetite, peptic discomforts,** such as mild spasms of the gastrointestinal tract, feeling of fullness, and flatulence.

Blessed Thistle (Cnicus benedictus, syn. Carduus benedictus, syn. Centaurea benedicta)

Blessed thistle is part of the Asteraceae family and is closely related to thistle (Carduus). It originates from the Mediterranean, but has been cultivated and also grows wild in Germany

Its leaves are mucronate and end abruptly in a short stiff point that is a continuation of the midrib. The upper leaves surround the flower heads like a hood, which makes this plant easy to recognize (▶ Fig. 3.9).

Medicinal applications use the **blessed thistle herb** (dried leaves and upper stems, including inflorescence dried leaves; Cnici benedicti herba).

▶ **Pharmacology.** The blessed thistle herb contains 0.25% bitters, such as cnicin and other sesquiterpenes, and 0.3% volatile oil. Its bittering power of 1:1800 is significant. For this reason, blessed thistle must be classified as a bitter, even if this plant is also associated with carminatives and gallbladder remedies.

Because of its bitter action, the blessed thistle herb is frequently used in herbal liqueurs.

▶ **Research.** Vanhaelen-Fastré demonstrated antibiotic actions for blessed thistle essential oil. The oil showed bacteriostatic effects against *Staphylococcus aureus* and *Staphylococcus faecalis*, but not against *Escherichia coli*. This may be interpreted as an indicator for the carminative component of the oil's effect.

Preparations

- **Tea**
  Add 1 cup of boiling water to 1 teaspoon of the finely chopped drug, then strain.
  Drink 1 cup before each meal.
- **Decoction**
  Add 1 teaspoon of the finely chopped drug to 1 cup of cold water. Bring to a brief boil, then strain.
  Drink 1 cup before each meal.
- **Tincture (1:5)**
  Add 20–30 drops to ½–1 glass of water.
  Drink 15–30 minutes before meals.

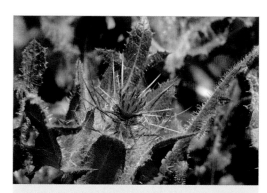

Fig. 3.9 Blessed Thistle, Cnicus benedictus. Photo: Dr. Roland Spohn, Engen.

▶ **Indications.** Blessed thistle is recommended for **lack of appetite**.

Preparations

- **Tea**
  Add 1 cup of boiling water to 2 teaspoons of the drug. Steep covered for 30 minutes, then strain.
  Drink 2–3 cups 15–30 minutes before meals.
- **Tincture (1:5)**
  Take 10–30 drops diluted in a shot glass of water several times a day.

Calamus (Sweet Flag) (Acorus calamus)

Calamus (▶ Fig. 3.10) is part of the monotypic Acoraceae family, which only encompasses the genus Calamus (Acorus).

In Germany, calamus grows wild and plentifully along creeks, riverbanks, and edges of ponds. Calamus is easy to overlook because it looks like grass or reeds and is hardly ever found in bloom. However, its wide, sheathlike leaves, which are reddish pink at the base, are easy to recognize.

Calamus is very popular in some areas of Germany as a symbol of Pentecost.

Medicinal applications use the **calamus rootstock** (Calami rhizome). Calamus roots and the entire calamus plant have a very pleasant scent and pungent aroma.

▶ **Pharmacology.** The flavor of calamus is predominantly bitter, but not exclusively, as with tonic bitters. In addition to the bitter component (acorin), calamus rootstock contains 1.5–3.5% volatile oil and tannin.

▶ **Indications.** Calamus is strongly tonifying for the stomach and promotes stomach secretions. It

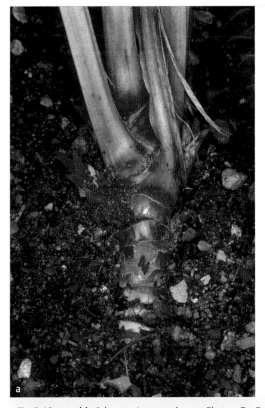
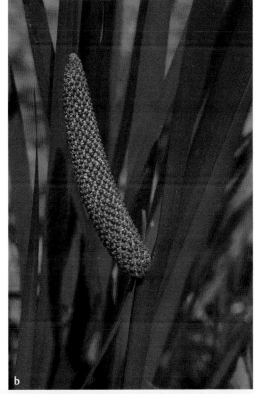

Fig. 3.10 **a and b** Calamus, Acorus calamus. Photos: Dr. Roland Spohn, Engen.

is also a significant appetite stimulant. Calamus tea is a popular prescription for **lack of appetite**. It has been known to be effective for lack of appetite owing to cancer.

Calamus's reputation has been tainted by tetraploid varieties of calamus originating in India and China. This type of calamus contains a large amount of beta-asaron and has been shown to have **carcinogenic potential** in long-term animal trials. The Commission E therefore decided to issue a negative monograph for calamus because safe and equally effective alternatives are available.

It is typically advised to avoid the administration of this drug to children. In the past, calamus root was used as a treatment during teething: A few pieces of calamus root were tied into a linen bag and given to children to suck on. Today, the root stock of orris root (Iris × germanica [Iridaceae]) can be used instead for this indication. This plant has a violet-like scent, but is a member of the iris family.

In the meantime, studies have shown that diploid calamus varieties originating in North America do not contain the problematic beta-asaron. Therefore, this plant may continue to be used medically **without concern** and reservation as a plant medicine.

Preparations

- **Tea**
  Add 1 cup of boiling water to ½ teaspoon of the drug. Steep covered for 5 minutes, then strain.
  Drink 1 cup before each meal.
- **Tincture**
  Take 20–30 drops 3 × a day diluted in 1 glass of water.

Wormwood (Artemisia absinthium)

For more information about this plant, see Wormwood (p. 111).

Preparation

- **Tea**
  Add 1 cup of boiling water to 1 teaspoon of the finely chopped drug. Steep covered for 5 minutes, then strain. Drink 1 cup before each meal.

Acrid Bitters

Ginger (Zingiber officinalis)

Ginger is primarily known as a spice plant, but it has been used medicinally for millennia.

The horizontally creeping, bulbous, and succulent ginger rootstock develops annual multileaved reedlike shoots that can grow up to 1 m in height from individual bulb segments. The multileaved shoots carry inflorescences up to 24 cm in length, while the narrow primary leaves on sterile shoots are lancet shaped that can grow up to 16 cm in length. The distal flower spike consists of imbricated, obovate bracts that overlap like roof shingles. Greenish-yellow tubular florets with brownish-violet dots are located in the leaf axils.

According to the German physician Gerhard Madaus (1890–1942), this plant, which originates from South Asia, probably no longer grows in the wild.

Medicinal applications use the **ginger rootstock** (Zingiberis rhizome).

▶ **Pharmacology.** Ginger root contains 2.5–3% volatile oil and pungent principles such as gingerol. As with all bitters, pungent principles promote saliva and gastric secretions. They also **increase** intestinal tonus and **peristalsis**. A placebo-controlled study involving 24 healthy males showed significant increases in the speed of gastric emptying (Wu et al.).

Serotonin antagonist actions have been verified pharmacologically for the ginger constituents 6-shogaol and gingerol. They dampen autonomous centers in the central nervous system (CNS) without showing any effect on the vestibular system. In any case, substances comprised of such small molecules can easily cross the blood-brain barrier.

▶ **Indications.** In clinical trials, ginger was shown to have antiemetic effects. This has been demonstrated in clinical, experimental, and controlled studies to be helpful for motion sickness.

▶ **Research.** Many studies have shown potential indications for ginger that will need to be assessed for future clinical relevance. Animal experiments showed antitumor effects for various ginger constituents or for alcoholic extracts. A combination extract of ginger and ginkgo biloba (Zingicomb) was shown to have anxiolytic effects in animal experiments. Schuhbaum and Franz compiled a very good overview of ginger. Ernst and Pittler showed in their review that ginger's antiemetic effect was well documented in several randomized trials. Vutyavanich et al. and Smith et al. showed ginger's antiemetic effect for nausea and vomiting during pregnancy in evidence-based studies, with a highly significant difference compared to placebos ($p < 0.001$).

Preparations

Tinctures are used most frequently, while tea preparations are used less often.

- **Tincture (1:5)**
  Add 10–20 drops to ½–1 glass of water.
  Take 15–30 minutes before meals.
- **Tea**
  Add 1 cup of hot water to 1 teaspoon of the coarsely powdered drug. Steep covered for 5–10 minutes, then strain.
  Drink 1 cup several times a day, 15–30 minutes before meals.

Galangal (Alpinia officinarum)

Galangal belongs to the ginger family (Zingiberacerae) and its main native habitat is China. Its long, creeping, slender, cylindrical rootstock is heavily branched and grows up to about 2 cm in diameter. It is covered with a multitude of large, light brown scales that leave white scars after they drop off. The rootstock produces up to 40 stalks that feature either flowers and leaves or only leaves. Flower stalks can grow 60–150 cm in height, and its flowers form dense terminal clusters. The white corolla is trilobate and tubular below. The fruit is shaped almost like a spherical capsule.

Medicinal applications use the **galangal rootstock** (Galangae rhizoma).

▶ **Pharmacology.** Galangal rootstock contains pungent principles, 0.5–1% volatile oil, and flavonoids.

Galangal's action is primarily **spasmolytic**, but antiphlogistic and antibacterial actions have also been described. Its spasmolytic action develops very rapidly and is strong enough to help in the early stages of biliary colic.

▶ **Indications.** The main indication for galangal is **spastic functional epigastric symptom,** in conjunction with severe meteorism, also known as **Roehmheld syndrome**.

Preparations

- **Tea**
  Add 1 cup of boiling water to 1 teaspoon of the finely chopped or coarsely powdered drug. Steep covered for 5–10 minutes, then strain. Drink 1 cup several times a day 15 minutes before meals.
- **Tincture**
  Add 10 drops to a small amount of lukewarm water.
  Take 15 minutes before meals.

Demulcents

Demulcents are characterized by their high **mucilage** content. Mucilage covers and protects inflamed mucosa, including the stomach. Mucilage also binds gastric acid and decomposition products that can irritate mucous membranes. However, herbal demulcents are of relatively limited use with chronic stomach disorders.

Iceland Moss (Cetraria islandica)

Botanically, Iceland moss is not a moss but a lichen with the botanical binomen Cetraria islandica. This explains its pharmacopoeial name, Lichen islandicus. Lichens are a symbiotic union of specific fungi and algae. Threads of mycelial hyphae closely surround green single-cell algae. The flat Icelandic moss thallus forks into two equal branches (dichotomous) (▶ Fig. 3.11). Small piles of fruiting bodies of the fungus (apothecia) are frequently found at the tips.

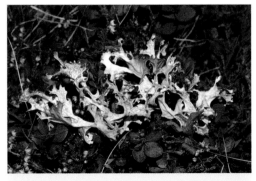

Fig. 3.11 Iceland Moss, Cetraria islandica. Photo: Dr. Roland Spohn, Engen.

In Germany, Iceland moss grows in pine forests and in heath areas, primarily in the Northern Lowland and in the Central Uplands. In North America, its range extends from Arctic regions from Alaska to Newfoundland south to the Rocky Mountains down to Colorado and east to the Appalachian Mountains of New England.

▶ **Note.** Iceland moss should not be confused with reindeer moss (Cladonia rangiferina), which looks completely different and is often used to make gray, weatherproof wreaths for decorating graves.

▶ **Pharmacology.** Iceland moss is a bitter as well as a demulcent, which lends it a special significance. It contains very high amounts, up to 40%, of moss starch (lichenin) which can be extracted from Iceland moss as a pure, white powder. It also contains 2–3% cetraric acid, which can be isolated as a white, needlelike substance. The mucilage contained in Iceland moss is digestible in the intestines, which is why this medicinal plant was also used as food in times of scarcity.

▶ **Indications.** Its combination of bitters and mucilage make Iceland moss useful for treating **chronic stomach disorders.** The bitters are a pronounced stomach tonic and are suitable as a general tonic. Alcoholic extractions of this drug, which largely lack mucilage, may be used as a tonic bitter.

Preparation

Iceland moss is most often prescribed as a tea in combination with other stomach remedies.
- **Tea**
  Add 1 cup of boiling water to 1–2 teaspoons of the finely chopped drug, then strain.
  Drink 1 cup several times a day before meals.

▶ **Therapy Recommendations.** For use with stomach disorders, Iceland moss should not be boiled. Instead, it should be covered with boiling water, then strained, or, preferably, macerated in cold water. This primarily dissolves the bitter principle and leaves the starch undissolved.

If a combination of bitter and demulcent action is desired, Iceland moss is boiled in water, and the cooking water is then poured off and used as a medicine.

Usnea (Usnea barbata)

Usnea barbata, also called "old man's beard," is the most commonly used tree lichen for medicinal purposes. In Germany, it grows plentifully in mountain forests.

▶ **Pharmacology.** Usnea contains plentiful bitters and lichen acids such as usnic acid. Usnic acid has been shown to have significant bacteriostatic effects even at higher dilution rates. So far, no clinically supported indications have been demonstrated.

▶ **Indications.** Usnea barbata is primarily used as an **aperitif.**

Flax (Flaxseed) (Linum usitatissimum)

Flax is an ancient cultivated plant that can be traced back several thousand years in history. Today, this annual or biannual plant is cultivated agriculturally as a field crop on all continents. The original native habitat of this plant is not known. Fiber (linen) produced from the long flax stalks is used for textiles.

Flax stalks can grow to about 1 m, are densely covered with linear, lanceolate leaves, and bear paniculate flower buds. The five-pedaled flower is usually strikingly blue and contains large ciliate corollar leaves (▶ Fig. 3.12). The fruit is a spherical or ovoid capsule of about 8 mm in length that contains about ten seeds.

Medicinal applications that use **flaxseeds** (Lini semen) were mentioned as far back as Hippocrates.

▶ **Pharmacology.** Flaxseeds contain fiber, such as hemicellulose, cellulose, and lignin. They also contain fatty oils consisting of 52–78% linolenic acid esters as well as protein, linustatin, and linamarin.

▶ **Indications.** Their high mucilage content makes flaxseeds suitable for treatment of chronic gastritis (inflammation of the stomach mucosa). Flaxseeds are especially indicated for subacute and chronic **gastritis** and **enteritis.** The Commission E

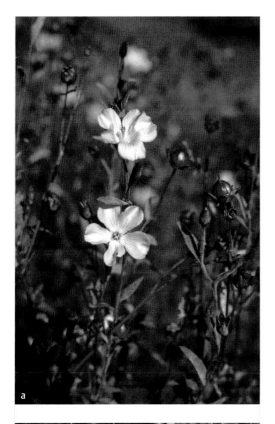

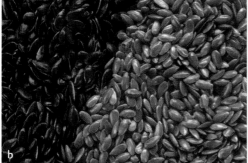

Fig. 3.12 a and b Flax, Linum usitatissimum. Photo: Dr. Roland Spohn, Engen.

monograph also lists a demulcent preparation of flaxseeds for these indications.

▶ **Research.** Grützner et al. confirmed the proven application of a flaxseed demulcent preparation for epigastric disorders.

Preparation

- **Flaxseed Demulcent Preparation**
  Macerate a daily dose of ground or chopped flaxseeds (for example, 1–2 tablespoons) overnight in 250–500 mL water that has first been boiled and then left to reach room temperature. In the morning, bring to a brief boil. Then strain, for example, through cheesecloth, to separate the mucilage from the seed hulls.
  Drink or eat (with a spoon) 1 cup several times a day.

Proven Prescriptions: Stomachic Teas

Prescriptions

Tea with Strong Bitter Effect
Rx
Centaurii herb. (centaury herb)
Trifolii fibrini fol. (bogbean leaves)
Calami rhiz. āā 20.0 (calamus rootstock)
M. f. spec.
Add 1 tablespoon of the blend to 1 L of water.
Boil for 15 minutes, then strain.
D.S.
Drink 1 cup of warm tea 1 hour before each main meal.

Prescriptions

Tea with Carminatives and Antispasmodics

For severe dyspepsia and tendency toward colic and meteorism.

Rx
Menth. pip. fol. (peppermint leaves)
Anisi fruct. (anise seeds)
Calami rhiz. āā 20.0 (calamus rootstock)
M. f. spec.
Add 1 cup of hot water to 1 tablespoon of the blend. Steep covered for 1 hour, then strain.
D. S.
Drink 1 cup of warm tea 1 hour before each main meal.

Prescriptions

Rx
Cnici benedicti herb. (blessed thistle herb)
Absinthii herb. (wormwood herb)
Melissae fol. āā 20.0 (lemon balm leaves)
M. f. spec.
Add 1 cup of hot water to 1 teaspoon of the blend. Steep covered for 20 minutes, then strain.
D. S.
Drink 1 cup 3 × a day.

Stomachic Tinctures

Prescriptions

Tea for Chronic Gastritis

Rx
Menth. pip. fol. (peppermint leaves)
Melissae fol. (lemon balm leaves)
Calami rhiz. (calamus rootstock)
Foeniculi fruct. āā 20.0 (fennel seeds)
M. f. spec.
Add 1 cup of boiling water to 1 teaspoon of the blend. Steep covered for 10 minutes, then strain.
D. S.
Drink 1 cup warm in small sips 2–3 × a day.

Prescriptions

Tea for Anacidity, Achylia, Anorexia

Rx
Absinthii herb. (wormwood herb)
Menth. pip. fol. āā 30.0 (peppermint leaves)
M. f. spec.
Add 1 cup of boiling water to 1 teaspoon of the blend. Steep covered for 10 minutes, then strain.
D. S.
Drink 1 cup 2 × a day slowly in small sips before meals.

Prescriptions

Tincture Blend for Dyspeptic Conditions

For long-term tea regimen.

Rx
Tinct. Gentianae (gentian tincture)
Tinct. Absinthii āā 20.0 (wormwood tincture)
Tinct. Menth. pip. 10.0 (peppermint tincture)
D. S.
Add 30 drops of the blend to 1 glass of water and drink right before meals.

Prescriptions

Bitters with Belladonna

Rx
Tinct. Belladonnae 5.0 (belladonna tincture)
Tinct. Gentianae (gentian tincture)
Tinct. Absinthii āā 20.0 (wormwood tincture)
D. S.
Add 30 drops of the blend to 1 glass of water and drink right before meals.

Prescriptions

Rx
Tinct. Belladonnae 2.0 (belladonna tincture)
Tinct. Menth. pip. 10.0 (peppermint tincture)
Tinct. Gentianae 20.0 (gentian tincture)
D. S.
Take 10–15 drops of the blend 3 × a day

Stomachic Mixtures

Prescriptions

Centaury Mixture

Rx

Extr. Centaurii fluid. 15.0 (centaury fluid extract)

Acid. hydr. dil. 3.0 (dilute hydrochloric acid, 12.5% HCl in H_2O)

Sir. simpl. 2.0 (simple syrup: 64 g sucrose dissolved in 36 mL water)

Aqu. dest. ad 200.0 (distilled water)

D. S.

Take 1 tablespoon of the blend 3 × a day.

Bibliography

Amann K, Maiwald L. Wie beeinflussen Bitterstoffe die Pepsin- und Säuresekretion im Magen? NaturaMed. 1988; 112:38–41

Czygan FC. Engelwurz oder Angelikawurzel—Angelica archangelica L. Z Phytother. 1998; 19(6):342–348

Ernst E, Pittler MH. Efficacy of ginger for nausea and vomiting: a systematic review of randomized clinical trials. Br J Anaesth. 2000; 84(3):367–371

Grützner KJ, Müller A, Schöllig HP. Wirksamkeit einer Schleimzubereitung aus Leinsamen bei funktionellen Oberbauchbeschwerden. Z Phytother. 1997; 18(5):263–269

Schuhbaum H, Franz G. Ingwer. Gewürz- und vielseitige Arzneipflanze. Z Phytother. 2000; 21:203–209

Smith C, Crowther C, Willson K, Hotham N, McMillian V. A randomized controlled trial of ginger to treat nausea and vomiting in pregnancy. Obstet Gynecol. 2004; 103(4):639–645

Vanhaelen-Fastré R. Constitution et proprietes antibacteriennes de l'huile essentielle de Cnicus benedictus [Constitution and antibiotical properties of the essential oil of Cnicus benedictus]. Planta Med. 1973; 24(2):165–175

Vutyavanich T, Kraisarin T, Ruangsri R. Ginger for nausea and vomiting in pregnancy: randomized, double-masked, placebo-controlled trial. Obstet Gynecol. 2001; 97(4):577–582

Wagner H, Wiesenauer M. Phytotherapie: Phytopharmaka und pflanzliche Homöopathika. 2nd ed. Stuttgart: Wissenschaftliche Verlagsgesellschaft; 2003

Wegener T. Anwendung eines Trockenextraktes aus Gentianae luteae radix bei dyspeptischem Symptomenkomplex. Z Phytotherapie. 1998; 19(3):163–164

Weiss RF. Phytotherapie der Magenleiden. Ärztez Naturheilverfahren. 1982; 23(3):149–154

Willuhn G. Der Lein oder Flachs—Linum usitatissimum L. Z Phytother. 1999; 20(2):120–126

Wu KL, Rayner CK, Chuah SK, et al. Effects of ginger on gastric emptying and motility in healthy humans. Eur J Gastroenterol Hepatol. 2008; 20(5):436–440

Questions

1. Which two main active principles are used in phytotherapy for treating chronic gastritis?
2. How do bitter medicinal plants differ in their effects?
3. What is the bittering power of gentian?
4. Which constituent of calamus is potentially carcinogenic and should not be used in phytopharmaceuticals?
5. Name one or two acrid bitters.
6. Name some typical demulcents.
7. Formulate a tea prescription for treating chronic gastritis.

Answers (p. 421) for Chapter 3.2.3

3.2.4 Gastric and Duodenal (Peptic) Ulcers

Medicinal Plants

Licorice, Glycyrrhiza glabra
Licorice root, Liquiritiae radix
German Chamomile, Matricaria recutita
German Chamomile flowers, Matricariae flos
Belladonna, Atropa belladonna
Belladonna root and leaves, Belladonnae radix et folium

The preceding chapters mentioned ulcer disorders several times. However, treatment of gastric and duodenal (peptic) ulcers requires a separate and more in-depth discussion because they are one of the most prevalent stomach and duodenal disorders and one with which many practitioners are constantly confronted. Peptic ulcers are also a typical example for the alternative or adjuvant use of plant medicines. They are disorders that are well understood and well defined, even if they exhibit individual characteristics, and a large number of effective synthetic drugs are available to treat these disorders. Critics of phytotherapy may claim that because of the potency and number of modern synthetic drugs available, phytotherapeutic alternatives are not necessary, particularly for peptic ulcer treatment.

The following intends to illustrate that in terms of efficacy, tolerability, and economic considerations, phytotherapeutic concepts do not compete with but are complementary to modern pharmacotherapy for the treatment of peptic ulcers. A wealth of experience and modern studies confirmed three main medicinal plants as especially suitable in this context: **licorice** (Liquiritiae radix), **belladonna** (Atropa belladonna), and **German chamomile** (Matricaria recutita). Chamomile has already been discussed in detail in earlier sections of this book (p. 42).

One basic understanding in this context should be that in addition to any pharmacotherapy, all peptic ulcer treatments need to include **dietary measures** and must address the psychosocial situation of the patient.

During the past few decades, important discoveries have been made regarding the **etiology** of peptic ulcers. For a long time, the pathogenic view was that peptic ulcers were caused by an imbalance between aggressive mucosal factors (primarily acid, pepsin, and biliary acids) and protective or defensive mucosal factors (primarily mucus and sufficient mucosal blood flow and mucosal regeneration). This imbalance was thought to be caused by psychogenic (psychosomatic) factors. Since then, epidemiologic observation has shown chronic gastritis caused by the persistent presence of **Helicobacter pylori** in the gastric mucosa to be another key factor—possibly the decisive factor—in the development of peptic ulcers. This led to an expansion of the existing therapy concept that focused mostly or entirely on blocking acids with H_2-antagonists, omeprazole, or antacids. The problems with this concept were twofold: A high recidivism rate when these drugs are stopped and known undesirable side effects of these drugs that made long-term or ongoing therapy problematic.

Since then, eradication of Helicobacter pylori by a combination of acid blockers, antibiotics, and in some cases, a bismuth preparation, has become an integral component in the **treatment of peptic ulcers** if Helicobacter is found in the gastric mucosa. The expectation is that truly successful eradication of Helicobacter pylori will also decrease the recidivism rate.

Another known ulcerogenic factor is the frequent use of certain drugs, especially salicylates and nonsteroidal anti-inflammatory drugs (NSAIDs). These drugs are known to be ulcerogenic and are now the most frequent cause of acute bleeding in the upper gastrointestinal tract. Theoretically, these **iatrogenic types of peptic ulcers** could be treated by stopping the use of these drugs and providing the appropriate therapy to heal the peptic ulcers. However, with heart and rheumatic diseases, these drugs are often essential and cannot simply be discontinued. The question is how complementary therapy can strengthen and protect mucous membranes against ulcerogenic factors to allow the continuation of important drug therapies without damaging gastric mucosa.

Plants for Treatment

Licorice (Glycyrrhiza glabra)

Licorice is an herbaceous perennial with a strong, woody, sweet-tasting rootstock that is brown on the outside and muddy yellow on the inside. Its stoloniferous (running) roots are about the thickness of a finger. Its upright, branched stalks can grow up to 1 m in height. Licorice branches are round at the bottom and angular at the top. The stalks bear three to seven pairs of ovoid, entire, and pinnate leaves that are arranged in an alternate binate pattern and are about 2–5 cm long and 1–2.5 cm wide (▶ Fig. 3.13). The leaf surface is glabrous, and the bottom of the leaf is sticky (viscid). The purple, white-tipped flowers are long-stemmed and bunched into clusters. Their calyx is bilabiate. The

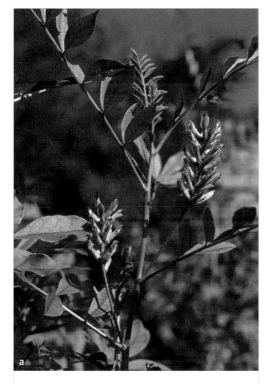

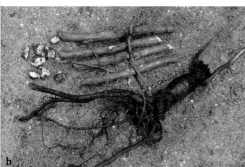

Fig. 3.13 a and b Licorice, Glycyrrhiza glabra. Photos: Dr. Roland Spohn, Engen.

two calyx lobes of the upper lip are coalesced, and the three lobes of the lower lip are free.

Licorice is native to southern Europe, where it grows in grassy and sunny brush areas. It is widely cultivated in southern Italy. A thick juice called licorice extract (Succus liquiritiae) is extracted from the dried, unpeeled roots.

Medicinal applications use the **licorice root** (Liquiritiae radix).

Traditional East Asian medical systems like Traditional Chinese Medicine or Japanese Kampo use the distinct but closely related species Glycyrrhiza uralensis (Chinese liquorice) in conjunction with generally equivalent indications. Nevertheless, the two species should not be confused.

▶ **Pharmacology.** Licorice root contains a minimum of 4% glycyrrhizin (glycyrrhizic acid) and 25% water-soluble components. In addition to the potassium salts and calcium salts contained in the glycyrrhizic acid, licorice contains a number of flavonoids of the flavanone and isoflavone group. Licorice has also been shown to contain phytosterols and coumarin. Glycyrrhetinic acid, the aglycone of glycyrrhizic acid, protects the mucous membranes in the gastrointestinal tract. Applied topically, it is strongly antiphlogistic.

Licorice also inhibits pepsin activity and increases stomach mucus viscosity.

Glycyrrhizin is viewed as the active principle in licorice that determines its efficacy.

▶ **Research.** In the 1970s, carbenoxolone, a pharmacologically developed drug containing a glycyrrhetinic acid derivative (sodium salt of succinic ester) revolutionized ulcer therapy. However, it was found to produce severe side effects, such as edema, hypokalemia, and high blood pressure (hyperaldosteronism), and, consequently, carbenoxolone was no longer recommended for use in ulcer therapy. The **pseudohyperaldosteronism** induced by carbenoxolone was attributed to glycyrrhizic acid. However, a clinical study of patients who experienced serious side effects from carbenoxolone showed that these same patients tolerated a standardized deglycyrrhizinated licorice extract without experiencing those side effects. At the same time, the healing rate of peptic ulcers was definitely comparable to that of carbenoxolone (Kleist et al.).

The modern history of licorice as a medicinal plant is based on the keen observations of a Dutch pharmacist, F.E. Revers. His discoveries laid the groundwork for subsequent research. Revers noticed that the people in his district who had stomach disorders highly praised a special product that contained licorice root extract. They reported that taking this product provided them with more reliable and sustained relief than anything else they tried. Revers deserves special credit for following up on this observation and engaging the interest of a Dutch university institute. Borst wrote about this in the *Lancet*. As far back as 1946, Revers reported that licorice tolerability and the development of undesirable effects were dose dependent. He found that patients with stomach disorders who took the licorice preparation longer term developed facial bloating after their gastric symptoms improved. There was an obvious connection between side effects, therapy duration, and amount of the preparation taken.

In 1998, Bielenberg compiled and critically assessed the entire pharmacologic literature about licorice. This produced a multitude of surprising results and indicated a much wider range of applications for licorice in practical phytotherapy than previously thought. In Japan, licorice has been used for a long time to treat viral hepatitis (B and C). In Germany, in 1994, Wildhirt tested this indication with very good results.

The **action profile** of licorice researched to date shows antiviral, interferon stimulating, antiphlogistic, and anti-inflammatory actions. Licorice also protects against cytotoxic damage and stabilizes liver lysosomes. Of particular interest is the fact that licorice inhibits DNA and RNA viruses. Antiallergic and secretolytic actions have also been shown. Animal trials also found anticarcinogenic actions. Overall, licorice appears to have substantial therapeutic potential that can encompass a multitude of indications.

For this discussion of peptic ulcers, the **antiulcerogenic** effects of licorice are especially relevant. Bielenberg hypothetically attributes these to the interaction between licorice and the level and metabolism of ascorbic acid, a process that is supported by many research results. This may also explain the positive therapeutic effects of licorice in ulcers induced by acetylsalicylic acid (ASA), since at typical dosages, ASA significantly lowers ascorbic acid levels. Similar effects have been observed with *Helicobacter pylori* infections. Of importance in this context is research showing that *in vitro*, glycyrrhetinic acid has a strong **bactericidal** effect

on different strains of *Helicobacter pylori*, and that this effect is dependent on dosage and duration of use. This included *Helicobacter pylori* strains that were resistant to the antibiotic clarithromycin or metronidazole (Ullmann et al.).

These results make licorice an interesting adjuvant to the therapies practiced today for peptic ulcers in the upper gastrointestinal tract. Long-term epidemiologic studies are needed to show if licorice is suitable for preventing the recurrence of peptic ulcers in long-term or continuous therapy without provoking undesirable effects. Studies are also needed to test if urgently needed ulcerogenic drugs such as ASA or NSAIDs can be prescribed long term without causing ulcers if they are taken concurrently with appropriately dosed licorice root preparations.

▶ **Indications.** The most important indication for licorice is **peptic ulcers of the stomach and duodenum**. In addition, its mucous membrane protecting action makes licorice suitable for all conditions that impact mucous membranes and lead to gastritis or irritable stomach.

The Commission E monograph for licorice root lists the indications catarrhs of the upper respiratory tract and gastric/duodenal ulcers.

Preparations

- **Tea**
  Add 1 cup of boiling water to ½ teaspoon of the finely chopped drug or add the drug to cold water and bring to a brief boil. Steep covered for 15 minutes, then strain. Drink 1 cup several times a day.
- **Fluid Extract (contains 4–6% glycyrrhizic acid)**
  Take 1 teaspoon diluted in a small amount of water several times a day.
- **Licorice "Juice" (Succus Liquiritiae)**
  Take 1.5–3 g diluted in a small amount of water before meals.

Ideally, practitioners should prescribe licorice preparations with standardized and reduced glycyrrhizic acid content. Future long-term studies are needed to show if this will assure adequate tolerability as well as therapeutic efficacy.

▶ **Therapy Recommendation.** Standardized, finished pharmaceutical licorice products should be used in the treatment of peptic ulcers.

German Chamomile (Matricaria recutita)

For more information about this plant, see German Chamomile (p. 42).

German chamomile is the **number one classic therapeutic** for mucous membranes. Its natural antiphlogistic principle is unsurpassed, but it is generally not sufficient as the only medicinal for treating manifest peptic ulcers.

Preparation 👉

- **Tea**
  Add 1 cup of hot water to 2 teaspoons of the drug. Steep covered for 5–10, then strain. Drink, while warm, in small sips.

▶ **Therapy Recommendations.** The chamomile tea "rolling regimen" (p. 45) is recommended for treating manifest peptic ulcers. This treatment distributes German chamomile tea slowly and evenly across the entire gastric mucosa. It also provides psychotropic effects for ulcer patients, who are often tense and stressed. This treatment allows them to start their day with a few minutes of rest, quietude and, hopefully, also relaxation.

Fluid extracts or ready-made chamomile preparations can be used if there is not enough time in the morning to freshly prepare chamomile tea. A sufficient dose, for example, 30–50 drops, is added to 1 glass of warm water and drunk.

Belladonna (Atropa belladonna)

Belladonna, also known as deadly nightshade, is one of many highly toxic plants in the nightshade (Solanaceae) family. It is a widely distributed plant that is native to Europe, North Africa, and western Asia, and it has been introduced and has naturalized in North America. In Germany, it grows in the central and southern regions. This herbaceous, perennial plant prefers deciduous forests and shaded areas. Its bluntly squared, densely branched stalk can grow to a height of 1 m and has fine, glandular hairs on the upper part (▶ Fig. 3.14).

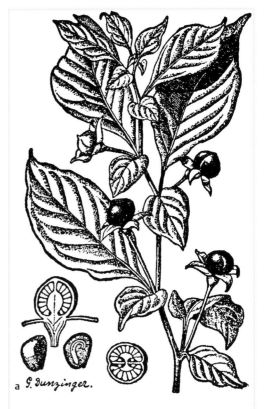

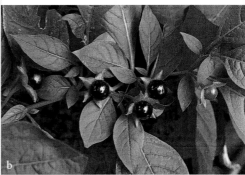

Fig. 3.14 a and b Belladonna, Atropa belladonna. Photo: Prof. Dr. Volker Fintelmann, Hamburg.

Belladonna has relatively delicate, elliptical, acuminate leaves that identify it as a shade plant. Its small leaves fill in the gaps between the larger leaves. This creates a leaf mosaic that allows the plant to make full use of light. Its individually pedicelled, drooping flowers are bell-shaped and brownish-red on the outside and muddy yellow on the inside, with purple veins. Its fruit is a spherical berry about the size of a cherry that is green initially and then turns a shiny black. The fruit contains a purple juice and many ovoid seeds. This fruit concentrates the highly toxic poison that is also found in the leaves.

Medicinal applications use the **belladonna leaves** (Belladonnae folium) as well as the **belladonna root** (Belladonnae radix).

▶ **Pharmacology.** Belladonna leaves contain a minimum of 0.3% alkaloids, including atropine, scopolamine, and L-hyosziamine. Dried belladonna root contains a higher concentration of alkaloids, with a minimum of 0.5%,

Belladonna's action is **parasympatholytic/anticholinergic** via the competitive inhibition of the neuromuscular transmitter acetylcholine at the receptor. This acetylcholine antagonism involves primarily the muscarinic and, to a lesser degree, the nicotinic effect of belladonna on the ganglia and neuromuscular end plate. Belladonna preparations, therefore, have peripheral effects on the autonomic nervous system and on smooth muscles as well as effects on the central nervous system (CNS).

Belladonna's parasympatholytic action induces the relaxation of smooth muscle organs and improves spastic conditions, especially in the gastrointestinal and biliary tracts. Its effect on the heart is positive dromotropic and positive chronotropic. With its action on the CNS, belladonna can affect muscle tremors and muscle rigidity in Parkinson's disease.

▶ **Note.** The increasing integration of phytotherapy and modern pharmacotherapy could lead to a renaissance for herbal extract preparations of belladonna–instead of isolated alkaloids–as this "natural" combination of different constituents can produce a therapeutic summation effect that is greater than the effect of its individual constituents.

Belladonna alkaloids are also antiemetic. This makes them suitable for treating nausea and vomiting in motion sickness disorders.

▶ **Indications.** The main indication for belladonna is **stomach colic associated with peptic ulcer disease**.

The Commission E monograph for belladonna lists the following indications: spasms and colic-like pain in the gastrointestinal and biliary tracts.

Side effects for belladonna include dry mouth, decreased sweat gland secretion, disturbed accommodation, reddened and dry skin, tachycardia, micturition disorders, hallucinations, and convulsions, especially in overdose situations. Belladonna increases the anticholinergic effects of the tricyclic antidepressants amantadine and quinidine.

Caution

Belladonna is contraindicated with tachycardia arrhythmias, benign prostatic hyperplasia (BPH) urine retention, narrow-angle glaucoma, acute pulmonary edema, and mechanical stenosis in the gastrointestinal area.

Preparations

- **Standardized Belladonna Powder**
  (Belladonnae pulvis normatus, according to the German Pharmacopoeia, DAB)
  Total alkaloid content: 0.28–0.32% (in accordance with the German Pharmacopoeia, DAB 10). Maximum daily dose: 0.6 g of the drug is equivalent to 1.8 mg total alkaloids (calculated as hyoscyamine). Single dose: 0.05–0.1 g; maximum single dose: 0.2 g.
- **Extract**
  Total alkaloid content: 1.3–1.45% (in accordance with the German Pharmacopoeia, DAB 10). Maximum daily dose: 0.15 g is equivalent to 2.2 mg total alkaloids (calculated as hyoscyamine).
  Single dose: 0.01 g; maximum single dose: 0.05 g
- **Standardized Belladonna Tincture** (according to the German Pharmacopoeia, DAB)
  Take 5–8 drops diluted in water 3 × a day.
- **Antispastic Tincture** (Tinctura antispastica, according to the German Prescription Formulas, DRF)

Prescriptions

Rx

Tinct. Belladonnae (belladonna tincture)

Tinct. Valerianae (valerian tincture)

Spir. Menth. pip. āā ad 30.0 (spirit of peppermint)

D.S.

Take 8–10 drops diluted in a small amount of water 3 × a day.

Preparations

- **Belladonna–Chamomile Combination**
  Add 5 drops of belladonna tincture to 1 cup of chamomile tea.
- **Belladonna–Lemon Balm Combination**
  Add 5 drops of belladonna tincture to 1 cup of lemon balm tea. This combination benefits from the mildly sedative effect of lemon balm.

▶ **Therapy Recommendations.** Herbal extract preparations of belladonna with a standardized alkaloid content should be used instead of isolated alkaloids. Extracts without a standardized alkaloid content are not safe and should be avoided. The practitioner is tasked with finding the best individual dosage for each patient. Tinctures are especially suitable for this purpose. The dosage must be low enough to prevent undesirable effects, but high enough to achieve the desired therapeutic effect. Prescribing this differentiated and highly active drug requires very precise dosage instructions.

Bibliography

Baas EU, Holtermüller KH, Sinterhauf K, Walter U. Das Verhalten von Gastrin, Renin, Aldosteron und Elektrolyten nach deglycyrrhizi-niertem Succus liquiritiae und Carbenoxolon bei Gesunden [Behavior of gastrin, renin, aldosterone and electrolytes after administration of deglycyrrhizinized liquorice and carbenoxolone in healthy subjects]. Z Gastroenterol. 1976; 14(2):273–276

Bielenberg J. Die Süßholzwurzel. Z Phytother. 1998; 19(4):197–208

Bielenberg J. Isoflavonoide aus der Süßholzwurzel. Ärztez Naturheilverfahren. 2001; 42(10):720–727

Borst JGG, Teuttolt SP, De Vries LA, Molhuysen JA. Synergistic action of liquorice and cortisone in Addison's and Simmonds's disease. Lancet. 1953(264):656–663

Fintelmann V. Phytopharmaka in der Gastroenterologie. Z Phytother. 1994; 15:137–141

Kleist von S, Stopik D, Kleist von D, Hampel KE: Klinische Studie zur Therapie des peptischen Ulkus mit deglycyrrhiziniertem Succus Liquiritiae (Caved-S®) bei bestehender relativer Kontraindikation gegen Carbenoxolon-Natrium. Aktuelle Gastroenterologie. 1978; 7:175–180

List PH, Weil E, Schmid W. Reinsubstanz oder galenische Zubereitung? Versuch einer Klärung am Beispiel des Bellan-Extraktes! Therapiewoche. 1967; 17:2040–2044

Maier K. Ergebnisse bei endoskopisch kontrollierter Therapie des Ulcus ventriculi, Ulcus duodeni und Ulcus pepticum jejuni mit dem Präparat Caved-S®. Aktuelle Gastroenterologie. 1976; 5:183–190

Revers FE. Heeft succus liquiritiae een genezende werking op ce maagzweer? [Question of therapeutic action of licorice juice on gastric ulcer]. Ned Tijdschr Geneeskd. 1946; 90:135–137

Ullmann U, Krausse R, Bielenberg F. Keimhemmende Effekte von Glycyrrhetinsäure gegenüber Helicobacter pylori. Ärztez Naturheilverfahren. 2003; 44:267–274

Wildhirt E. Experience in Germany with glycyrrhizinic acid for the treatment of chronic viral hepatitis. In: Nishioka K, Suzuki H, Mishiro S, Oda T, eds. Viral Hepatitis and Liver Disease. Tokyo: Springer; 1994: 658–661

Questions

1. Do you know a plant medicine that has been proven to have bactericidal effects on *Helicobacter pylori*?
2. Which spasmolytic principle was originally derived from belladonna?

Answers (p. 421) for Chapter 3.2.4

3.3 Gastroenterological Disorders

Some of the most frequently diagnosed gastroenterological disorders include **functional bowel disorders** such as irritable bowel syndrome (IBS), meteorism, diarrhea, and constipation. These conditions are difficult to treat and present a problem even for strictly science-oriented and evidence-based medicine because of the small number of effective synthetic drugs available. This provides yet another opportunity for plant medicines to close a therapeutic gap.

This chapter also discusses the use of phytotherapeutics to treat the **rectal disorders** proctitis and hemorrhoids.

3.3.1 Irritable Bowel Syndrome (IBS)

> ### Medicinal Plants
>
> **German Chamomile, Matricaria recutita**
> German Chamomile flowers, Matricariae flos
> **Fennel, Foeniculum vulgare**
> Fennel seeds (fruit), Foeniculi fructus
> **Caraway, Carum carvi**
> Caraway seeds (fruit), Carvi fructus
> **Peppermint, Mentha piperita**
> Peppermint leaves, Menthae piperitae folium

Irritable bowel syndrome (IBS) is one of the most prevalent bowel disorders. It primarily presents as imbalances in vegetative tonicity in conjunction with emotional lability. Examinations of the abdomen often do not produce any objective findings. Sometimes, the abdomen—especially the upper abdomen—seems distended. Frequently, however, the abdomen is soft and pliable. The most certain pathognomonic sign for IBS is spastic colon, especially of the descending colon. When palpated, the contracted colon rolls across the fingertips like an elastic pipe.

IBS is differentiated into three basic types: IBS with constipation, IBS with diarrhea, and a combination of these two conditions. IBS is found in about 10 to 15% of the population in the Western world. Its causes have not been determined definitively, but some of the causes being discussed are increased sensitivity to visceral stimuli, changes in

central pain processing, and impaired colon mobility, especially with development of spasms.

Treating IBS is complex. Peppermint oil is a key phytotherapeutic remedy that has been shown to be effective in many evidence-based studies. In addition, carminatives and—depending on type—either laxatives or antidiarrheal remedies may be used. Van Rensen provides an excellent update on this topic.

Diagnosing IBS requires a thorough history that encompasses the patient's entire medical condition, including the often variable stages of the disorder and the many and insufficient prior treatment attempts. Even though this condition is benign, it can impact patients profoundly, which presents practitioners with both diagnostic as well as therapeutic challenges. Most patients will present as very anxious and fearful and should be educated in detail about the persistent, but benign, nature, of their disorder to counter their very frequent fears about developing cancer.

One little known and often misdiagnosed special type of IBS is **Proctalgia fugax,** also known as levator ani syndrome. It presents as sudden, very painful spastic conditions in the anal area. However, the pain is located significantly higher than in sphincter spasms associated with hemorrhoids. The pain is usually fairly brief, from a few minutes to a quarter of an hour, but it can occur repeatedly. It frequently develops at night during sleep. The patient's description of this pain is usually sufficient to diagnose this condition. The pain is always associated with anxiety, which indicates psychosomatic factors. However, even if a definitive clinical diagnosis of this condition has been made, a proctoscopy should be done to exclude organic causes such as rectal cancer. Calming or antispasmodic suppositories are not needed because the pain usually subsides before these remedies become effective. Except for this aspect, the treatment of this condition is the same as for IBS.

▶ **Note.** IBS is a pathogenically oriented umbrella term for many conditions formerly referred to as spastic colitis, mucous colitis, intestinal myxoneurosis, chronic enteritis, and chronic colitis. It also encompasses diagnoses such as dyspepsia, dysbacteria, or chronic spastic constipation. Even most cases diagnosed as cholecystopathy and biliary tract dyskinesia are actually persistent spasms of the colon in the right colic flexure area.

Plants for Treatment

German Chamomile (Matricaria recutita)

For more information about this plant, see German Chamomile (p. 42).

see German Chamomile (p. 42).

> **Preparations**
>
> - **Tea**
>   Add 1 cup of hot water to 2–3 teaspoons of the drug. Steep covered for 5–10 minutes, then strain.
>   Drink 1 cup 3–4 × a day as a course of therapy. Chamomile tea therapy needs to be longer term.
> - **German Chamomile Tea with Fennel and Caraway**
>   This carminative tea combining equal parts of German chamomile, fennel, and caraway has been shown to be very effective. Preparation is the same as for chamomile tea above.
>   Drink 1 cup after meals, in the morning, midday, and in the evening.
> - **German Chamomile Tea with Belladonna**
>   Add 5 drops of belladonna tincture to 1 cup of German chamomile tea.
>   This tea is indicated for very painful conditions.

Fennel (Foeniculum vulgare)

For more information about this plant, see Fennel (p. 76).

see Fennel (p. 76).

> **Preparations**
>
> - **Tea**
>   Add 1 cup of hot water to 1 teaspoon of freshly crushed seeds. Steep covered for 5 minutes, then strain.
>   Drink 1 cup several times a day.
> - **German Chamomile Tea with Fennel and Caraway**
>   For preparation, see instructions above.

Caraway (Carum carvi)

For more information about this plant, see Caraway (Carum carvi) (p. 75).

see Caraway (Carum carvi) (p. 75).

> **Preparations**
>
> - **Tea**
>   Add 1 cup of hot water to 1 teaspoon of freshly crushed caraway seeds. Steep covered for 5 minutes, then strain.
>   Drink warm 3 × a day with meals.
> - **German Chamomile Tea with Fennel and Caraway**
>   For preparation, see instructions above.

Peppermint (Mentha piperita)

For more information about this plant, see Peppermint (p. 46).

see Peppermint (p. 46).

The significance of peppermint essential oil and its main active constituent, menthol, has been discussed in a previous section of this book. See Peppermint (Mentha × piperita) (p. 46).

Pure peppermint oil as indicated for the treatment of irritable bowel syndrome (IBS) was established by studies conducted at a university clinic in England (Rees, Somerville): 0–2 mL of peppermint oil was placed in gelatin capsules, which were then coated with a cellulose acetate-phthalate solution to prevent disintegration within the stomach. This preparation provided remarkably fast and sustained improvements even in refractory, treatment-resistant cases.

▶ **Therapy Recommendation.** Rub peppermint oil into the skin of the abdomen in the morning and in the evening.

For references corresponding to the preceding section, see Bibliography following 3.3.2 (p. 81).

3.3.2 Meteorism, Roemheld Syndrome

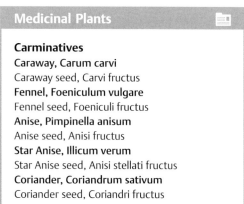

> **Medicinal Plants**
>
> **Carminatives**
> **Caraway, Carum carvi**
> Caraway seed, Carvi fructus
> **Fennel, Foeniculum vulgare**
> Fennel seed, Foeniculi fructus
> **Anise, Pimpinella anisum**
> Anise seed, Anisi fructus
> **Star Anise, Illicum verum**
> Star Anise seed, Anisi stellati fructus
> **Coriander, Coriandrum sativum**
> Coriander seed, Coriandri fructus

Meteorism is one of the most frequent disorders seen in clinical practice. It can be caused by very different underlying disorders with varying degrees of impact. Upper abdominal meteorism is the most prevalent condition. As a rule, the stomach and the intestines are equally involved in the development of this condition. In many cases, the intestines play the leading role, as with intestinal dyspepsia fermentation or isolated chronic enteritis.

The German physician Ludwig Roemheld (1871–1938) described a **gastric cardia symptom complex** now known as Roemheld syndrome. Minor or major meteorism can also frequently be one of the symptoms of arteriosclerosis. The vascular system and the blood supply of abdominal organs play an important role in the development of excessive gas in the upper abdomen (sclerosing mesenteritis). The main cause of meteorism in this condition is not so much the accumulation of gas, for example, as a result of increased fermentation, but primarily the insufficient resorption of gas.

The connection between meteorism and **biliary tract disorders** is as important as the cardiac connection. Stomach distension with bloating, pressure, and belching are characteristic symptoms of latent, masked, or manifest cholecystopathy. In some cases, meteorism can be caused by food allergies. Severe meteorism is also frequently seen in patients with advanced pulmonary emphysema.

Despite its wide range of causes, meteorism requires symptomatic treatment. We need to prescribe treatments that rapidly decrease abdominal bloating and provide at least temporary relief, regardless of the actual disorder that is causing this agonizing condition. Patients experience abdominal bloating as profoundly distressing. Even if they are not in pain, except for the occasional colic, they are extremely uncomfortable, and this seriously impacts their mood, appetite, and sleep. Eliminating meteorism also relieves the strain on the heart and vessels.

Treatment requires causal intervention at a decisive point in the disease process.

In addition to the carminatives described next, many **antidyspetic** remedies are also indicated for this condition.

Plants for Treatment: Carminatives

Simple herbal remedies have always played in important role in the treatment of meteorism. The plants used in those remedies are referred to as carminatives. This name derives from the Latin *carminare*, which means to cleanse. The actions of carminatives are not as strong as those of specific antispasmodics or antibiotics, but they provide proven relief for this disorder, which is primarily functional in nature.

The group of herbal carminatives includes a large number of plants, predominantly those that contain volatile oils and have shown spasmolytic and antimicrobial effects on the muscles of the gastrointestinal tract. **Caraway** (Carum carvi), **fennel** (Foeniculum vulgare), and **anise** (Pimpinella anisum) are primarily carminative; and this is why they are referred to as carminatives. Their fruits (seeds) are very similar, but they differ in potency. In the following, they are presented in order of potency, with caraway exhibiting the highest potency.

The carminatives caraway, fennel, and anise belong to the Umbelliferae family. They represent a notable transition from medicinal plants to spices and occupy a peculiar intermediate position. Their spicy flavor also makes them suitable as food supplements.

Chamomile, peppermint, lemon balm, and angelica also have carminative effects. However, they are primarily important stomach remedies and are discussed in the chapter dealing with gastric disorders (see Chapter 3.2 "Gastric Disorders" (p. 42)).

▶ **Research.** Despite their frequent use, carminatives have been fairly marginalized in scientific literature, with a few exceptions. This may be because pharmacologic research about the effects of carminatives did not seem to make economic sense. Volatile oils are mainly responsible for the action of carminatives, but not all volatile oils are equally carminative. The adsorption rate of charcoal or kaolin clay and their countless variants can be precisely determined and calculated, and they are useful for removing toxic intestinal contents. However, they do not come close to the efficacy of carminative plant medicines for relieving intestinal gas.

An older experimental study by Creamer is worth mentioning in this context. He showed that esophageal reflux and ejection of gas or fluids from the stomach occurs within 5 to 15 minutes following the administration of a carminative. This effect persists for about 5 minutes. Gastroscopic studies have shown that the stomach mucosa exhibits increased reddening and its folds become more prominent following the administration of a carminative. This leads to hyperemia of the stomach mucosa caused by the axon reflex. According to Creamer, the main effects of carminatives on the stomach are based on stimulation of the muscularis mucosae and of the mucosa, which increases their tonus. This also explains why carminatives are not effective if the mucosa is seriously atrophied and no longer presents a point of application, for example, in cases of chronic atrophic gastritis.

Glatzel showed the strong physiological effects of spices in numerous studies. They stimulate digestive secretion that in turn stimulates intestinal peristalsis and even blood pressure and heart function. The addition of capsicum spices (paprika, chili) to rice stimulates adrenal gland activity and corticosteroid production. Similar effects have been demonstrated for mustard. Foods seasoned with mustard, especially those high in fat, such as sausages, are digested more quickly and more thoroughly. In addition, mustard accelerates stomach emptying and intestinal passage. Bitters such as gentian and wormwood have similar beneficial effects.

Caraway (Carum carvi)

Caraway is an umbelliferous plant in the Apeaceae family, with white or reddish flowers that are small and inconspicuous. As with many umbelliferous plants, its leaves are bipinnate (▶ Fig. 3.15). One characteristic makes caraway easy to recognize and differentiate from other members of the Apeaceae family: the lower pair of bipinnate leaves of each leaf is far apart from the next pair and attached crosswise to the stalk. These lower pairs of leaves appear to be stipels.

Caraway is one of the most frequent plants found growing in the wild in Germany. It grows along the edges of paths, in ditches along rural roads, and in meadows. Caraway plant medicine is derived almost exclusively from cultivated plants, not from wild caraway.

Caraway is one of our most reliable and strongest carminatives and it is very well tolerated. It has no known undesirable effects.

Medicinal applications use the **caraway seeds** (fruit, Carvi fructus).

▶ **Note.** Caraway is an important spice that is highly valued because of its carminative effects.

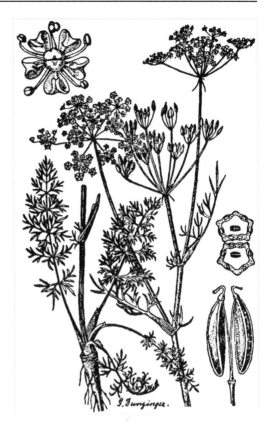

Fig. 3.15 Caraway, Carum carvi.

This is the reason caraway is primarily added to foods that cause flatulence, especially cabbage dishes.

The fruit (seed) of the dill plant (Anethum graveolens) tastes similar to caraway. Only the green parts of the dill plant are generally used in cooking. Dill seeds are also carminative, but less potent than caraway. Dill seeds are primarily used as a spice.

▶ **Pharmacology.** Caraway seeds contain a minimum of 3% volatile oil (Carvi aetheroleum) and also fatty oil. Caraway oil contains 50–65% d-carvone.

▶ **Indications.** The Commission E monograph for caraway seeds and caraway oil lists the following indications: dyspeptic problems such as mild gastrointestinal tract spasms, bloating, and fullness. Its main indication is meteorism.

Preparations

- **Tea**
  Add 1 cup of hot water to 1 teaspoon of freshly crushed caraway seeds. Steep covered for 5 minutes, then strain.
  Drink warm 3 × a day with meals.
- **Caraway Essential Oil**
  Add 2–3 drops to a small amount of water and drink with meals.

▶ **Therapy Recommendations.** In cases of severe and painful abdominal bloating, an emulsion of 10% caraway oil and 90% carrier oil (for example, olive oil) can be rubbed into the skin of the abdomen in a circular pattern. The navel should be omitted.

Caraway oil volatilizes easily and needs to be stored in a well-sealed container at all times.

Fennel (Foeniculum vulgare)

Fennel is an umbelliferous plant, like caraway, but it looks very different. It can grow up to 1–2 m in height. Its leaves are very finely articulated and very long and its flowers are yellow (▶ Fig. 3.16).

Fennel originates from southern Europe and is cultivated in some areas of Germany. It can occasionally be found in the wild, but it is not naturalized there. It has naturalized in many areas of North, Central, and South America and around the Pacific. There are a number of subspecies and varieties of fennel being cultivated. In the Mediterranean and Balkan regions and in California, fennel is cultivated as an agricultural field crop.

Fennel is not as strong a carminative as caraway. However, its special flavor is advantageous. It is used as an excellent flavor corrigent for carminative tea blends and its own carminative action supports the effect of tea blends.

Medicinal applications use the **fennel seeds** (fruit, Foeniculi fructus).

▶ **Pharmacology.** Fennel seeds contain a minimum of 4% volatile oil, including anethole and fenchone, and fatty oil. Fennel essential oil (Oleum Foeniculi or Foeniculi aetheroleum) is a colorless to pale yellow liquid.

▶ **Indications.** Fennel tea is especially recommended for dyspepsia and diarrhea in infants. During an initial fasting period, the infant is given only

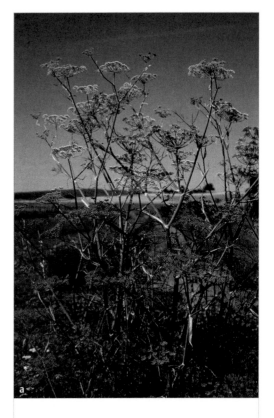
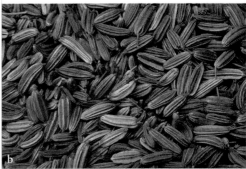

Fig. 3.16 a and b Fennel, Foeniculum vulgare. Photos: Dr. Roland Spohn, Engen.

fennel tea. This provides hydration and the carminative effects of the tea reduce **meteorism** and **intestinal spasms**.

The Commission E monograph for fennel lists the same indications as for caraway (p. 73): dyspeptic problems such as mild gastrointestinal tract spasms, bloating, and fullness. Its main indication is meteorism.

Preparations

- **Tea**
  Add 1 cup of hot water to 1 teaspoon of freshly crushed fennel seeds. Steep covered for 5 minutes, then strain.
  Drink 1–2 cups several times a day.
- **Fennel Essential Oil**
  Add 2–4 drops to a small amount of water. Several times a day.

Anise (Pimpinella anisum)

Anise is an umbelliferous plant in the Apeaceae family, like caraway and fennel. The plant grows to about 0.5 m in height and has a pungent odor and small, white flowers. Its lower leaves are undivided and heart shaped to round, and its upper leaves are frequently trifid. Anise originates from the Middle East and Asia. It is cultivated in some areas of Germany and has naturalized in some areas of North America.

Medicinal applications use the **anise seeds** (fruit, Anisi fructus).

▶ **Pharmacology.** Anise seeds contain a minimum of 2% volatile oil and fatty oil. The main constituent of the volatile is trans-anethole.

▶ **Indications.** Anise is a fairly effective carminative and an even better flavor corrigent. Its carminative action is much weaker than caraway and fennel.

The Commission E monograph for anise seeds lists the following indications: dyspeptic complaints (internal use only) and catarrhs of the respiratory tract (internal and external use).

Preparations

- **Tea**
  Add 1 cup of boiling water to 1 heaping teaspoon of the crushed or coarsely powdered drug. Steep covered for 10–15 minutes, then strain.
  Drink 1 cup several times a day.
- **Anise Essential Oil**
  Add 3 drops to 1 cube of sugar.
  Let dissolve in month; repeat several times a day.

Other Carminatives

Star Anise (Illicum verum)

Despite the similarity in name, star anise, compared to anise, is a very different plant botanically. Star anise is an evergreen tree that grows in East Asia and belongs to the Schisandraceae family.

Medicinal applications use the **star anise fruit** (Anisi stellati fructus).

▶ **Pharmacology.** Star anise fruit contain 5–6% volatile oil, fatty oil, and tannins. Its action is largely identical to that of anise seeds (Pimpinella anisum); star anise does not offer any particular advantages.

Preparation

- **Star Anise Essential Oil**
  Add 3 drops to 1 cube of sugar.
  Let dissolve in month; repeat several times a day.

Coriander (Coriandrum sativum)

Coriander is commonly used in herbal medicine prescriptions. This small and delicate plant is also in the Umbelifferae/Apiaceae family and originates from southeast Europe.

Coriander fruit (seeds), **Coriandri fructus**, are larger than caraway fruit (seeds) and are spherical (▶ Fig. 3.17), which makes it easy to differentiate them. Coriander seeds have a weak carminative effect. Their predominant use is as a spice and as a flavor corrigent in tea blends.

Preparation

- **Tea**
  Add 1 cup of boiling water to 2 teaspoons of the crushed drug. Steep covered for 10 minutes, then strain.
  Drink 1 cup several times a day between meals.

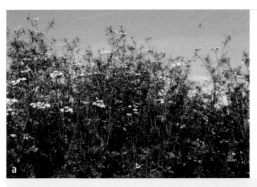
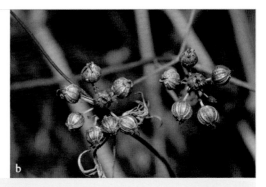

Fig. 3.17 **a and b** Coriander (cilantro), Coriandrum sativum. Photos: Dr. Roland Spohn, Engen.

Proven Prescriptions: Carminative Teas

- **Anise-Fennel-Coriander Tea**
  This blend of equal parts of anise, fennel, and coriander is very effective.
  The seeds are prescribed "contused," which in this context means crushed or ground. This allows the water to permeate the seeds and to extract their active constituents. Crushed seeds do not stay fresh as long as whole seeds and lose a portion of their volatile oil over time. This tea blend can be stored for several weeks.
  Since this tea contains volatile oil, it should not be boiled, but instead infused with boiling water.

Prescriptions

Rx
Carvi fruct. cont. (crushed caraway seeds)
Foeniculi fruct. cont. (crushed fennel seeds)
Anisi fruct. cont. āā 20.0 (crushed anise seeds)
M. f. spec.
Add 1 cup of boiling water to 1 teaspoon of the tea blend. Steep covered for 20 minutes, then strain.
D.S.
Drink 1 cup warm after each meal.

- **Combination with Spasmolytic and Sedative Medicinal Plants**
  Adding additional plants, especially those listed for acute gastritis (see Section 3.2.1 "Acute Gastritis" (p. 42)), is often helpful because of their additional spasmolytic and sedative effects:

Prescriptions

Rx
Carvi fruct. (caraway seeds)
Foeniculi fruct. āā 20.0 (fennel seeds)
Menth. pip. fol. (peppermint leaves)
Melissae fol. āā 30.0 (lemon balm leaves)
M.f. spec.
Add 1 cup of boiling water to 1 teaspoon of the tea blend. Steep covered for 15 minutes, then strain.
D.S.
Drink 1 cup warm several times a day.

Prescriptions

Rx
Carvi fruct. (caraway seeds)
Foeniculi fruct. āā 20.0 (fennel seeds)
Matricariae flos ad 100.0 (German chamomile flowers)
M.f. spec.
Add 1 cup of boiling water to 1 teaspoon of the tea blend. Steep covered for 15 minutes, then strain.
D.S.
Drink 1 cup several times a day.

- **"Four Winds Tea"**
  The following prescription is very effective. Its name derives from the four constituents used in the tea blend.

Rx
Carvi fruct. (caraway seeds)
Foeniculi fruct. (fennel seeds)
Menth. pip. fol. (peppermint leaves)
Matricariae flos āā ad 100.0 (German chamomile flowers)
M. f. spec.
Add 1 cup of boiling water to 1–2 teaspoons of the tea blend. Steep covered for 10 minutes, then strain.
D.S.
Drink warm in small sips.

- **Combination with Bitters or Cholagogues for Meteorism with Severe Dyspeptic Symptoms**

Rx
Carvi fruct. (caraway seeds)
Foeniculi fruct. (fennel seed)
Absinthii herb. (wormwood herb)
Millefolii herb. āā ad 100.0 (yarrow herb)
M. f. spec.
Add 1 cup of boiling water to 1 teaspoon of the tea blend. Steep covered for 15 minutes, then strain.
D.S.
Drink 1 cup warm before each meal.

- **Combination with Laxatives for Meteorism with Gastric Cardia Symptom Complex (Roehmheld syndrome) and Insufficient Fecal Evacuation**

Rx
Carvi fruct. (caraway seeds)
Foeniculi fruct. āā 20.0 (fennel seeds)
Menth. pip. fol. (peppermint leaves)
Sennae fol. āā 30.0 (senna leaves)
M. f. spec.
Add 1 cup of boiling water to 1–2 teaspoons of the tea blend. Steep covered for 20 minutes, then strain.
D.S.
Drink 1 cup in the morning and in the evening.

Carminative Tinctures

Carminative tincture blends usually combine essential oils with additional tinctures. Caraway essential oil (Oleum Carvi) is the most effective herbal carminative. It is helpful to add a tincture that contains some ether, for example, valerian essential oil tincture or ether spirit, as a solvent to improve extraction and absorption of the essential oil.

- **Carminative Tincture (Tinct. carminativ.)**
  Tinctura carminativa is a blend of 16 parts zedoary rhizome (Curcuma zedoaria),
  8 parts calamus rhizome (Acorus calamus),
  8 parts galangal rhizome (Alpinia galanga),
  4 parts caraway seeds (Carum carvi), 4 parts anise seeds (Pimpinella anisum), 4 parts Roman chamomile flowers (Chamaemelum nobile), 2 parts laurel leaves (Laurus nobilis), 2 parts cloves (Syzgium aromaticum), 2 parts mace (Myristica fragrans), 1 part bitter orange peel (Citrus × aurantium) and 100 parts each of peppermint (Mentha × piperita) hydrosol and grape alcohol (spirit of wine).
  In addition to carminatives, this blend contains many spices and aromatic flavors. Its carminative action is weak and likely not sufficient on its own. However, it is well suited as an adjuvant to tincture blends.

- **Potent Carminative Tincture**

Rx
Ol. Carvi 5.0 (caraway essential oil)
Tinct. carminativ. (see Carminative Tinctures (p. 79))
Tinct. Valerian. aeth. āā 20.0 (ethereal valerian tincture)
D.S.
Add 20 drops to a small amount of water and take after meals, 3 × a day.

- **"Caraway Drops"** (according to the German Prescription Formulas, DRF)

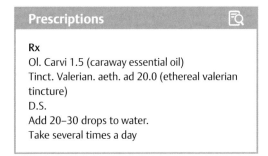

Prescriptions

Rx
Tinct. carvi. comp. ("caraway drops," according to the German Prescription Formulas, DRF) 20.0
D.S.
Add 20–30 drops to water.
Take 3 × a day.

- **Combination with Valerian**

Prescriptions

Rx
Ol. Carvi 1.5 (caraway essential oil)
Tinct. Valerian. aeth. ad 20.0 (ethereal valerian tincture)
D.S.
Add 20–30 drops to water.
Take several times a day

- **Even More Potent Blend**

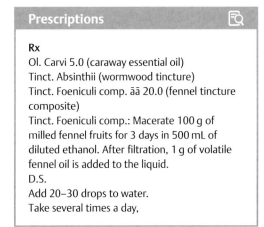

Prescriptions

Rx
Ol. Carvi 5.0 (caraway essential oil)
Tinct. Absinthii (wormwood tincture)
Tinct. Foeniculi comp. āā 20.0 (fennel tincture composite)
Tinct. Foeniculi comp.: Macerate 100 g of milled fennel fruits for 3 days in 500 mL of diluted ethanol. After filtration, 1 g of volatile fennel oil is added to the liquid.
D.S.
Add 20–30 drops to water.
Take several times a day,

- **Combinations with Cardiac and Vascular Remedies**
  For conditions involving significant cardiac symptoms, carminatives can be combined with cardiovascular remedies.
  The following combination has been shown to be helpful for the gastric cardia symptom complex (Roemheld syndrome):

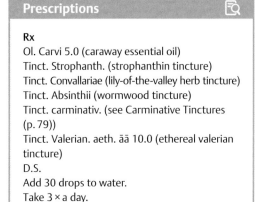

Prescriptions

Rx
Ol. Carvi 5.0 (caraway essential oil)
Tinct. Strophanth. (strophanthin tincture)
Tinct. Convallariae (lily-of-the-valley herb tincture)
Tinct. Absinthii (wormwood tincture)
Tinct. carminativ. (see Carminative Tinctures (p. 79))
Tinct. Valerian. aeth. āā 10.0 (ethereal valerian tincture)
D.S.
Add 30 drops to water.
Take 3 × a day.

- **"Caraway Drops" and Belladonna for Spastic Symptoms**

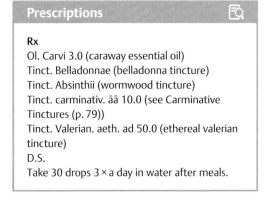

Prescriptions

Rx
Ol. Carvi 3.0 (caraway essential oil)
Tinct. Belladonnae (belladonna tincture)
Tinct. Absinthii (wormwood tincture)
Tinct. carminativ. āā 10.0 (see Carminative Tinctures (p. 79))
Tinct. Valerian. aeth. ad 50.0 (ethereal valerian tincture)
D.S.
Take 30 drops 3 × a day in water after meals.

▶ **Therapy Recommendations.** For patients who are uncomfortable with the high caraway content of these prescriptions, the amount of caraway should be reduced.

It is also important to consider the quality of caraway essential oils. Very fresh caraway oil will have a much more pronounced caraway odor and taste than older caraway oil.

Carminative Hydrosols

- **Carminative Hydrosol** (Aquae Carminativae, see Carminative Tinctures (p. 79))
Take 1 tablespoon 3–4×a day after or between meals. This excellent remedy tends to be undeservedly underutilized. It is a pleasant tasting, colorless liquid distilled from German chamomile, Roman chamomile, fennel, caraway, coriander, and bitter orange peel (Citrus × aurantium).
- **Combinations**
Carminative hydrosol is an excellent combination for mixtures, infusions, and decoctions, see example below.

Prescriptions

Rx
Tinct. Belladonnae 2.0 (belladonna tincture)
Aqu. carminativ. (see Carminative Tinctures (p. 79))
Aqu. Chamomillae āā ad 100.0 (chamomile hydrosol)
D.S.
Take 1 tablespoon 3 × a day

Fennel hydrosol, peppermint hydrosol, or valerian hydrosol may be substituted for Aqu. Chamomillae. For special indications, parsley hydrosol, sage hydrosol, or Aqu. Tiliae may be added.

- **Aqua Tiliae**
100 g dried flowers (or better, 500 g fresh flowers) of the linden tree (Tilia platyphyllos or Tilia cordata) are powdered, filled into a small sack, and distilled via steam distillation until 1 L of liquid has been recondensed.

Bibliography

Creamer B. Oesophageal reflux and the action of carminatives. Lancet. 1955; 268(6864):590–592

Dew MJ, Evans BK, Rhodes J. Peppermint oil for the irritable bowel syndrome: a multicentre trial. Br J Clin Pract. 1984; 38(11–12): 394–398, 398

Dieterich E. Neues Pharmazeutisches Manual. 8th ed. Berlin: Verlag von Julius Springer; 1901:32

Frerichs G, Arends G, Zörnig H. Hagers Handbuch der Pharmazeutischen Praxis. Vol. 1, 2nd ed. Berlin: Verlag von Julius Springer; 1938:1306

Glatzel H. Gewuerze und Organfunktionen, Ergebnisse neuerer Untersuchungen. MMW Munch Med Wochenschr. 1965; 107 (7):332–342

Rees WDW, Evans BK, Rhodes J. Treating irritable bowel syndrome with peppermint oil. BMJ. 1979; 2(6194):835–836

Rensen van I. Pfefferminzöl beim Reizdarmsyndrom – ein Update. Z Phytother. 2009; 30:129–134

Somerville KW, Richmond CR, Bell GD. Delayed release peppermint oil capsules (Colpermin) for the spastic colon syndrome: a pharmacokinetic study. Br J Clin Pharmacol. 1984; 18(4):638–640

Wagner H, Wiesenauer M. Phytotherapie: Phytopharmaka und pflanzliche Homöopathika. 2nd ed. Stuttgart: Wissen-schaftliche Verlagsgesellschaft; 2003

Weiss RF. Phytotherapie der Magenleiden. Ärztez Naturheilverfahren. 1982; 23(3):149–154

Wildgrube HJ. Untersuchung zur Wirksamkeit von Pfefferminzöl auf Beschwerdebild und funktionelle Parameter bei Patienten mit Reizdarm-Syndrom (Studie). Naturheilpraxis. 1988; 5:2–5

Zoch E. Über die Inhaltsstoffe des Handelspapains [Contents of commercial papain]. Arzneimittelforschung. 1969; 19(9):1593–1597

3.3.3 Inflammatory Bowel Disease (IBD)

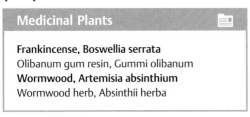

Medicinal Plants

Frankincense, Boswellia serrata
Olibanum gum resin, Gummi olibanum
Wormwood, Artemisia absinthium
Wormwood herb, Absinthii herba

In general, inflammatory bowel disease (IBD) and its symptoms are not considered to be within the treatment scope of phytopharmaceuticals. The unambiguous and clearly defined standard treatment for this disorder has been glucocorticoids and mesalazine. However, this therapy is primarily symptomatic and antiphlogistic and cannot be considered a truly satisfactory approach. Finding alternative treatments for this disorder must be of great interest, especially if these alternatives are well tolerated in long-term treatment.

Meanwhile, many IBS patients are reporting about their own experience with the complementary use of phytopharmaceuticals. Well-documented research results are now available for frankincense, wormwood, and a combination remedy that contains myrrh, chamomile, and coffee charcoal. These are important plant medicines for adjuvant therapy or secondary prevention. Langhorst has compiled a good overview on this topic.

Plants for Treatment

Frankincense (Boswellia serrata)

The resin obtained from the Indian **frankincense** tree (Boswellia serrata) has long been highly valued in Ayurvedic medicine. The Commission E has not compiled a monograph on frankincense because this medicinal plant has not traditionally been used in German phytotherapy.

▶ **Pharmacology.** Frankincense, also known as olibanum gum resin (Gummi olibanum), contains several boswellic acids plus 4–8% volatile oil with monoterpenes. The boswellic acids directly impact inflammation by specifically inhibiting 5-Llipoxygenase. However, they do not impact cyclooxygenase. Experimental studies have also shown analgesic, immunosuppressive, and antimicrobial effects for frankincense.

▶ **Indications.** Ayurvedic medicine uses frankincense as adjuvant therapy for **polyarthritis** and for **remission therapy during acute inflammatory episodes** of ulcerative colitis and Crohn's disease.

The recommended daily dose is 400 to 1200 mg of a standardized dried frankincense extract (Olibanum extractum siccum).

▶ **Research.** A randomized, double-blind parallel group comparison study tested a boswellia extract (H 15) for efficacy and safety compared to mesalazine in patients with active Crohn's disease. The daily dosage given was 3.6 g H 15 or 4.5 g mesalazine. Treatment efficacy was assessed using the Crohn's Disease Activity Index (CDAI). The extract H 15 reduced the CDAI by 80 or 90 points and mezalazine by 62 or 53 points. This provided statistical proof for the noninferiority of H 15. Patients given H 15 showed significantly higher rates of clinical improvement than patients given mesalazine, but this difference was not statistically significant ($p = 0.061$); 16 of 44 patients given H 15 achieved complete remission (36.4%), compared to 12 of 39 patients given mesalazine (30.8%). Tolerability of H 15 was higher than that of mesalazine.

Gerhardt et al. state several times that the results of this study show the noninferiority of boswellia serrata extract (H 15) compared with standard mesalazine therapy. Ammon presents a more recent overview of boswellia.

▶ **Therapy Recommendation.** Boswellia therapy for this indication should only use a standardized, finished pharmaceutical boswellia product in a sufficient dosage.

Wormwood (Artemisia absinthium)

For more information about this plant, see Wormwood (p. 111).

▶ **Indications.** Research has shown antiviral effects for wormwood in Crohn's disease. However, the results of the following, evidence-based study should not be overrated. They do present an interesting perspective for developing new options to treat this serious, eminently chronic intestinal disorder.

▶ **Research.** A randomized, double-blind, placebo-controlled trial tested the impact of a powdered wormwood drug on the activity of Crohn's disease and if it would allow for a reduction of conventional antiphlogistic drugs. The impetus for this study was information about the **antiviral effects** of wormwood especially on DNA viruses.

Forty adult patients on standard therapy received 3 × 2 capsules a day of a standardized, powdered wormwood drug, or a placebo, in addition to their standard therapy. The patients' dosage of 5-aminosalicylates, azathioprine, and methotrexate was to remain constant, while the dosage of prednisone was to be tapered from 40 mg a day to 0 mg. After week 11, prednisone treatment could be resumed if needed. All scores that documented the activity of the disease showed the superiority of wormwood compared to placebo at all control points of the study ($p < 0.01$). Only 2 of the patients in the wormwood group, but 16 patients in the placebo group, needed to resume prednisone after 10 weeks (Omer et al.).

Combination of Myrrh, Chamomile, and Coffee Charcoal

A traditional, fixed-combination drug that contains 100 mg myrrh, 70 mg dry extract of chamomile flowers (4–6:1), and 50 mg coffee charcoal is approved for "supporting gastrointestinal function." The antiphlogistic effects of myrrh and chamomile and the absorptive effect of coffee charcoal seemed to indicate that this fixed combination drug may also be suitable for treating chronic inflammatory bowel disorders, especially ulcerative colitis. Langhorst et al. tested this combination in comparison with mesalazine in a randomized, prospective double-blind, double-dummy study to assess its potential for maintaining remission in ulcerative colitis. The results of the study showed equal efficacy for both parameters and noninferiority of the phytopharmaceutical remedy. There were no significant differences in recidivism rates, onset of recidivism, inflammation activity, and tolerability. This showed this fixed combination drug to be a potential alternative to the standard therapy for Crohn's disease.

Bibliography

Ammon HPT. Indian Boswellia oder die Renaissance des Olibanums in der westlichen Welt. Z Phytother. 2013; 34(2):70–73

Gerhardt H, Seifert F, Buvari P, Vogelsang H, Repges R. Therapie des aktiven Morbus Crohn mit dem Boswellia-serrata-Extrakt H 15. Z Phytother. 2001; 22:69–75

Langhorst J, Varnhagen I, Schneider SB, et al. Randomised clinical trial: a herbal preparation of myrrh, chamomile and coffee charcoal compared with mesalazine in maintaining remission in ulcerative colitis—a double-blind, double-dummy study. Aliment Pharmacol Ther. 2013; 38(5):490–500

Langhorst J. Phytotherapie bei chronisch-entzündlichen Darmerkrankungen. Z Phytother. 2013; 34:274–278

Omer B, Krebs S, Omer H, Noor TO. Steroid-sparing effect of wormwood (Artemisia absinthium) in Crohn's disease: a double-blind placebo-controlled study. Phytomedicine. 2007; 14(2–3):87–95

3.3.4 Diarrhea

Medicinal Plants

Tormentil, Potentilla tormentilla
Tormentil root, Tormentillae rhizoma
Bilberry, Vaccinium myrtillus
Bilberry fruit, Myrtilli fructus
Blackberry, Rubus fruticosus
Blackberry leaves, Rubi fruticosi folium
Common Oak (Quercus robur), Sessile Oak
(Quercus petraea)
Oak bark, Quercus cortex
Uzara, Xysmalobium undulatum
Uzara root, Xysmalobii rhizoma
Poppy, Papaver somniferum
Opium tincture, Tinctura Opii

Diarrhea is a symptom of many different disorders. It is the guiding symptom of bacterial or viral infectious diseases, including **summer diarrhea**, which is frequently caused, for example, by salmonella, shigella, or yersinia. Diarrhea is also a symptom of **allergic enteropathy**, an intestinal condition that could be called "hay fever of the small intestine," and that is not easy to diagnose. It causes food to pass through extremely quickly, which typically looks like "snow showers" on X-rays of the small intestine. Its macroscopic presentation during endoscopy is severely swollen mucosa; histolog shows high eosinophil counts. Often, this condition is diagnosed *ex juvantibus* based on knowledge about a general allergic predisposition.

Functional intestinal disorders with hypermotility and hypersecretion, especially in the small intestine, is a third main cause of diarrhea. Diarrhea as a symptom of ulcerative colitis should also be mentioned to complete the picture. It is important to remember that diarrhea may be a concomitant symptom of other organic disorders, for example, hyperthyroidism. Diarrhea is also a typical symptom of chronic alcohol abuse.

Only a few of the abovementioned causes for diarrhea can be effectively treated. However, herbal antidiarrheals can provide symptomatic treatment. The two primary remedies are both medicinal plants with predominantly tannic actions: **tormentil** (Potentilla tormentilla) and **bilberry** (Vaccinium myrtillus).

Severe bacterial enterocolitis should be treated with **antibiotics** or antibacterial chemotherapeutics.

▶ **Note.** Salmonellosis, a common infection, is only treated with antibiotics if the condition becomes septic. It has been shown that the use of antibiotics as a standard treatment is not advantageous because it does not shorten the course of the disease and frequently creates chronic carrier patients. No antivirals can be recommended for viral enteritis.

Diarrhea associated with hyperthyroidism or ulcerative colitis requires treatment of the underlying disorder. However, a symptomatic costive agent is usually required. For a long time, opium tincture (Tinctura Opii normata Ph.Eur.) was used to treat these conditions, but today, the synthetic drug loperamide hydrochloride is the remedy of choice. The disadvantage of opium tincture is that it requires a specific type of prescription (see US Uniform Controlled Substances Act, for example), but loperamide also has some restrictions for its use. It should not be used for conditions where inhibition of peristalsis needs to be avoided. It is not suitable as a monotherapeutic in acute dysentery. Severe liver disorders inhibit the metabolization of loperamide and may negatively impact plasma electrolyte balance.

Plants for Treatment

Tormentil (Potentilla tormentilla, Potentilla erecta)

Tormentil is a small and inconspicuous member of the rose family (Rosacea). Its thick rootstock grows a number of basal leaves that have three to five lobes and several leafed stalks that bear numerous yellow flowers. A distinct characteristic of tormentil is that its flower corolla features only four leaves (▶ Fig. 3.18). This rare floral trait differentiates tormentil from other Potentilla species. Cutting the rootstock reveals its red interior.

In Germany, tormentil is widespread and found in lowland forests and in moors and mountainous areas. These two habitats are very different: wet hill moors and boggy mountain forests on the one hand, and arid pine forests and heaths with poor, sandy soil on the other hand. In boggy regions, tormentil grows smaller and more stout, with numerous stalks arising from one rootstock and small flowers. In arid pine forests, tormentil grows larger, and its rootstock grows fewer stalks with larger leaves and flowers.

In both habitats, tormentil can absorb only a small amount of water. Even in a boggy area, the plant cannot absorb a lot of water because the water is acidic and not well tolerated by the plant

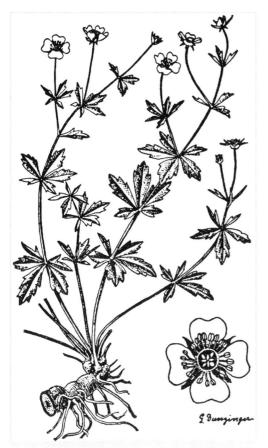

Fig. 3.18 Tormentil, Potentilla tormentilla (Potentilla erecta).

in large amounts. The German botanist A.F.W. Schimper (1856–1901) called this condition "physiologic dryness."

Medicinal applications use only the **tormentil rootstock** (Tormentillae rhizoma).

▶ **Pharmacology.** In Germany, tormentil is the most important and most productive tannin-bearing herb. Its tannin content is 15–20% (Latté).

▶ **Note.** Rhatany root (Ratanhia) only contains 10% tannins, and other imported tannin-bearing plant medicines such as catechu contain even less tannin.

▶ **Indications.** Its high tannin content makes tormentil rootstock an astringent. Tormentil root is suitable for treating all cases of diarrhea that are not an indication for antibiotic or chemotherapeutic treatment. This includes **acute and subacute enteritis** and **enterocolitis**, **summer diarrhea**, and, with some limitations, diarrhea with functional causes. The best results are achieved with acute and subacute enteritis and colitis.

Astringents are less effective with persistent, chronic colitis, but plant medicines that contain tannins can also be helpful in certain phases of this disorder.

The Commission E monograph for tormentil root lists the following indications: unspecified diarrhea disorders and mild mucous membrane inflammations of the mouth and pharynx.

Preparations

- **Tea**
  Add 1 teaspoon of the chopped drug to 1 cup of cold water. Bring to a brief simmer and strain immediately.
  Drink 1 cup 3 × a day.
- **Tincture**
  Take 10–30 drops in a shot glass of water several times a day, or—with acute symptoms—every hour.

Tormentil tincture is easily combined with other tinctures to create individualized remedies.

- **Simple Costive Drops for Diarrhea**

Prescriptions

Rx
Tinct. Tormentillae (tormentil tincture)
Tinct. carminativ. āā 25.0 (see Carminative Tinctures (p. 79))
D.S.
Add 30–40 drops to warm chamomile tea.
Drink 3–5 × a day.

- For Diarrhea with Spasms and Colic

Rx
Tinct. Tormentillae 30.0 (tormentil tincture)
Tinct. Belladonnae 5.0 (belladonna tincture)
Tinct. carminativ. ad 50.0 (see Carminative Tintures (p. 79))
D.S.
Add 30 drops to a small amount of water.
Drink 3 × a day.

- For Torpid Gastroenteritis

Rx
Tinct. Tormentillae 30.0 (tormentil tincture)
Tinct. Absinthii (wormwood tincture)
Tinct. Gentianae āā 10.0 (gentian tincture)
D.S.
Add 30 drops to a small amount of water.
Drink 3 × a day.

Bilberry (European Blueberry, Huckleberry) (Vaccinium myrtillus)

In Germany, bilberry (▶ Fig. 3.19) grows everywhere in forests and moors. Both its leaves (**Myrtilli folium**) and its berries (**Myrtilli fructus**) are used medicinally.

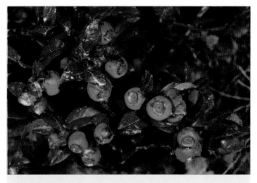

Fig. 3.19 Bilberry, Vaccinium myrtillus. Photo: Dr. Roland Spohn, Engen.

▶ **Pharmacology.** Only the berries are used as an antidiarrheal. They contain 7% tannins, plus anthocyans and flavone glycosides. The main action results from their tannin content.

▶ **Indications.** Dried bilberries are a reliable antidiarrheal. Bilberry teas or concentrated aqueous decoctions provide three healing modalities: astringent, antiseptic, and adsorptive.

These remedies result in stools becoming acidic, and stool odor changing from unpleasant to aromatic.

Dried bilberry fruit are also a reliable remedy for mild summer diarrhea and other kinds of nonspecific diarrhea.

Fresh bilberries eaten in large amounts in late summer have laxative effects and are contraindicated for diarrhea.

In some areas, dried bilberries are chewed as a remedy for diarrhea. This therapy is also effective, but it introduces the coarser cellulose parts of the berries (peels, seeds) into the intestines. This can cause irritations of sensitive gastric mucosa.

- **Tea**
  Add 3 tablespoons of the drug to 500 mL of water. Boil for 10 minutes, covered, then strain.
  Drink one glass, warm, several times a day.
- **Decoction**
  Add 2–3 tablespoons of dried bilberries to 500 mL of water. Bring to a boil and boil for 30 minutes, covered, then strain.
  Take 1 tablespoon several times a day.

Blackberry (Rubus fruticosus)

Medicinal applications use the **blackberry leaves harvested and dried while the plant is flowering** (Rubi fructicosi folium). Their tannin content makes them a plausible astringent for mucous membranes. However, their therapeutic efficacy is far less than that of the classic tannin medicinals tormentil and bilberry.

▶ **Indications.** Blackberry leaves are primarily indicated for mild, nonspecific, **acute diarrhea**, such as travel or summer diarrhea.

Preparation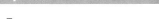

- **Tea**
  Add 1 cup of boiling water to 1 heaping teaspoon of the finely cut drug. Steep covered for 10–15 minutes, then strain. Drink 1 cup several times a day between meals.

Common Oak (Quercus robur), Sessile Oak (Quercus petraea)

For more information about this plant, see Oak (p. 287).
　　Medicinal applications use the **oak bark** (Quercus cortex). The bark of young twigs and young growths from the stump are collected and dried in the spring.

▶ **Pharmacology.** Oak bark contains tannins and flavonoids (for example, quercetin) and combines the astringent effects of tannins with the antiphlogistic effects of flavonols.

Preparation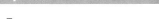

- **Tea**
  Add ½ teaspoon of the finely cut or coarsely powdered drug to 1 cup of cold water. Bring to a brief boil, steep covered for 5 minutes, then strain.
  Drink 1 cup warm several times a day 30 minutes before meals.

Uzara (Xysmalobium undulatum)

Uzara (Xysmalobium undulatum) is a member of the subfamily of Asclepiadoideae. Its native habitat is South Africa. Medicinal applications use the dried subterranean parts of 2- to 3-year-old uzara plants, the **uzara root** (Uzarae radix). Traditional healers of the Xhosa people use this root to prepare a remedy

called "Uzara," which is primarily used for digestive disorders. The European plant name and its indication are derived from this remedy.

▶ **Pharmacology.** Uzara root contains glycosides with a cardenolide structure.

Caution

Uzara root inhibits small intestine motility and, in high doses, is thought to be similar in its effects to digitalis. For this reason, uzara root should not be used concurrently with cardioactive glycosides.

Poppy (Papaver somniferum)

Poppy's (▶ Fig. 3.20) native habitat is the Middle East, but it can also be cultivated in central Europe. Its labor-intensive cultivation would require substandard wage labor for it to be profitable in an legitimate commercial context. Each seed capsule of the plant needs to be tended by hand to cut the capsule and collect the raw, milky juice (raw opium).
　　Poppy (p. 355) supplies opium, which is the most effective and most well-known costive. It is derived from the dried milky juice harvested from unripe poppy seed capsules. Its main alkaloid is morphine.

▶ **Indications.** Opium's pure alkaloids are not needed for treating diarrhea. Its costive and anticolic effects are most pronounced in whole extracts. However, the tincture referred to as opium drops (Tinctura Opii normata Ph.Eur.) is the most effective remedy for **severe acute diarrhea with spastic pain**.

Preparations

- **Tincture** (according to the German Pharmacopoeia, DAB 10)
  This tincture contains a minimum of 1% morphine.
  A single dose consisting of 5–10 drops is equivalent to 1–2 mg morphine. The daily maximum dose is 5.0 g and is equivalent to 50–60 mg morphine.

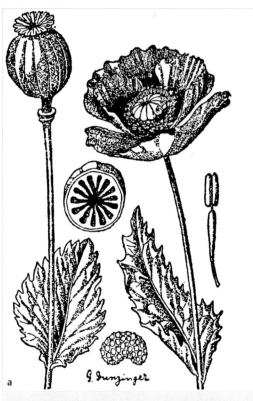
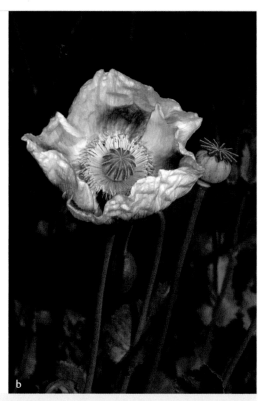

Fig. 3.20 **a and b** Poppy, Papaver somniferum. Photo: Dr. Roland Spohn, Engen.

• Combination with Belladonna and Tormentil

For special indications, opium tincture can be combined with other plant tinctures, see below for example.

Prescriptions

Rx
Tinct. Opii 5.0 (opium tincture)
Tinct. Belladonnae 10.0 (belladonna tincture)
Tinct. Tormentillae 20.0 (tormentil tincture)
D.S.
Take 10 drops in water 2–3 × a day.

▶ **Therapy Recommendations.** Opium tincture requires a specific type of prescription in Germany and in North America (see US Uniform Controlled Substances Act, for example). It should only be prescribed for very severe diarrhea that does not respond to any other treatment.

Opium tincture should only be prescribed for a few days. Diarrhea that persists beyond that requires urgent comprehensive diagnostics to determine its cause.

For references corresponding to the preceding section, see Bibliography following 3.3.5 (p. 97).

3.3.5 Chronic Slow Transit Constipation

Medicinal Plants

Antiabsorptive and Hydragogue Laxatives

Senna, Senna alexandrina, syn. Cassia acutifolia, syn. Cassia angustifolia
Senna leaves, fruit, and pods, Sennae folium et fructus et folliculi
Rhubarb, Rheum palmatum/officinale
Rhubarb root, Rhei rhizoma
Aloe Vera, Aloe vera
Aloe Vera extract, Extractum aloes
Alder Buckthorn, Rhamnus frangula
Alder buckthorn bark, Frangulae cortex
Cascara Sagrada, Frangula purshiana, Rhamnus purshiana
Cascara Sagrada bark, Rhamni purshianae cortex

Bulk-Forming Laxatives and Lubricants

Flax, Linum usitatissimum
Flaxseeds, Lini semen
Psyllium black/blond, Plantago psyllium/ovata
Psyllium seeds (black/blond), Plantaginis psyllii seu ovatae semen
Castor Bean, Ricinus communis
Castor Bean seeds, Ricini semen

The use of laxatives to treat constipation presents a number of issues.

In addition to a few synthetic laxatives, there are a large number of plant-based laxatives. These are divided into two main groups: **antiabsorptive/hydragogue laxatives** and **bulk-forming laxatives**. The first group is primarily suitable for short-term treatment and should never be used long term. Bulk-forming laxatives are suitable for long-term use. Both types can be combined to treat mixed forms of constipation.

Short-term use of laxatives is necessary in preparation for radiologic or endoscopic examinations of the intestines. They are also useful for acute constipation, for example due to changes in environment or resulting from the use of costive drugs.

Long-term use of lubricants and bulk-forming laxatives is also useful. However, practitioners should make sure that prescribing laxatives as the only treatment for constipation is a temporary measure while patients make more general modifications in their lifestyle and diet. Laxative prescriptions should always be targeted toward restoring intestinal autoregulation.

The tendency toward **abuse of laxatives** should not be underestimated. Laxative abuse often produces substantial side effects. The most serious side effect is electrolyte imbalance, especially a tendency toward hypokalemia. Chronic intestinal motility disorders are also being posited. Extended use of laxatives that contain anthranoid can cause *pseudomelanosis coli*. This condition was previously viewed by some authors as precancerous but is now predominantly viewed as benign.

Many patients self-medicate using laxatives. Practitioners and pharmacists should pay attention to this fact and talk to their patients about laxative use because the side effects of laxatives are not common knowledge. This is especially important if patients present with electrolyte imbalances. On the other hand, the option for patients to self-medicate by using laxatives should not be contested.

> **Caution** ⚠
>
> Laxatives should not be prescribed long term without thorough diagnostics, especially to exclude possibly serious organic causes such as obturations caused by intestinal tumors.

Plants for Treatment

Antiabsorptive and Hydragogue Laxatives

Antiabsorptive and **hydragogue** laxatives, also sometimes called drastic laxatives, such as senna, rhubarb, alder buckthorn (Rhamnus frangula, syn. Frangula alnus), cascara sagrada (Frangula purshiana, Rhamnus purshiana), common buckthorn (Rhamnus cathartica), and aloe vera (Aloe vera), derive their laxative effects from their anthranoid content. Anthranoids are structurally based on anthracene, which derives its laxative effects from 1,8-dehydroxylation.

Anthranoids increase motility and are antiabsorptive. They inhibit the resorption of electrolytes and water from the colon and increase both volume and filling pressure of fecal bulk. This initiates propulsive contractions that stimulate colon motility. In addition, anthranoids stimulate active chloride secretion, which releases water and electrolytes into the colon. The pharmacokinetics and pharmacodynamics of anthranoid laxatives have been well documented, but its modes of action have not been fully explained. Possible mutagenic and carcinogenic effects of anthranoid laxatives have been posited. However, this discussion is primarily based on results of animal studies of the synthetic anthranoid drug danthron (dantron), which does appear to increase the incidence of colon carcinoma. No such effects have been observed with naturally occurring anthranoids.

We therefore continue to maintain that the plants described in this chapter are useful and effective laxatives primarily suitable for **short-term use** because of their known drastic effects. We also show that medically appropriate long-term therapies for constipation include complementary concepts or different concepts altogether, rather than the exclusive use of antiabsorptive and hydragogue anthranoid laxatives.

▶ **Research.** Anthranoids were originally called emodins. This term referred to derivatives of 1,8-dihydroxy-9,10-anthraquinones (Koch). When additional anthracene derivatives were discovered, they were called anthraquinones. However, since they are not actually responsible for the laxative effect, more neutral terms were used, such as anthracene derivatives, hydroanthracene derivatives, and anthroglycosides. In the end, the term anthranoids was introduced by Lemli and became the standard name.

Despite the fact that many toxicology studies—for example by Rudolph and Mengs—showed that sennosides can be considered relatively low toxicity substances without mutagenic or carcinogenic effects, the discussion was rekindled by an article published by Siegers et al. In response, the German Federal Ministry of Health initiated a graduated process to assess the safety of sennosides. In a study published earlier, Sieger presented the results of a retrospective study of 3,049 colonoscopies (1981–1987) that correlated the incidence of *melanosis coli*—a typical result of anthranoid laxatives—with pathological colorectal changes in mucosa. Melanosis coli was found in 3.13% of patients with unremarkable mucosa, 1.89% of colitis patients, 4.98% of diverticulosis patients, 8.64% of patients with adenomas and—surprisingly—in only 3.29%

of patients with **colorectal carcinomas** (6 of 152). A prospective follow-up study of 1,095 patients was conducted from October 1989 to March 1991. This study asked the physicians performing the colonoscopy to document all incidences of *melanosis coli* and to record those associated with colorectal tumors (adenomas and carcinomas). The results of this study produced some surprising deviations from those of the previous retroactive study. They show a correlation with *melanosis coli* in 6.9% of patients with unremarkable mucosa, 9.8% for adenomas, and 18.6 (!)% instead of 3.29% in the retrospective study for colorectal carcinomas. The only category that showed the same correlation in both studies was for patients with colitis: 2.3 or 1.89%. According to Siegers, these newer results document a high cancer risk for long-term use of anthranoid-containing laxatives. In Germany, this theory of anthranoid drug carcinogenicity was also strongly defended by a working group led by Westendorf.

However, this theory strongly contradicts the experience of gastroenterologists and the results of other epidemiological studies such as the Melbourne Colorectal Cancer Study. This study of a large number of patients was not able to find a correlation between laxative use and colorectal cancer (Kune et al.).

In a 2-year carcinogenicity study on rats, Lydén-Sokolowski et al. showed no link between sennosides and an increased incidence of colorectal carcinoma. There is also a remarkable difference between women and men in frequency of laxative use (10:1), but the ratio of colorectal cancer in women and men is about 1:1. Loew (1994a) presented the results of another study that examined the link between *melanosis coli*, anthranoid laxative use, and colorectal tumor incidence. He also found a significant difference in the rate of *melanosis coli* in women and men of 8.7% and 1.8%, respectively. This ratio was found in patients who were older than 70 years (9.1%) and younger than 70 years (3.8%). A comparison of the rate of *melanosis coli* in colorectal carcinoma patients and in the control group showed a correlation of 6.1 and 4.2%, respectively, for a total of 945 patients studied. These results show that there is no significant difference. It is also worth noting that *melanosis coli* occurs primarily in the upper section of the colon, near the beginning of the small intestine.

Most cancers typically occur at the other end of the colon, in the rectal area.

It would appear that from the point of view of practical medicine, these results settle the discussion in favor of anthranoid laxatives. This demonstrates once again the dilemma of toxicology in medicine. To what extent can the results of *in vitro* trials, especially pertaining to mutagenicity, be transferred to the complex human organism in a way that at least achieves a probability bordering on certainty? Is it possible that such trials completely ignore the many natural repair mechanisms in the human organism?

Loew (1994b) compiled an overview of this controversial discussion in which he cites the critical restraint of one of the most renowned scientists in this field, Bruce Nathan Ames. According to Ames, at any given moment, oxidative damage occurs in the normal human metabolism and the organism seems to know how to counteract this damage. Critics of phytotherapy as a component of modern pharmacotherapy have increasingly cited toxicity, mutagenicity, and carcinogenicity risks of medicinal herbs in order to discredit the entire field of phytotherapy. Some examples include Aristolochia clematitis (birthwort), pyrrolizidine alkaloids, and quercetin. This makes it all the more important to have a fair and **objective discussion** about these topics and not to choose research models that do not reflect the reality of the biological organism to which the research results will be applied. Of course, the toxicology risks of plant medicines need to be assessed, but this requires the development of **adequate research models**. These models will certainly examine different questions than those that apply to synthetic single constituent drugs. The question of carcinogenicity is primarily a question about epidemiology, and this is an area that modern medicine has very much neglected in the past.

Senna (Senna alexandrina, Cassia acutifolia, Cassia angustifolia)

Senna derives from two types of cassia: Tinnevelly senna, also known as Cassia angustifolia, which primarily originates from India, and the North African Alexandrian or Khartum senna, also known as Cassia acutifolia (▶ Fig. 3.21). Cassia shrubs are members of the legume family Fabacea. Both types of cassia have pinnate leaves. The current nomenclature for both

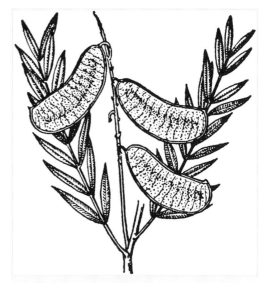

Fig. 3.21 Senna, Senna alexandrina, syn. Cassia acutifolia, syn. Cassia angustifolia.

types of cassia is Senna alexandrina, syn. Cassia acutifolia, syn. Cassia angustifolia.

Medicinal applications use the stripped pinnate parts of **senna leaves** (leaflets, Sennae folium) as well as **senna fruit** (Sennae fructus) and **senna pods** (Sennae folliculi).

The action of senna fruit and senna pods is milder than that of the leaflets, even though their sennoside content is higher.

▶ **Pharmacology.** Senna's active principle derives from anthranoids, also referred to as anthraquinone glycosides. As **sennoside A** and **B**, they primarily act on the colon. Senna also contains about 10% mucilage, plus tartaric acid salts. The anthranoids contained in senna leaves and fruit are antiabsorptive and hydragogue and inhibit resorption of electrolytes and water from the colon. This increases fecal bulk and filling pressure, which in turn stimulates intestinal motility by causing propulsive contractions. In addition, senna stimulates active chloride secretion and increases the secretion of water and electrolytes.

▶ **Indications.** Senna is a reliable and fairly strong laxative. The Commission E indication for senna is simply **constipation**.

Preparation

- **Tea**
  Add 2 teaspoons of the chopped drug to 1 cup of cold water. Soak for 6–12 hours, then strain.
  Drink 1–2 cups in the evening.

- **Combination with Caraway, Fennel, and Peppermint**

Prescriptions

Rx
Carvi fruct. (caraway seeds)
Foeniculi fruct. (fennel seeds)
Menth. pip. fol. (peppermint leaves)
Sennae fol. āā ad 100.0 (senna leaves)
M. f. spec.
Add 250 mL of hot water to herb blend (2 teaspoons to 1 tablespoon). Steep covered for 15 minutes, then strain.
D.S.
Drink 1 cup in the morning and evening.

▶ **Therapy Recommendations.** Short-term applications of laxatives should use standardized finished pharmaceutical products that have been tested for efficacy. Tea prepared solely from senna leaves should only be prescribed in special cases, for example, when severe, acute constipation needs to be unblocked in patients with otherwise healthy intestinal tracts.

Senna tea prescriptions do not offer any advantages over finished pharmaceutical products and the tea's effects are unpredictable. Small doses of 1–2 g will cause soft stools in 5–7 hours. Higher doses of 2–4 g act more quickly, but often cause watery evacuation accompanied by abdominal pain. Even higher doses of 8–12 g produce even more severe side effects and can cause severe colic, nausea, and vomiting.

The poor tolerability and colic-like effects of larger doses of senna leaves is primarily caused by their resin content. If senna leaves are soaked in cold water, less resin is dissolved into the tea. This makes the tea more tolerable, but it also decreases the tea's laxative effect. For this reason, senna leaf tea prepared using cold water maceration should only be used in case of a very irritable colon.

Rhubarb (Rheum palmatum, R. officinale)

The two types of rhubarb used medicinally are Rheum palmatum var. tanguticum (▶ Fig. 3.22) (also called turkey rhubarb) and Rheum officinale. They both belong to the Polygonaceae family and originate in the high mountains of China. Rhubarb that is equal in quality to Chinese rhubarb is also cultivated in the German state of Bavaria and in other regions.

Medicinal applications use the thick **rhubarb rootstock** (Rhei rhizome).

▶ **Note.** The types of rhubarb used medicinally are not the same as the rhubarb grown in most gardens, which is primarily Rheum rhaponticum and Rheum rhabarbarum. The stalks of the latter are used in cooking (stewed fruit, rhubarb pie). Their rhizome contains the same substances as the medicinal types of rhubarb, but in much smaller quantities.

▶ **Pharmacology.** The active substances in rhubarb are anthranoid **laxatives**, for example, rhein (cassic acid), rheum emodin, chrysophanol and tannins, flavones, resins, starch, and salts. The tannins and bitters contained in rhubarb are **costive** and this gives rhubarb a peculiar dual role. In small amounts, the tannic and bitter actions predominate and make rhubarb an aperitif and mild tonic bitter. When taken in larger amounts, the laxative actions of anthranoids predominate and in those higher dosages, make rhubarb the laxative it is generally known for.

Rhubarb is popular as an adjuvant and has been shown to be effective for supporting the choleretic

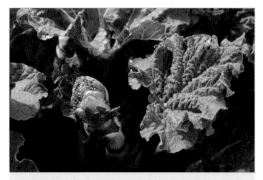

Fig. 3.22 Rhubarb, Rheum palmatum. Photo: Dr. Roland Spohn, Engen.

and cholekinetic effects of gallbladder or liver remedies. For this reason, rhubarb is found in many combination remedies.

Preparations ☞

- **Tea**
  Add 1 cup of hot water to 1 teaspoon of the coarsely powdered drug. Steep covered for 10 minutes, then strain.
  Drink 2 cups in the evening.
- **Aqueous Rhubarb Tincture** (Rhei tinctura aquosa, according to the German Pharmacopoeia, DAB 6)
  Take 1 tablespoon 1–3 × a day.

Aloe Vera (Aloe vera)

The concentrated juice of **Aloe barbadensis Miller** contains a minimum of 28% hydroxyanthracene derivatives, calculated as anhydrous barbaloin (aloin). The concentrated juice of **Aloe vera** (▶ Fig. 3.23) contains a minimum of 18% hydroxyanthracene derivatives, calculated as anhydrous aloin.

Aloe vera is marketed as a brownish mass that is processed in various ways. This plant is primarily a laxative, but also a choleretic.

Medicinal applications should only use finished **pharmaceutical aloe vera products**. Aloe vera is also frequently found combined with other laxative drugs.

Caution ⚠

High doses of aloe vera have drastic and abortifacient effects. Aloe vera laxatives should not be used during pregnancy.

Alder Buckthorn (Rhamnus frangula)

Alder buckthorn is a shrub in the Rhamnaceae family. It grows wild throughout Germany in alder groves, in damp forests, and along the edges of streams, and it is found throughout Europe. It has been introduced and has naturalized in the Midwest and Northeast America. Alder buckthorn's greenish-white flowers are small and inconspicuous and grouped in small clusters in the leaf axils. Its leaves are not very large, and they are elliptical and entire.

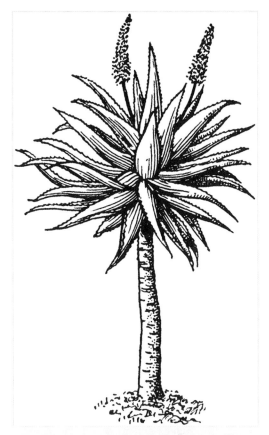

Fig. 3.23 Aloe vera, Aloe vera.

The shrub is thornless and is frequently found as dense underbrush in damp forests, together with alders, spindle trees, snowball bushes, and other shrubs. Its bark features distinctive whitish dots and stripes, which makes it easy to recognize (▶ Fig. 3.24). The color of its small fruit is another recognizable characteristic: they start out red and then turn black.

Medicinal applications use the alder **buckthorn bark** (Frangulae cortex).

▶ **Note.** Buckthorn should not be confused with **bird cherry** (Prunus padus). This shrub is often included in the buckthorn family, but it is a very different plant and has no medicinal value. Bird cherry grows in the same locations as buckthorn. As its name indicates, it is a member of the cherry family, has pretty white flowers that hang down in clusters, and emits a strong, somewhat unpleasant, fetid sweet odor. Buckthorn and bird cherry are easy to tell apart.

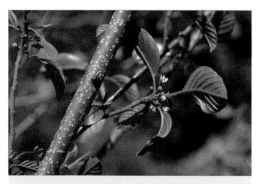

Fig. 3.24 Alder Buckthorn, Rhamnus frangula. Photo: Dr. Roland Spohn, Engen.

▶ **Pharmacology.** Buckthorn bark contains anthranoids and bitters. While it is fresh, the bark has emetic effects and needs to age for 1 year before it can be used medicinally. The fermentation process that takes place during that time destroys the emetic frangula glycoside frangulin. Buckthorn bark used for medicinal applications should contain a minimum of 6% hydroxyanthracene derivatives.

▶ **Indications.** Buckthorn, like rhubarb, is a mild to moderate laxative with little irritating effects on the intestines. The actions of senna and aloe vera are stronger.

Since buckthorn is only mildly colic inducing, it can be used for spastic constipation. Habituation occurs much more slowly with buckthorn than with senna. This makes buckthorn especially suitable for treating patients with **habitual constipation** who require a laxative to help their colon return to normal function.

Preparations

- **Tea**
  Add 1 cup of boiling water to 1 teaspoon of the chopped drug. Steep covered for 10 minutes, then strain.
  Drink 1 cup on the evening at bedtime.
- **Fluid Extract** (according to the German Pharmacopoeia, DAB)
  Take 20–40 drops in the evening.

Cascara Sagrada (Frangula purshiana, Rhamnus purshiana)

Cascara sagrada, or North American buckthorn (Rhamnus purshiana), is native to North America and a close relative of alder buckthorn (Rhamnus frangula). As with buckthorn, medicinal applications use the **cascara sagrada bark** (Rhamni purshianae cortex).

Cascara sagrada is a stronger laxative than buckthorn. There are no other essential differences between the two plants.

Preparation

- **Tea**
  Add 1 cup of boiling water to 1 teaspoon of the finely chopped drug. Steep covered for 10 minutes, then strain.
  Drink 1–2 cups in the evening at bedtime.

Proven Prescriptions

Practitioners can choose from a wide spectrum of remedies to create individualized treatments for constipation. Anthranoids, with their variety of actions provide a range of options. Senna is the strongest and most drastic laxative, aloe vera less so and North American buckthorn (Rhamnus purshiana) and rhubarb are even less strong. Low doses of North American buckthorn (Rhamnus purshiana) and rhubarb may even be used as tonics.

The following **basic formula** should guide the composition of a good, mild, and effective laxative tea. The colic-stimulating effect of the laxative component needs to be balanced by adding carminatives and antispasmodics. This means that all laxative teas should contain components from two groups of medicinal plants. The task of the practitioner is to choose a mixture that meets the patient's individual needs. Patients with very irritable colons and a tendency toward spasms need teas that contain more carminative and spasmolytic and less laxative actions. Patients with severe, atonic constipation need the opposite combination.

Prescriptions

Laxative Tea with Caraway and Peppermint
Rx
Carvi fruct. 20.0 (caraway seeds)
Menth. pip. fol. 30.0 (peppermint leaves)
Sennae fol. 10.0 (senna leaves)
Frangulae cort. 30.0 (buckthorn bark)
M. f. spec.
Add 1 cup of boiling water to 1–2 teaspoons of the tea blend. Steep covered for 10 minutes, then strain.
D.S.
Drink 1 cup in the evening.

Prescriptions

Laxative Tea with Chamomile and Fennel
Rx
Matricariae flos (German chamomile flowers)
Foeniculi fruct. (fennel seeds)
Frangulae cort. (buckthorn bark)
Sennae fol. āā ad 100.0 (senna leaves)
M. f. spec.
Add 1 cup of boiling water to 1–2 teaspoons of the tea blend. Steep covered for 10 minutes, then strain.
D.S.
Drink 1 cup in the evening.

These effective and pleasant tasting laxative teas meet all requirements. If necessary, the amount of senna leaves may be reduced somewhat in favor of more buckthorn bark.

Prescriptions

Combination of Buckthorn Fluid Extract and Belladonna for Spastic Constipation
Rx
Extr. Belladonnae 0.3–0.5 (belladonna extract)
Extr. Frangulae fluid. ad 30.0 (buckthorn bark fluid extract)
D.S.
Take 20–40 drops in water in the evening.

Prescriptions

Combination of Buckthorn and Rhubarb to Increase Laxative Effect
Rx
Extr. Frangulae fluid. 60.0 (buckthorn bark fluid extract)
Extr. Rhei fluid. 40.0 (rhubarb fluid extract)
D.S.
Take ½–1 teaspoon in water in the evening.

Prescriptions

Combination for Spastic Constipation and Flatulence
Rx
Ol. Carvi 2.0 (caraway essential oil)
Extr. Frangulae fluid. 6.0 (buckthorn bark fluid extract)
Tinct. Foeniculi 8.0 (fennel tincture)
Tinct. Belladonnae ad 30.0 (belladonna tincture)
D.S.
Take 20 drops 3 × a day.

Bulk-Forming Laxatives and Lubricants

Bulk-forming laxatives and lubricants are not true laxatives, but they are very useful for treating chronic constipation because they do not cause any irritation. Their action is based solely on **mechanical bulking of intestinal contents (increasing fecal bulk)**. This causes a stretch reflex and stimulates intestinal peristalsis. When used to treat diarrhea, these substances can normalize bowel transit time by increasing fluid retention. Bulk-forming laxatives and lubricants work more slowly than chemical laxatives and drastic plant laxatives (anthranoid drugs). They require some time, usually a few days, to produce results. However, this also makes them very suitable for **long-term or continuous use**.

▶ **Therapy Recommendations.** Bulking agents require sufficient fluid in the intestines. They should always be prescribed in combination with at least 1 glass of water or tea.

Even though bulk-forming laxatives and lubricants are practically without side effects, they can sometimes cause abdominal pain at the beginning of treatment. If that happens, the dosage should be reduced and slowly increased until full tolerability is achieved.

Flax (Linum usitatissimum)

For more information about this plant, see Flax (p. 62).

Flaxseeds, the seeds of the flax plant, are both bulking and lubricating. Flaxseeds have a bulking factor of 6. Their mucilage content makes them a good lubricant and increases fecal bulk. This causes a stretch reflex that stimulates intestinal peristalsis. The fatty oil content of flaxseeds provides additional lubrication for the increased fecal bulk. These two actions of flaxseeds are complementary.

Side effects for the use of flaxseeds are unlikely. Even the trace amounts of hydrocyanic acid and its derivatives found in flaxseeds do not cause harm. They may even increase therapeutic efficacy because they have mildly tonic effects and improve the flavor of flaxseeds.

▶ **Note.** The **flaxseed cake** that remains after flaxseeds are pressed to produce flaxseed oil (Placenta Lini seminis) contains primarily mucilage. Flaxseed cake is used externally as a cataplasm and should be used instead of crushed whole flaxseeds for this application because it does not require the precious flaxseed oil.

▶ **Indications.** Flaxseeds are one of the best remedies for **chronic constipation** and are suitable for continuous use. The Commission E lists the following indications for the internal use of flaxseeds: chronic constipation, colons damaged by abuse of laxatives, irritable colon, diverticulitis, and as mucilage for gastritis and enteritis. For external use, it is approved as a cataplasm for local inflammation.

Preparations

- **Flaxseeds**
  Take 1–2 tablespoons of flaxseeds 2–3 × a day with plenty of fluids.
- **Crushed Flaxseeds**
  Crushed or ground flaxseeds are more effective and may be easier to use.

Prescriptions

Rx
Lini sem. cont. 200.0 (crushed flaxseeds)
M. f.
Stir 2–4 tablespoons into stewed fruit or similar type of food.
D.S.
Take 1–2 × a day.

▶ **Using Crushed or Ground Flaxseeds.** Crushed or ground flaxseeds are available in pharmacies and health food stores. This easy way of using flaxseeds is recommend provided the following rules are followed.

Definition

Rules for using crushed or ground flaxseeds:
- The amount of flaxseeds used must be sufficient to create the desired effect. The minimum single dose is 1 tablespoon. At the beginning, in the morning and in the evening, 1–2 tablespoons of crushed flaxseeds should be stirred into applesauce or milk, or better yet, into granola, raw oats, or oatmeal and quark or yogurt to create a kind of porridge. At least 1 teaspoon of honey should be added.
- Inform the patient that flaxseeds need to be taken for many weeks or months. Unlike conventional laxatives, flaxseeds cannot be expected to produce sufficient bowel movements after only 1 to 2 days. It may take 3 or more days to see any effects. Instruct patients not to reach for their previous laxatives if they do not see the desired effects after 1 to 2 days. If necessary, patients can use enemas or clysters in the interim. In a short time, the daily amount of flaxseeds can be reduced to a single dose of at least 1 tablespoon (or 2 or more, if necessary) in the morning.
- Ready-to-use crushed or ground flaxseeds must be used within 1 week. If stored for longer, the flaxseed oil contained in the seeds begins to become rancid. This changes the flavor of the seeds, and they can become irritating to the stomach.

Psyllium (Plantago psyllium/ovata)

Psyllium seeds are similar to flaxseeds in their effects. Black psyllium seed (Plantago psyllium) consists of the dried, ripe **seeds** of a type of plantain that grows in southern Europe. Blond psyllium **seed husks** (Plantago ovata) consist of the epidermal layer and adjacent collapsed seed layers of a plant that grows widely in India and Iran. Plantago psyllium has a swelling index of at least 10 and Plantago ovata has an even greater swelling index.

▸ **Note.** Blond psyllium **seed husks** (Plantago ovata) were valued highly by Persian and Arabic physicians during the Middle Ages.

▸ **Therapy Recommendation.** After taking psyllium preparations, patients should drink 1–2 glasses of water, up to about 1–2 L a day.

Castor Bean (Ricinus communis)

The castor bean (or castor oil) tree, also sometimes called palm of Christ or palma Christi, is native to East Africa and belongs to the family of Euphorbiaceae. It is cultivated in India, China, and Brazil for oil production (Büechi). Its seeds are pressed to produce castor oil, **Ricini semen**, which contains 80% triricinolin, the triglyceride of ricinoleic acid. In Europe, castor oil has been used as a laxative since the 18th century. In addition to the oil, castor beans also contain proteins, including the toxic lectin ricin. Cold-pressed castor oil (Oleum Ricini), as described in the European Pharmacopoeia, does not contain ricin.

Castor oil is a reliable laxative of remarkable therapeutic scope. Its dosage is easily adaptable, and its efficacy is well documented. In high doses, castor oil is used as a bowel cleanse before endoscopies or radiologic diagnostics. In low doses, it is used as a laxative. Children generally do not like the taste of castor oil, but it is an especially suitable laxative for children.

Bibliography

Büechi S. Rizinusöl. Z Phytother. 2000; 21:312–318

Classen B. Rubus fruticosus agg. L.—Portät einer Arzneipflanze. Z Phytother. 2008; 29:47–50

Ewe K, Lemli J, Leng-Peschlow E, Sewing KF, Eds. Senna – 2nd International Symposium, Konstanz, April 1993: Proceedings. Pharmacology 1993; 47 (Suppl 1)

Fintelmann V, Giesel B. Durchfallerkrankungen im Kleinkind- und Schulkindalter. Klin Padiatr. 2005; 11:44–46

Fintelmann V. Neues über Anthranoid-Laxanzien und karzinogenes Risiko. Z Phytother. 1993; 14(2):72–73

Gardiner JS, Walker SA, MacLean AJ. A retrospective mortality study of substituted anthraquinone dyestuffs workers. Br J Ind Med. 1982; 39(4):355–360

Koch A, Kraus L. Pflanzliche Laxanzien mit Anthranoiden als Wirkstoffen. Dtsch Apoth Ztg. 1991; 28:1459–1466

Kune GA, Kune S, Field B, Watson LF. The role of chronic constipation, diarrhea, and laxative use in the etiology of large-bowel cancer. Data from the Melbourne Colorectal Cancer Study. Dis Colon Rectum. 1988; 31(7):507–512

Latté KP. Potentilla erecta—Porträt einer Arzneipflanze. Z Phytother. 2006; 27:198–206

Lemli J. Metabolismus der Anthranoide. Z Phytother. 1986; 7:127–129

Loew D. Anthranoidlaxanzien. Ursache für Kolonkarzinom? Dtsch Apoth Ztg. 1994b; 34:3180–3183

Loew D. Pseudomelanosis coli durch Anthranoide. Z Phytother. 1994a; 15:321–328

Lydén-Sokolowski A, Nilsson A, Sjöberg P. Two-year carcinogenicity study with sennosides in the rat: emphasis on gastrointestinal alterations. Pharmacology. 1993; 47 Suppl 1:209–215

Mori H, Sugie S, Niwa K, Takahashi M, Kawai K. Induction of intestinal tumours in rats by chrysazin. Br J Cancer. 1985; 52(5): 781–783

Rudolph RL, Mengs U. Electron microscopical studies on rat intestine after long-term treatment with sennosides. Pharmacology. 1988; 36 Suppl 1:188–193

Siegers CP, von Hertzberg-Lottin E, Otte M, Schneider B. Anthranoid laxative abuse—a risk for colorectal cancer? Gut. 1993; 34(8):1099–1101

Westendorf J, Marquardt H, Poginsky B, Dominiak M, Schmidt J, Marquardt H. Genotoxicity of naturally occurring hydroxyanthraquinones. Mutat Res. 1990; 240(1):1–12

Westendorf J, Poginsky B, Marquardt H, Kraus L, Marquardt H. Possible carcinogenicity of anthraquinone-containing medical plants. Planta Med. 1988; 54(6):562

3.3.6 Proctitis

Medicinal Plants

German Chamomile, Matricaria recutita
Chamomile Flowers, Matricariae flos
Calamus, Acorus calamus
Calamus rootstock, Calami rhizoma
St.-John's-wort, Hypericum perforatum
St.-John's-wort herb, Hyperici herba

There are no specific medicinal plants for the treatment of proctitis. Treatment usually encompasses **anti-inflammatory remedies**, primarily chamomile, as well as **astringents** and **spasmolytics**. Tormentil is a suitable astringent due to its high tannin content. A **mild laxative** such as buckthorn or rhubarb (p. 92) is often needed to prevent fecal stasis.

Plants for Treatment

German Chamomile (Matricaria recutita)

For more information about this plant, see German Chamomile (p. 42).

Preparation

- **Tea**
  Add 1 cup of hot water to 2–3 teaspoons of the drug. Steep covered for 5–10 minutes, then strain.
  Drink 1 cup 3 × a day.

- **Combination of Chamomile and Demulcents**, e.g., Mallow Flowers or Flaxseed Mucilage, for **Acute Irritation**

Prescriptions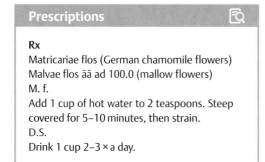

Rx
Matricariae flos (German chamomile flowers)
Malvae flos āā ad 100.0 (mallow flowers)
M. f.
Add 1 cup of hot water to 2 teaspoons. Steep covered for 5–10 minutes, then strain.
D.S.
Drink 1 cup 2–3 × a day.

- **Combination of Chamomile and Astringents,** e.g., **Tormentil Root or Potentilla Herb, for Subacute and Chronic Conditions**

Prescriptions

Rx
Matricariae flos (German chamomile flowers)
Tormentillae rhiz. (tormentil rootstock)
Frangulae cort. āā ad 100.0 (buckthorn bark)
M. f.
Add 1 cup of hot water to 2 teaspoons of the blend. Steep covered for 10 minutes, then strain.
D.S.
Drink 1 cup in the morning and in the evening for several weeks.

▶ **Therapy Recommendation.** Localized treatment using retention enemas or suppositories is recommended. Retention enemas contain about 20 mL of chamomile tea. Other plants (demulcents, astringents, tonics) may be added to the tea, depending on proctitis type and symptoms.

Calamus (Acorus calamus)

For more information about this plant, see Calamus (p. 59).

In some cases, tonics may be needed to stimulate mucosal secretions and to improve intestinal smooth muscle tone.

Preparations

- **Tea**
  Add 1 cup of boiling water to ½–1 teaspoon of the drug. Steep covered for 5 minutes, then strain.
  Drink 1 cup with each meal.
- **Tincture**
  Add 20–30 drops to 1 cup of chamomile tea.

St.-John's-wort (Hypericum perforatum)

For more information about this plant, see St.-John's-wort (p. 264).

3.3.7 Hemorrhoids

Medicinal Plants

Butcher's-broom, Ruscus aculeatus
Butcher's-broom root, Rusci aculeati rhizoma
Witch Hazel (Common, American),
Hamamelis virginiana
Witch Hazel leaves and bark, Hamamelidis folium et cortex
Quaking Aspen, Populus tremula
Quaking Aspen bud, Populi gemma
Tormentil, Potentilla tormentilla
Tormentil Root, Tormentillae rhizoma
German Chamomile, Matricaria recutita
German Chamomile flowers, Matricariae flos
Arnica, Arnica montana
Arnica flowers, Arnicae flos
Common Oak (Quercus robur), Sessile Oak (Quercus petraea)
Oak bark, Quercus cortex

It is important to note that there is no phytotherapeutic for treating the cause of hemorrhoids.

The following is recommended to provide **symptomatic treatments** for the subjective burdensome symptoms caused primarily by inflammation or thrombosis of the hemorrhoid knots. If applied in the early stages, appropriate phytotherapeutic treatment reduces subjective symptoms and is **preventive**.

Caution

Bleeding associated with hemorrhoids requires a medical examination to exclude organic causes masked by hemorrhoids, such as adenomas or tumors.

▶ **Therapy Recommendation.** The initial treatment for **acute inflamed hemorrhoids** is moist chamomile or arnica compresses. Ointments constitute only supportive therapy.

Compresses should be cool, at most, room temperature. Cold compresses could cause more harm than good because they are more likely to stimulate spasms.

Plants for Treatment

Butcher's-broom (Ruscus aculeatus)

Butcher's-broom originates from the Mediterranean and is experiencing a revival in attention and use. This thorny evergreen subshrub belongs to the asparagus (Asparagaceae) family. It grows wild on the dry, sunny slopes of macchie (maquis) in the entire Mediterranean region. Like garden asparagus (Asparagus officinalis), butcher's-broom has very small, almost scalelike leaves (▶ Fig. 3.25). It develops leaflike phylloclades next to these leaf remnants. In garden asparagus, these phylloclades are roundish, needle-shaped, and resemble leaves. In butcher's-broom, the phylloclades are larger, leaflike, and leathery, and terminate in a sharp-tipped spine. Butcher's-broom (also known as sweet broom) derives its name from the likeness of its phylloclades to the brush of the tool (broom) used for sweeping and brushing.

Medicinal applications use the thick, fleshy **butcher's-broom rootstock** (Rusci aculeati rhizome).

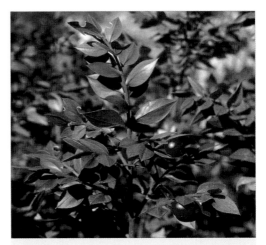

Fig. 3.25 Butcher's-broom, Ruscus aculeatus. Photo: Dr. Roland Spohn, Engen.

▶ **Pharmacology.** The active constituents of butcher's-broom include steroid saponin glycosides such as ruscogenin and neoruscogenin. Two derivatives of neoruscogenin predominate in terms of amounts: the spirostanol ruscin and the furostanol ruscoside. Its steroid structure is similar to that of adrenal cortex steroids, but without the cortisone-like effects.

Animal experiments have shown butcher's-broom to have a tonifying effect on veins as well as anti-exudative, antiphlogistic, and mild diuretic effects.

▶ **Note.** Decoctions of butcher's-broom rootstock boiled in water or wine were used for centuries to treat gynecologic disorder and several other disorders, and as a diuretic. Van Rensen published a review of the history, pharmacology, and clinical applications of butcher's-broom with extensive references.

▶ **Indications.** Butcher's-broom rootstock is a therapeutic for veins and a reliable medicinal for treating **anorectal syndrome** and **hemorrhoids**. It reduces swelling of inflamed hemorrhoid knots, tonifies blood vessels in that area, and provides subjective relief.

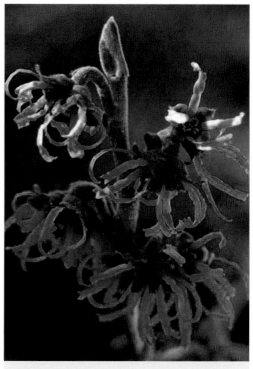

Fig. 3.26 Witch hazel (Common), Hamamelis virginiana. Photo: Naturfoto Franke Heckler, Panten-Hammer.

Witch Hazel (Common, American) (Hamamelis virginiana)

One of the most useful hemorrhoid ointments is derived from the North American witch hazel (also known as common), Hamamelis virginiana (▶ Fig. 3.26). This shrub is also frequently cultivated in gardens. It gets its name from the bright yellow (i.e., hazel-colored) leaves that often appear in early spring when there is still snow on the ground.

Medicinal applications use the **witch hazel leaves** (Hamamelidis folium) and the **witch hazel bark (Hamamelidis cortex)**.

▶ **Pharmacology.** The most important constituents of witch hazel leaves are tannins (3–8%), primarily gallotannins, flavonoids, and volatile oil. Witch hazel bark contains a minimum of 4% tannins. Witch hazel characteristic components include hamamelitannins, gamma-hamamelitannins, ellagitannin, catechin derivatives, and free gallic acid. These constituents are astringent, anti-inflammatory, and locally hemostatic.

Arnica (Arnica montana)

For more information about this plant, see Arnica (p. 144).

Arnica provides rapid relief for inflamed hemorrhoids because it also acts as a vein decongestant in the area to which it is applied.

Preparation

- **Tincture**
  For compresses, add 1–2 teaspoons of arnica tincture to 500 mL water.
  Apply compresses for at least 1 hour in the morning and evening, and midday, if possible.
  Compresses can be followed by application of one of the hemorrhoid ointments described earlier, preferably witch hazel.

Other Plants for Treating Hemorrhoids

Quaking Aspen (Populus tremula)

Medicinal applications use the **quaking aspen buds** (Populi gemma). They contain salicyl alcohol derivatives, volatile oil, and flavonoids.

Hemorrhoid ointment prepared from crushed fresh aspen buds is decongesting, soothing, and relieves itching. It has undeservedly faded into obscurity.

> **Preparations**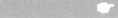
>
> - **Quaking Aspen Ointment, Unguentum Populi**
> - **Quaking Aspen Suppositories** (Suppositoria Populi, according to the German Prescription Formulas, DRF)

Tormentil (Potentilla tormentilla, Potentilla erecta)

For more information about this plant, see Tormentil (p. 84).

▶ **Indications.** This plant is primarily indicated for **anal fissures**.

> **Preparation**
>
> - **Ointment**

Belladonna can be added to reduce spasms.

> **Prescriptions**
>
> Rx
> Extr. Tormentill. 5.0 (tormentil extract)
> Extr. Belladonnae 0.5 (belladonna extract)
> Ungt. moll. ad 50.0 (white soft paraffin)
> M. f. ungt.
> D.S.
> Apply the ointment 1–3 × a day.

German Chamomile (Matricaria recutita)

For more information about this plant, see German Chamomile (p. 42).

▶ **Indications.** This treatment is primarily indicated for **acutely inflamed hemorrhoids**.

> **Preparations**
>
> - **Tea**
>   For moist compresses, add 1 cup of hot water to 2–3 teaspoons of the drug. Steep covered for 5–10 minutes, then strain.
>   For sitz baths, add 50 g of the drug to 10 L of warm water.
> - **Fluid Extract**
>   For moist compresses, add 1 teaspoon to 500 mL of water at room temperature.
> - **Chamomile Suppositories** (Suppositoria Chamomillae, according to the German Prescription Formulas, DRF)
>   Chamomile suppositories are suitable for follow-up treatment.

Common Oak (Quercus robur), Sessile Oak (Quercus petraea)

For more information about this plant, see Oak (p. 287).

▶ **Indications.** This treatment is primarily suitable for additional **inflammation of the anal skin surrounding hemorrhoids**.

> **Preparation**
>
> - **Decoction**
>   For compresses or sitz baths, add a small handful of the drug to 1 L of water. Boil covered for 15 minutes, then strain. Use at room temperature.

Proven Prescriptions

The composition of a "hemorrhoid tea" for relieving hemorrhoids symptoms is the same as for a standard laxative tea that is a laxative, anti-inflammatory, and antispasmodic. A tonic bitter is added to tonify the hemorrhoidal portal vessels and to relieve the hemorrhoidal plexus. In some cases, a hemostatic is also added.

Prescriptions

Rx
Matricariae flos (German chamomile flowers)
Calami rhiz. (calamus rootstock)
Foeniculi fruct. (fennel seeds)
Sennae fol. (senna leaves)
Frangulae cort. āā ad 100.0 (buckthorn bark)
M. f. spec.
Add 1 cup of boiling water to 1–2 teaspoons of the blend. Steep covered for 10 minutes, then strain.
D.S.
Drink 1 cup in the morning and in the evening.

Bibliography

van Rensen I. Der stechende Mäusedorn—Ruscus aculeatus L. Z Phytother. 2000; 21(5):271–286

Questions

1. What are carminatives?
2. Name some typical carminatives.
3. Formulate a prescription for a medicinal tea to treat meteorism.
4. Are there plant medicines for adjuvant treatment of chronic inflammatory bowel disorders (IBDs)?
5. What are typical phytotherapeutics for treating diarrhea?
6. What are typical phytotherapeutics for treating constipation?
7. Formulate a prescription for a "mild" laxative tea.

Answers (p. 421) for Chapter 3.3

3.4 Hepatic and Biliary Disorders

3.4.1 Hepatic Disorders

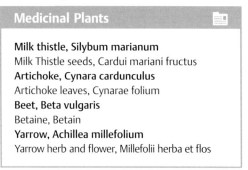

Medicinal Plants

Milk thistle, Silybum marianum
Milk Thistle seeds, Cardui mariani fructus
Artichoke, Cynara cardunculus
Artichoke leaves, Cynarae folium
Beet, Beta vulgaris
Betaine, Betain
Yarrow, Achillea millefolium
Yarrow herb and flower, Millefolii herba et flos

There are two large categories of acute and chronic liver disorders: **viral inflammatory disorders** and **toxic metabolic disorders**.

There are now well established treatments for viral hepatitis using newly developed antivirals. Cure rates for chronic conditions have risen significantly and are now at about 90%, depending on the type of virus. However, these treatments have significant undesirable drug side effects and do not work for a residual group of nonresponders. This calls for complementary medicine strategies such as phytotherapy. Milk thistle, for example, can be helpful in treating chronic hepatitis C.

The situation is different for **hepatotoxicity**. There are no known chemically defined drugs to successfully treat toxic liver disorders. Modern medicine treats these disorders by recognizing the noxa and eliminating them, if possible. The main noxa for liver damage continues to be alcohol and synthetic drugs. Alcohol damages the liver metabolically, which leads to the development of alcoholic fatty liver disease. It can also cause **alcoholic hepatitis**, a much more dangerous disease that can develop into alcoholic cirrhosis. The liver can largely recover and heal during all stages of liver damage caused by alcohol if alcohol consumption is stopped completely. However, abstinence is often not accepted in the patient's environment and is difficult to implement. **Hepatotoxic drugs**, such as tuberculostatic and cytostatic drugs, synthetic estrogen, antimalarials, and certain sulfonamides, are often indispensable for treating serious diseases. Moderate liver disorders as a potential outcome of these treatments are viewed as an acceptable risk.

Despite these therapeutic dilemmas, the **possibilities offered by phytotherapy** for the treatment of hepatic disorders have not been fully recognized and taken advantage of to date. Practitioners who feel a sense of responsibility in this field will search for rational therapies that are subjectively and objectively effective, even if these therapies are not accepted by pharmacologists, who base their acceptance entirely on "active substance" thinking. The plants described in this chapter—milk thistle, artichoke, beet, and yarrow—have a long tradition for the treatment of hepatic disorders and have been proven in many ways, including by impeccable scientific studies.

Medicinal plants work holistically, and it is not always possible to clearly differentiate their effect on the liver from their effect on the gallbladder. For this reason, there will be overlaps between the discussion of hepatic and biliary disorders. However, hepatic disorders are the main indication for the plants discussed in this chapter.

▶ **Note.** Essential phospholipids derived from soybeans are not considered phytotherapeutics. This class of substances was therefore evaluated by the Commission B, which is responsible for chemically defined substances, and not assessed by the Commission E, which is responsible for phytotherapy.

The German physician and founder of modern organopathy, Johann Gottfried Rademacher (1772–1849), who was a contemporary of the physician Christoph Wilhelm Hufeland (1762–1836), referred to liver disorders as hepatopathies. This undifferentiated term is currently being replaced by differentiated and more specific disease names as a result of the development of modern laboratory diagnostics, a significantly improved and more differentiated histological assessment of liver tissue, and modern imaging techniques.

Plants for Treatment

Milk Thistle (Silybum marianum)

Milk thistle is a large plant in the Asteraceae family. It has large purple-red flowers, and glossy, wavy, spiny-edged leaves with peculiar white veins (▶ Fig. 3.27). The leaves look like they are sprinkled with chalk. Milk thistle originates from the Mediterranean and is cultivated throughout Germany, where it is also frequently grown as an ornamental garden plant.

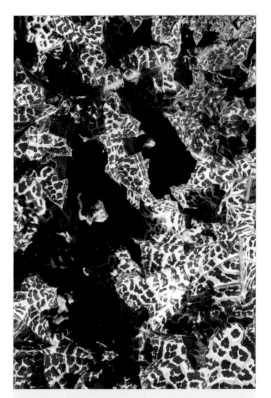

Fig. 3.27 Milk thistle, Silybum marianum. Photo: Thieme Verlagsgruppe, Stuttgart.

Medicinal applications use the ripe **milk thistle seeds** (fruit) that are freed from the pappus (Cardui mariani fructus).

▶ **Pharmacology.** Milk thistle is one of the phytotherapeutics for which a large body of excellent pharmacology and corresponding proof of clinical efficacy has been developed. Wagner et al. describe silymarin as the liver-protecting compound of milk thistle. This active compound consists of three components: silibinin, silidianin, and silichristin. They make up about 2–3% of the dried drug and are an isomeric mixture in the flavonolignan class. Until their discovery in milk thistle, flavonolignans were not known to exist in plants.

We also now have reliable information about the pharmacokinetics of milk thistle. Studies of 14-C-labeled silibinin in dogs and rats showed that peroral application of silymarin results in about 50% absorption and that about 10% of the applied amount reaches enterohepatic circulation. The primary route for silymarin elimination is biliary excretion of sulfate and glucuronide conjugates.

Definition

Silymarin—primarily through **silibinin**, its main active constituent—acts therapeutically on the following areas of liver cells:

- Silymarin stimulates **RNA polymerase I activity** in the cell nucleus. This increases ribosomal **protein synthesis** in liver cells via rRNA synthesis and promotes the liver's regenerative capacity (Sonnenbichler and Zetl).
- Silymarin stabilizes the **lipid structures** of liver cell membranes. This action may apply to cells in general, which would extend silymarin's effect beyond the liver.
- Silymarin's **antiperoxidative effect** makes it a **free radical scavenger** (Fehér et al.).
- Silymarin's **antifibrotic effect** is used for treating chronic liver disorders with a strong tendency toward fibrogenesis (Boigk et al.; Schuppan et al.).

▶ **Indications.** The main indication for silymarin is **hepatotoxicity** caused primarily by chronic and excessive alcohol use, liver-damaging drugs, and numerous industrial and environmental toxins (Fintelmann 1986). The finished pharmaceutical silymarin product Legalon, which is marketed as a patented drug in Germany, Austria, and Switzerland, has been shown to be very effective as an **adjuvant** therapy for chronic inflammatory liver disorders resulting from various **viral hepatitis infections** (Kiesewetter et al.).

For alcohol-induced liver damage, silymarin should be prescribed for a limited period in addition to abstinence from alcohol to increase the rate of liver regeneration and restore liver function as a vital component of overall health. In cases where the use of liver-toxic drugs is required to treat serious diseases, adjuvant use of silymarin as a potential liver protection factor can either prevent, or at least significantly limit, toxic liver damage. The same applies to chemically induced liver damage that is usually work-related, for example, by chlorinated cyclic or halogenated hydrocarbons.

The objection that treatment of hepatotoxicity involves only the removal of the damaging noxa has no basis in fact. Silymarin has been shown to improve liver generation following the removal of noxa (Filip et al.; Fintelmann and Albert; Kurz-Dimitrowa; Saba et al.; Salmi and Sarna). If removal of noxa is not possible, the adjuvant use of silymarin as a curative and preventive remedy is absolutely indicated.

The Commission E monography approved the general effect of milk thistle for dyspeptic complaints. Silymarin formulations (standardized to at least 70–80% silymarin) are approved for toxic liver damage and for supportive treatment in chronic inflammatory liver disease and hepatic cirrhosis.

A special indication exists for the specific intravenous silymarin preparation, Legalon SIL, a water-soluble derivative of silibinin-C-2',3-dihydrogen succinate, disodium salt in vial form. It is viewed today as the safest antidote for life-threatening **amanita mushroom** (Amanita phalloides, death cap) **poisoning.**

Large multicentric studies show that Legalon SIL can lower the mortality rate from > 20% to < 10% compared with the previously used intensive therapy that included high doses of penicillin G (Floersheim et al.). Legalon SIL infusions within 24 hours of diagnosing amanita mushroom poisoning can lower mortality rates to almost zero.

▶ **Research.** Milk thistle seeds have been used for a long time to treat various disorders, for example "hydrops." Milk thistle's special indication for liver disorders was not known until it was discovered by the German physician, Johann Gottfried Rademacher. Rademacher studied many medicinal plants and developed a milk thistle seed tincture that came to be known as Tinctura Rademacheri.

Starting in 1970, milk thistle acquired a completely new role in the treatment of liver disorders. The finished pharmaceutical silymarin product Legalon (Madaus) was introduced for the treatment of toxic liver disease and quickly gained high renown from physicians and patients. Animal experimental trials that began around 1970 primarily examined the preventive and curative effects of silymarin on toxic liver damage in rats. The outcome of these trials showed previously unknown **preventive** and **curative effects.** The most intensively studied subject was liver intoxication induced by alpha-amanitin, the main toxin in amanita mushrooms (Amanita phalloides, death cap). Other liver-damaging substances, such as carbon tetrachlorides, N-galactosamine, or thioacetamide, were also

studied and showed equally good results (Vogel et al.). Clinical experience confirmed the efficacy of Legalon in humans (Ferenci et al.; Filip et al.; Fintelmann; Fintelmann and Albert; Floersheim et al.). Within the first 2 weeks of treatment, patients begin to feel better overall. Gastrointestinal symptoms, meteorism, and upper abdominal distension are reduced. Increased appetite and physical stamina are also frequently observed.

The Vienna cirrhosis study (Ferenci et al. 1989) provides impressive proof that the median survival rate of patients with toxic alcoholic liver cirrhosis who were treated with silymarin was significantly higher than in the placebo group. It is thought that this is primarily due to the **protein synthesis increasing effects** of silymarin.

Studies have also shown **antifibrotic effects** for silymarin, which are used specifically for chronic liver disorders with a strong tendency toward fibrosis, especially for chronic hepatitis B and C (Boigk et al.; Schuppan et al.).

In 2008, Ferenci et al. published the results of studying the use of intravenous silibinin infusions in patients with chronic hepatitis C who did not respond to the standard therapy of pegylated interferon and ribavirin. He was able to demonstrate a drastic virus load reduction and good therapy tolerability. Since then, this action of silymarin/silibinin has been studied in many centers as well as clinically. Without a doubt, silibinin has antiviral properties that have been demonstrated to extend beyond the hepatitis C virus. It prevents this virus from replicating, clearly influences membrane function to prevent the hepatitis C virus from invading liver cells, and appears to have anti-inflammatory effects. So far, these very interesting research results have not yet been replicated for oral use of silymarin. However, clinical experience has shown that silymarin is very useful as an adjuvant therapy for conventional hepatitis therapy by stimulating liver regeneration. In the author's experience, it is essential. Reviews by Pohl (2013) provide answers for the questions raised in this context and also include current data.

Legalon serves as an example that the efficacy of a phytotherapeutic remedy with indications based on traditional medical usage can effectively be proven using modern criteria of experimental pharmacology and clinical studies equivalent to those that have been established for synthetic, chemically defined substances.

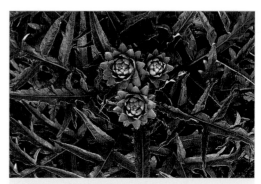

Fig. 3.28 Artichoke, Cynara cardunculus (Cynara scolymus). Photo: Prof. Dr. Volker Fintelmann, Hamburg.

▶ **Therapy Recommendations.** A milk thistle extract containing a standardized amount of silibinin is recommended for treating defined liver disorders.

In case of strong suspicion of amanita mushroom (Amanita phalloides, death cap) poisoning, Legalon SIL should be given intravenously as an infusion as soon as possible. The recommended daily dose of silibinin is 20 mg/kg divided into four 2-hour infusions, with attention paid to fluid balance.

Artichoke (Cynara cardunculus, Cynara scolymus)

Artichokes have been taxonomically renamed as Cynara cardunculus L. ssp. flavescens Wiklund. Many texts however still refer to it as Cynara scolymus.

Like milk thistle, artichokes are thistlelike plants that belong to the Asteraceae family. The plant can grow to a height of 2 m and has large purple flower heads (▶ Fig. 3.28).

Artichokes are primarily known as a vegetable in the Mediterranean and are increasingly popular as such in Germany. In North America, artichokes are cultivated agriculturally in California. The lower parts of the fleshy flower tepals and the flower receptacle are eaten as vegetables. These are valued for their pleasantly bitter flavor derived from cynaropicrin. This bitter compound is found only in the green parts of the plant. It is at its highest level shortly before the plant flowers and when the seeds ripen.

Medicinal applications use the **artichoke foliar leaves** (Cynarae folium).

▶ **Pharmacology.** One of the known constituents of artichokes—**cynaropicrin**, a sesquiterpene lactone—has already been mentioned. The bittering power of artichoke leaves is listed as 11,500. Cynarine, identified as 1,5-dicaffeoylquinic acid, is another therapeutically relevant constituent of artichokes. Artichoke extracts contain only traces of cynarine as a genuine constituent. It develops during galenic preparation via transesterification of 1,3-dicaffeoyl-quinic acid. Other known artichoke constituents include coffeic acid (another hydroxycinnamic acid), luteolin, and the luteolin glycosides scolymoside and cynaroside (flavonoids).

The pharmacological action of artichokes likely results from a combination of polyphenol compounds. According to current research, artichoke leaves are **choleretic, antioxidant,** and **lipid lowering**.

▶ **Research.** Gebhardt (1995b) identified **luteolin** as a lipid-lowering constituent of artichoke leaves. The results of a double-blind, placebo-controlled study also confirmed this lipid-lowering effect. This randomized, double-blind, multicentric study involved 143 patients with total cholesterol levels of > 280 mg/dL. These patients received a daily dose of 1800 mg of a dry artichoke extract derived from fresh artichoke leaves (Valverde Artischocke, coated tablets) compared with placebo for 6 weeks. The artichoke extract showed a significant superiority ($p < 0.0001$) over placebo. Total cholesterol was lowered by 18.5% compared with 8.9% in the placebo group. Low density lipoprotein (LDL) cholesterol was lowered by 22.9% compared with 6.3%. Tolerability was excellent (Englisch et al.).

Artichoke's **choleretic effects** were shown by Hammerl and Pichler and by Kirchhoff et al. (1994) in double-blind studies and confirmed experimentally in isolated perfused rat livers (Matuschowski et al.). A pressed juice of fresh artichoke leaves that was nonconformant with the Commission E monograph for artichoke produced long-lasting and sustained increases in bile flow as well as bile acid clearance. These effects were shown to be derived in large part, but not exclusively, from the phenolic fraction of the constituents. This was confirmed for individual isolated phenols. These quantitative as well as qualitative choleretic effects provide a plausible explanation for the clinical efficacy of artichoke preparations.

Hammerl and Pichler also showed connections between artichoke and arteriosclerosis prevention. Maros et al. (1966; 1967) showed that artichoke extracts promote rat liver regeneration. These studies were not followed up systematically until recently, when they were largely confirmed by modern experimental and clinical studies using a standardized aqueous dry extract of artichoke leaves (Kirchhoff et al. 1994).

Study results presented by Gebhardt (1995a) using primary hepatocyte cultures also confirmed the highly effective reduction of hepatic *de novo* synthesis of cholesterol. **Inhibition of cholesterol biosynthesis** was proven beyond a doubt by measuring the incorporation of 14-C acetate into the nonsaponifiable lipid fraction. Since artichoke juice also reduces intrahepatic cholesterol via choleretic increases in cholesterol excretion, both mechanisms may contribute to a reduction of serum cholesterol and possibly of other lipids.

Gebhardt (1995d) also showed pronounced **antioxidant effects** for artichoke extract in molecular and cellular test systems. Artichoke extract was shown to inhibit malondialdehyde (MDA) production induced by exposure of hepatocyte cultures to the oxidant tert-butylhydroperoxide (t-BHP). The results of this study show unusually high antioxidant activity for the extract tested. It significantly inhibited MDA production in concentrations as low as 1 µg/mL.

When one considers the special pathogenic role of oxidized LDL cholesterol in the development of arteriosclerosis, the free radical scavenging effects of artichoke leaves could be viewed as a possible third aspect of artichoke's effect on fat metabolism. This provides an astoundingly comprehensive theoretical and experimental explanation for the clinically proven lipid-lowering effects of artichoke leaves. It supports the conclusion that artichoke is more **lipid regulating** than lipid lowering.

In another study, Gebhardt (1995c) also confirmed the liver generation-promoting, **hepatoprotective effects** of artichoke shown in earlier studies. He demonstrated that artichoke extract can significantly reduce the rate of cell death in hepatocytes exposed to carbon tetrachloride. The author points out that this strong antioxidant effect is likely not confined to liver cells, but this point needs to be studied more generally. This makes artichoke extract even more interesting for future studies. In that study, Gebhardt also showed **anticholestatic effects** in liver cells with artichoke leaf extract.

▶ **Indications.** The Commission E monograph for artichoke leaves only lists **dyspeptic problems**, which is plausible given artichoke's content of bitters and its choleretic effect. This indication has been well documented in traditional use and by clinical, controlled studies (Kirchhoff et al. 1993). In addition to carminative, spasmolytic, and appetite-stimulating and lipid-lowering effects, artichoke leaves also have notable antiemetic effects. This special indication sets it apart from other hepatic and biliary remedies.

Of the documented application areas, artichoke's **lipid-lowering effect** is probably the most important. On the one hand, lipometabolic disorders and hyperlipidemia are very common and considered to be a major cofactor for the development of arteriosclerosis. On the other hand, currently available synthetic lipid-lowering drugs have considerable undesirable effects. Having an alternative phytotherapeutic treatment option that is very well tolerated is certainly welcomed by practitioners and patients.

▶ **Research.** A comprehensive, yearlong observational study (Fintelmann 1996) of 52 investigators and 533 patients and an average treatment duration of 6 weeks showed a highly significant reduction of typical symptoms of dyspeptic disorders in the following order: vomiting, nausea, pain spasms in the right upper abdomen, general abdominal pain, lack of appetite, constipation, meteorism, and fat intolerance. The correlation between the assessment by treating physicians and by treated patients was very high.

107

Another important result of this study was proof of the lipid-lowering effects of artichoke leaf extract. A minimum of two cholesterol and triglyceride values were available for 302 patients. Statistical analysis showed significant reductions of total cholesterol ($p < 0.001$) from 264.24 mg/dL (median: 266 mg/dL) to 233.91 mg/Ll (median: 232 mg/dL). Similar positive results were obtained for triglycerides.

These results were fully confirmed by a follow-up study. The goal of this observational study of 203 patients was to determine whether the lipid-lowering effects shown in the previous study were transient or persisted long term. During the average application period of 23 weeks, the study showed continual improvements for about 4 months. At that point, maximum efficacy seemed to have been reached and was maintained at that level. The drug was very well tolerated long term (Fintelmann 1998). A subsequent randomized, double-blind, placebo-controlled, evidence-based study confirmed these lipid-lowering effects (Englisch et al.). In this study, total cholesterol was lowered from 18.5% compared with 8.6% in the placebo group (a difference of $p < 0.0001$). Another subsequently published randomized, placebo-controlled, double-blind study conducted in the United Kingdom also demonstrated these lipid-lowering effects of artichoke extract (Bundy et al.).

Artichoke's **antioxidant effects** have not been as well studied clinically as its proven antidyspeptic and lipid-lowering effects. Artichoke leaves appear to have similar efficacy as silymarin derived from milk thistle seeds. It has already been mentioned that the antioxidant properties of artichokes are likely not confined to the liver. This represents an open, highly interesting, and very promising area for future research.

▶ **Therapy Recommendation.** Medicinal applications should give preference to finished **pharmaceutical artichoke products**.

Beet (Beta vulgaris)

Betaine, a phytochemical compound prevalent in beets (Beta vulgaris), was discovered by French authors in the 19th century to have effects similar to milk thistle. This white sweet tasting substance interacts with the methylation cycle inside liver cells by acting as a methyl donor. This is viewed as supporting liver cell regeneration and conversion of triglycerides into transport fat.

Betaine is one of the essential hepatotropic and lipotropic amino acids, similar to methionine. It does not have any damaging effects, is very well tolerated, and is a fitting plant medicine for the liver. However, there are currently no recent studies about the efficacy of beets that are comparable to studies about milk thistle or artichoke.

Yarrow (Achillea millefolium)

Yarrow is one of the most abundant plants in Germany. It grows in dry meadows, pastures, and along agricultural fields. Its leaves are narrow, delicate, and bipinnatipartite. Yarrow flowers are small and its colors range from white to pale yellow to red. Large numbers of flowers form dense clusters (▶ Fig. 3.29).

Medicinal applications use **yarrow herb** (fresh or dried above-ground parts, Millefolii herba) and **yarrow flowers** (Millefolii flos).

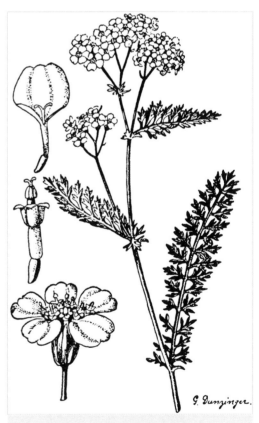

Fig. 3.29 Yarrow, Achillea millefolium.

▸ **Pharmacology.** Yarrow contains bitter sesquiterpene lactones, flavonoids, tannins, and 0.1–0.5% volatile oil.

During steam distillation, yarrow develops proazulene oil that is very similar in its effects to blue chamomile oil. Like chamomile, yarrow is **antiphlogistic**. However, unlike chamomile, this effect does not determine the overall effect of yarrow.

▸ **Note.** The proazulene or blue oil content of yarrow varies widely and should be stated on the label of medicinal yarrow products (Orth and Kempster). Some types of yarrow contain practically no volatile oil.

▸ **Indications.** The indication of yarrow for liver disorders is not as clearly defined as for the other plants in this chapter. Yarrow is primarily a tonic bitter with a few additional anti-inflammatory, carminative, and spasmolytic properties. This makes yarrow useful for treating **upper abdominal symptoms** in patients with liver disorders.

Its combination of active constituents makes yarrow applicable for biliary disorders. Its predominant bitter effects also make it useful for atonic gastric disorders. The Commission E monograph for yarrow lists the following indications: loss of appetite and dyspeptic ailments, such as mild, spastic symptoms in the gastrointestinal tract.

Preparation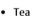

- **Tea**
  Add 1 cup of hot water to 1 teaspoon of the finely chopped drug. Steep covered for 5 minutes, then strain.
  Drink 1 cup several times a day.

▸ **Therapy Recommendation.** Practical experience has shown that moist warm liver compresses made with yarrow tea are quite effective. Yarrow's spasmolytic effects help to reduce unpleasant symptoms of bloating in patients with chronic liver disorders. They are best used midday, when patients with chronic liver disease should take a rest and lie down, or in the evening, at bedtime.

Bibliography

Boigk G, Stroedter L, Herbst H, Waldschmidt J, Riecken EO, Schuppan D. Silymarin retards collagen accumulation in early and advanced biliary fibrosis secondary to complete bile duct obliteration in rats. Hepatology. 1997; 26(3):643–649

Bundy R, Walker AF, Middleton RW, Wallis C, Simpson HCR. Artichoke leaf extract (Cynara scolymus) reduces plasma cholesterol in otherwise healthy hypercholesterolemic adults: a randomized, double-blind placebo-controlled trial. Phytomedicine. 2008; 15(9):668–675

Englisch W, Beckers C, Unkauf M, Ruepp M, Zinserling V. Efficacy of Artichoke dry extract in patients with hyperlipoproteinemia. Arzneimittelforschung. 2000; 50(3):260–265

Fehér J, Csomos G, Vereckei A. Free Radical Reactions in Medicine. Berlin: Springer; 1987

Ferenci P, Dragosics B, Dittrich H, et al. Randomized controlled trial of silymarin treatment in patients with cirrhosis of the liver. J Hepatol. 1989; 9(1):105–113

Ferenci P, Scherzer TM, Kerschner H, et al. Silibinin is a potent antiviral agent in patients with chronic hepatitis C not responding to pegylated interferon/ribavirin therapy. Gastroenterology. 2008; 135(5):1561–1567

Filip J, Brodanova M, Chlumsky J. Weitere Möglichkeiten der Anwendung von Legalon in der Behandlung von Lebererkrankungen. In: Csomos G, ed Aktuelle Hepatologie. Hamburg: Hanseatisches Verlagskontor; 1977

Fintelmann V, Albert A. Nachweis der therapeutischen Wirksamkeit von Legalon® bei toxischen Lebererkrankungen im Doppelblindversuch. Therapiewoche. 1980; 30:5589–5594

Fintelmann V, Petrowicz O. Langzeitanwendung eines Artischocken-Extraktes bei dyspeptischem Syndrom. Naturamed. 1998; 13: 17–26

Fintelmann V. Antidyspeptische und lipidsenkende Wirkungen von Artischockenextrakt. Ergebnisse klinischer Untersuchungen zur Wirksamkeit und Verträglichkeit von Hepar SL® forte an 533 Patienten. Z Allgemeinmed. 1996; 72:48–57

Fintelmann V. Der toxisch-metabolische Leberschaden und seine Behandlung. Z. f. Phytotherapie. 1986; 7:65–73

Fintelmann V. Postoperatives Verhalten der Serumcholinesterase und anderer Leberenzyme [Postoperative behavior of serum cholinesterase and other liver enzymes]. Med Klin. 1973; 68(24):809–815

Fintelmann V. Zur Therapie der Fettleber mit Silymarin. Therapiewoche. 1970; 20:1055–1062

Floersheim GL, Weber O, Tschumi P, Ulbrich M. Die klinische Knollenblätterpilzvergiftung (Amanita phalloides): prognostische Faktoren und therapeutische Massnahmen. Eine Analyse anhand von 205 Fällen [Clinical death-cap (Amanita phalloides) poisoning: prognostic factors and therapeutic measures. Analysis of 205 cases]. Schweiz Med Wochenschr. 1982; 112 (34):1164–1177

Gebhardt R. Artischockenextrakt: In-vitro-Nachweis einer Hemmwirkung auf die Cholesterin-Biosynthese. Med Welt. 1995a; 46:348–350

Gebhardt R. Inhibition of cholesterol biosynthesis by artichoke (Cynara scolymus L.) extracts. Secondary Products—Physiologically Active Compounds, 43rd Annual Congress, Soc. Med. Plant. Res., Halle, 03.–07.09.1995; 1995 b

Gebhardt R. In-vitro-Nachweis der Hepatoprotektion durch Artischockenblätterextrakt am Beispiel von Tetrachlorkohlenstoff. Pharm Ztg. 1995c; 140:34–37

Gebhardt R. Protektive antioxidative Wirkungen von Artischocken-Extrakt an der Leberzelle. Med Welt. 1995d; 46:393–395

Hammerl H, Pichler O. Untersuchungen über den Einflusseines Artischockenextraktes auf die Serumlipide im Hinblick auf die Arterioseprophylaxe. Wien Med Wochenschr. 1959; 109: 853–855

Kiesewetter E, Leodolter I, Thaler H. Ergebnisse zweier Doppelblindstudien zur Wirksamkeit von Silymarin bei chronischer Hepatitis [Results of two double-blind studies on the effect of silymarine in chronic hepatitis]. Leber Magen Darm. 1977; 7(5):318–323

Kirchhoff R, Beckers C, Kirchhoff B, Trinczek-Gärtner H, Petrowicz O, Reimann HJ. Steigerung der Cholerese durch Artischockenextrakt—Ergebnisse einer placebokontrollierten Doppelblindstudie. Arztl Forsch. 1993; 40(6):1–12

Kirchhoff R, Beckers C, Kirchhoff GM, Trinczek-Gärtner H, Petrowicz O, Reimann HJ. Increase in choleresis by means of artichoke extract. Phytomedicine. 1994; 1(2):107–115

Kurz-Dimitrowa D. Leberschutzbehandlung psychiatrisch-neurologischer Patienten bei Langzeittherapie mit Psychopharmaka. Zeitschrift für Präklininische Geriatrie. 1971; 9:275

Maros T, Rácz G, Katonai B, Kovács VV. Wirkungen der Cynara Scolymus-Extrakte auf die Regeneration der Rattenleber [Effects of Cynara Scolymus extracts on the regeneration of rat liver]. 1. Arzneimittelforschung. 1966; 16(2):127–129

Maros T, Seres-Sturm L, Rácz G, Rettegi C, Kovács VV, Hints M. Wirkungen der Cynara scolymus-Extrakte auf die Regeneration der Rattenleber [Effects of Cynara scolymus-extracts on the regeneration of rat liver]. 2. Arzneimittelforschung. 1968; 18(7):884–886

Matuschowski P, Nahrstedt A, Winterhoff H. Pharmakologische Untersuchungen eines Frischpflanzenpresssaftes aus Cynara scolymus auf choleretische Wirkung. Z Phytother. 2005; 26:14–19

Orth M, Kempster M. Neues über die uralte Arzneipflanze Schafgarbe. Z Phytother. 1998; 19(3):156–160

Orth M. Zusammensetzung und Biologie der ätherischen Öle von Achillea millefolium L. Z Phytother. 1999; 20(6):345–346

Pohl RT. Silibinin wirksam bei Hepatitis C. NaturaMed. 2013; 6:40–46

Pohl RT. Wie Silibinin das Hepatitis-C-Virus bekämpft. Z Phytother. 2013; 34(5):221–226

Polyak SJ, Ferenci P, Pawlotsky JM. Hepatoprotective and antiviral functions of silymarin components in hepatitis C virus infection. Hepatology. 2013; 57(3):1262–1271

Saba P, Galeone F, Salvadorini F, Guarguaglini M, Troyer C. Therapeutische Wirkung von Silymarin bei durch Psychopharmaka verursachten chronischen Hepatitiden. Gazz Med Ital. 1976; 135(4):236–251

Salmi HA. Sarna S. Effect of silymarin on chemical, functional, and morphological alterations of the liver. A double-blind controlled study. Scand J Gastroenterol. 1982; 17(4):517–521

Schuppan D, Stösser W, Burkard G, Walosek G. Verminderung der Fibrosierungsaktivität durch Legalon bei chronischen Lebererkrankungen. Z Allgemeinmed. 1998; 74:577–584

Sonnenbichler J, Zetl I. Untersuchungen zum Wirkungs-mechanismus von Silibinin. V. Einfluss von Silibinin auf die Synthese ribosomaler RNA, mRNA und tRNA in Rattenlebern in vivo [Mechanism of action of silibinin. V. Effect of silibinin on the synthesis of ribosomal RNA, mRNA and tRNA in rat liver in vivo]. Hoppe Seylers Z Physiol Chem. 1984; 365(5):555–566

Vogel G, Trost W, Braatz R, et al. Untersuchungen zur Pharmakodynamik, Angriffspunkt und Wirkungsmechanismus von Silymarin, dem antihepatotoxischen Prinzip aus Silybum marianum (L.) Gaertn. 1. Mitteilung: Akute Toxikologie bzw. Verträglichkeit, allgemeine und spezielle (Leber-)Pharmakologie. [Pharmacodynamics, site and mechanism of action of silymarin, the antihepatoxic principle from Silybum mar. (L) Gaertn. 1. Acute toxicology or tolerance, general and specific (liver-) pharmacology].. Arzneimittelforschung. 1975; 25(1):82–89

Wagner H, Hörhammer L, Münster R. Zur Chemie des Silymarins (Silybin), des Wirkprinzips der Früchte von Silybum marianum (L.) Gaertn. (Carduus marianus L.) [On the chemistry of silymarin (silybin), the active principle of the fruits from Silybum marianum (L.) Gaertn. (Carduus marianus L.)]. Arzneimittelforschung. 1968; 18(6):688–696

Wichtl M, Ed. Teedrogen und Phytopharmaka. 5. ed Stuttgart: Wissenschaftliche Verlagsgesellschaft; 2008

Winter Y, Wegener T. Zuverlässige Wirkungen des Presssaftes aus Artischockenblütenknospen bei Verdauungsbeschwerden. Z Phytother. 2009; 30(3):111–116

3.4.2 Biliary Dyskinesia

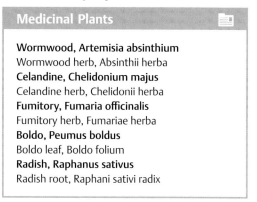

Medicinal Plants

Wormwood, Artemisia absinthium
Wormwood herb, Absinthii herba
Celandine, Chelidonium majus
Celandine herb, Chelidonii herba
Fumitory, Fumaria officinalis
Fumitory herb, Fumariae herba
Boldo, Peumus boldus
Boldo leaf, Boldo folium
Radish, Raphanus sativus
Radish root, Raphani sativi radix

Many gastroenterologists strictly deny that biliary dyskinesia exists because it is diagnosed based on subjective complaints and by excluding organic changes. Patients complain about **nonspecific symptoms** in the right upper abdomen that can radiate to the back or to the right shoulder and can develop into mild colic. Weiss included fat intolerance or worsening of symptoms caused by fatty meals into this symptoms complex. Laboratory tests do not show cholestasis. Test meals to show gallbladder response are inconclusive because many people who are nonsymptomatic also show no or very little gallbladder response to test meals. The patient's symptoms may also be caused by irritable bowel disorders because the gallbladder and the bile duct are located in the same area as the right colic flexure (hepatic flexure).

The biliary system may also frequently contribute to dyspeptic symptoms. This comprehensive term describes the complex interactions in the upper digestive tract. It is subject to complicated hormonal regulation that assures synergistic cooperation between all organs that play a significant role in the digestive process. If one organ does not participate or reacts too slowly, the entire system becomes imbalanced. The medicinal plants and remedies used to treat functional dyspepsia are discussed below (see Chapter 3.5 (p. 121) "Functional Dyspepsia" (p. 121)).

There is much discussion about phytotherapeutic remedies that are specific to the biliary system. Clinical specialists consider phytotherapeutic cholagogues as unnecessary. Practitioners, however, frequently prescribe these remedies—usually as combination drugs (Hänsel 1985; Maiwald 1985; Schilcher 1995; Seifert).

Prescribing **plant-based cholagogues** can certainly address the patient's subjective feeling of being ill. Disdain and references to placebo effects are countered by manifold studies that show objective results. Maiwald (1969; 1983; 1985; 1991), who has conducted and published many comprehensive studies of bile-active phytotherapeutics, has demonstrated choleretic and spasmolytic effects for plant-based cholagogues. These remedies can also stimulate pancreatic secretions. In any case, patients experiencing biliary dyspepsia symptoms have the right to be taken just as seriously as, for example, patients diagnosed with symptomless cholecystolithiasis.

Specific cholecystokinetic effects have been shown primarily for turmeric (p. 122). Artichoke leaf extract (p. 106), which is discussed in detail in the previous chapter (p. 106), has proven choleretic effects. These remedies are covered in the chapters that discuss their main indications.

▶ **Note.** Weiss attempted to differentiate between choleretics and cholagogues: cholagogues stimulate bile production and choleretics increase bile flow. However, he also admitted that it is not possible to draw a clear line between these two types of remedies. In practical use, the term cholagogues is now used as a kind of umbrella term for all remedies that promote an increased flow of bile.

Plants for Treatment
Wormwood (Artemisia absinthium)

Wormwood is a member of the Asteraceae family, with small, inconspicuous yellow flowers, and whitish-gray pannose pinnatipartite leaves (▶ Fig. 3.30). It grows wild along fences, roads, and in waste disposal areas and can reach a height of up to 1 m. It is also easily cultivated in gardens.

The plant has a strong and pungently aromatic odor.

Medicinal applications use the **wormwood herb** (fresh or dried upper shoots and leaves, or fresh or dried basal leaves, or a mixture of these plant parts, Absinthii herba), harvested during the flowering season.

▶ **Pharmacology.** The wormwood herb contains a minimum of 0.3% (w/v) volatile oil (Oleum Absinthii), α-thujone, β-thujone, thujyl alcohol, monoterpenes, and sesquiterpenes. It also contains

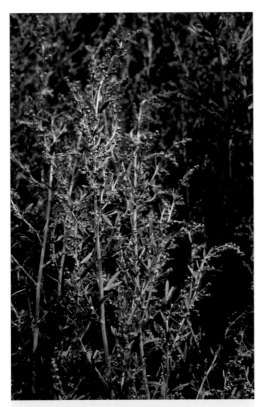

Fig. 3.30 Wormwood, Artemisia absinthium. Photo: Dr. Roland Spohn, Engen.

sesquiterpene lactone bitters, primarily absinthin and anabsinthin, plus flavones, ascorbic acid, and tannins. Bitter is by far the dominating principle in wormwood. Its bittering power is a minimum of 15,000.

Unlike wormwood oil (Oleum Absinthii), which contains thujone, the bitter constituents in the wormwood herb are largely nontoxic. Wormwood oil is used in the manufacture of absinthe, a blend of wormwood oil and alcohol that is especially popular as an aperitif in France. In Germany, special legislation made the making of absinthe illegal in 1923 because of its toxic effect on the central nervous system (CNS) with excessive use. In 1998, absinthe became available on the market again, but with much lower limits for its thujone content. The usual standardized finished pharmaceutical wormwood products contain so little of the

dangerous wormwood oil (Oleum Absinthii) that no damaging effects are to be expected.

Isolated wormwood essential oil is not used because of its toxicity.

▶ **Indications.** Wormwood is a typical aromatic bitter. It is also a pronounced **carminative** and **choleretic**. In addition to its bitter effects, wormwood has a stimulating psychedelic effect on the CNS that is balancing and regulating. This differentiates wormwood from other bitter drugs. One cup of wormwood tea can often be more helpful for lack of concentration than a cup of coffee.

Wormwood is a very reliable gastric and biliary remedy. It helps with minor symptoms of atonic and achylic gastric conditions that are often a sign of **biliary system hypofunction** and with digestion of foods that cause bloating and meteorism. Wormwood is one of the best remedies for **biliary dyskinesia**. Countless people with biliary disorders can improve their symptoms again and again using a simple wormwood tincture. However, wormwood fails to help with severe biliary colic. For this reason, wormwood is described in this chapter even though it could have been included in the section on Bitters (amara) (p. 52).

The Commission E lists the following indications in its monograph for wormwood: loss of appetite, dyspepsia caused by bile excretion problems of the gallbladder, and biliary dyskinesia.

Preparations

- **Tea**
  Add 1 cup of boiling water to 1 teaspoon of the finely chopped drug. Steep covered briefly, for 1–2 minutes, then strain.
  Drink 15 to 30 minutes after meals.
- **Tincture**
  Add 10–30 drops to plenty of water, since the bitter taste improves with increasing dilution.
  Drink 3 × a day.

▶ **Therapy Recommendations.** People suffering from gallbladder disorders should always carry a bottle of **wormwood tincture** when traveling. This allows them to treat problems that might occur when deviating from their usual diet. Because of the higher thujone content of the tincture as compared with aqueous extractions, the maximum daily dose for wormwood tincture should not exceed 60 drops a day, and regular use should be limited to a few weeks.

Wormwood tea is best drunk some time after meals to stimulate primarily the gallbladder rather than the stomach. Its bitter taste is best tolerated if the tea is consumed while still comfortably warm.

It does not make sense to sweeten the bitter wormwood tea because sweet and bitter flavors do not harmonize. Surprisingly, many patients grow accustomed to and develop a genuine liking for the bitter flavor of wormwood tea.

Wormwood tea regimens should last no longer than 3–4 weeks. If gallbladder symptoms subsequently worsen again—for example, as a result of poor dietary choices, anxiety, or physical strain—the tea can be used again occasionally.

Celandine (Chelidonium majus)

Celandine belongs to the Papaveraceae (poppy) family. Like the opium poppy (Papaver somniferum), celandine contains an orange-yellow milky juice that can be found in the entire plant, including the roots. Its medium-size flowers are bright golden yellow. The plant has many branches and lyrate, pinnate leaves (▶ Fig. 3.31).

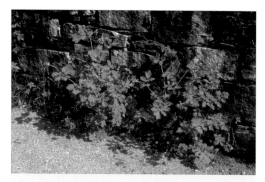

Fig. 3.31 Celandine, Chelidonium majus. Photo: Dr. Roland Spohn, Engen.

Celandine is a typical ruderal species and consequently prefers to grow near human settlements. It can be found along fences, roads, as a weed in the garden, and even in cities.

Medicinal applications use the **celandine herb** (dried above-ground parts, Chelidonii herba) that is collected and dried while the plant is in bloom.

▶ **Pharmacology.** The celandine herb contains a minimum of 0.6% total alkaloids (chelidonine) based on the dry drug. The main alkaloid, according to recent studies, is coptisine (Schilcher 1997). Chelidonine is primarily concentrated in the roots. The main alkaloid components are benzophenan-thridine (including chelidonine) and protoberberines (including coptisine and protopine).

During the flowering stage, celandine's total alkaloid content seems to be on the lower side. For this reason, the regulation by the German Pharmacopoeia (DAB) to harvest the plant during bloom should be questioned (Schilcher 1997).

▶ **Research.** As far back as 1939, Daniel and Schmaltz showed in animal experiments that 2 mg/kg chelidonine increased bile production by 60%. Baumann et al. found slow, but continuous increases in bile flow in animal experiments. They attributed these increases more to celandine's choleretic than its cholekinetic effect.

More recently to those studies, induction of toxic hepatitis by celandine was not confirmed clinically and was also largely ruled out by experimental *in vitro* trials (Adler et al.).

▶ **Indications.** About 30 alkaloids have been documented for celandine. They are mild analgesics, CNS sedatives, and spasmolytics. The spasmolytic effect acts directly on smooth muscles. Celandine's overall mild sedative, cholagogic (choleretic/cholecystokinetic), and spasmolytic actions make it suitable for treating **spasm in the gastrointestinal tract**, including biliary tract and gallbladder spasms.

The Commission E monograph for celandine lists the following indications: spastic discomfort of the bile ducts and gastrointestinal tract.

Preparations

Celandine is well suited for combining with other cholagogues because of its alkaloid content and resulting cholekinetic and spasmolytic actions. When celandine is used by an experienced practitioner, it can be a very effective therapeutic for treating conditions that primarily focus on the drug's spasmolytic action. However, belladonna is a much more potent drug for these conditions.

- **Tea**
  Add 1 cup of hot water to 2 teaspoons of the finely chopped drug. Steep covered for 5–10 minutes, then strain.
  Drink warm 3 × a day between meals for 3 weeks.
- **Tincture**
  Add 20 drops to a small amount of water. Drink 3 × a day.

- **Cholagogue Tincture** (Tinctura cholagoga, according to the German Prescription Formulas, DRF)

Prescriptions

Rx
Tinct. Cardui Mariae 10.0 (milk thistle tincture)
Tinct. Chelidonii (celandine tincture)
Tinct. Strychni āā 5.0 (nux vomica tincture, Strychni semen)
D.S.
Add 30 drops to a small amount of water. Drink 3 × a day.

- **Strong Cholagogue Tincture** (Tinctura cholagoga fortis, according to the German Prescription Formulas, DRF)
  This tincture is stronger than the cholagogue tincture (DRF) above because it includes the spasmolytic influence of belladonna and the choleretic influence of peppermint:

Prescriptions

Rx
Ol. Menth. pip. 1.0 (peppermint essential oil)
Tinct. Belladonnae 4.0 (belladonna tincture)
Tinct. Chelidonii (celandine tincture)
Tinct. Cardui Mariae āā ad 30.0 (milk thistle tincture)
D.S.
Add 40 drops to a small amount of water. Drink 3 × a day.

Fumitory (Fumaria officinalis)

Fumitory is an old medicinal plant. It is part of the Papaveraceae family that includes poppy (Papaver somniferum) and celandine.

This annual herbaceous plant with bipinnate tender leaves and small, calcarate, purplish pink flowers with crimson tips is a common weed in agricultural fields. It is found throughout Europe and grows wild along roads, in poor soil, and as a weed in the garden (▶ Fig. 3.32).). Its name is derived from the Latin *fumus*, meaning smoke, and refers to the fact that when fumitory is burned, the smoke is irritating to the eyes. Its French name is *fumeterre* or earth smoke.

Medicinal applications use the **fumitory herb** (dried above-ground parts, Fumariae herba), harvested during the flowering season.

▶ **Pharmacology.** Like other members of the Papaveraceae (poppy) family, fumitory is a rich source of alkaloids. Fumitory also contains isoquinoline alkaloids, for example, fumarin.

▶ **Indications.** Fumarin is primarily spasmolytic, similar to the effects of papaverine derived from poppy. This effect has been shown to act on the biliary and gastrointestinal tract. Fumitory is considered an amphocholeretic because studies have shown that it increases insufficient bile secretion and inhibits overly active choleresis (Fiegel). Its gallbladder regulating function makes it suitable as a general cholagogue. Fumitory's specific indications, however, are **spastic symptoms** in the gallbladder and biliary tract area and in the upper

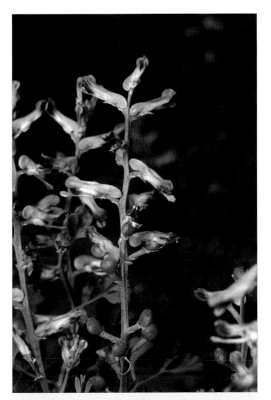

Fig. 3.32 Fumitory, Fumaria officinalis. Photo: Dr. Roland Spohn, Engen.

slender branches, and its bark is light brown. Its leaves are attached by short petioles and are leathery, elliptical, and covered in tufts of hair. Boldo blooms all year.

Medicinal applications use the **boldo leaves** (Boldo folium).

▶ **Pharmacology.** Boldo leaves contain 0.2–0.5% alkaloids in methanol extractions. Its main alkaloid, boldine, is a benzylisoquinoline alkaloid in the aporphine class. Other components include polyphenols and a volatile oil. Ascaridol, one of the constituents of boldo volatile oil, is a reactive endoperoxide considered to be somewhat toxic. It was, for example, used as an anthelmintic. It is, however, poorly water-soluble and aqueous boldo leaf extracts are considered quite safe toxicologically. Boldo leaves have antioxidant, anti-inflammatory, hepatoprotective, and cholagogue effects (Latté).

▶ **Indications.** Boldo leaf extracts are spasmolytic and choleretic and increase gastric juice secretion. They are indicated for dyspeptic disorders, especially if accompanied by **spastic symptoms**.

Their comparatively milder action makes boldo leaves especially suitable for combining with other biliary system remedies discussed here. Relevant clinical studies are not yet available.

gastrointestinal tract. These are also the indications listed for fumitory in the Commission E monograph.

Fumitory is well suited for combining with other cholagogues and antidyspeptics.

▶ **Note.** Fumitory's spasmolytic action is also thought to affect the sphincter of Oddi (Wagner).

Preparation

- **Tea**
  Add 1 cup of hot water to 2 teaspoons of chopped fumitory herb. Steep covered for 10 minutes, then strain.
  Drink 1 cup several times a day with meals.

Boldo (Peumus boldus)

Boldo is a shrub or tree that can grow to a height of 6 m. Its main native habitat is Chile. Boldo has

---

Preparations

- **Tea**
  Add 1 cup of boiling water to 2 teaspoons of the finely chopped drug. Steep covered for 10 minutes, then strain.
  Drink 1 cup 2–3 × a day.
- **Fluid Extract**
  Add 20 drops, for example, to a cup of chamomile tea.
  Drink 3 × a day.

Radish (Raphanus)

Radish is a cultivated plant that originates from Asia and has many cultivars, from the small red breakfast radish to the giant daikon.

Radish plants can grow to more than 1 m in height. Its leaves are lyrate and pinnately cleft. Its flowers are pale violet to white with violet veins

(▶ Fig. 3.33). Radishes are in the Brassicaceae family along with mustard, cabbage, and rape (canola).

Medicinal applications primarily use **fresh radish root juice** (Raphani sativi radix) derived from the black Spanish radish (Raphanus sativus ssp. niger).

▶ **Indications.** Application areas for radish are **chronic biliary dyskinesia** and tendency toward dyspeptic symptoms with constipation.

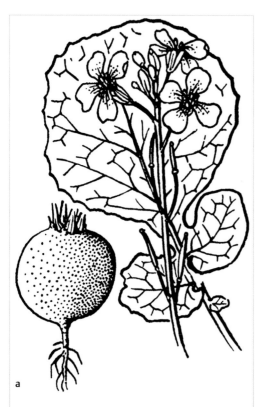

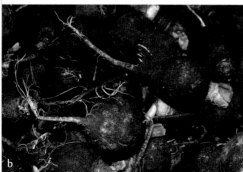

Fig. 3.33 a and b Radish, Raphanus sativus. Photo: Dr. Roland Spohn, Engen.

Radish is an old folk remedy for biliary disorders. However, many studies have shown that radish juice is not a bile stimulant, but an intestinal tonifier. It mildly stimulates peristalsis and promotes fecal transit. It can even cause mild diarrhea. Radish's positive impact on the biliary system and the liver, therefore, is indirect via its influence on the intestines. The tonifying effect of radish possibly also acts on the smooth muscles of the biliary system and improves bile flow.

> ## Caution
>
> Many people do not tolerate radish juice well and develop gastric symptoms with acid reflux and belching. When this happens, it indicates that radish juice is causing too much irritation in the stomach and that a different remedy should be chosen.

> ## Preparation
>
> - **Freshly Pressed Juice**
>   Peel and chop or grate white or black radish. Juice by using a manual press, juicer, or a blender and strainer. Refrigerate the juice for a few hours to neutralize its initially pungent flavor. A small amount of sugar or, better yet, some flaxseed gruel can be added just before consumption.
>   One medium-size radish supplies a generous daily dose of about 250 mL of juice.

▶ **Therapy Recommendation.** Radish juice needs to be used long term as a **regimen** to develop its effect. The average daily dose is 100 to 150 mL, divided into individual portions. After every 4 or 5 days of drinking the juice, there should be a 2- or 3-day break.

Proven Prescriptions: Cholagogue Teas

Functional biliary disorders are complex, often with very individualized symptoms. This makes them very suitable for treatments using tea or tincture mixture prescriptions.

There are many plants to choose from and treatment should be focused on plants that meet all requirements. Determining the main individual indication is key. Is it stimulating bile flow, or is it the carminative and spasmolytic or tonifying effects? Most patients with biliary system disorders also need mild, balanced stimulation of their digestion and the addition of a mild laxative may make sense.

- **Basic Prescription with Four Components** (that provide phytotherapeutic synergism)

Prescriptions

Rx
Menth. pip. fol. 50.0 (peppermint leaves)
(= cholagogue main component)
Melissae fol. 20.0 (lemon balm leaves)
(= sedative adjuvant [supplement])
Foeniculi fruct. 20.0 (fennel seeds)
(= supplemental carminative)
Frangulae cort. 10.0 (buckthorn bark)
(= mild laxative)
M. f. spec.
Add 1 cup of hot water to 1–2 teaspoons of the blend. Steep covered for 1–2 minutes, then strain.
D.S.
Drink 1 cup 3 × a day in small sips while still comfortably warm (after meals and at bedtime).

- **Tea to Stimulate Bile Flow**

Prescriptions

Rx
Cnici benedicti herb. (blessed thistle herb)
Absinthii herb. (wormwood herb)
Menth. pip. fol. (peppermint leaves)
Cardui Mariae fruct. (milk thistle seeds)
Taraxaci rad. c. herb. āā ad 100.0 (dandelion root and herb)
M. f. spec.
Add 1–2 cups of boiling water to 1 teaspoon of the blend. Steep covered for 20 minutes, then strain.
D.S.
Drink 3 cups a day for 3–4 weeks.

- **Predominantly Carminative and Mild Laxative Tea**

Prescriptions

Rx
Carvi fruct. (caraway seeds)
Foeniculi fruct. āā 10.0 (fennel seeds)
Menth. pip. fol. 30.0 (peppermint leaves)
Millefolii herb. (yarrow herb)
Stoechad. flos āā 20.0 (sandy everlasting flowers, Helichrysum arenarium)
Sennae fol. 15.0 (senna leaves)
M. f. spec.
Add 1 cup of hot water to 1–2 teaspoons of the blend. Steep covered for 15 minutes, then strain.
D.S.
Regularly drink 1 cup in the morning and in the evening.

If the above tea does not provide sufficient laxative effects, senna can be increased up to double the given amount. Initially, it can be helpful to start with 1 tablespoon of the herb blend and 1 cup of water instead of 1–2 teaspoons. The tea derives a pleasant color from the use of sandy everlasting (Helichrysum arenarium), also referred to as "Stoechado flos." This tea should not be taken for more than 4 weeks.

- **Bitter Tea That Provides Good Biliary Tonification as well as Carminative and Mild Laxative Effects**

Prescriptions

Rx
Carvi fruct. 10.0 (caraway seeds)
Menth. pip. Fol (peppermint leaves)
Absinthii herb. āā 30.0 (wormwood herb)
Frangul. cort. (buckthorn bark)
Sennae fol. conc. āā 15.0 (chopped senna leaves)
M. f. spec.
Add 1 cup of hot water to 1–2 teaspoons of the blend. Steep covered for 10 minutes, then strain.
D.S.
Drink 1 cup in the morning and in the evening.

The prescription above is a time-tested excellent tea, and patients request it again and again.

However, it should only be prescribed for short periods because of its laxative component.

- **Strongly Bitter and Bile-Stimulating Tea**

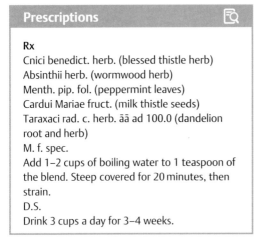

Prescriptions

Rx
Cnici benedict. herb. (blessed thistle herb)
Absinthii herb. (wormwood herb)
Menth. pip. fol. (peppermint leaves)
Cardui Mariae fruct. (milk thistle seeds)
Taraxaci rad. c. herb. āā ad 100.0 (dandelion root and herb)
M. f. spec.
Add 1–2 cups of boiling water to 1 teaspoon of the blend. Steep covered for 20 minutes, then strain.
D.S.
Drink 3 cups a day for 3–4 weeks.

▶ **Therapy Recommendation.** The flavor of all biliary teas can be improved by adding sugar or honey. Diabetics or calorie-conscious patients can use artificial sweeteners.

Cholagogue Tinctures

As with teas, there is a large selection of tinctures to choose from. Adding belladonna tincture can increase spasmolytic effects. If mild laxative effects are desired, tea mixtures should be the treatment of choice.

- **Strongly Carminative and Sedative Tincture Blend**

Prescriptions

Rx
Ol. Carvi 5.0 (caraway essential oil)
Tinct. Absinthii (wormwood tincture)
Tinct. carminativ. (see Carminative Tinctures (p. 79))
Tinct. Belladonnae āā 10.0 (belladonna tincture)
Tinct. Valerian. aeth. 15.0 (ethereal valerian tincture)
D.S.
Take 30 drops 3 × a day after meals.

- **Strong Bitter, Tonifying Tincture Blend for Stimulating Appetite**

Prescriptions

Rx
Tinct. Cardui Mariae (milk thistle tincture)
Tinct. Absinthii āā 15.0 (wormwood tincture)
Spir. Menth. pip. 20.0 (spirit of peppermint)
D.S.
Add 20 drops to a small amount of water. Drink shortly before meals, 2 × a day.

- **Antispasmodic Tincture Blend**

Prescriptions

Rx
Ol. Carvi 5.0 (caraway essential oil)
Tinct. Belladonnae (belladonna tincture)
Tinct. Chelidonii (celandine tincture)
Tinct. Cardui Mariae āā 10.0 (milk thistle tincture)
Tinct. Valerian. aeth. 15.0 (ethereal valerian tincture)
D.S.
Take 20 drops 3 × a day.

- **Antispasmodic, Carminative, and Bitter Tincture Blend**

Prescriptions

Rx
Tinct. Belladonnae (belladonna tincture)
Tinct. Absinthii (wormwood tincture)
Tinct. Cardui Mariae (milk thistle tincture)
Tinct. Foeniculi comp (p. 79). (fennel tincture composite)
Tinct. Chamomillae āā 10.0 (German chamomile tincture)
D.S.
Take 20 drops in a small amount of water after midday and evening meals.

▶ **Therapy Recommendation.** Cholagogic (bile-stimulating) tinctures are important for treating acute symptoms. Patients with biliary system disorders should always carry these tinctures with them and use them at the first sign of symptoms after eating large meals or any foods that cause severe bloating.

For references corresponding to the preceding section, see Bibliography following 3.4.3.

3.4.3 Gallstones, Postcholecystectomy Syndrome

Gallstones that are causing symptoms are clearly an indication for surgery. Minimally invasive surgery techniques are constantly being perfected and make a **cholecystectomy** possible even for high-risk or very old patients. Surgical removal of asymptomatic, so-called silent gallstones continues to be more controversial. It is being justified primarily as a preventive to avoid possible complications from obstructive jaundice or potential development of gallbladder cancer. The latter is found in about 10% of cholecystolithiasis patients.

The decision should be made between the physician and the patient on a case-by-case basis and should include a detailed consideration of the potential complications of surgery. This particularly includes postsurgical postcholecystectomy syndrome.

Patients who have undergone a cholecystectomy frequently experience the same postsurgery symptoms they had presurgery and that led to the decision to have surgery in the first place (Seifert). Sometimes, postsurgery symptoms are even more severe than they were presurgery. This is rarely attributable to genuine postoperative complications like biliary tract blockages or choledocholithiasis not identified during surgery. The most frequent reason for the recurrence of symptoms postsurgery is that gallstones were not the cause of the upper abdominal symptoms that led to the surgery. Functional postcholecystectomy symptoms require the same cholagogue therapy as biliary tract dyskinesia (see "Biliary Dyskinesia" (p. 111)).

▶ **Research.** Older studies by Gracie and Ransohoff show that a majority of 3,326 patients examined between 1956 and 1969 due to asymptomatic gallstones and observed over the course of years remained symptomless for more than 15 years. The results of this study indicate that the risk of developing symptoms decreases in longer term. The few cases in which patients developed complications were preceded by warning symptoms. The authors'

summary assessment was very clear: Let resting gallstones rest.

According to Koslowski, no "objective" cause was found for the development of biliary symptoms in about two-thirds of patients with postcholecystectomy syndrome. These patients were eventually diagnosed with biliary tract dyskinesia and functional or psychovegetative disorders following, often times, extensive diagnostics. Seifert concludes that these symptoms were the same as the presurgery symptoms that were falsely attributed to existing, but silent gallstones.

Plants for Treatment

For more information about treating postcholecystectomy syndrome, see Biliary Dyskinesia (p. 111). All plants discussed in that chapter are also applicable to this indication.

Proven Prescriptions

See Proven Prescriptions: Cholagogue Teas (p. 116).

Bibliography

Adler M, Appel K, Canal T, et al. Wirkung von Schöllkrautextrakten an humanen Hepatozyten in vitro. Z Phytother. 2006; 27–P01:19

Baumann JC, Heintze K, Muth HW. Klinisch-experimentelle Untersuchungen der Gallen-, Pankreas- und Magensaftsekretion unter den phytocholagogen Wirkstoffen einer Carduus marianus-Chelidonium-Curcuma-Suspension [Clinico-experimental studies on the secretion of bile, pancreatic and gastric juice under the influence of phyto-cholagogous agents of a suspension of Carduus marianus, Chelidonium and Curcuma]. Arzneimittelforschung. 1971; 21(1):98–101

Daniel K, Schmaltz D. Das Schöllkraut. Stuttgart: Hippokrates; 1939

Fiegel G. Die amphocholeretische Wirkung der Fumaria officinalis [.Amphocholeretic effect of Fumaria officinalis]. Z Allg Med. 1971; 47(34):1819–1820

Gracie WA, Ransohoff DF. The natural history of silent gallstones: the innocent gallstone is not a myth. N Engl J Med. 1982; 307 (13):798–800

Hänsel R. Pflanzliche Cholagoga. Dtsch Apoth Ztg. 1985; 125:1373–1378

Hänsel W. Die Gelbwurzel—Curcuma domestica Val., Curcuma xanthorrhiza Roxb. Z Phytother. 1997; 18:297–306

Koslowski L. Gibt es eine chronische Appendizitis mit der Indikation zur Operation. Med Welt. 1983; 34:393–394

Latté KP. Boldoblätter. Die Blattdroge von Peumus boldus Molina. Z Phytother. 2014; 35(1):40–46

Maiwald L, Hengstmann D. Objektivierung einer gebesserten Cholerese. Therapiewoche. 1969; 19:1661

Maiwald L, Schwantes PA. Curcuma xanthorrhiza Roxb., eine Heilpflanze tritt aus dem therapeutischen Schattendasein. Z Phytother. 1991; 12:435–445

Maiwald L. Pflanzliche Cholagoga. Z Allgemeinmed. 1983; 59:1304

Maiwald L. Pflanzliche Choleretika und Cholagoga. Der Kassenarzt. 1985; 25(7):40–44

Schilcher H. Pharmazeutische Aspekte pflanzlicher Gallentherapeutika. Z Phytother. 1995; 16:211–222

Schilcher H. Schöllkraut—Chelidonium majus L. Z Phytother. 1997; 18(6):356–366

Seifert E. Postcholezystektomiesyndrom und endoskopische retrograde Cholangiopankreatographie nach Cholezystektomie. Therapiewoche. 1982; 32:2793–2798

Wagner H, Wiesenauer M. Phytotherapie: Phytopharmaka und pflanzliche Homöopathika. 2nd ed. Stuttgart: Wissenschaftliche Verlagsgesellschaft; 2003

Wichtl M. Pflanzliche Cholagoga. Erfahrungsheilkunde. 1978; 27: 329–332

Questions

1. What are the pharmacologically defined effects of silymarin?
2. What is the botanical name for artichoke?
3. Which plant family does artichoke belong to?
4. What are the pharmacologically defined effects of artichoke?
5. What is biliary tract dyskinesia?
6. Write a prescription for a predominantly spasmolytic biliary tea.

Answers (p. 421) for Chapter 3.4

3.5 Functional Dyspepsia

Medicinal Plants

Turmeric, Curcuma longa
Turmeric root, Curcumae longae rhizoma
Artichoke, Cynara cardunculus
Artichoke leaves, Cynarae folium
Dandelion, Taraxacum officinale
Dandelion root and herb, Taraxaci radix cum herba
Wormwood, Artemisia absinthium
Wormwood herb, Absinthii herba
Milk Thistle, Silybum marianum
Milk Thistle seeds, Cardui mariani fructus
Peppermint, Mentha piperita
Peppermint leaves, Menthae piperitae folium
Bitter Candytuft, Iberis amara
Haronga, Harungana madagascariensis
Haronga leaves and bark, Harongae folium et cortex
Papaya, Carica papaya
Papaya fruit, Caricae papayae fructus
Pineapple, Ananas comosus
Bromelain, Bromelainum

Definition

Definition of functional dyspepsia according to the 1998 Multinational Working Teams to Develop Diagnostic Criteria for Functional Gastrointestinal Disorders—Rome Committees (Drossmann et al.)
1. Persistent and recurring pain centered primarily in the upper abdomen or discomfort, such as
   - early satiety
   - fullness
   - bloating in the upper abdomen
   - nausea
   that existed for at least 12 weeks in the preceding 12 months.
2. No indication for organic diseases that can explain the symptoms.
3. Pain or discomfort is not exclusively relieved by defecation and/or is not associated with a change in bowel pattern (frequency or consistency).

The term "functional dyspepsia" derives from a multinational consensus decision. It results from efforts that began in 1991 to develop an internationally recognized definition of functional gastrointestinal disorders.

The Commission E chose the umbrella term "dyspeptic disorders" in the 1980s for a large number of medicinal plants applicable for gastrointestinal therapy. This term was viewed at the time as a kind of "secret weapon" because classically defined indications do not apply to most of these phytotherapeutics. They are primarily suitable for treating functional gastrointestinal tract disorders.

Nowadays, gastroenterologists also recognize this common functional disorder as existent. Up to 30% of the general population suffer from this disorder and about one-quarter of them seek medical advice because of persistent and severe symptoms. These patients suffer almost exclusively from subjective symptoms. There are no objective and measurable findings to prove functional dyspepsia.

Functional dyspepsia is a combination of motor and secretion disorders with psychosomatic and frequently also dietary causes, including, for example, irregular or hastily eaten meals and excess calorie consumption. However, dyspeptic symptoms also indicate a more generally dysfunctional digestive system. Digestive function depends on the finely coordinated activity of various organ systems. This activity is regulated and controlled by more than 120 known hormones that act on the gastrointestinal system. It involves primarily the stomach, small intestine, liver, pancreas, and biliary system. Each of these organ systems can initiate the dysfunction, and each organ dysfunction can initiate other organ dysfunctions. This is why dyspeptic symptoms are so difficult to treat with synthetic monodrugs and why typical phytotherapeutic combination remedies or symptom-oriented combinations of phytotherapeutics are so successful.

Some effective and suitable antidyspeptics include bitters (p. 52) or carminatives (p. 74). These medicinals and their main indications are described in the respective chapters. This chapter introduces a few typical **antidyspeptics** with substance compositions that reflect the complexities of the human digestive system especially well. We also discuss **plant-based "enzyme preparations"** such as papain and bromelain, which stimulate pancreatic secretions and support the pancreas through enzyme supplementation. These treatments are based on the assumption that the pancreas disorder is functional in nature and that no manifest, morphologically diagnosable organ damage (chronic pancreatitis) is involved.

The plant remedies used to treat functional dyspepsia can easily be combined to target the most dominant symptoms. This often produces additive effects. A few examples: bitter drugs for decreased gastric juice secretion; pineapple and haronga leaves or bark for endocrine pancreatic insufficiency; carminatives and spasmolytics for colic symptoms and bloating; cholagogues or spasmolytics for reduced bile production or biliary tract dyskinesia.

▶ **Note.** The diagnosis of pancreatitis is still made far too often and too quickly in clinical practice whenever a patient presents with nonspecific and undiagnosed upper abdominal symptoms. Numerous studies have shown that in the vast majority of cases, this diagnosis is a kind of "stop gap" made to satisfy the desire and expectations of patients for an explanation of their symptoms, but it is not very satisfactory for the physician.

Chronic pancreatitis is a separate disorder with a clearly delineated histology and nosology. It is nearly identical to chronic gastritis. As in chronic gastritis, a slow atrophic process develops over the course of years and eventually results in complete atrophy and cessation of function of the exocrine pancreatic glands. This chronic, progredient pancreatitis is characterized by severe, often almost unbearable pain in the left and/or central upper abdominal region that radiates toward the back and by increasing steatorrhea. There are no really effective treatments for this disorder. Treatment is symptomatic and involves pain relievers and large amounts of pancreatic enzyme supplementation to make the condition somewhat bearable. Plant medicines are not able to provide a cure for this condition either. Their effect is also symptomatic and substitutive.

For references corresponding to the preceding section, see Bibliography following 3.5.1 (p. 127).

3.5.1 Dyspeptic Symptoms

Plants for Treatment

Turmeric (Curcuma longa, C. domestica)

Turmeric originates from and is today cultivated on a large scale in India. This plant is often referred to as "curry," but curry is a blend of many spice plants that includes turmeric, which provides the yellow color to the mix. Turmeric is an herbaceous, upright plant that grows from a rootstock. Its spiral leaves grow to about 1 meter in length and are similar to banana leaves. Its strobiliform inflorescence is located at the end of the stem (▶ Fig. 3.34).

Medicinal applications use the **turmeric rootstock** (Curcumae longae rhizome).

▶ **Pharmacology.** The most important constituents of turmeric are curcuminoids and 2–7% volatile oil. Curcuminoids provide turmeric's characteristic yellow color. They contain a total of 3–5% curcumin, desmethoxycurcumin, and bidesmethoxycurcumin.

Turmeric's cholagogic action has been confirmed in experimental animal studies. Studies have also shown antioxidant effects that explain turmeric's hepatoprotective, antihepatotoxic, anti-inflammatory, and antitumor effects, which have also been proven experimentally (Fintelmann and Wegener).

▶ **Indications.** The Commission E monograph for turmeric lists only one indication: dyspeptic conditions. However, turmeric is also well suited to treating biliary tract dyskinesia due to its cholagogic action, especially when combined with been confirmed by an observational study (Fintelmann and Wegener).

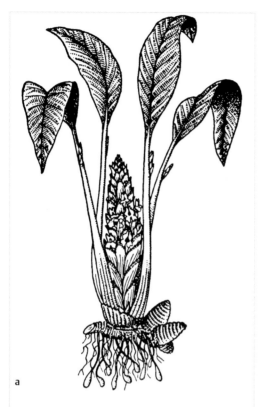

> **Caution**
>
> Turmeric can irritate gastric mucosa and can increase symptoms of gastric hypersensitivity and especially hyperacidity.

▶ **Research.** In an observational study with 440 patients by Kammerer and Fintelmann, a curcuma extract finished pharmaceutical product was used. Typical functional dyspepsia symptoms were assessed using a four-step scaled evaluation. Global efficacy and tolerability were also assessed using a five-step scaled evaluation by physicians and patients. After 4 weeks of therapy, patients displayed a significant average decrease of symptoms of 63.5%. The most pronounced effect was observed with nausea and vomiting. More than 85% of patients and physicians rated treatment efficacy as good to very good. No undesirable effects were observed (Kammerer and Fintelmann).

Preparations

- **Tea**
  Add 1 cup of hot water to 1–2 teaspoons of the finely chopped drug. Steep covered for 5 minutes, then strain.
  Drink 1 cup before meals.
- **Tincture**
  Add 10–15 drops to a small amount of water. Drink 3 × a day.
- **Turmeric Infusion** (Infusum Curcumae, according to the German Prescription Formulas, DRF)

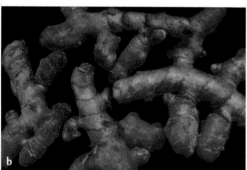

Fig. 3.34 a and b Turmeric, Curcuma longa. Photo: Dr. Roland Spohn, Engen.

the spasmolytic effects (p. 113) of celandine (Chelidonium majus).

Turmeric also influences fat metabolism, and its lipid-lowering effects have been well documented in older studies. This makes turmeric a good choice for successfully treating the symptoms complex of **bloating, nausea,** and **upper abdominal pain** caused by eating high-fat foods. This indication has

Prescriptions

Rx
Infus. Curcumae rhiz. 6.0/180.0 (turmeric rootstock infusion)
Aqu. Menth. pip. ad 200.0 (peppermint hydrosol)
D.S.
Take 1 tablespoon 3 × a day.

▶ **Therapy Recommendation.** Standardized turmeric extract preparations should be the first choice for treatment.

Artichoke (Cynara cardunculus, Cynara scolymus)

For more information about this plant, see Artichoke (p. 106).

Artichokes are considered a traditional liver remedy. In addition to hepatoprotective and lipid-regulating effects, artichoke also has typical cholagogic properties that make it a suitable antidyspeptic.

▶ **Indications.** Artichoke is similar to turmeric rootstock in its effect on dyspeptic symptoms. Both are most effective with dyspeptic symptoms that appear in conjunction with fat intolerance or **fat digestion disorders.** Artichoke's effect appears to be somewhat weaker, probably because turmeric triggers a stronger secretory effect.

▶ **Therapy Recommendation.** As with turmeric, standardized artichoke extract preparations should be the first choice for treatment.

Dandelion (Taraxacum officinale)

Dandelion is a well-known meadow plant and a member of the Asteraceae family. Its single stalk rises from a basal rosette of runcinate leaves and bears a single yellow flower (▶ Fig. 3.35). These bright yellow flowers lend color to meadows and fields in the spring. During cloudy periods, dandelion

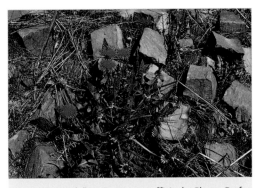

Fig. 3.35 Dandelion, Taraxacum officinale. Photo: Prof. Dr. Volker Fintelmann, Hamburg.

flower heads close up and become inconspicuous. These flower heads mature into spherical seed heads called blowballs, which are popular with children and contain many fruits (seeds). Each seed is attached via a long stem to a pappus of fine hairs that allows the wind to disperse the seeds.

Dandelion taproots reach deep into the soil. Its leaves are a popular salad constituent in the spring. They taste pleasantly bitter and aromatic and are often eaten together with cress and other spring plants. They are a major component of traditional spring regimens.

Medicinal applications use the chopped **entire dandelion plant,** gathered while flowering, Taraxaci planta tota.

▶ **Pharmacology.** Important dandelion constituents include bitters such as lactucopicrin (taraxacin), triterpenoids, and phytosterols. Dandelion has a bittering power of 600.

▶ **Indications.** Dandelion is known to have cholagogic and mild diuretic effects. It is typically used for dyspeptic symptoms and lack of appetite.

Preparation
• **Tea** Add 1–2 teaspoons of the finely chopped drug to 1 cup of cold water. Bring to a brief boil and steep covered for 15 minutes, then strain. Drink 1 cup each in the morning and in the evening for 4–6 weeks.

Wormwood (Artemisia absinthium)

For more information about this plant, see Wormwood (p. 111).

▶ **Indications.** Wormwood is a typical aromatic bitter with additional carminative and choleretic actions. This makes wormwood effective for **dyspeptic symptoms,** especially in conjunction with **lack of appetite.** The Commission E also lists biliary tract dyskinesia as an indication for wormwood.

Wormwood is one of the best examples to illustrate that the recognized efficacy of a biliary remedy is not necessarily determined by its choleretic and cholekinetic potency. Peppermint, turmeric, and other plants are much more potent in this regard than wormwood.

In fact, wormwood occupies a special place among the remedies for treating dyspeptic upper abdominal symptoms. It acts in the same way on primarily atonic conditions of the stomach and of the biliary tract. Ptosis and atony of the stomach present as the typical gastroptosis (downward displacement of stomach). The gallbladder can also be atonic and ptotic, which presents as enlarged in size with a lack of contraction following a test meal and can be seen via ultrasound or X-rays.

In general, this condition is constitutional in asthenic **psychovegetatively labile personalities**. These patients may experience long periods without symptoms interrupted by brief or longer periods of dyspeptic symptoms that are always accompanied by lack of appetite and aversion to many foods. Patients presenting with these symptoms are weak, depressed, and worried about cancer. **Constitutional arterial hypotension** presents a similar picture and is often associated with a "weak" stomach. Wormwood—preferably as a tincture—is an excellent remedy in these cases, which are fairly common, refractory, and difficult to treat. It can be used regularly and for longer periods to treat these conditions.

Preparations

- **Tea**
  Add 1 cup of boiling water to 1 teaspoon of the finely chopped drug. Steep covered for 1–2 minutes, up to a maximum of 5 minutes, then strain.
  Drink 1 cup before meals several times a day.
- **Tincture**
  Take between 10 to 30 drops in plenty of water, depending on the severity of the symptoms, 3 × a day. Maximum daily dosage should not, however, exceed 60 drops.

▶ **Additional Therapy Options**

Milk Thistle (Silybum marianum, Carduus marianus)

For more information about this plant, see Milk Thistle (p. 103).

Preparation

- **Tea**
  Add 1 cup of hot water to 1 teaspoon of milk thistle seeds. Steep covered for 10–15 minutes, then strain.
  Drink 1 cup 3 × a day.

Peppermint (Mentha piperita)

For more information about this plant, see Peppermint (p. 46).

Peppermint is especially indicated for conditions where **pain** is the dominant symptom. It is well suited for individualized prescriptions.

Preparation

- **Tea**
  Add 1 cup of hot water to 1–2 teaspoons of the drug. Steep covered for 10–15 minutes, then strain.
  Drink 1 cup several times a day.

Bitter Candytuft (Iberis amara)

Nowadays, this mildly bitter drug is used only in combination remedies.

▶ **Indications.** Iberogast is a pharmaceutically manufactured combination remedy that contains extracts of bitter candytuft (Iberis amara), angelica roots (Angelicae radix), milk thistle seeds (Silybi mariani fructus), celandine herb (Chelidonii herba), caraway seeds (Carvi fructus), licorice root (Liquiritiae radix), peppermint leaves (Menthae piperitae folium), lemon balm leaves (Melissae folium), and chamomile flowers (Matricariae flos). Many studies thoroughly document the efficacy of Iberogast for **dyspeptic symptoms** and **irritable colon**. More recent studies confirm the efficacy of Iberogast, which is likely one of the most prescribed phytotherapeutic gastrointestinal remedies.

▶ **Research.** Iberogast contains nine partner extracts and the contribution of each extract to the remedy's overall effect cannot be determined.

In a randomized, double-blind study, Madisch et al. (2001) tested a version of this combination that contained only six of the nine extracts (angelica, celandine, and milk thistle seeds were removed). The efficacy of this reduced combination was far superior to placebo, but was somewhat weaker than the efficacy achieved in earlier studies that included the original nine-extract preparation. This combination remedy, therefore, needs to be viewed as a holistic "unit."

More recent placebo-controlled and double-blind studies in 60 patients with functional dyspepsia showed the significant superiority of Iberogast compared with placebo (Madisch et al. 2004). Holtmann et al. systematically analyzed the available evidence for Iberogast.

Another overview of Iberogast was compiled by Ottillinger et al. This phytotherapeutically labeled combination remedy can be considered one of the most well-documented phytopharmaceuticals for treatment of functional dyspepsia and irritable stomach.

Antidyspeptics for Excretory Pancreatic Function

Haronga (Harungana madagascariensis)

The haronga tree grows to a height of 2–12 m. It is in the same Hypericaceae family as St.-John's-wort (Hypericum perforatum). Medicinal applications use the **haronga leaves and bark** (Harungae folium et cortex).

▶ **Note.** Preparations using haronga leaves and bark are popular folk remedies for gastrointestinal disorders in Madagascar and in some parts of the central African continent.

▶ **Pharmacology.** Haronga contains dimer 1,8-dihydroxyanthracene derivatives. The leaves primarily contain hypericin and pseudohypericin. The bark contains harunganin and madagascin.

Haronga stimulates pancreas and stomach secretions. It also has cholagogic and cholecystokinetic properties.

▶ **Indications.** Its pharmacodynamics make haronaga suitable for treating **dyspepsia** and as an **adjuvant treatment for pancreatic insufficiency.** However, haronga does not usually replace

enzyme substitution, which is needed in most cases.

> **Caution**
>
> The constituents of haronga leaves and bark can cause photosensitivity in very light-skinned and light-sensitive people.
>
> Haronage is contraindicated for acute and chronic recurring pancreatitis, severe functional liver disorders, and for biliary and urinary tract disorders, especially if they involve symptomatic stones.

Papaya (Carica papaya)

Papaya is cultivated in India, Sri Lanka, Pakistan, Brazil, and other tropical countries. It is native to Mexico and northern South America and has become naturalized in California, the Caribbean islands, Florida, Hawaii, and Texas. Papaya grows to a height of 4–6 m. Its wood is spongy, and its trunk is crowned by a tuft of large, hand-shaped, seven-lobed leaves. Female papaya trees develop melon-like fruit that can weigh up to 7 kg and turn yellow when ripe. The orange fruit pulp has a pleasant aroma.

Medicinal applications use the **papaya fruit** (Caricae papayae fructus).

Scarifying the unripe fruit produces a clear latex (raw papain, Papainum crudum) that dries quickly when exposed to air. This latex is collected and dried and used to produce papain, with protease as its active principle. Papaya leaves contain less papain.

▶ **Pharmacology.** Papain primarily cleaves peptide bonds that involve alkaline amino acids. The optimum pH is 6.5. Depending on the quality of papain products, they can digest from 35 to 250 times their weight of coagulated chicken egg white protein. Papain oxidizes easily and is destroyed relatively quickly by the stomach acid (Wagner and Wiesenauer).

Zoch presents research about the constituents of papain. He documented the enzymatic activity of papain and thereby confirmed its **antidyspeptic efficacy.**

▶ **Indications.** Papain has been known for a long time as a valuable remedy for dyspeptic symptoms and is frequently used in the tropics. It promotes fermentative digestion, primarily by ferment substitution (supplementation).

Its proteolytic action seems to also make papain suitable as an constituent in enzyme supplements for digestive disorders caused by exocrine pancreatic insufficiency.

> **Caution**
>
> Increased fibrinolysis resulting from papain treatment may cause increased bleeding in patients with blood clotting disorders or who are taking anticoagulants. Therefore, papain is contraindicated in cases of known bleeding disorders. Papain may also cause allergic reactions, including asthma attacks.
>
> Papain has been shown to have embryotoxic and teratogenic effects in humans and unripe papaya fruit is a known abortifacient. Therefore, papain should be avoided during pregnancy.

▶ **Therapy Recommendation.** Only finished pharmaceutical papain products with a standardized enzyme content should be prescribed.

Pineapple (Ananas comosus)

Pineapple is a member of the Bromeliaceae family and contains a proteolytic enzyme similar to papaya. Acetone is used to extract **raw bromelain** (Bromelainum crudum)—a genuine mix of proteolytic enzymes—from juice obtained by pressing pineapple stems. Its optimum pH is between 4.5 and 5.

▶ **Pharmacology.** Experimental studies showed bromelain to have **antiphlogistic effects**. It was also shown to effect blood coagulation by prolonging prothrombin and bleeding time as well as thromboelastography response rates and inhibiting platelet (thrombocyte) aggregation. Animal experiments also showed that proteolytic

enzymes like bromelain can be enterally resorbed, most likely via the lymphatic system.

▶ **Indications.** The main application areas for bromelain are **dyspepsia** and **digestive disorders in conjunction with pancreatic disorders**.

Bromelain can be combined with other digestive enzymes.

> **Caution**
>
> Drugs or preparations that contain bromelain can increase bleeding tendency in patients, especially if they are concurrently taking anticoagulants.

▶ **Therapy Recommendation.** Only pharmaceutically manufactured pineapple preparations should be used.

Bibliography

Drossmann DA, Corazziari E, Talley NJ, Thompson WG, Withehead WE, Eds. Rome II: A multinational consensus document on functional gastrointestinal disorders. Gut 1999;45(II):1–81

Fintelmann V, Petrowicz O. Langzeitanwendung eines Artischocken-Extraktes bei dyspeptischem Syndrom. Naturamed. 1998; 13: 17–26

Fintelmann V, Wegener T. Curcuma longa—eine unterschätzte Heilpflanze. Dtsch Apoth Ztg. 2001; 141:3735–3743

Fintelmann V. Antidyspeptische und lipidsenkende Wirkungen von Artischockenextrakt. Ergebnisse klinischer Untersuchungen zur Wirksamkeit und Verträglichkeit von Hepar SL® forte an 533 Patienten. Z Allgemeinmed. 1996; 72:48–57

Holtmann G, Adam B, Vinson B. Evidenz-basierte Medizin und Phytotherapie bei funktioneller Dyspepsie und Reizdarmsyndrom: Eine systematische Analyse der verfügbaren Evidenz zum Präparat Iberogast [Evidence-based medicine and phytotherapy for functional dyspepsia and irritable bowel syndrome: a systematic analysis of evidence for the herbal preparation Iberogast]. Wien Med Wochenschr. 2004; 154(21–22):528–534

Kammerer E, Fintelmann V. Curcuma-Wurzelstock bei dys-peptischen Beschwerden—Ergebnisse einer Anwendungs-beobachtung an 440 Patienten. Naturamed. 2001; 16(8):18–24

Madaus G. Lehrbuch der biologischen Heilmittel. Reprint Hildesheim: Verlag Georg Olms; 2021

Madisch A, Holtmann G, Mayr G, Vinson B, Hotz J. Treatment of functional dyspepsia with a herbal preparation. A double-blind, randomized, placebo-controlled, multicenter trial. Digestion. 2004; 69(1):45–52

Madisch A, Melderis H, Mayr G, Sassin I, Hotz J. Ein Phytotherapeutikum und seine modifizierte Rezeptur bei funktioneller Dyspepsie. Ergebnisse einer doppelblinden plazebokontrollierten Vergleichsstudie [A plant extract and its modified preparation in functional dyspepsia. Results of a double-blind placebo-controlled comparative study]. Z Gastroenterol. 2001; 39(7):511–517

Ottillinger B, Storr M, Malfertheiner P, Allescher HD. STW 5 (Iberogast®)–a safe and effective standard in the treatment of functional gastrointestinal disorders. Wien Med Wochenschr. 2013; 163(3–4):65–72

Wagner H, Wiesenauer M. Phytotherapie: Phytopharmaka und pflanzliche Homöopathika. 2nd ed. Stuttgart: Wissenschaftliche Verlagsgesellschaft; 2003

Zoch E. Über die Inhaltsstoffe des Handelspapains [Contents of commercial papain]. Arzneimittelforschung. 1969; 19(9):1593–1597

Questions

1. What constitutes "functional dyspepsia"?
2. List its main symptoms.
3. Which plant medicines are typically used to treat it?
4. How many components does the well-studied finished pharmaceutical product Iberogast contain?
5. Which plant gave this drug its name?

Answers (p. 421) for Chapter 3.5

3.6 Endocrine and Metabolic Disorders

Endocrine and metabolic disorders are characterized by the dominance of either "too much" (hyperactivity) or "too little" (hypoactivity) activity. Medical treatment primarily focuses on suppression or supplementation. Surgical procedures are a second important treatment option. Treatments that address the underlying causes of the disorder are the exception.

The primary phytotherapeutic remedies for metabolic disorders also focus on **substitution (supplementation) or suppression**. Phytotherapy, however, does offer alternatives to conventional therapy, for example, for treating hyperthyroidism or lipometabolic disorders. The phytotherapeutics used to treat these conditions are designated as category 2 and 3 remedies, as discussed in Chapter 1 (see ▶ Table 1.3). They offer alternatives to synthetic drugs or can support synthetic drug therapy.

Insufficient treatment of indications such as diabetes, hyperproteinemia, dyslipoproteinemia, or hyperthyroidism can lead to serious **secondary disorders** such as generalized arteriosclerosis or thyrotoxicosis. Therefore, this chapter will also provide judicious information about the role that complementary phytotherapeutics can play with each of these disorders.

3.6.1 Glucose Metabolism Disorders (Diabetes mellitus)

Medicinal Plants

Kidney Bean, Phaseolus vulgaris
Kidney bean pods (without seeds), Phaseoli fructus sine semine

Diabetes mellitus is the most common glucose metabolism disorder. It requires very precise medical guidance with the goal of rebalancing the carbohydrate metabolism. Diabetes is not a uniform disorder. Type 1 diabetes (previously known as juvenile-onset diabetes) and type 2 (previously known as adult-onset diabetes) are very different in terms of their etiology and pathogenesis. Diabetes also has a preliminary stage referred to as impaired glucose tolerance (preciously known as latent or prediabetes). There are no studies to show if traditional phytotherapeutics during these early stages, along with dietary and lifestyle modifications, can delay or even prevent diabetes. In recognition of the possibilities provided by phytotherapeutics, these questions should be taken seriously and give rise to long-term studies on these topics in the future.

The phytotherapeutics discussed here certainly do not replace insulin or oral antidiabetic drugs. However, they can be **supportive** in the early stages of manifest diabetes or for stages of diabetes treated only by dietary metabolic regulation. Clinical practice has shown repeatedly that patients receiving supportive phytotherapeutic treatment can make do with surprisingly low doses of insulin or oral antidiabetic drugs. However, adjuvant phytotherapeutic treatment of diabetes requires practitioners to be very familiar with this disease and its standard therapies and to be very experienced in the use of phytotherapeutics.

Traditional phytotherapeutics recommended primarily native (European) plants to treat diabetes mellitus, for example, **bilberry leaves (Myrtilli folium)**), **bean pods** (Leguminae phaseoli), **golden cinquefoil tops** (Potentilla aurea), and **goat's rue** (Galega officinalis) herb (dried, above-ground parts, harvested during the flowering season) and seeds. More recently, (European) nonnative plants such as **thorny or prickly burnet** (Poterium spinosum, Sarcopoterium spinosum) or **copalchi** (Hintonia latiflora, syn. Coutarea latifolia) were added.

There are no positive Commission E monographs available for these phytotherapeutics. In fact, goat's rue and bilberry leaves received a negative monograph because there is no research that documents its efficacy and in extremely high doses and long-term use, bilberry leaves have been observed to cause intoxications. However, these drugs are listed here as adjuvant treatment options because they can be used for type 2 diabetes that does not require pharmaceutical treatment and is being managed by dietary measures. There is data from experimental studies on animals of Galega officinalis that supports its traditional indication for diabetes and metabolic syndrome (Palit et al.). Other treatment options and adjuvant drugs are shown in an overview of therapy options for type 2 diabetes (Kraft). This overview includes cinnamon, which has been the subject of controversy.

Plants for Treatment

Kidney Bean (Phaseolus vulgaris)

Medicinal applications use the **bean pods without seeds** (Leguminae phaseoli).

This plant contains glucose, amino acids, allontoin, potassium salts, and silicic acid. The basis for its efficacy is unknown.

Weiss had good success with a combination of Phaseolus vulgaris and other native (European) plants that he referred to as "diabetes tea." This tea prescription is likely to be of a more historical nature because galegae seeds are not readily available in pharmacies anymore.

More recently, cinnamon is also used as a dietary supplement to support the treatment of type 2 diabetes. However, no definitive clinical study results are available to document its efficacy.

Preparations

- **Tea**
  Add a handful of the drug to 500 mL of water. Boil until liquid is reduced by half. Drink in 2 portions in the morning and in the evening.
- **"Diabetes Tea" (according to R. F. Weiss)**

Prescriptions

Rx
Myrtilli fol. (bilberry leaves)
Phaseoli legumin. concis. (chopped kidney bean pods)
Galegae herb. (goat's rue herb)
Galegae sem. (goat's rue seeds)
Menth. pip. fol. āā ad 200.0 (peppermint leaves)
M. f. spec.
Add 1 cup of hot water to 2 tablespoons of the blend. Steep covered for 20 minutes, then strain.
D.S.
Drink 1 cup 3–4 × a day.

Important Medicinal Plant Components: Inulin

Inulin, guar gum, and acarbose are plant-derived substances used as adjuvant diabetes treatments. They can be classified as phytotherapeutics with some limitations.

Inulin, a polysaccharide, is an important part of diabetes treatment. It serves as an energy reserve for some plants, primarily elecampane root (Inula helenium), from which it derives its name. This flavorless or slightly sweet substance promotes satiety but has no nutritional value and does not raise blood glucose levels.

Inulin also occurs in other well-known plants, such as artichoke, black salsify, burdock, and sunflowers. For this reason, some of these plants are used as vegetables in diabetic dietary treatment. One plant that is especially high in inulin is Jerusalem artichoke (Helianthus tuberosus), a close relative of sunflowers (Helianthus annuus). Jerusalem artichoke bulbs are used as a vegetable. The sweet tasting juice derived from Jerusalem artichokes can be used by diabetics as a substitute for artificial sweeteners.

Guar Gum

Guar gum is a rubbery substance derived from the seeds of guar gum beans (Cyamopsis tetragonoloba), which originates from India and Pakistan. In water, this substance quickly forms a viscous colloidal solution. This high swelling effect makes guar gum a dietary fiber that delays stomach emptying and thereby slows the absorption of carbohydrates in the intestines. This leads to a more efficient use of endogenous insulin and balancing of blood glucose levels.

Guar gum is especially suitable for **adipose diabetics** because it quickly creates satiety. Guar gum flower is used as a thickening and binding agent. The disadvantages of guar gum include unpleasant aftertaste and frequent flatulence and meteorism.

Acarbose

Acarbose is a pseudotetrasaccaride. Chemically, it is a complex oligosaccharide consisting of two glucose molecules, one amino sugar molecule and one cyclitol molecule. When acarbose is taken orally, it is minimally processed in the intestines and only 20% of it is resorbed. Its action is based on inhibition of amylase and saccharase in the small intestine (enzyme inhibitor). This delays the release of glucose from foods and glucose resorption.

The therapeutic effects of acarbose are similar to that of guar gum: improved blood glucose profile, reduction in postprandial increases in blood glucose levels, and reduced reactive hypoglycemia. Its disadvantages also include flatulence and meteorism, and more rarely, diarrhea.

Bibliography

Kraft K. Phytotherapeutische Optionen bei Diabetes mellitus Typ 2. Z Phytother. 2013; 34(1):6–11

Palit P, Furman BL, Gray Al. Novel weight-reducing activity of Galega officinalis in mice. J Pharm Pharmacol. 1999; 51(11): 1313–1319

3.6.2 Lipometabolic Disorders (Hyperlipoproteinemia, Dyslipoproteinemia)

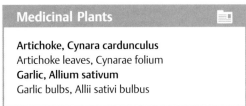

Medicinal Plants

Artichoke, Cynara cardunculus
Artichoke leaves, Cynarae folium
Garlic, Allium sativum
Garlic bulbs, Allii sativi bulbus

Lipometabolic disorders are very common today in the industrialized world. Because of their substantial contribution to the development of generalized atherosclerosis and arteriosclerosis, any normalization of lipid metabolism contributes toward the prevention of these disorders.

Diet plays such a major role in the etiology and pathogenesis of lipometabolic disorders that **nutritional guidance** or—in the case of manifest hyperlipidemias—special **diets** should be the main therapy component. Practitioners are tasked with helping their patients to move away from a hypercaloric diet that contains too many or the wrong kinds of fat and carbohydrate components. Only when these dietary measures cannot sufficiently normalize lipometabolic disorders is the use of medications justified. The first and primary treatment is to transition patients to an individually appropriate diet that allows their lipid metabolism to rebalance itself. The use of medications is a second step.

Plants for Treatment

Artichoke (Cynara cardunculus, C. scolymus)

For more information about this plant, see Artichoke (p. 106).

▶ **Pharmacology.** Artichoke's lipid-lowering effects were demonstrated in older studies and confirmed in more recent clinical studies. Gebhardt provided impressive experimental data showing multiple and complementary effects of artichoke (p. 106) on lipid metabolism.

Primarily clinical studies showed that the choleretic action of artichoke leaf extracts contribute toward increased elimination of cholesterol. Gebhardt showed that a standardized artichoke leaf extract (p. 106) inhibits the biosynthesis of cholesterol in liver cells.

▶ **Note.** The results presented here were achieved using finished pharmaceutical artichoke products that have also been useful in clinical practice. Other artichoke leaf extracts have not been tested for lipid-lowering effects to date.

▶ **Indications.** One of the main aspects of the use of artichoke to treat lipid metabolism disorders is its excellent tolerability, which has been confirmed in several observation trials. Unlike the known side effects of synthetic lipid-lowering (antilipidemic) drugs, artichoke does not cause any liver changes. In fact, it has been shown to be hepatoprotective and promote liver cell regeneration. This makes artichoke especially suitable for long-term or continuous use in the treatment of **mixed hyperlipemia** (type IIa, IIb, IV).

However, artichoke is not a substitute for synthetic lipid-lowering drugs like nicotinic acid, fibrates, bile acid sequestrants, or HMG-CoA reductase inhibitors (statins), but is used as an adjuvant treatment. Artichoke's primary indication is as a **supplemental medication** for lipid metabolism disorders managed entirely by diet.

▶ **Therapy Recommendation.** Only finished pharmaceutical artichoke products containing sufficient amounts of active constituents should be used to treat lipid disorders.

Garlic (Allium sativum)

For more information about this plant, see Garlic (p. 154).

▶ **Indications.** Garlic's lipid-lowering action is indicated for the treatment of **hyperlipoproteinemia** and **dyslipoproteinemia** when dietary measures are not sufficient to normalize lipid metabolism. Garlic needs to be prescribed until serum lipids are normalized.

There are no reliable studies to confirm if the lipid-lowering action of garlic persists beyond cessation of garlic therapy and for how long.

Garlic has more side effects than artichoke. Studies have shown diarrhea, kidney function disorders, asthma attacks, nausea and vomiting, and contact dermatitis as side effects (Siegers). Garlic's strong odor, which many people find objectionable, is accepted by many because of its proven efficacy.

Garlic has a long tradition in **folk medicine** as a preventive antiaging remedy. Modern phytochemical and pharmacological studies have confirmed that garlic is a possible preventive against generalized arteriosclerosis. However, as with artichoke, long-term epidemiological studies are needed to support reliable conclusions.

▶ **Research.** Garlic's lipid-lowering effects have been well documented in several clinical studies. In a multicentric, double-blind, placebo-controlled study of 261 patients (134 verum, 127 placebo), Mader showed that a daily dose of 800 mg of dried garlic powder lowered mean cholesterol from 266 to 235 mg/dL ($\hat{=}$ 12%) and mean triglycerides from 226 to 188 mg/dL ($\hat{=}$ 17%). The difference compared with the placebo group was highly significant ($p < 0.001$). Garlic was most effective in lowering cholesterol in patients with initial total cholesterol levels between 250–300 mg/dL. Numerous other studies have confirmed these results, showing cholesterol reductions ranging from 5% to a maximum of 23% (Auer et al.; Brewitt et al.).

▶ **Therapy Recommendation.** Treatments should use standardized, finished pharmaceutical garlic products for which lipid-lowering effects have been demonstrated.

Bibliography

Artichoke

Englisch W, Beckers C, Unkauf M, Ruepp M, Zinserling V. Efficacy of Artichoke dry extract in patients with hyperlipoproteinemia. Arzneimittelforschung. 2000; 50(3):260–265

Fintelmann V, Petrowicz O. Langzeitanwendung eines Artischocken-Extraktes bei dyspeptischem Syndrom. Naturamed. 1998; 13: 17–26

Fintelmann V. Antidyspeptische und lipidsenkende Wirkungen von Artischockenextrakt. Ergebnisse klinischer Untersuchungen zur Wirksamkeit und Verträglichkeit von Hepar SL® forte an 533 Patienten. Z Allgemeinmed. 1996; 72:48–57

Fröhlich E, Zigler W. Über die lipidsenkende Wirkung von Cynarin. Subsid Medica. 1973; 25:5–12

Gebhardt R. Artischockenextrakt: In-vitro-Nachweis einer Hemmwirkung auf die Cholesterin-Biosynthese. Med Welt. 1995; 46:348–350

Hammerl H, Pichler O. Untersuchungen über den Einfluss eines Artischockenextraktes auf die Serumlipide im Hinblick auf die Arteriosklerosepprophylaxe. Wien Med Wochenschr. 1959; 109: 853–855

Schwandt P, Richter WD. Fettstoffwechselstörungen. Stuttgart: Wissenschaftliche Verlagsgesellschaft; 1992

Garlic

Auer W, Eiber A, Hertkorn E, et al. Hypertonie und Hyperlipidämie: In leichteren Fällen hilft auch Knoblauch. Multizentrische und placebokontrollierte Doppelblindstudie zur lipid- und blutdrucksenkenden Wirkung eines Knoblauchpräparates. Allgemeinarzt. 1989; 11:205–209

Brewitt D, Lehmann B. Lipidregulierung durch standardisierte Naturarzneimittel. Multizentrische Langzeitstudie an 1209 Patienten. Kassenarzt. 1991; 5:47–55

Brosche T, Siegers CP, Platt D. Auswirkungen einer Knoblauch-Therapie auf die Cholesterinbiosynthese sowie auf Plasma- und Membranlipide. Med Welt. 1991(Suppl 7a):10–11

Gebhardt R. Multiple Wirkung von Knoblauchextrakten auf die Cholesterin-Biosynthese. Med Welt. 1991; 7a:12–13

Mader FH. Treatment of hyperlipidaemia with garlic-powder tablets. Evidence from the German Association of General Practitioners' multicentric placebo-controlled double-blind study. Arzneimittelforschung. 1990; 40(10):1111–1116

Sendl A, Schliack M, Löser R, Stanislaus F, Wagner H. Inhibition of cholesterol synthesis in vitro by extracts and isolated compounds prepared from garlic and wild garlic. Atherosclerosis. 1992; 94(1): 79–85

Siegers O. Toxikologische Bewertung von Knoblauch und Knoblauchinhaltsstoffen. Dtsch Apoth Ztg. 1989; 129 Suppl 15: 11–13

General Overview

Kraft K. Phytotherapeutische Optionen bei Fettstoffwechselstörungen. Z Phytother. 2013; 34(1):12–15

3.6.3 Hyperthyroidism

> ### Medicinal Plants
>
> **Bugleweed, Lycopus virginicus/europaeus**
> Bugleweed herb, Lycopi herba
> **Motherwort, Leonurus cardiaca**
> Motherwort herb, Leonuri cardiacae herba

Hyperthyroidism is the only endocrine disorder—aside from female hormone disorders—that is sufficiently treatable according to modern requirements by phytotherapeutics. State-of-the-art thyroid function diagnostics enable metabolic disorders, including latent hyperthyroidism, to be diagnosed in their latent stages. In this latent stage, patients may experience pronounced symptoms even though serum levels of T_3 and T_4 are normal while basal TSH (thyroid-stimulating hormone) is frequently maximally suppressed. The author's many years of practical experience have shown that this constellation can be very successfully treated using **plant-based antithyroid remedies** and that the treatment is well tolerated.

Plants for Treatment

Bugleweed (Lycopus virginicus/ europaeus)

Bugleweed is a member of the Lamiaceae family and is native to North America and Europe, where it frequently grows in damp meadows, along streambeds, and in ditches.

As with all Lamiacea, bugleweed's opposite leaves are lanceolate, roughly incised and toothed, and decussate. Its small, inwardly flowers are white with crimson red dots.

Medicinal applications use the **bugleweed herb** (fresh or dried above-ground parts, Lycopi herba).

▶ **Pharmacology.** Bugleweed contains hydrocinnamic acid and caffeic acid derivatives, lithospermic acid, and flavonoids.

Aqueous bugleweed extracts are antithyrotropic, as they inhibit iodine transport, release preformed thyroid hormones, and inhibit TSH. They also lower prolactin levels (Kleemann et al.; Wagner et al.).

▶ **Research.** Newer pharmacological studies compared the cardiac effects of bugleweed with the beta-blocker atenolol. Both drugs were administered perorally to thyroxine-treated hyperthyroid rats. Even very small doses of bugleweed reduced significant typical effects of induced hyperthyroidism such as raised body temperature and elevated beta-adrenoceptor density in heart tissue. While the beta-blocker was more effective in lowering the heart rate and blood pressure, bugleweed was more effective in lowering body temperature and cardiac hypertrophy. These results confirm bugleweed's efficacy for treating cardiac symptoms of hyperthyroidism (Vonhoff and Winterhoff).

▶ **Indications.** Bugleweed is suitable for treating mild and especially **latent hyperthyroidism**. It is also an excellent remedy for treating **autonomic nervous disorders** that present as hyperthyroidism symptoms but without measurable thyroid dysfunction. Patients should be advised about the frequently observed sedative effects of bugleweed in the early stages of treatment and to consider possible impacts on driving or operating machinery. Combining bugleweed with motherwort (see p. 135) is especially useful for autonomic nervous disorders.

The Commission E monograph for bugleweed lists the following indications: mild thyroid hyperfunction with disturbances of the autonomic nervous system. Tension and pain in the breast (mastodynia).

The results of a three-arm cohort study confirmed the efficacy of bugleweed (Elling et al.).

> ### Caution ⚠
>
> Long-term use of bugleweed in higher doses can result in goiter development. Discontinuation of bugleweed preparations can cause rebound phenomena with increased TSH and prolactin secretion. Bugleweed therapy can interfere with thyroid diagnostic procedures using radioactive isotopes by blocking iodine.

▶ **Therapy Recommendations.** Therapy should primarily make use of finished pharmaceutical bugleweed products.

The average dose stated on the label of the particular preparation should be reached very gradually. Clinical subjective symptoms in particular—along with objective hormone levels—provide feedback about when the optimal individual dosage is reached.

Bugleweed treatment should be withdrawn slowly by gradually reducing the dosage.

Motherwort (Leonurus cardiaca)

For more information about this plant, see Motherwort (p. 173).

▶ **Pharmacology.** Motherwort contains stachydrine and bitter glycosides. It is mildly negatively chronotropic, hypotensive, and sedative.

▶ **Indications.** Unlike bugleweed, motherwort is not antithyrotropic. Motherwort's traditional use in combination with bugleweed likely derives from motherwort's primary indication of **vegetative functional cardiac symptoms**, which are frequently the primary subjective symptoms of hyperthyroidism. This makes motherwort an effective complement to the antithyrotropic action of bugleweed in treating these disturbing subjective symptoms.

The Commission E monograph for motherwort lists the following indications: nervous cardiac disorders and as an adjuvant for thyroid hyperfunction.

Preparation

- **Tea**
  Add 1 cup of hot water to 1 teaspoon of the finely chopped drug. Steep covered for 5 minutes, then strain.
  Drink 2–3 cups a day.

Bibliography

Elling R, Wieland V, Niestroj M. Besserung der Symptome einer leichten Schilddrüsenüberfunktion mit einem Trockenextrakt aus Wolfstrappkraut (Thyreogutt® mono). Wien Med Wochenschr. 2013; 163:95–101

Kleemann S, Winterhoff H, Noetzel S, Gumbinger HG, Kemper FH. Inhibition of TSH-effects by plant extracts and phenolic plant constituents—in vitro studies. Planta Med. 1986; 52(6):550–551

Scheck R, Biller A. Wolfstrappkraut—eine Alternative zu synthetischen Thyreostatika? Naturamed. 2000; 15:31–36

Vonhoff C, Winterhoff H. Kardiale Effekte von Lycopus europaeus L. im Tierexperiment. Z Phytother. 2006; 27(3):110–119

Wagner H, Hörhammer L, Frank U. Lithospermsäure, das antihormonale Wirkprinzip von Lycopus europaeus L. (Wolfsfuss) und Symphytum officinale L. (Beinwell) [Lithospermic acid, the antihormonally active principle of Lycopus europaeus L. and Symphytum officinale. 3. Ingredients of medicinal plants with hormonal and antihormonal-like effect]. Arzneimittelforschung. 1970; 20(5):705–713

Questions

1. Are there defined antidiabetic phytotherapeutics?
2. Are there defined phytotherapeutic remedies for treating dyslipoproteinemia?
3. Which plant has been shown conclusively to have antithyrotropic effects?

Answers (p. 422) for Chapter 3.6

4 Heart and Circulatory System Disorders

The heart, circulatory system, and vessels are a functional unit and cannot be viewed separately. Any disturbance in even a single important location within this unit impacts the entire organism. Many cardiac plant medicines support this holistic approach by providing much more comprehensive therapeutic effects than synthetic drugs with their often selective effects. In this chapter, you will learn about the therapeutic and preventive applications of medicinal plants for heart and circulatory disorders, especially well illustrated by hawthorn (Crataegus) as a prime example.

Heart and circulatory system disorders are the most frequent cause of death in the modern mechanized world today and cause enormous economic impacts. Despite the fact that modern science-based cardiology has achieved great efficiencies in diagnostics and therapy, this has not resulted in improved morbidity rates. The primary reason for this lack of improvement may be that for many decades not much attention was paid to prevention, a concept that only more recently moved into the focus of discussion. Heart and circulatory system disorders are an especially good example for illustrating how the very mechanistic orientation of medical science does not recognize disease states until an organ system is so manifestly damaged that the only treatment options are surgical correction or drug substitution.

Until now, modern cardiology has considered phytotherapeutics to be absolutely unnecessary for its area of specialty. This may be understandable with regards to highly effective drugs such as synthetic digitalis drugs, selective beta-blockers, calcium antagonists, or angiotensin-converting enzyme (ACE) inhibitors, especially when the concept of prevention is not considered. However, long-term studies of coronary heart disease have shown that the old medical wisdom that "prevention is better than cure" is still valid. It will likely be a long time until modern cardiology will seriously consider the manifold offerings of phytotherapy for a comprehensive pharmacotherapy of heart and circulatory system disorders.

However, the possibilities and limitations of phytotherapy described in this chapter are designed to inspire all those whose work with patients is guided by the principle that disease is not a "technical defect," but an expression of the psychosomatic unit "human being." One of the grandiose misunderstandings of modern medicine is to mistake the heart and circulatory system for a mechanical pump system. The dependence of the heart and the circulatory system on, for example, emotions can no longer be overlooked or denied. In the future, this holistic view will completely revise the significance of cardiac plant remedies and demonstrate their unique role, especially in the area of **prevention**.

This chapter focuses on degenerative diseases. It also discusses typical vascular disorders, heart arrhythmia, and functional heart and circulatory disorders.

Medicinal Plants

Coronary Heart Disease
Hawthorn, Crataegus laevigata/monogyna
Arnica, Arnica montana
Bishop's weed, Ammi visnaga
Galangal, Alpinia officinarum

Congestive Heart Failure (Cardiac Insufficiency)
Hawthorn, Crataegus laevigata/monogyna
Squill (sea onion), Drimia maritima, syn. Scilla maritima, syn. Urginea maritima
Lily-of-the-Valley, Convallaria majalis
Pheasant's Eye, Adonis vernalis
Oleander, Nerium oleander
Strophanthus kombe, Strophanthus kombe
Smooth Strophanthus, Strophanthus gratus

Peripheral Vascular and Cerebrovascular Disorders
Garlic, Allium sativum
Wild Garlic (Ramson), Allium ursinum
Onion, Allium cepa
Ginkgo, Ginkgo biloba
Periwinkle, Vinca minor

Heart Arrhythmias
Scotch Broom, Cytisus scoparius, syn. Sarothamnus scoparius
Yellow Jessamine, Gelsemium sempervirens
Motherwort, Leonurus cardiaca

Arterial Hypertension
Yohimbe, Rauwolfia serpentina
Mistletoe, Viscum album
Olive, Olea europaea

Arterial Hypotension
Rosemary, Rosmarinus officinalis
Motherwort, Leonurus cardiaca
Camphor, Cinnamomum camphora

Venous Disorders
Horse Chestnut, Aesculus hippocastanum
Sweet Clover, Melilotus officinalis
Common Grape Vine, Vitis vinifera

4.1 Degenerative Heart and Vascular Disorders

This term describes all types of noninflammatory heart and vascular disorders. Damage due to aging is the predominant cause of these disorders by far. The term **coronary heart disease** encompasses degeneration of the heart muscle resulting in long-term congestive heart failure (cardiac insufficiency) as well as arteriosclerotic degeneration of the coronary arteries causing symptoms of angina pectoris and cardiac infarction. **Arteriosclerosis** describes the degeneration of arteries that manifests as peripheral artery occlusive disease (PAOD), also known as peripheral arterial disease (PAD) and its classic symptom, Charcot's syndrome (Claudicatio intermittens, intermittent claudication). In the central area of the arteries that supply the brain, it can lead to cerebral vascular insufficiency and apoplexy. By applying a comprehensive etiology of "sclerosis," these different disorders can be combined into one chapter from a holistic point of view and then subdivided according to their differentiated treatment options.

Timely diagnosis of degenerative heart and circulatory system disorders, treatment in their early stages and prevention, if possible, is one of the most urgent tasks of our time. Phytotherapy can make substantial contributions in this area.

The outstanding role of hawthorn has already been mentioned. **Arnica, garlic, ginkgo** and the **digitalis (heart) glycosides** (lily-of-the-valley, squill, pheasant's eye), to mention just the most important ones, accompany and complement hawthorn.

4.1.1 Coronary Heart Disease

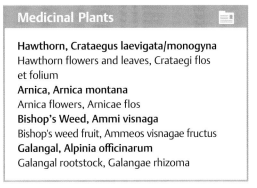

Medicinal Plants

Hawthorn, Crataegus laevigata/monogyna
Hawthorn flowers and leaves, Crataegi flos et folium
Arnica, Arnica montana
Arnica flowers, Arnicae flos
Bishop's Weed, Ammi visnaga
Bishop's weed fruit, Ammeos visnagae fructus
Galangal, Alpinia officinarum
Galangal rootstock, Galangae rhizoma

Coronary heart disease is the most common type of heart disorder today. It has become extremely common primarily in the Western world as an expression of a modern, hectic, performance-driven lifestyle. It remains to be seen if the "heartlessness" that characterize the mindset of an **achievement-oriented society** and the frequently cited mobbing are much more important in the development of coronary heart disease then the so-called **risk factors** that dominate the current discussion, such as hyperlipoproteinemia, hypertension, nicotine abuse, and obesity. Answers to these questions can be provided when medical science goes beyond defining disease factors in terms of chemical and physical measurements and also considers factors such as feelings and emotions. Not until these factors are considered in addition to diagnostic findings will the comprehensive therapeutic significance of, for example, the universal heart remedy hawthorn, be truly understood.

Plants for Treatment

Hawthorn (Crataegus laevigata, Crataegus monogyna)

English hawthorn (Crataegus laevigata) and **common hawthorn** (Crataegus monogyna) are shrubs in the Rosaceae family. These two types of hawthorn look very similar and are common in Germany. The leaves of English hawthorn have three to five lobes that are unevenly serrated, and their

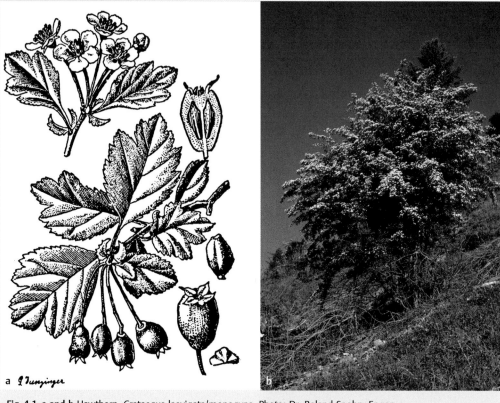

Fig. 4.1 a and b Hawthorn, Crataegus laevigata/monogyna. Photo: Dr. Roland Spohn, Engen.

segments are more oval in shape (▶ Fig. 4.1). Its leaves, twigs, and pedicels are bare. The plant usually bears two pistils, and more rarely, only one, or even three pistils. Common hawthorn has only one pistil. Its leaves are more deeply lobed, and the lobes are pointed. Its twigs are bare but its pedicels are covered with hair. Both types of hawthorn are equally effective and used in medicine.

Medicinal applications of hawthorn use the **flowers** (Crataegi flos) and the **leaves** (Crataegi folium).

▶ **Note.** Pink hawthorn differs from the other two types of hawthorn only in its red flowers. It is not used medicinally. Several other types of hawthorn that have been imported into Germany, especially from North America, also have no medicinal significance.

▶ **Pharmacology.** Hawthorn is one of most pharmacologically studied and documented phytotherapeutics. The following summarizes the results of these pharmacological studies. Literature references

are provided to enable the reader to learn more about the results of each of these studies.

Important constituents of hawthorn include dehydrocatechins of the flavan type with a low degree of polymerization that are referred to as oligomeric procyanidins. Monomeric flavonoids such as hyperoside, quercetin, and vitexin rhamnoside are another important group of substances found in hawthorn. Other important constituents include biogenic amines, triterpene acids, sterols, purines, and catechinic tannins.

Flavonoids and oligomeric procyanidins are considered to be the most important constituents of hawthorn. Both have been separately pharmacologically studied, showing that flavonoids may be more important for myocardial metabolism, and oligomeric procyanidins may be more important for coronary circulation. However, these pharmacologic studies of the isolated constituents once again showed that the composition of the whole extract is more important than its individual constituents.

Recent studies of hawthorn confirmed medical experience that the onset of the effects of hawthorn is slow to develop and usually takes up to 8 weeks. On the other hand, the effects of hawthorn on the heart muscle or on coronary blood flow rates can be pharmacologically shown to persist for many weeks after hawthorn preparations are stopped.

The frequent discrepancy between pharmacologic effects and traditional medical indications for phytotherpeutics does not apply to hawthorn.

Definition

Gabard and Trunzler summarize the **pharmacology profile** of hawthorn as follows:

- Increased coronary blood flow and myocardial circulation
- Improved heart muscle contractility (mildly positive inotropy)
- Eurhythmic effects on certain types of electrical heart instabilities
- Increased myocardial tolerance for oxygen deficiency
- Increased cardiac output, lowering of peripheral vascular resistance (as a measure of afterload), and improved cardiac performance

---

Hawthorn was the first drug assessed in detail by the Commission E and has, since 1978, been the subject of much controversy and discussion for years (Steinhoff, Anonymous). Notable was the discrepancy between the voluminous, careful pharmacologic studies, and the rather sparse literature on clinical efficacy. The detailed monograph presented by Ammon and Händel contains an astounding number of pharmacologic effects. The therapeutic efficacy that can be derived from these effects was known and described in traditional phytotherapy, but the medical, clinical studies comparable to the pharmacologic studies were missing.

In the meantime, many valid controlled studies have proven hawthorn's clinical efficacy. However, hawthorn still has not gained the role it deserves in modern cardiology. Most certainly, the primary reason is the one-sided overemphasis in this field on immediate measurable results versus clinical efficacy that also takes into consideration how the patient feels.

▶ **Research.** Many experimental animal studies have shown that hawthorn increases the coronary flow rate by inhibiting tissue phosphodiester activity followed by a subsequent increase in cyclical adenosine monophosphate (cAMP). Hawthorn's effect on improving heart muscle contractility has also been well documented by a multitude of predominantly animal experimental studies. These studies showed that hawthorn's effect is not due to a digitalis-like effect. Unlike digitalis glycosides, which impact myocardial contractility, hawthorn affects the myocardial **energy metabolism**. This also explains why the effects of digitalis occur quickly whereas hawthorn requires long-term treatment to be effective, provided the myocardium is still able to respond.

Hawthorn's **regulating effect on heart rhythm** has also been documented pharmacologically. Standardized hawthorn extracts demonstrated positive chronotropic and dromotropic effects as well as negative bathmotropic effects.

Studies of hypoxia using a nitrogen/oxygen mix (10% oxygen) showed that hawthorn increases myocardial tolerance to oxygen deprivation. There are also numerous animal experiments showing pharmacologically that hawthorn increases cardiac output, lowers peripheral vascular resistance, and increases cardiac performance.

Animal experimental studies showing the **heart-protective effects** of hawthorn are also very interesting. Preventive administration of a standardized, high-dosage hawthorn extract preparation was shown to significantly reduce heart muscle hypoxia that was artificially induced by coronary ligature in rats. Almost 50% of the animals in the control group died whereas all animals that received the hawthorn preparation survived (Chatterjee et al.). Preventive long-term hawthorn therapy also appears to inhibit arteriosclerosis (Tauchert 1997).

▶ **Indications.** Hawthorn is an especially good example for illustrating the special characteristics of phytotherapeutic remedies compared with modern synthetic drugs. From the perspective of modern phytotherapy, hawthorn is a **universal cardiac remedy** with a specific connection to the human heart and a broad spectrum of indications for treating functional and organic heart disorders.

The therapeutic efficacy achieved by hawthorn is based on its combination of different, pharmacologically proven effects. These cannot be matched by a single synthetic drug but would instead always require prescriptions of multiple substance groups with differing effects. Synthetic drugs also typically are not administrable until objective and therefore massive, often irreversible changes of the heart and the coronary arteries have taken place. On the other hand, hawthorn's strength is its **preventive** possibilities. Timely treatment prevents the later stages of coronary heart disease from developing in the first place. From an economic perspective, this would give a preeminent role to hawthorn for the treatment of degenerative heart disorders.

The author's practical experience has shown hawthorn to be a heart remedy of first choice for treating the **aging heart**. This term describes physiologic or possibly pathologic degenerative changes of the heart that present as decreased stamina, slightly increased blood pressure, angina pectoris symptoms, and arrhythmia. These symptoms are frequently accompanied by the subjective experience of excessively strong or arrhythmic heart beats that frequently do not correlate with measurable pulse rates or ECG results. These symptoms, commonly referred to as heart palpitations, often impact patients more than schematic objective findings, probably because palpitations are always also associated with fear and chest tightness.

Hawthorn has also been shown to be very beneficial in the treatment of **cor pulmonale**. This condition is known to be sensitive and even refractory to digitalis. In the past, intravenous administration of hawthorn achieved very good immediate results. It provided astoundingly rapid relief of the dyspnea (cardiac asthma) experienced most profoundly during the night and spontaneously initiated diuresis. Hawthorn can be combined with mild synthetic diuretics. Parenteral preparations are no longer available because it has been shown pharmacologically that enteral administration can reliably produce lasting effects. Achieving the therapeutic effects of hawthorn described here therefore requires more patience. Its outstanding tolerability makes hawthorn an excellent choice in preventive long-term treatment.

> **Definition**
>
> The 1983 Commission E monograph provides the best comprehensive description of the **efficacy of hawthorn**. It lists the following indications:
> - Decreasing functional capacity of the heart corresponding to class I and II of the NYHA (New York Heart Association) Functional Classification
> - Pressure and tightness in the heart area
> - Aging heart not yet requiring digitalis
> - Mild forms of bradycardia cardiac arrhythmia

Cardiomyopathy, which is observed more and more frequently, is another important indication for hawthorn therapy. These most likely toxic myocardial disorders, especially dilated cardiomyopathy, are a profound therapeutic challenge for which hawthorn represents another treatment option. In practice, long-term treatment using a high-dose hawthorn preparation, also in combination with a synthetic drug, has shown to be effective for advanced stages of this disorder. Milder versions of **postinfection heart failure** also respond very well to hawthorn.

The tolerability of digitalis glycosides can also be increased by concomitant administration of hawthorn. This method significantly improved congestive heart failure, especially in older patients with severe digitalis intolerance, using extremely low digitalis doses.

The following study results impressively document the possibilities of using hawthorn for treating **mild congestive heart failure** and **angina pectoris**. It must be emphasized again that hawthorn's effects go beyond the narrowly defined questions researched in these studies. Hawthorn's full potential will not be realized until the changing feelings and emotional states of heart patients receive the same serious scientific focus as the registration of the changing findings. Hawthorn has both preventive and curative efficacy and is therefore a true heart-healing remedy.

▶ **Research.** Many studies focus on the treatment of congestive heart failure and sometimes also on improving coronary blood flow. This lead the Commission E to reformulate its hawthorn monograph, first published in 1983 and slightly revised in 1988, and to focus its indication areas entirely on **congestive heart failure as defined by NYHA II**. While recognizing the value of these studies, it must be emphasized that this indication limitation does not do justice to hawthorn at all. These studies use the possibilities of modern cardiology to demonstrate the effects of hawthorn on mild stages of congestive heart failure using modern study designs. However, limiting the potential of hawthorn to the effects examined in these studies would be shortsighted. From the perspective of pharmacology and medical experience, it is obvious that hawthorn has much more comprehensive therapeutic efficacy.

As far back as 1981, Iwamoto et al. published a study of 120 patients that tested the efficacy of hawthorn compared to placebo for **congestive heart failure NYHA I and II**. The results of this study showed significant differences in favor of the hawthorn group regarding symptoms such as dyspnea and heart palpitations.

A randomized, controlled, double-blind study by Hanak and Brückel compared the effects of 180 mg/d hawthorn extract in 60 patients with stable **angina pectoris** to placebo. Therapeutic efficacy was assessed by a standardized ergometer stress test. The outcome of the study showed improvement or normalization of pathologic ECG results prior to the study of hawthorn. These improvements were as significant increase in exercise tolerance as an expression of increased coronary blood flow and more efficient myocardial oxygen use. The study showed significant differences compared to placebo.

Meanwhile, numerous new studies show the application of new testing procedures for hawthorn, as illustrated by the following examples.

In a placebo-controlled, double-blind study Schmidt et al. (1994) examined working capacity as measured using an ergometer bicycle in 78 patients with congestive heart failure defined as NYHA functional class II. The study showed that by the 56th treatment day, 600 mg/d of hawthorn extract increased working capacity by more than one exercise step (+28 W) on the ergometer while working capacity in the placebo group remained nearly unchanged (+5 W). The hawthorn group also exhibited significant decreases in systolic blood pressure, heart rate, and rate pressure product.

In 1998, Schmidt et al. published the results of an observational study of 3,664 patients with congestive heart failure (defined as NYHA functional class I and II) who were treated for a minimum of 8 weeks with 900 mg of hawthorn extract. A total of 940 physicians in private practice participated in this observational study. The results showed that 1,476 patients who were treated exclusively with the hawthorn preparation confirmed that hawthorn was well tolerated. The study examined the rate pressure product, working capacity, and symptom score of nine symptoms typically seen in congestive heart failure.

In a randomized, double-blind study of 72 patients with congestive heart failure, Förster et al. tested the duration of working capacity using ergospirometry and showed that 900 mg/d of hawthorn extract increased duration by a statistical average of 30 seconds compared to less than 2 seconds in the control group.

Tauchert et al. (1997; 2002) compared 900 mg/d of hawthorn extract with 3 × 12.5 mg in a multicentric, double-blind comparative study. None of the target parameters (bicycle ergometry, rate pressure product, score assessment of five typical symptoms) showed significant differences between the two preparations. Treatment needed to be stopped for one patient due to side effects.

In a clinical study of 20 patients with compensated congestive heart failure defined as NYHA functional class II and a left ventricular ejection fraction (LVEF) of < 55% as confirmed by angiography, Eichstädt et al. showed that 4 weeks of 560 mg/d of hawthorn extract significantly increased resting LVEF from 40.18 to 43.50% and exercise LVEF from 41.51 to 46.56%. Resting and exercise blood pressure was significantly lowered, the heart rate did not show any significant change during exercise and working capacity increased from 703.75 to 772.11 W/min.

Weikl and Noh, using the same preparation as above, studied 7 patients with global congestive heart failure (defined as NYHA functional class II and III), with the ejection fraction determined by angiography, and showed that hawthorn increased the ejection fraction of the arithmetic median from 29.8% to 40–45% without changes in heart rate. Various symptom scores also showed significant improvements.

In a crossover, double-blind study, O'Conolly et al. examined 36 elderly patients with multiple morbidities (median age of 74) with stenocardiac symptoms and decreasing cardiac capacity as defined by NYHA I–II. These patients received 3 × 1 film-coated tablets of a Crataegus extract preparation or a placebo per day for 6 weeks. Patients receiving hawthorn showed significant median decreases in resting heart rate and rate pressure product. Exercise loads of 25 and 50 W for 2 minutes showed median values for heart rate, systolic and diastolic arterial blood pressure and rate pressure product to be significantly lower than for the placebo group. At the same time, patients receiving hawthorn had fewer stenocardiac symptoms and showed significantly superior psychological stabilization on psychological assessment scores, improved sleep, and lack of appetite observed before the study.

Two other studies document hawthorn's superior cardiac efficacy. A 3-year cohort study confirmed hawthorn to be extremely well tolerated, even with long-term use. Compared to conventional therapy of congestive heart failure, patients receiving hawthorn (preparation WS 1442) registered significant improvement of symptoms and experienced a higher quality of life (Eggeling et al. 2006).

Another prospective, multicentric cohort study involving pharmacies showed that self-medication guided by pharmacists using the same hawthorn extract WS 1442 produced profound improvements in physical stamina assessed as being limited by early-stage congestive heart failure with excellent application safety (Belgardt et al.).

Tauchert (2002) published the results of a prospective, randomized, double-blind study in 2002 that examined patients with congestive heart failure in stage NYHA II who received 900 mg/1 800 mg hawthorn extract WS 1442 or a placebo in addition to standard therapy. Both doses of hawthorn extract showed significant superiority compared to placebo.

A very comprehensive prospective study of the efficacy of hawthorn extract for congestive heart failure (CHF) was begun as part of the **SPICE Study** WS 1442 in CHF (SPICE stands for Survival and Prognosis: Investigation of Crataegus Extract). This international, randomized, placebo-controlled double-blind study was conducted in 2,300 patients with congestive heart failure NYHA II–III (LVEF < 35%) in 120 study centers.

This study began in 1998 and concluded in 2006. Its results were first presented by Christian J.F. Holubarsch at the i2 Summit/56th American College of Cardiology Annual Scientific Session in New Orleans in March 2007. Inclusion criteria for the study were patients with cardiologist assessed congestive heart failure NYHA class II or III and LVEF ≤ 35%. In addition to individualized standard therapy (85% diuretics, 83% ACE inhibitors, 64% beta-blockers, 57% heart glucosides, and 56% nitrates) patients received either 2 × 450 mg of the hawthorn extract WS 1442 or a placebo. The primary endpoints of the study were a composite of cardiac death, myocardial infarction, or hospitalization due to the progression of heart failure. The secondary endpoints were cardiac death and sudden cardiac death as well as assessment of all other cardiac events and assessment of safety parameters. Treatment lasted for 24 months.

A total of 2,681 patients in stage NYHA III were enrolled in the study (1,338 WS 1442; 1,343 placebo) in 156 centers in 13 European countries. Of total study participants, 84% were male. Total morbidity was significantly reduced by WS 1442 at 6 and 18 months and tendentially reduced at 12 and 24 months. Frequency of sudden cardiac death was reduced compared to placebo for patients with LVEF < 25%. Adverse events were less frequent in the WS 1442 group than in the placebo group (Holubarsch et al.).

A Cochrane meta-analysis of 10 evidence-based (placebo-controlled double-blind) studies showed clear advantages for treating patients with congestive heart failure with hawthorn. Compared to placebo, hawthorn significantly improved cardiac output (LVEF), exercise tolerance, cardiac oxygen consumption during exercise and typical subjective symptoms of congestive heart failure (Pittler et al.). Eggeling (2012) provides a good overview of the data that shows evidence for the use of hawthorn with congestive heart failure.

The author's practical experience of many years with hawthorn extract preparations can be summarized as follows: Hawthorn extracts provide long-term and sustained improvements in heart muscle capacity. Hawthorn extracts work remarkably well in conjunction with standard cardiac drugs. Without a doubt, high-dosage hawthorn extracts, when prescribed early, profoundly improve the prognosis for survival and quality of life for patients with congestive heart failure.

However, selectively improving the prognosis for manifest congestive heart failure as an adjuvant for conventional therapy is not the true profile for hawthorn. Its most important therapeutic effectiveness is to be found in prevention. It should be prescribed at the earliest signs of myocardial insufficiency (NYHA I–II) because its cardinal effectiveness is the capacity to restore healthy heart function, and not the role of adjuvant in cases of manifest and irreversible damage.

used for the indications of manifest disorders described here.

Other preparations may be used primarily for very **early prevention** and should not be eliminated from practical medicine by one-sided phytochemical thinking. Simple teas or tinctures can be successful in combination with other medicinal plants. This applies especially for functional heart disorders. For this reason, some of R.F. Weiss's prescriptions are included here.

Proven Prescriptions

Preparations

- **Tea**
  Medicinal applications use the hawthorn flowers and/or leaves.
  Add 1 cup of hot water to 2 teaspoons of the drug. Steep covered for 20 minutes, then strain.
  Drink 1 cup in the morning and 1 cup in the evening, and initially, also 1 cup midday.
  Sweetening the tea with 1–2 teaspoons of honey is advisable because hawthorn tea tastes fairly bland. Sugar consumption is considered beneficial for heart disorders. In the past, cardiologists successfully administered a combination of glucose and strophanthin intravenously.
- **Tincture**
  Take 10–20 drops 3 × a day.
- **Fluid Extract**
  Take 10 drops 3 × a day.
- **Cardiac Tincture** (Tinctura cardialis, according to the German Prescription Formulas, DRF)
  This tincture consists of hawthorn fluid extract (Extr. Crataegi fluid. 10.0) and lily-of-the-valley tincture (Tinct. Convallariae 20.0).
  Take 20 drops 3 × a day.

▶ **Therapy Recommendations.** Only standardized extract products that are prominent in current clinical studies of hawthorn efficacy should be

Prescriptions

Combination with Lemon Balm
Rx
Crataegi flos (hawthorn flowers)
Crataegi fol. (hawthorn leaves)
Melissae fol. āā ad 100.0 (lemon balm leaves)
M. f. spec.
Add 1 cup of hot water to 1 teaspoon of the drug. Steep covered for 10 minutes, then strain.
D.S.
Drink 1 cup in the morning and 1 cup in the evening.

Lemon balm leaves improve the flavor of the tea and are a mild sedative.

Prescriptions

Combination with Mistletoe
Rx
Crataegi flos (hawthorn flowers)
Crataegi fol. (hawthorn leaves)
Visci albi herb. āā ad 100.0 (mistletoe herb)
M. f. spec.
Add 1 cup of hot water to 1–2 teaspoons of the blend. Steep covered for 10 minutes, then strain.
D.S.
Drink 1 cup in the morning and 1 cup in the evening.

The mistletoe component is intended to also lower blood pressure.

Prescriptions

Tea for Raised Blood Pressure and Angina Pectoris

Rx
Visci albi herb. (mistletoe herb)
Crataegi flos (hawthorn flowers)
Matricariae flos (German chamomile flowers)
Valerian. rad. āā ad 100.0 (valerian root)
M. f. spec.
Add 1 cup of hot water to 2 teaspoons of the blend. Steep covered for about 12 hours, then strain.
D.S.
Drink 1 cup in the morning and 1 cup in the evening for several months.
German chamomile acts as a carminative and valerian as a sedative.

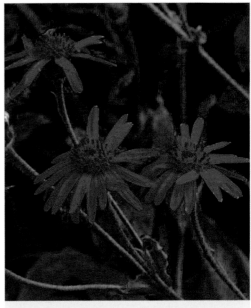

Fig. 4.2 Arnica, Arnica montana. Photo: Naturfoto Franke Heckler, Panten-Hammer.

Arnica (Arnica montana)

This ancient medicinal plant, sometimes called mountain tobacco, is a member of the sunflower family (Asteraceae). Arnica montana grows wild on mountain meadows and was abundant in Germany in the past. Today it has become so rare in Germany that it has received protective status as an endangered plant. Its orange flowers with replicate ray florets and its opposite, smooth, longitudinally veined leaves are easy to recognize (▶ Fig. 4.2).

Medicinal applications use the **arnica flowers** (Arnicae flos).

▶ **Pharmacology.** Arnica flowers contain sesquiterpene lactones of the helenanolid type as well as flavonoids, such as isoquercetin, astragalin, and luteolin-7-glucoside, plus volatile oil with thymol and thymol derivatives, phenol carbonic acid, such as chlorogenic acid, cynarin, caffeic acid, and coumarins, such as umbelliferone and scopoletin.

▶ **Indications.** The most important indication for arnica is **angina pectoris symptoms**. Even though arnica can improve blood flow to the heart through the coronary vessels in a similar manner as hawthorn, arnica's action differs from hawthorn

in significant ways. Arnica's action is characterized by its fast-acting stimulating effect. For this reason, arnica is preferred for **acute cardiac debilities** and angina pectoris. Hawthorn is preferred for long-term treatment of coronary heart disease. This difference between the actions of arnica and hawthorn should also be a consideration in the treatment of the aging heart that has not yet reached the stage of heart muscle insufficiency (heart failure). If the objective is short-term treatment of cardiac debility, the remedy to consider is arnica. If the objective is prevention or amelioration of more minor symptoms, hawthorn is the remedy of choice.

Allergic reactions are typical for Asteraceae, in general (Hausen). However, they are not a justification for contraindications. This is especially true for arnica. Very high doses of arnica can cause intoxication, dizziness, tremor, tachycardia, arrhythmia, and even collapse. In most cases, however, internal use of arnica is well tolerated. In the author's experience, even with very frequent prescriptions of arnica, no such acute side effects have been observed to date. Studies and a review by Merfort also confirm the rather low allergy risk for arnica.

> **Caution**
>
> For patients with an existing history or indications of an allergic reaction to Asteraceae or arnica, this plant should be very carefully dosed, or a different drug should be chosen.

▶ **Note.** Arnica is one of the important medicinal plants that are no longer sufficiently recognized for their comprehensive efficacy even in phytotherapy. The Commission E monograph for arnica only contains its numerous **external applications**, especially trauma edema, hematoma, distortions, bruises, and muscular arthritis (myositis). Arnica certainly provides an excellent remedy for these conditions.

Internal applications of arnica, for example, for the indication of coronary heart disease or acute treatment of angina pectoris, which Goethe considered extremely valuable (Eckermann), are no longer listed. One of the reasons, in the opinion of the authors, is the overemphasis on the extreme sensitivity of a few individuals to arnica.

> **Preparations**
>
> - **Tea**
>   Add 1 cup of boiling water to 2 teaspoons of arnica flowers. Steep covered for about 10 minutes, then strain.
>   Drink 1 cup twice a day slowly, in small sips. This tea is used for mild symptoms or as a preventive.
> - **Tincture**
> - **Add** 5–10 drops to a small amount of warm water. This dosage is helpful for mild symptoms or as a preventive.
>   For moist and warm compresses to be placed on the heart area, dilute this tincture 3 to 10 times with water.
>   For acute angina pectoris symptoms, add 50 drops to 1 glass of lukewarm water and drink slowly within 15 minutes.

Additional Therapy Options

Bishop's weed (Ammi visnaga)

For more information about this plant, see Bishop's-weed on p. 202.

▶ **Pharmacology.** Bishop's weed causes spasmolysis of the smooth vascular and bronchial muscles. There are strong indications that of the two bishop's weed constituents, khellin acts more strongly on bronchial muscles and visnadin acts more strongly on vascular muscles.

Bishop's weed has also been shown to have mild positive inotropic effects and can increase coronary circulation.

▶ **Indications.** Bishop's weed is less effective than hawthorn and arnica, but it provides a good therapy alternative if treatment with these two other plants does not achieve sufficient results. Bishop's weed also seems to have specific preventive long-term effects for angina pectoris symptoms. In the author's opinion, bishop's weed fruit should be one of the therapy options for **coronary heart disease**, especially as a preventive and adjuvant treatment.

The Commission E issued a negative monograph for bishop's weed based on its risk assessment.

> **Caution**
>
> Bishop's weed fruit is not suitable for self-medication. Prescribers of this remedy must be aware of the stated risks and must monitor these risks during treatment.

Galangal (Alpinia officinarum)

For more information about this plant, see Galangal (p. 61).

▶ **Indications.** This pungent drug has strong spasmolytic effects on smooth muscles. In the author's clinical experience, it can provide rapid relief for **primarily functional, spastic angina pectoris symptoms**.

Bibliography

Anonymus. Goethe und die Arnika. MMW Munch Med Wochenschr. 1961; 23:XLVII

Ammon HTT, Händel M. Crataegus. Toxikologie und Pharmakologie. Teil I: Toxizität. Planta Med. 1981; 43:105–120

Anonymus. Bekanntmachung über die Zulassung und Registrierung von Arzneimitteln. Monographie: Crataegus (Weißdorn). Bundesanzeiger (Nr. 1)1984

Belgardt C, Fintelmann V, Schubert-Zsilavecs M, Funk P, Niestroj M. Crataegus in der Empfehlung des Apothekers. Dtsch Apoth Ztg. 2007; 147:81–86

Chatterjee SS, Koch E, Jaggy H, Krzeminski T. In-vitro- und In-vivo-Untersuchungen zur kardioprotektiven Wirkung von oligomeren Procyanidinen in einem Crataegus-Extrakt aus Blättern mit Blüten [In vitro and in vivo studies on the cardioprotective action of oligomeric procyanidins in a Crataegus extract of leaves and blooms]. Arzneimittelforschung. 1997; 47(7):821–825

Eckermann JP. Gespräche mit Goethe in den letzten Jahren seines Lebens. Vol. 1. Leipzig: Philipp Reclam; 1836:11–13

Eggeling T, Aubke W, Regitz-Zagrosek V, Ernen C, Rychlik R. Langzeitergebnisse einer 3-Jahres-Kohortenstudie zur Behandlung der Herzinsuffizienz mit Crataegus. Hausarzt. 2006; 15 Suppl 1:1–5

Eggeling T. Die Evidenz spricht für Weißdorn-Spezialextrakt. Erfahrungsheilkunde. 2012; 61(03):133–139

Eichstädt H, Bäder M, Danne O, Kaiser W, Stein U, Felix R. Crataegus-Extrakt hilft dem Patienten mit NYHA-II-Herzinsuffizienz. Therapiewoche. 1989; 39:3288–3296

Fintelmann V. Crataegus-Spezialextrakte bei Patienten mit chronischer Herzinsuffizienz. Z Phytother. 2004; 25:27–34

Fintelmann V. Weißdorn schont und stärkt das Altersherz. Arztl Prax. 1991; 86:11–14

Forschergruppe Klostermedizin. Bergwohlverleih - Arnica montana L. (Asteraceae). http://www.klostermedizin.de/index.php/heilpflanzen/historische-monographien/41-bergwohlverleih-arnica-montana-l-asteraceae. (Accessed 9 March 2022)

Förster A, Förster K, Bühring M, Wolfstädter HD. Crataegus bei mäßig reduzierter linksventrikulärer Auswurffraktion. Ergospirometrische Verlaufsuntersuchung bei 72 Patienten in doppelblindem Vergleich mit Placebo. Munch Med Wochenschr. 1994; 136 Suppl 1:21–26

Gabard B, Chatterjee SS. Cerebral edema induced by triethyltin in the rat: effect of an extract of ginkgo biloba. Naunyn Schmiedebergs Arch Pharmacol. 1980; 311 Suppl:R68

Gabard B, Trunzler G. Zur Pharmakologie von Crataegus. In: Rietbrock N, Schnieders B, Schuster J, eds. Wandlungen in der Therapie der Herzinsuffizienz. Braunschweig, Wiesbaden: Vieweg; 1983

Hanak T, Brückel MH. Behandlung von leichten stabilen Formen der Angina pectoris mit Crataegutt® novo. Therapiewoche. 1983; 33:4331–4333

Hausen BM. Allergiepflanzen – Pflanzenallergene. Landsberg: Ecomed; 1988: 26–30

Holubarsch CJF, Colucci WS, Meinertz T, Gaus W, Tendera M, Survival and Prognosis: Investigation of Crataegus Extract WS 1442 in CHF (SPICE) trial study group. The efficacy and safety of Crataegus extract WS 1442 in patients with heart failure: the SPICE trial. Eur J Heart Fail. 2008; 10(12):1255–1263

Iwamoto M, Sato T, Ishizaki T. Klinische Wirkung von Crataegutt bei Herzerkrankungen ischämischer under/oder hypertensiver Genese [The clinical effect of Crataegutt in heart disease of ischemic or hypertensive origin. A multicenter double-blind study]. Planta Med. 1981; 42(1):1–16

Kaul R. Der Weißdorn. Stuttgart: Wissenschaftliche Verlagsgesellschaft; 1998

Krzeminski T, Chatterjee SS. Ischemia and early reperfusion induced arrhythmias: beneficial effects of an extract of Crataegus oxyacantha L. Pharm Pharmacol Lett. 1993; 3:45–48

Loew D. Crataegus—Spezialextrakte bei Herzinsuffizienz. Gesicherte pharmakologische und klinische Ergebnisse. Der Kassenarzt. 1994; 15:43–50

Mävers WH, Hensel H. Veränderungen der lokalen Myokarddurchblutung nach oraler Gabe eines Crataegusextraktes bei nichtnarkotisierten Huden [Changes in local myocardial blood circulation following oral administration of a Crataegus extract in non-narcotized dogs]. Arzneimittelforschung. 1974; 24(5):783–785

Merfort I. Arnika—aktueller Stand hinsichtlich Wirksamkeit, Pharmakokinetik und Nebenwirkungen. Z Phytother. 2010; 31(4):188–192

O'Conolly M, Bernhöft G, Bartsch G. Behandlung älterer, multimorbider Patienten mit stenocardischen Beschwerden. Therapiewoche. 1987; 37:3587–3600

Pittler MH, Guo R, Ernst E. Hawthorn extract for treating chronic heart failure. Cochrane Database Syst Rev. 2008; 1(1):CD005312

Schmidt U, Albrecht M, Podzuweit H, Ploch M, Maisenbacher J. Hochdosierte Crataegus-Therapie bei herzinsuffizienten Patienten NYHA-Stadium I und II. Z Phytother. 1998; 19:22–30

Schmidt U, Kuhn U, Ploch M, Hübner WD. Wirksamkeit des Extraktes Li 132 (600 mg/Tag) bei achtwöchiger Therapie. Placebokontrollierte Doppelblind-Studie mit Weißdorn an 78 herzinsuffizienten Patienten im Stadium II nach NYHA. Munch Med Wochenschr. 1994; 136 Suppl 1:13–19

Steinhoff B. : Vom Arzneibuch und der Kommisson E bis zu ESCOP und der WHO. Weissdorn im Spiegel der Monographien Pharm Unserer Zeit. 2005; 34(1):14–21

Tauchert M, Ploch M, Hübner WD. Wirksamkeit des Weißdorn-Extraktes Li 132 im Vergleich mit Captopril. Multizentrische Doppelblind-Studie bei 132 Patienten mit Herzinsuffizienz im Stadium II nach NYHA. Munch Med Wochenschr. 1994; 136 Suppl 1:27–33

Tauchert M. Efficacy and safety of crataegus extract WS 1442 in comparison with placebo in patients with chronic stable New York Heart Association class-III heart failure. Am Heart J. 2002; 143(5):910–915

Tauchert M. Weißdornextrakt zur Prävention der schweren Herzinsuffizienz. Fortschr Med. 1997; 115(55)

Trunzler G, Gabard B.. Neue Erkenntnisse zur Crataegus-Pharmakologie und ihre Bedeutung für die Herztherapie in der Praxis. Ärztez Naturheilverfahren. 1983; 8:407–412

Trunzler G, Schuler E. Vergleichende Studien über die Wirkungen eines Crataegus-Extraktes, von Digitoxin, Digoxin und g-Strophantin am isolierten Warmblüterherzen. Arzneimittelforschung. 1962; 12:198

Weikl A, Noh HS. Der Einfluß von Crataegus bei globaler Herzinsuffizienz. Herz und Gefäße. 1992; 12:516–524

Weinges K, Kloss P, Trunzler G, Schuler E. Über kreislaufwirksame dimere und oligomere Dehydro-Catechine. Planta Med. 1971; 19 Suppl:61–65

4.1.2 Congestive Heart Failure

Medicinal Plants

Hawthorn, Crataegus laevigata/monogyna
Hawthorn flowers and leaves, Crataegi flos et folium
Squill, Drimia maritima, syn. Scilla maritima, syn. Urginea maritima
Squill bulb, Drimia maritima bulbus (Scillae bulbus)
Lily-of-the-Valley, Convallaria majalis
Lily-of-the-Valley herb, Convallariae herba
Pheasant's Eye, Adonis vernalis
Pheasant's Eye herb, Adonidis herba
Oleander, Nerium oleander
Oleander leaves, Oleandri folium
Strophanthus Kombe, Strophanthus gratus
Strophanthus seeds, Strophanthi semen

Congestive heart failure in need of treatment often results from degenerative heart disorders, especially coronary heart disease. This is illustrated by the terms "Myodegeneratio cordis" or "sclerotic heart disease" formerly used to describe this disorder. Congenital congestive heart failure or birth defects of the heart are indications for early surgical corrections and play a minor role compared to degenerative causes. Cardiomyopathies are a third possible cause for congestive heart failure. The etiology and pathogenesis of these disorders are not yet well researched. They may be caused by inflammation or cardiotoxic processes or may frequently be idiopathic.

In the past, congestive heart failure was a domain of **digitalis preparations**. In principle, foxglove is classified as a powerful phytotherapy (forte) and is no longer used in phytotherapy. Standard digitalis therapy involves the isolated, usually synthetically derived substance digitoxin or digoxin. These substances are less and less frequently derived from the actual foxglove plant. More typically, these substances are partly synthetically manufactured from similar substances in other plants. It is likely that it is only a matter of time before digitalis glycosides are genetically engineered. This will sever any remaining connection with the plant. Therefore, it is not the intent of this book to provide a detailed discussion of the possibilities of digitalis therapy, which is part of every physician's standard expertise. Other synthetic

drugs used to treat congestive heart failure are **ACE inhibitors**. Phytotherapy cannot and does not want to compete with these drugs. However, phytotherapy does offer treatment possibilities of which the practitioner should be aware.

One of these phytotherapeutics is **hawthorn**, which is discussed in detail earlier in this chapter. It does not contain glycoside constituents. **Lily-of-the-valley**, **squill**, **pheasant's eye**, and **oleander** are other options. These are often somewhat misleadingly referred to as digitaloids because their constituents are similar to foxglove glycosides. Strophanthus is also discussed here, even though its position is similar to foxglove.

The isolated partially synthesized k-strophanthin or g-strophanthin (ouabain) can no longer be called phytotherapeutics. Cardiology no longer views these substances as important, primarily because of the insufficient enteral resorption and elimination rate, which has been documented by studies.

In 1997, Loew and Loew published a very good overview of phytotherapy for congestive heart failure.

Plants for Treatment

Hawthorn (Crataegus laevigata, Crataegus monogyna)

If digitalis glycosides and strophanthin are not options for the reasons discussed above, the treatment of first choice for congestive heart failure is hawthorn (p. 137), which is discussed in detail earlier in this chapter.

▶ **Indications.** Recent studies show that hawthorn can be used to treat congestive heart failure up to class **NYHA III** (for overview, see Fintelmann). **Cor pulmonale** (pulmonary heart disease) is another special indication for hawthorn.

▶ **Therapy Recommendation.** The above indications should be treated only with sufficiently dosed, especially standardized, high-dose extract preparations (600–900 mg/d). See Therapy Recommendations.

Squill (Drimia maritima, Scilla maritima, Urginea maritima)

Squill (▶ Fig. 4.3) is a member of the subfamily Scilloideae in the Asparagaceae family (formerly the Hyacinthaceae family) that grows on the

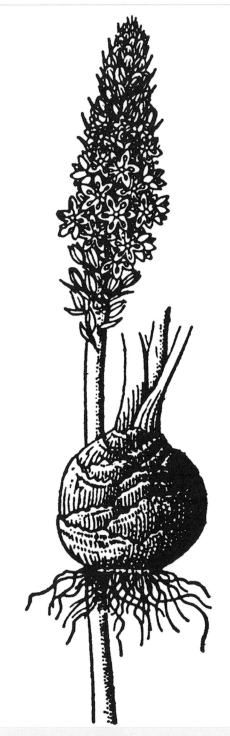

Fig. 4.3 Squill, Drimia maritima (syn. Scilla maritima, syn. Urginea maritima).

coastal regions of the Mediterranean Sea. It has been used since ancient times to successfully treat edema and heart disorders. Squill comes in a red or a white version, depending on the color of the bulb. Medicinal applications of squill primarily use the white version. The effects of squill are similar to digitalis, but weaker.

Medicinal applications use the **dried scales** of the squill bulbs (Scillae bulbi) of the white variety of squill (Drimia maritima, syn. Scilla maritima, syn. Urginea maritima). These are collected after the plant has flowered and are sliced into horizontal and vertical strips.

▶ **Pharmacology.** The scales of squill bulbs contain glycosides of the bufadienolide type. Its main glycosides are scillaren A and proscillaridin A. The drug also contains flavonoids and anthocyanins. Proscillaridin is the crystalized pure squill glycoside. It is remarkably fast acting and is therefore similar to strophanthin. Its resorption rate is 20–30%.

Squill glycosides are largely conjugated by glucuronic and sulfuric acids and excreted via the biliary tract, which makes them independent of kidney function. This is an area of similarity with digitoxin.

▶ **Indications.** Squill is indicated for all types of **mild congestive heart failure**, especially to achieve increased diuresis. Squill's diuretic effect is substantial, and this differentiates it from other glycoside drugs.

The Commission E monograph for squill indicates mild forms of congestive heart failure (also with decreased kidney function).

Squill exhibits the same side effects that are typical for heart glycosides. However, its elimination rate of 30–50% makes these quickly reversible. As with digitalis, squill can cause nausea, vomiting, and stomach problems as well as diarrhea. It can also cause heart arrhythmia.

Contraindications and interactions for squill are comparable to those of digitalis.

▶ **Note.** The assertion made in the past that squill is especially effective for cor pulmonale (pulmonary heart disease) and that it is therefore especially indicated for emphysema patients suffering from cor pulmonale has been disproven.

Likewise, no special efficacy for squill with coronary sclerosis has been documented.

> ### Preparation
>
> - **Tincture**
>   Prescribed as part of a prescription formulation (p. 151) together with other cardioactive (cardiac glycoside) plants.

▶ **Therapy Recommendation.** Finished pharmaceutical products should be given preference.

Lily-of-the-Valley (Convallaria majalis)

Lily-of-the-valley (▶ Fig. 4.4) grows in forests, especially in the somewhat more humid deciduous forests.

Medicinal applications use the **lily-of-the-valley dried herb** (above-ground parts of the plant, Convallariae herba) harvested during flowering.

▶ **Pharmacology.** Lily-of-the-valley is one of the cardenolide plants and contains 0.1–0.5% cardiac glycosides. Forty cardenolides have been isolated and identified for this plant. Its main glycosides are convallatoxin, convalloside, and lokundjoside (Loew and Loew). Even though convallotoxin is easily water-soluble, its resorption rate is only 10%. Its metabolized glycosides are eliminated via the renal as well as the biliary system. Its elimination rate is 40–50%.

The glycoside action of lily-of-the-valley is not comparable to that of digitalis and is certainly also less than that of squill.

▶ **Indications.** Lily-of-the-valley extracts are primarily suitable for the treatment of **mild congestive heart failure**. Its advantage is that it is fast acting and has a high elimination rate. This means that for all practical purposes, lily-of-the-valley glycosides do not accumulate. They also do not impact the heart impulse conduction system and arrhythmia is not a concern. This makes lily-of-the-valley an especially good therapeutic for **bradycardia types** of congestive heart failure. It complements the action of hawthorn in the treatment of the aging heart.

Weiss referred to lily-of-the-valley as a **cardiosedative** that is especially well suited for the treatment of functional heart disorders.

The overall rare and rather weak side effects of cardiac glycosides, such as nausea and vomiting, also apply to lily-of-the-valley. Its interactions and contraindications are the same as for digitalis and squill.

> ### Preparation
>
> - **Tincture**

▶ **Therapy Recommendation.** Finished pharmaceutical products with standardized glycoside content should be given preference.

Pheasant's Eye (Adonis vernalis)

Pheasant's eye (▶ Fig. 4.5) primarily grows in Eurasia. It is native to the steppes north of the Black Sea in southern Russia. From there, it spread to the

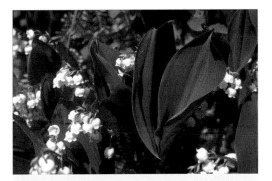

Fig. 4.4 Lily-of-the-Valley, Convallaria majalis. Photo: Dr. Roland Spohn, Engen.

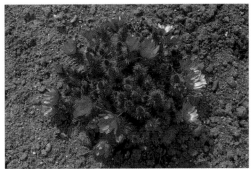

Fig. 4.5 Pheasant's Eye, Adonis vernalis. Photo: Dr. Roland Spohn, Engen.

eastern parts of Germany, traveling along a south-ern hiking trail through Hungary and Bohemia to Thuringia and the Harz Mountains. A few known locations are found along the slopes of the Oder River valley.

Meanwhile, pheasant's eye has become native to Germany, but it is rare. It has protected status and may not be collected in large amounts.

The shiny, golden, large flowers of pheasant's eye blooming on dry slopes in the spring are a beautiful sight to behold.

Medicinal applications use the **pheasant's eye herb** (dried above-ground parts; Adonidis herba) gathered during the flowering season.

▶ **Pharmacology.** The drug contains 0.2–0.8% cardiac glycosides of the cardenolide type, with cymarin and adonitoxin occurring in the largest amount. Nowadays, cymarin is the lead substance. Its resorption rate is 15–37%. Adonis glycosides are primarily eliminated via the renal system and have an elimination rate of 28–39%.

The pharmacokinetics of pheasant's eye place it in the middle of the range of digitaloids.

▶ **Indications.** Weiss rated pheasant's eye as a **cardiosedative**, with an even stronger action than lily-of-the-valley. He termed it a mistake to place pheasant's eye's mild cardiotonic action in the same category as digitalis or squill.

The main indications for pheasant's eye, according to Weiss, are **functional heart disorders** with nervous tachycardia, extrasystoles and **postinfectious cardiac insufficiency (heart failure)**.

Oleander (Nerium oleander)

This plant is listed to complete the discussion of cardiac glycoside plants. Oleander is a well-known decorative plant with evergreen, leathery leaves, and beautiful bundles of white to red flowers. It is native to the Mediterranean. In cooler climates, it is grown as a potted plant that is moved outside in summer and brought inside, for example, into a greenhouse, in the winter.

Medicinal applications use the **oleander leaves** (Oleandri folium) (▶ Fig. 4.6).

▶ **Pharmacology.** Oleander leaves contain 1–2% cardiac cardenolide glycosides. Oleandrin consti-tutes about 83% of the total glycoside content of oleander extracts. Its resorption rate of 65–86% is the highest of all digitaloids. Oleander glycosides are quickly eliminated via the renal and biliary pathways at an elimination rate of 41%.

▶ **Indications.** Oleander does not offer any thera-peutic advantages. Weiss considered it dispensable compared to other digitaloids.

The Commission E issued a negative monograph for oleander because its clinical efficacy is not suf-ficiently documented and preparations without precisely dosed glycoside content, for example, teas, can easily cause intoxication.

Proven Prescriptions for Digitaloids

Drugs that contain cardiac glycosides are combined with hawthorn, sedatives and/or carminatives.

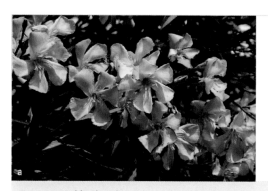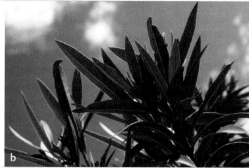

Fig. 4.6 **a and b** Oleander, Nerium oleander. Photos: Dr. Roland Spohn, Engen.

Prescriptions

Hawthorn and Squill Tincture (Tinctura Crataegi cum Scilla, according to the German Prescription Formulas, DRF)
Rx
Tinct. Scillae 5.0 (squill tincture)
Tinct. Crataegi 10.0 (hawthorn tincture)
Tinct. Valerianae ad 30.0 (valerian tincture)
D.S.
Take 15 drops 3 × a day.

Prescriptions

Tincture for mild congestive heart failure with severe heart palpitations
Rx
Tinct. Convallariae 5.0 (lily-of-the-valley tincture)
Tinct. Crataegi 10.0 (hawthorn tincture)
Tinct. Valerian. 15.0 (valerian tincture)
D.S.
Take 20–30 drops 3x a day after meals.

Prescriptions

Composite for Arteriosclerosis With Angina Pectoris Symptoms and Gastrocardia Symptom Complex (Roemheld Syndrome)
Rx
Ol. Carvi 5.0 (caraway essential oil)
Tinct. Convallariae (lily-of-the-valley tincture)
Tinct. Crataegi (hawthorn tincture)
Tinct. carminativ. āā 10.0 (see Carminative Tinctures (p. 79))
D.S.
Take 20 drops 3x a day.

Prescriptions

Composite for Primarily Functional Heart Disorders
Rx
Extr. Adonidis fluid. (pheasant's eye fluid extract)
Tinct. Convallariae (lily-of-the-valley tincture)
Tinct. Valerianae āā 10.0 (valerian tincture)
D.S.
Take 30 drops 3x a day.

Strophanthus kombe (Strophanthus gratus)

Strophanthus plants are vines that grow in the tropical jungles of Africa. They provide the dreaded arrow poison that can cause cardiac arrest and death if even small amounts of this poison enter the bloodstream of the body through small injuries.

Medicinal applications use the **strophanthin seeds** (Strophanthi semen) (▶ Fig. 4.7).

▶ **Pharmacology.** Both types of strophanthus growing wild in the tropics contain strophanthin glycoside. The purified compound is a crystalline powder. K-strophanthin derived from strophanthus kombe and g-strophanthin (ouabain) have largely

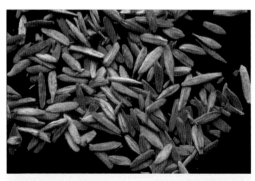

Fig. 4.7 Strophanthus, Strophanthus kombe. Photo: Dr. Roland Spohn, Engen.

identical effects. Cymarin, or k-strophanthin-α, occurs in both types of strophanthus.

▶ **Indications.** Strophanthin can be viewed as the **most effective acute cardiac remedy.** Intravenous injections of strophanthin are extremely fast acting. Its effect is reflected by the pulse within a few minutes and even during the slow injection. Subjective effects, especially on dyspnea, quickly become apparent. There is hardly any accumulation of the drug in the heart. Stropanthin's enteral resorption is only 3–5% and its renal elimination rate is 40–50%. Intravenous strophanthin treatment has largely been replaced by digitalis glycosides.

Peroneal administration of strophanthin tincture is very different from intravenous strophanthin injection. It must not be viewed as a substitute for intravenous applications under any circumstances. Peroneally administered strophanthin is largely eliminated. However, to conclude that strophanthin tincture has no effects would be erroneous and based on unrealistic expectations for strophanthin's potential. Strophanthin is a mild cardiotonic that works very well primarily with functional conditions involving little myocardium or coronary damage.

Preparation

- Tincture
  According to Weiss, strophanthin tincture is very suitable for combining with other cardiotonic, sedative or antispasmodic tinctures, for example, with lily-of-the-valley tincture, valerian tincture, or belladonna tincture. These combinations need to be administered for several months or longer, with breaks.
  A combination with caraway oil and Carminative Tincture (see Carminative Tincture (p. 79)) is indicated for arteriosclerosis patients presenting with meteorism as well as for younger vagotonia patients.
  A combination with belladonna tincture is indicated for younger patients with vagotonia and vegetative dysregulation as well as for patients with gastrointestinal disorders to complement the action of belladonna with a mild cardiotonic.

Proven Prescriptions

Prescriptions

Tincture Blend for Vagotonia, Extrasystoles, and Arterial Hypertension
Rx
Tinct. Strophanthi (strophanthin tincture)
Tinct. Belladonnae āā 10.0 (belladonna tincture)
Tinct. Valerianae 20.0 (valerian tincture)
D.S.
Take 30 drops 3 × a day.

Prescriptions

Caraway Oil Combination for Gastrocardia Symptom Complex
Rx
Ol. Carvi 5.0 (caraway essential oil)
Tinct. Strophanthi (strophanthin tincture)
Tinct. Belladonnae āā 10.0 (belladonna tincture)
Tinct. Valerian. aeth. 20.0 (ethereal valerian tincture)
D.S.
Take 30 drops 3 × a day.

Prescriptions

For Functional Heart Disorders
Rx
Tinct. Strophanthi (strophanthin tincture)
Tinct. Convallariae (lily-of-the-valley tincture)
Tinct. Nuc. Vomicae (Nux Vomica tincture)
Tinct. Valerianae āā 10.0 (valerian tincture)
D.S.
Take 30 drops 3 × a day.

Bibliography

Fintelmann V. Crataegus-Spezialextrakte bei Patienten mit chronischer Herzinsuffizienz. Z Phytother. 2004; 25 Suppl 1:27–34

Hempelmann FW, Heinz N, Flasch H. Lipophilie und enterale Resorption bei Cardenoliden [Lipophilicity and enteral absorption of cardenolides]. Arzneimittelforschung. 1978; 28 (12):2182–2185

Lauterbach F. Enterale Resorption, biliäre Ausscheidung und enterohepatischer Kreislauf von Herzglykosiden bei der Ratte. Naunyn Schmiedebergs Arch Exp Pathol Pharmakol. 1964; 247: 391–411

Loew D. Phytotherapie bei der Herzinsuffizienz. Z Phytother. 1997; 18(2):92–96

Loew DA, Loew AD. Pharmakokinetik von herzglykosidhaltigen Pflanzenextrakten. Z Phytother. 1994; 15(4):197–202

Rietbrock N, Vöhringer HF, Kuhlmann J. Der Metabolismus herzwirksamer Glykoside. Herz/Kreisl. 1977; 9:825–832

Schwinger RH, Erdmann E. Die positiv inotrope Wirkung von Miroton. Z Phytother. 1992; 13(3):91–95

4.1.3 Peripheral and Cerebral Vascular Disorders

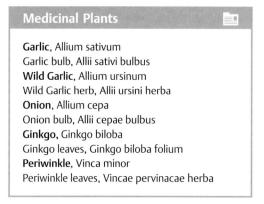

Medicinal Plants

Garlic, Allium sativum
Garlic bulb, Allii sativi bulbus
Wild Garlic, Allium ursinum
Wild Garlic herb, Allii ursini herba
Onion, Allium cepa
Onion bulb, Allii cepae bulbus
Ginkgo, Ginkgo biloba
Ginkgo leaves, Ginkgo biloba folium
Periwinkle, Vinca minor
Periwinkle leaves, Vincae pervinacae herba

In addition to degenerative heart diseases, **peripheral and cerebral vascular disorders**—or generalized arteriosclerosis—represent another large group of common disorders in the industrialized world. Peripheral occlusive disease (POD) and its main symptom of intermittent claudication are very common disorders seen with excessive tobacco consumption. It has led to expansive development of vascular surgery. Physicians who believe in phytotherapy and its remedies must make it clear that phytotherapeutics can be very useful as preventives before the development of later stages of this disorder, also from an economic perspective. The cost of dealing with advanced stages of peripheral arterial vascular disorders are high and can hardly be calculated.

The same applies for **cerebral circulation disorders** resulting from arteriosclerotic vascular disorders, which lead to cerebrovascular insufficiency and apoplexy. The tragic experience of a stroke with loss of language and paralysis on one side of the body provides justification for any therapy attempt—even it if has not yet been conclusively scientifically proven—that holds out hope for preventing this end stage of a disorder that develops slowly, over a long period of time. It also begs the question if we can even still afford to always delay scientific recognition of therapies until it is too late. The renowned physician Carl Gustav Carus (1789–1869) stated this very aptly in the 19th century: "It would certainly be absurd arrogance of science (which would then no longer deserve to be called science) for a physician—whose highest task and ultimate goal, after all, is always to benefit his

patients—to reject anything because his immediate sharp reasoning and individual opinion does not provide sufficient reason for its application" (Carus 1859).

The literature on garlic and ginkgo has expanded dramatically during the past decades. This illustrates the need—from our point of view—to change the thinking on how best to benefit patients.

Plants for Treatment

Garlic (Allium sativum)

Garlic is a member of the Amaryllidaceae family and a species in the onion genus (Allium). This ancient medicinal plant has a history of thousands of years of human use and is consumed today in great quantities. It occupies a peculiar intermediate position between spice and medicinal remedy.

Medicinal applications use the **garlic bulb** (Allii sativi bulbus). It consists of the fleshy, thickened leaves of the lower part of the stem, referred to as onion scales (▶ Fig. 4.8). What differentiates garlic from the culinary onion is that garlic consists of 6–15 partial bulbs called cloves. These cloves are seated in the basal part of the stem axil. Onions, therefore, are not roots, but fleshy underground stems.

▶ **Note.** A recipe for garlic in cuneiform characters dated 3000 BC demonstrates that the first indications for the use of garlic go back to the Stone Age. An ancient Egyptian papyrus dated 1600 BC reports that workers employed in building the pyramids went on strike because they did not receive sufficient amounts of garlic and onions for their daily meals. They workers evidently needed both to remain healthy and fit. It seems obvious that people in those days already knew what modern science has since then confirmed: that garlic is antimicrobial. The workers building the pyramids likely needed sufficient amounts of garlic as protection against amoebic dysentery, which was very common then. Garlic was used both for prevention and for therapy.

The most well-known representative of the onion genus is the common onion (Allium cepa). Chives (Allium schoenoprasum), leeks (Allium porrum), and shallots (Allium ascalonicum) also belong to this genus. Onion is also known to have significant health-promoting effects. The onion differs from garlic, in part, but the two are very complementary.

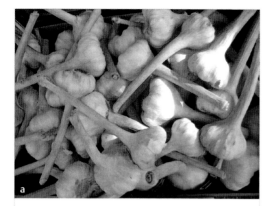

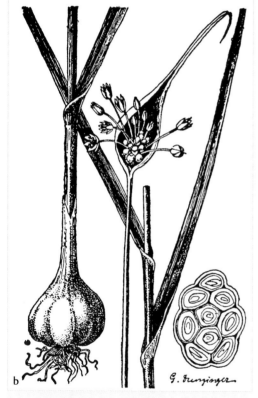

Fig. 4.8 a and b Garlic, Allium sativum. Photo: Thieme Verlagsgruppe, Stuttgart.

▶ **Pharmacology.** Despite the long history of garlic as a medicinal plant, pharmacology did not really study its constituents until the 20th century.

In 1944, the oil was first extracted and shown experimentally to have **antibacterial** and **antifungal** effects.

The next key step in the research into garlic's constituents was the discovery by the organic chemist Stoll (Stoll and Seebeek) that fresh garlic cloves contain a chemically very unstable, odorless substance that is enzymatically changed into the substance that gives garlic its characteristic odor after the clove is cut. He called this first odorless stage **alliin**, and the new substance that develops from alliin and gives garlic its odor, **allicin**. This second substance has also been shown to be chemically very unstable and continues to change into metabolites. One of those metabolites is **ajoene**, which was discovered later and is thought to be responsible for the aggregation inhibition of thrombocytes.

There is now extensive literature about garlic. The manufacturers of some new and popular garlic preparations have stimulated considerable pharmaceutical, pharmacologic, and clinical research. Koch and Hahn as well as Reuter created overviews about garlic in 1988 that are well worth reading.

Garlic chemistry has developed into its own area of research. The therapeutic efficacy of garlic derives from a combination of many constituents, including vitamins, nicotinic acid amide, hormones that are similar in effect to male and female sexual hormones, ferments, choline, thiocyanic acid, iodine, saponins, and others. Its full efficacy is derived from the sum of these constituents. So far, no uniform single substance has been isolated from garlic that can at least achieve its primary effect.

The intense interest in garlic derives from the following four main effects of garlic: antimicrobial, lipid lowering, fibrinolytic, and thrombocyte aggregation inhibiting.

▶ **Research.** Many studies have confirmed garlic's **antimicrobial** effects, which were known in traditional medicine, as discussed above. Garlic was found to have antibacterial and antimycotic actions. In addition, *in vitro* and *in vivo* studies showed that garlic is effective against protozoa and viruses (Wagner and Sendl). This antimicrobial activity is primarily derived from allicin. It is thought to be based on the inhibition of the sulfhydryl groups in certain enzymes of the microorganisms.

Allicin exhibits substantial antimicrobial activity. Even in dilutions of 1:85,000 to 1:125,000, it can completely inhibit the growth of grampositive and gram-negative bacteria. The antibiotic action of 1 mg of allicin corresponds to 15 iU of penicillin. When garlic is heated for longer periods or exposed to high heat, most of its antimicrobial potential is lost. Therefore, dry garlic extracts exposed to these conditions are largely ineffective for this indication.

Garlic's antimicrobial effect has not yet gained sufficient significance in its application. It seems that more extensive clinical studies are needed to determine whether garlic preparations can fill in therapeutic gaps for bacterial, viral or fungal infections.

Many *in vivo* and *in vitro* studies have shown the preventive and curative effects of garlic in **lowering lipids/cholesterol** in plasma (Gebhardt). Garlic prevented hypercholesterolemia provoked by feeding cholesterol to animals and minimized secondary induced atheromatous vascular changes. This effect is also attributed primarily to allicin. Its effect is not as pronounced as modern synthetic lipid-lowering drugs, which means garlic is probably recommended more for preventive application. Its use should also always be accompanied by appropriate dietary measures, and it should be emphasized that long-term treatment is required to see results.

Arteriosclerosis always also involves **lowered fibrinolysis activity**. Animal experiments as well as clinical studies have shown that garlic increases fibrinolysis activity. For example, it was shown to increase fibrinolysis in myocardial infarction patients by 130%, which is a significant effect compared to placebo. Which of the constituents of garlic is responsible for this increase in fibrinolysis activity is subject to conjectures. It is thought that the active principle is garlic's sulfur compounds. However, Song et al. isolated an anticoagulating substance in garlic that is possibly identical to phytic acid. This substance has intense fibrinolytic and coagulation inhibiting effects, prolongs prothrombin time, and precipitates calcium ions.

It is thought that a specific active constituent in garlic blocks thromboxane synthesis. Consumption of 100–150 mg/kg of fresh garlic almost completely **inhibits thrombocyte aggregation** for 1–2 hours. Finished pPharmaceutical garlic products may be completely ineffective in this respect. It is not yet known whether ajoene, mentioned above, or other polysulfides are the active principles involved (Jung et al. 1989; 1991).

▶ **Indications.** The various effects described above suggest a wide spectrum of indications for garlic. Garlic is often viewed as a universal remedy that can counteract all tribulations of aging. Others view it as the most overrated natural remedy.

The entire field of research into garlic indicates that its lipid-lowering, fibrinolytic activity increasing, and thrombocyte aggregation inhibiting effects make garlic a suitable therapeutic for **arteriosclerotic disorders**. Its use is especially important and appropriate in the **early stages** of these disorders and can have preventive effects. In the final stages of arteriosclerosis, garlic can, at best, provide symptomatic relief.

It was, however, shown that the early stages of plaque formation on arterial walls were not only effectively blocked by an aqueous extract of dried garlic powder, but newly formed plaque was dissolved (Grünwald).

The Commission E only shows indications for garlic as an adjuvant for increased lipid values and as a preventive for age-related vascular changes.

Side effects of garlic on the gastrointestinal system or allergic reactions are rare. The strong odor of garlic, however, does bother some patients, which is why sufficient doses of an effective garlic preparation or fresh garlic are rarely taken regularly over a long period of time.

▶ **Research.** Antidyspectic effects are certainly not one of the main actions of garlic. They were not adopted by the Commission E, especially because garlic causes gastrointestinal irritations in some people. The clinical impact of garlic's antimicrobial effectiveness remains completely open. There are no modern studies that show garlic preparations to be true alternatives to chemotherapeutics or antibiotics for microbially caused infectious diseases. Weiss viewed amoebic dysentery in the Mediterranean region and "bacterial dysentery" in the more northern European countries as indications for garlic, but those have not been sufficiently proven.

In the past, garlic was thought to **lower blood pressure**. No proof of this action was available when the Commission E compiled its monograph for garlic and this indication area was not included. Since then, a high daily dose of 900–1200 mg lyophilized garlic powder was shown to significantly lower diastolic blood pressure by four studies and systolic blood pressure by three studies. Garlic has been shown to have additive effects when combined with synthetic antihypertensive drugs. A traditional proven, fixed combination remedy pairs garlic with hawthorn. Petkov (1961; 1966) pointed out that garlic is thought to have detoxifying effects for chronic lead poisoning. He showed that the use of garlic provided a statistically significant reduction of the stippling of erythrocytes that is typical for intoxication.

However, there are no newer studies that confirm this indication. In 2015, Scheffler published a overview of the research on garlic.

This is certainly not the final word on garlic. There are no newer research results, largely because garlic's indication areas are covered by synthetics today. However, in the future, we may see a renaissance of garlic as a medicinal, especially in the area of prevention.

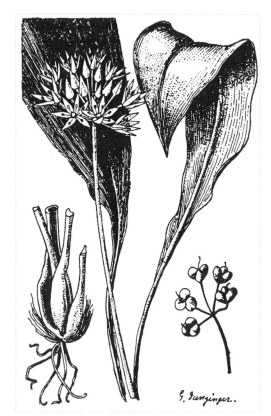

Fig. 4.9 Wild Garlic, Allium ursinum.

> ### Preparation ☞
>
> - **Tincture 20 drops**
>   Take 3 × a day.

Wild Garlic (Allium ursinum)

In Germany, wild garlic (▶ Fig. 4.9) grows wild and is a native inhabitant of shaded, deciduous forests. It always grows in large clusters and betrays its presence from afar with its strong, garlic-like odor. Its flowers are pure white and a decorative element of spring flora in the forests of the Central Uplands.

Medicinal applications use the **wild garlic herb** (Allii ursini herba).

▶ **Pharmacology.** According to studies by Wagner and Sendl, the constituents of wild garlic resemble those of Allium sativum, but with quantitative differences in alliin/allicin/ajoene fractions. Methyl and dimethyl homologues of ajoene have also been isolated from wild garlic.

▶ **Indications.** Wild garlic has similar effects as garlic. Its primary effect seems to be on the intestines. It provides effective therapy for **meteorism** and **dyspeptic conditions caused by fermentation**. Its effect on the **vascular system** is much less pronounced than that of garlic. A phytotherapeutically justified medicinal indication for wild garlic is not given.

> ### Preparation ☞
>
> - **Tea**
>   Add hot water to 1–2 teaspoons of the dried drug. Steep covered for 5 minutes, then strain.
>   Drink 1–2 cups in the morning and in the evening.

Ginkgo (Ginkgo biloba)

Ginkgo biloba—*biloba* is Latin for two lobes or bilobal—is an ancient plant that was traditionally planted near temples in China and Japan. It is the only living species in the division Ginkgophyta, which is related to conifers. The leaves of this dioecious tree of medium size are long-stemmed, bilobal, and have radiate, forked veins (▶ Fig. 4.10). The tree sheds its leaves in the autumn. As with conifers, the ginkgo pollen is dispersed by wind. Ginkgo's yellow fruit contains a woody core.

Ginkgo biloba no longer grows in the wild. Many fossils document that ginkgo trees were once widespread throughout the world in prehistoric periods.

Medicinal applications of ginkgo use the **leaves** (Ginkgo biloba folium).

Scientific interest in ginkgo biloba extracts (GBEs) has grown over the past decades, much as with hawthorn and garlic. This is the reason there is now extensive literature available about its

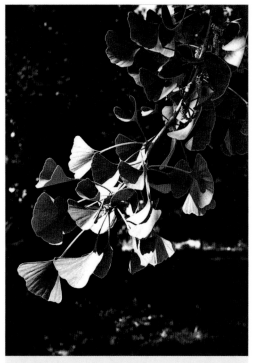

Fig. 4.10 Ginkgo, Ginkgo biloba. Photo: Prof. Dr. Volker Fintelmann, Hamburg.

pharmacology as well as its indications (see below).

▶ **Note.** Interest in GBEs was initially triggered by the introduction of special extracts and numerous other finished pharmaceutical products. This interest may have been enhanced by the fact that for a period in the 1980s, sales of GBEs were the second highest of all preparations in the German market. It is therefore no surprise that this gave rise to criticism from those who inherently object to medicinal products that show high sales, especially when the product is a phytotherapeutic. This criticism took the form of articles, which were often polemic.

▶ **Pharmacology.** Ginkgo biloba contains flavonoids, procyanidins, diterpenoids, ginkgolides, and bilobalide. The flavonoid content in GBEs account for its **free radical scavenging characteristics** being a predominant action. Each living organism constantly creates free radicals that need to be enzymatically scavenged and metabolized. Ischemia, hypoxia, and other metabolic disorders increase the production of free radicals. This creates a chain reaction that imbalances enzyme systems, cell membranes, and cell functions. The most important interaction in vascular physiology is between the eicosanoids (thromboxane, prostacyclin, prostaglandins, leukotrienes).

The dynamic balance between prostacyclin and thromboxane A_2 is of particular importance. Prostacyclin is responsible for vasodilation and inhibition of thrombocyte aggregation. Thromboxane A_2 is responsible for vasoconstriction and increasing thrombocyte aggregation. This balance can be disturbed by free radicals, for example, by lipid peroxides, which can cause a relative excess of thromboxane A_2. Studies have shown that GBEs can scavenge these radicals and thereby render them harmless.

The **flow characteristics of blood** are improved by decreasing thrombocyte and erythrocyte aggregation and by controlling blood viscosity. Hemorrelogic studies have shown that GBEs can improve blood flow *in vitro* and *in vivo*. GBEs also protect erythrocytes by protecting membranes from hemolysis. They maintain normal cell metabolism by enhancing oxygen and glucose uptake and utilization in the tissues. Studies have also shown antiedematous effects in the brain. The mechanism of this action is still the subject of debate.

Sancesario and Kreutzberg see connections with astrocyte activation, which is responsible for the phagocytosis myelin debris.

Another mechanism of action was found that is primarily based on the terpene lactones in GBEs, especially ginkgolide B. It was described as a very active antagonist of the platelet activating factor (PAF).

▶ **Research.** There has been an increase in studies and discussion of **toxic effects** for ginkgo biloba. The neurotoxic substance 4'-O-methylpyridoxine (MPN) contained primarily in the seeds, but also in the leaves, has caused intoxication with the main symptoms of tonic and tonic-clonic spasms, especially in Japan and China. However, the MPN content in pharmaceutically manufactured preparations used in Europe is far below the dose that led to intoxications in Asia, primarily as a result of consumption of raw seeds (Leistner and Arenz).

Ginkgolic acids are thought to be responsible for **allergic reactions**. According to the Commission E monograph, the ginkgolic acid content of finished pharmaceutical products should not exceed 5 ppm.

A **risk of bleeding** caused by ginkgo preparations reported in a few individual cases can now be excluded (Schulz 2006). A large, retrospective, epidemiological analysis of data from more than 300,000 patients did not show increases of bleeding events during ginkgo treatment. Bleeding risk was also not increased during concurrent treatment with aspirin or phenprocoumon; in fact, it was lower than expected. These conclusions are supported by another proband study (Jiang et al.).

▶ **Indications.** The pharmacologically studied effects of ginkgo mentioned earlier present a complex picture. However, they do reflect the clinical experience showing the main effects of GBE for disorders that result from arteriosclerotic changes in peripheral and central arterial vessels. Ginkgo has been shown to be an important medicinal plant for treating circulation disorders, especially in the brain.

The following main indications reflect decades of use and medical experience. In addition, a growing body of research results from controlled and double-blind studies has been developed for these indications during the past few years.

The indications for ginkgo in the Commission E monograph are described as follows:

- Symptomatic treatment of disturbed performance in organic brain syndrome within the regimen of a therapeutic concept in cases of dementia syndromes. The primary target groups are dementia syndromes, including primary degenerative dementia, vascular dementia, and mixed forms of both.
- Improvement of pain-free walking distance in peripheral arterial occlusive disease in stage II, according to Fontaine classification (intermittent claudication), in a regimen of physical therapeutic measures, in particular walking exercise.
- Vertigo.
- Tinnitus.

Brain disorders continue to challenge modern medicine. Time and again, drugs have been developed that were subsequently considered unnecessary. Terms such as "impure placebos" used by the pharmacologist Kuschinsky (1975a, 1975b) for drugs that increase circulation indicate skepticism toward and dismissal of these types of drugs. This is contrasted by the profound misery reflected in the feelings and emotions of such patients, especially in the early stages of cerebrovascular insufficiency.

Definition

The three main **applications areas** for ginkgo are:
- Brain disorders resulting from degenerative changes (dementia).
- Peripheral arterial circulation disorders presenting as symptoms of intermittent claudication.
- Vascular vertigo, tinnitus, and sudden hearing loss.

The following few examples represent a large number of studies with results that all point in the same direction. There is no question that GBEs provide effective improvements for the indications above and that it has established itself in the treatment of such vascular disorders.

▶ **Research.** In a randomized, double-blind study, Weitbrecht und Jansen showed that 60 patients with mild to moderately severe primarily **degenerative dementia** experienced significant improvements in their clinical condition and in the results of their psychometric tests compared to placebo following treatment with a GBE for 4 or 12 weeks.

In a randomized, placebo-controlled double-blind study of 40 outpatients diagnosed with mild to moderate **cerebrovascular insufficiency**, Halama et al. showed the effects of a GBE on the symptoms of this disorder. The differences in measured parameters were highly significant. The GBE was shown to have superior effects on short-term memory disorders, cognitive function, and vertigo. The GBE also significantly improved symptoms such as headaches and tinnitus, compared to placebo.

In a randomized, double-blind study of two groups of 50 patients with **cerebral insufficiency**, Vorberg showed that treatment with a GBE achieved significant improvements in the group given a GBE for concertation, memory, anxiety, vertigo, headaches, and tinnitus.

Le Bars et al. studied the effects of a GBE on 309 outpatients with **Alzheimer type dementia** as well as **vascular dementia** for 52 weeks in a randomized, placebo-controlled, double-blind trial. The outpatients given a GBE showed significant differences compared to the group given a placebo on cognition, daily living skills, and overall clinical impression. The group given the GBE achieved a significantly higher response rate and was rated low in side effects.

Kanowski et al. also conducted a double-blind, placebo-controlled, multicentric study, but using a higher dosage of GBE than Le Bars (240 mg instead of 120 mg per day). The study included senile Alzheimer type dementia patients and patients with mild to moderate multi-infarct dementia (MID). Treatment duration was 24 weeks. The improvements measured for several parameters were 32% for the group given a GBE and 17% for the group given a placebo, a statistically significant difference. These results are comparable to those achieved by acetylcholinesterase inhibitors (AChEI), but with far better tolerability.

Short-term therapy has also produced surprisingly good results, as was shown by Maurer et al. in a placebo-controlled, double-blind study of 20 patients with mild to moderate Alzheimer type dementia.

This sampling of research results reflects our current state of knowledge and indicates that ginkgo is exceptionally well suited for the treatment of brain disorders resulting from degenerative vascular changes.

Numerous studies also show the effects of GBE on **peripheral arterial occlusive disease (PAOD)** and confirm its efficacy for this indication.

As early as 1984, Bauer published the results of a randomized, double-blind study of 79 patients in Fontaine stage II B who were treated for 6 months with either GBE or placebo. His results regarding pain-free and absolute walking distance and plethysmography measurements clearly document the efficacy of GBE and its statistically significant superiority compared to placebo. The objective findings and clinical assessment of the examiner correlated with the subjective assessment of the patients treated.

In 1987, Rudofsky showed that GBE provides statistically significant improvements in ergometric exercise capacity and, at the same time, reduces the lactate:pyruvate ratio compared to placebo. Study parameters associated with blood flow characteristics also showed that GBE produced significant improvements compared to placebo.

In 1985, Hamann showed that a GBE can increase the known effects of **vestibular rehabilitation exercise.** This randomized, double-blind study included 35 patients with Meniere's disease, vestibular neuropathy. and posttrauma conditions who continued to have symptoms of vertigo despite previous conventional infusion therapy and other measures to increase circulation. The duration of these disorders averaged 3 to 4 years. All patients received vestibular rehabilitation. In addition, 17 patients received 160 mg of a GBE and 18 patients received a placebo, per day. The total treatment duration was 4 weeks. During treatment, body sway amplitude decreased by 22.2 mm (39%) for the group with vestibular rehabilitation treated with a GBE and by only 10.3 mm for those treated with placebo. This difference was highly significant. Subjective symptoms showed equal rates of improvement in the group given an GBE as well as in the placebo group.

In a pilot study of eight patients undergoing aortic coronary bypass surgery, Siegel et al., using extensive measurement parameters for 2 months, demonstrated the preventive effects of ginkgo against **arteriosclerotic vascular changes**. These effects were attributed to radical scavenging effects.

Studies also show decisive improvements for **tinnitus and co-existing symptoms,** such as vertigo and hearing disorders.

These symptoms were tested in a randomized, double-blind study (Meyer) in 210 older patients for a period of 12 weeks. Compared to placebo, the group that was given a GBE showed a significant decrease in symptom severity at the end of the treatment period. The group given a GBE showed improvements after an average of 70 days of treatment, whereas the group given placebo showed improvements after 119 days of treatment. These results were confirmed in another randomized multicentric study of 259 tinnitus patients (Tinnitus-Multicenter-Study).

Last, in a prospective, randomized, reference-controlled study of 80 sudden hearing loss patients, Hoffmann et al. showed in 1993 that infusions of GBEs in a 6% hydroxyl-ethylated starch solution (HAES) was marginally significantly superior to a therapy using naftidrofuryl in 6% HAES regarding the target parameter relative hearing gain ($p = 0.06$).

▶ **Therapy Recommendations.** The exclusive use of standardized extracts as finished pharmaceutical products is recommended. These are also the forms used for which the most extensive experimental and clinical study results are available.

GBE treatment should focus on the beginning of symptoms and not wait until the end stages of, for example, Alzheimer-type dementia or multi-infarct dementia.

Periwinkle (Vinca minor)

This plant, also known as lesser or dwarf periwinkle, must be included here. Periwinkle is a member of the Apocynaceae or dogbane family, which also includes Indian snakeroot (Rauwolfia serpentine). This plant—found in Germany in shady beech forests—is a low-growing groundcover with bare, elliptic, lanceolate leaves that are leathery and evergreen, with a shiny surface (▶ Fig. 4.11). Its solitary flowers are attached to long, tender stems, and are bluish purple, like violets.

Periwinkle is more common in central and southern Germany than in northern Germany. It is also frequently grown as a ground cover in shady garden areas. Medicinal applications use the dried **periwinkle herb** (above-ground parts of the whole plant, Vincae pervincae herba).

▶ **Note.** The name vinca is derived from the Latin *vincere* (= to conquer, to overcome), which could be an indication that the healing power of this plant was already known and valued a long time ago. Books about herbalism from the Middle Ages describe periwinkle as a remedy for headaches, vertigo, and memory loss. This plant no longer played a role in modern phytotherapy until French, Hungarian, and Italian physicians revisited and studied it.

Vince minor needs to be differentiated from Madagascar periwinkle (Vinca rosea, Catharanthus roseus). This plant originated on the East African island of Madagascar and is used to isolate vinblastine and vincristine, which are used as cytostatic drugs.

▶ **Pharmacology.** In 1953, Schnittler and Furlenmeier discovered the alkaloid vincamine as the main active constituent of periwinkle. Further pharmacologic and clinical research focused exclusively on this one isolated constituent, which cannot be considered a phytotherapeutic as we see it. Vincamine is listed as a recognized constituent for the manufacture of circulation enhancing remedies.

▶ **Indications.** The Commission E compiled a **negative monograph** for periwinkle because all newer research refers exclusively to vincamine. There was insufficient evidence of efficacy for the drug itself.

Bibliography

Carus CG. Erfahrungsresultate aus ärztlichen Studien und ärztlichem Wirken. Leipzig: Brockhaus; 1859: 67

Kuschinsky G. Homöopathie und ärztliche Praxis. Dtsch. Ärztebl.: Ärztl. Mitteilungen. 1975a; 8:496

Kuschinsky G. Homöopathie und ärztliche Praxis. Dtsch. Ärztebl.: Ärztl. Mitteilungen. 1975b; 20:1425–1429

Garlic

Gebhardt R. Multiple Wirkung von Knoblauchextrakten auf die Cholesterin-Biosynthese. Med Welt. 1991; 7a:12–13

Grünwald J. Knoblauchextrakt wirksam gegen arteriosklerotische Plaquebildung. Z Phytother. 2005; 26(5):239–240

Jung F, Kiesewetter H, Pindur G, Jung EM, Mrowietz C, Wenzel E. Thrombozytenfunktionshemmende Wirkung von Knoblauch. Med Welt. 1991; 7a:18–19

Jung F, Wolf S, Kiesewetter H, et al. Wirkung von Knoblauch auf die Fließfähigkeit des Blutes. Natur- und Ganzheitsmedizin. 1989; 7: 216–221

Koch HP, Hahn G. Knoblauch. Grundlagen der therapeutischen Anwendung von Allium Sativum L. Munich: Urban & Schwarzenberg; 1988

Petkov W. Pharmakologische und klinische Untersuchungen des Knoblauchs. Dtsch Apoth Ztg. 1966; 51:1861–1867

Petkov W. Über den Wirkungsmechanismus des Panax ginseng C. A. Mey. Zur Frage einer Pharmakologie der Reaktivität. 1. Mitteilung. Arzneimittelforschung. 1961; 3:288–295

Reuter HD. Spektrum Allium sativum. Basel: Aesopus; 1988

Scheffler K. Knoblauch zeigt vielfältige vasoaktive Effekte. NaturaMed. 2015; 1:16–20

Song CS, Kim JH, Rhee DJ. Blood anticoagulant substance from garlic extraction, and physical and chemical properties. Yonsei Med J. 1963; 114(3–4):17–20

Stoll A, Seebeck E. Chemical investigations on alliin, the specific principle of garlic. Adv Enzymol Relat Subj Biochem. 1951; 11: 377–400

Wagner H, Sendl A. Bärlauch und Knoblauch. Dtsch Apoth Ztg. 1990; 130:1809–1815

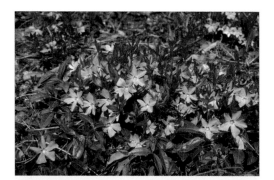

Fig. 4.11 Periwinkle, Vinca minor. Photo: Dr. Roland Spohn, Engen.

Walter-Matsui R. Antimikrobielle Wirkungen des Knoblauchs. Biol Med. 1988; 3:139–140

Winkler G, Lohmüller EM, Landshuter J, Weber W, Knobloch K. Schwefelhaltige Leitsubstanzen in Knoblauchpräparaten. Dtsch Apoth Ztg. 1992; 132:2312–2317

Ginkgo

Bauer U. 6-monatige randomisierte Doppelblind-Studie zur Wirkung von Extraktum Ginkgo Biloba im Vergleich zu Placebo bei Patienten mit peripheren chronisch arteriellen Verschlusskrankheiten [Month double-blind randomised clinical trial of Ginkgo biloba extract versus placebo in two parallel groups in patients suffering from peripheral arterial insufficiency]. Arzneimittelforschung. 1984; 34(I):716–720

Halama P, Bartsch G, Meng G. Hirnleistungsstörungen vaskulärer Genese. Randomisierte Doppelblindstudie zur Wirksamkeit von Ginkgo-biloba-Extrakt. Fortschr Med. 1988; 106:408–412

Hamann KF. Physikalische Therapie des vestibulären Schwindels in Verbindung mit Ginkgo-biloba-Extrakt. Therapiewoche. 1985; 35:4586–4590

Hoffmann F, Beck C, Schulz A, Ottermann P. Ginkgoextrakt EGb 761 (Tebonin®)/HAES versus Naftidrofuryl (Dusodril®)/HAES: Eine randomisierte Studie zur Hörsturztherapie. In: Reuter HD: Spektrum Ginkgo biloba. Basel: Aesopus; 1993: 5

Jiang X, Williams KM, Liauw WS, et al. Effect of ginkgo and ginger on the pharmacokinetics and pharmacodynamics of warfarin in healthy subjects. Br J Clin Pharmacol. 2005; 59(4):425–432

Kanowski S, Herrmann WM, Stephan K, Wierich W, Hörr R. Proof of efficacy of the ginkgo biloba special extract EGb 761 in outpatients suffering from mild to moderate primary degenerative dementia of the Alzheimer type or multi-infarct dementia. Pharmacopsychiatry. 1996; 29(2):47–56

Kleijnen J, Knipschild P. Ginkgo biloba. Lancet. 1992; 340(8828): 1136–1139

Krieglstein J, Oberpichler H. Ginkgo biloba und Hirnleistungsstörungen. Pharm Ztg. 1989; 134(38):9–19

Le Bars PL, Katz MM, Berman N, Itil TM, Freedman AM, Schatzberg AF. A placebo-controlled, double-blind, randomized trial of an extract of Ginkgo biloba for dementia. North American EGb Study Group. JAMA. 1997; 278(16):1327–1332

Leistner E, Arenz A. Toxikologische Sicherheit von Präparaten aus Ginkgo biloba. Z Phytother. 1997; 18(4):230–231

Maurer K, Ihl R, Dierks T, Frölich L. Clinical efficacy of Ginkgo biloba special extract EGb 761 in dementia of the Alzheimer type. J Psychiatr Res. 1997; 31(6):645–655

Meyer B. Etude multicentrique randomisée à double insu face au placebo du traitement des acouphénes par l'extrait de Ginkgo biloba [Multicenter randomized double-blind drug vs. placebo study of the treatment of tinnitus with Ginkgo biloba extract]. Presse Med. 1986; 15(31):1562–1564

Otani M, Chatterjee SS, Gabard B, Kreutzberg GW. Effect of an extract of Ginkgo biloba on triethyltin-induced cerebral edema. Acta Neuropathol. 1986; 69(1–2):54–65

Reuter HD. Spektrum Ginkgo biloba. Basel: Aesopus; 1993

Rudofsky G. Wirkung von Ginkgo-biloba-Extrakt bei arterieller Verschlusskrankheit. Randomisierte plazebokontrollierte Cross-over-Doppelblindstudie [Effect of Ginkgo biloba extract in arterial occlusive disease. Randomized placebo controlled crossover study]. Fortschr Med. 1987; 105(20):397–400

Sancesario G, Kreutzberg GW. Stimulation of astrocytes affects cytotoxic brain edema. Acta Neuropathol. 1986; 72(1):3–14

Schilcher H. Ginkgo biloba L. Untersuchungen zur Qualität, Wirkung, Wirksamkeit und Unbedenklichkeit. Z Phytother. 1988; 9:119–127

Schulz V. Ginkgo: Kein erhöhtes Blutungsrisiko. Z Phytother. 2006; 27(4):179–180

Schulz V. Ginkgo-biloba-Spezialextrakt. Erfolgsgeschichte eines rationalen Phytopharmakons. Z Phytother. 2004; 25 Suppl 1: 12–19

Siegel G, Schäfer P, Winkler K, Malmsten M. Ginkgo biloba (EGb 761) in arteriosclerosis prophylaxis. Wien Med Wochenschr. 2007; 157(13–14):288–294

Spegg H. Ginkgo biloba—Ein Baum aus Urzeiten, ein Phytopharmakon mit Zukunft. PTAheute. 1990; 4:576–583

Sticher O, Hasler A, Meier B. Ginkgo biloba – Eine Standortbestimmung. Dtsch Apoth Ztg. 1991; 131:1827–1835

Meyer B. Etude multicentrique des acouphènes. Epidémiologie et thérapeutique [A multicenter study of tinnitus. Epidemiology and therapy]. Ann Otolaryngol Chir Cervicofac. 1986; 103(3):185–188

Vorberg G. Ginkgo biloba extract (GBE) a long-term study of chronical cerebral insufficiency in geriatric patients. Clin Trials J. 1985; 22:149–157

Weitbrecht WU, Jansen W. Primär degenerative Demenz: Therapie mit Ginkgo-biloba-Extrakt. Plazebo-kontrollierte Doppelblind- und Vergleichsstudie [Primary degenerative dementia: therapy with Ginkgo biloba extract. Placebo-controlled double-blind and comparative study]. Fortschr Med. 1986; 104(9):199–202

Weitbrecht WU. Wirkungen und Wirksamkeit des Ginkgo-biloba-Extraktes. Perfusion. 1989; 2:40–44

Periwinkle

Schnittler E, Furlenmeier A. Vincamin, ein Alkaloid aus Vinca minor L. (Apocynaceae). Helv Chim Acta. 1953; 36(1):2017–2020

4.2 Heart Arrhythmia

4.2.1 Benign Cardiac Arrhythmia

> **Medicinal Plants**
>
> **Scotch Broom**, Cytisus scoparius
> Scotch Broom herb, Cytisi scoparii herba
> **Yellow Jessamine**, Gelsemium sempervirens
> Yellow Jessamine root, Gelsemii rhizoma
> **Motherwort**, Leonurus cardiaca
> Motherwort herb, Leonuri herba

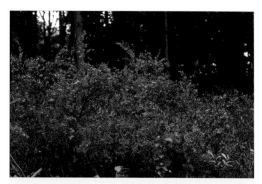

Fig. 4.12 Scotch Broom, Cytisus scoparius (Sarothamnus scoparius). Photo: Dr. Roland Spohn, Engen.

Cardiac arrhythmia can have many functional and organic causes. They range from benign paroxysmal tachycardia—which is harmless but severely impacts a patient's sense of well-being—to severe block formation in the cardiac conduction system (CCS), which can become indications for implantation of a pacemaker. Digitalis glycosides can, on the one hand, restore heart rhythm, especially with chronic heart failure. On the other hand, arrhythmia is also one of the side effects to be concerned about with digitalis. Many effective synthetic antiarrhythmia drugs are not effective, and, in some cases, they themselves can cause serious arrhythmia. They also frequently cause substantial undesired effects.

Regarding phytotherapeutic alternatives, antiarrhythmic properties have been attributed to hawthorn. This effect of hawthorn is pharmacologically documented. However, this special effect is part of the overall efficacy profile of hawthorn and is not a selective indication. This makes hawthorn different from Scotch broom (Cytisus scoparius, syn. Sarothamnus scoparius), which is certainly the most powerful plant-derived antiarrhythmic. Yellow jessamine (Gelsemium sempervirens) is another antiarrhythmic plant.

Both medicinal plants are not comparable to synthetic antiarrhythmic drugs. They are especially not suitable for emergency and acute therapy. They do, however, offer alternatives to practitioners for benign cardiac arrhythmia.

Plants for Treatment

Scotch Broom, Cytisus scoparius, syn. Sarothamnus scoparius

Scotch broom is one of the most widespread and beautiful plants of the flora of Germany (▶ Fig. 4.12).

It grows in heaths and arid pine forests as well as along sandy slopes and railroad embankments, and in June, the stands of Scotch broom develop bright yellow flowers. Many images document the beautiful regions of blooming Scotch broom that can be found, for example, at Hiddensee island, and in other heath regions. Scotch broom can grow as tall as an average human adult and can form dense thickets. Its large, yellow flowers attract many insects.

Medicinal applications use the **Scotch broom herb** (above-ground parts of the whole plant, Sarothamni scoparii herba)

▶ **Pharmacology.** Scotch broom is not a member of the group of digitalis-like medicinal plants. It occupies a special place because it contains alkaloids instead of glycosides. The most well known of these is sparteine but more than 20 other quinolizidine alkaloids have been identified. The minimum alkaloid content of the drug is 0.8%. These alkaloids are primarily located in the trunk of the plant and in the epidermis and subepidermis of the organs. Scotch broom also contains flavonoids, isoflavones, coumarins, caffeic acid derivatives, and traces of volatile oil. The seeds contain lectins.

The actions of the various alkaloids are sympathomimetic and vasoconstrictory. They also raise blood pressure. Sparteine is the most studied of these alkaloids and is considered antiarrhythmic. It inhibits sodium ion transport through cell membranes, which reduces increased excitability of the cardiac conduction system (CCS). It also normalizes pathologic changes to signal formation in the atrium of the heart. Unlike, for example, digitalis glycosides, sparteine has no positive inotropic effect, but does lengthen the diastole.

▶ **Indications.** The main indications for Scotch broom, in the opinion of the authors, are primarily **functional heart arrhythmias** of the more **tachycardia** type in combination with **blood pressure that tends to be low (hypotension).**

The Commission E monograph for Scotch broom only lists functional heart and circulatory system disorders. It did not consider the evidence for specific antiarrhythmic effects to be sufficient. In 2008 Wichtl refers to the improvement of circulatory system dysregulation.

Scotch broom is contraindicated for high blood pressure and during pregnancy because it can increase uterine tonus in pregnant women.

Caution

Due to Scotch broom's tyramine content, concurrent use of Scotch broom and monoaminoxidase (MAO) inhibitors should be avoided because this could cause a hypertensive crisis.

▶ **Note.** It is certainly problematic to label Scotch broom preparations as a cardiac antiarrhythmic drug without a differentiated description. With today's tightly defined indications, this is bound to lead to misunderstandings. However, there are good reasons to place Scotch broom in the chapter on cardiac arrhythmia. These types of arrhythmia have primarily functional causes and are therefore considered benign from the point of view of science-based cardiology. They do, however, profoundly impact a patient's sense of well-being. This justifies the use of an antiarrhythmic drug that is well documented for its good tolerability also in long-term and continuous use.

Preparation

- **Tea**
  Add 1 cup of boiling water to 1 teaspoon of the drug. Steep covered for 10 minutes, then strain.
  Drink 1 cup of freshly prepared tea 3–4 × a day.

Prescriptions

- **Infusion**
  Rx
  Infus. Sarothamni scop. herb. 2.5/180.0 (Scotch broom herb infusion)
  D.S.
  Take 1 tablespoon 3–4 × a day.

Motherwort (Leonurus cardiaca)

Motherwort is a member of the Lamiaceae family. It is easily recognizable by its tall stiff, growth and large leaves with five laciniate lobes. Its flowers are small, inconspicuous and pale red, and crowded into the leaf axils. Motherwort frequently grows in Germany in inhospitable locations near buildings, along the edges of village streets, and along fences.

Medicinal applications use the **motherwort herb** (above-ground parts of the whole plant; Leonuri cardiacae herba) gathered during flowering season.

▶ **Pharmacology.** The motherwort drug contains alkaloids, for example, stachydrine, and bitter glycosides.

In 2010, Ritter et al. published a detailed study of motherwort's pharmacology. It involved the use of a bioassay-guided extract fractionation procedure, resulting in the development of a cardioactive Leonurus cardiaca refined extract (LCRE) from the aqueous Soxhlet extraction of Leonurus cardiaca. Intracoronary application of this special extract in isolated rabbit hearts perfused according to the Langendorff technique prolonged the PQ interval and increased both the basic cycle length and the activation recovery interval. In concurrent voltage clamp experiments, LCRE exerted a calcium antagonistic activity (I(Ca.L) blockade, reduced the repolarizing current I(K.r), and prolonged the action potential (AP) duration. LCRE displayed only weak effects on the amplitude and voltage dependence of the I(f) amplitude of the adult guinea pig sinus node; and it significantly prolonged the activation time constant of I(f). I(Na) was not affected by the application of LCRE, which is a welcome result because this effect is associated with the risk of proarrhythmic side effects.

In addition to the above data, a study of the vector field similarity of the excitation propagation on the heart muscle surface by means of epicardial mapping indicates a strong antiarrhythmic potential for this drug. The natural decay of the vector field similarity in the myocardium treated by the special extract was reduced compared to the vehicle control experiment. Typically, the decay of the vector field similarity is sped up rather than slowed down by the application of drugs to hearts prepared according to the Langendorf technique. Therefore, these results for motherwort are extraordinary. This result is also of special clinical relevance because the decay of the vector field similarity of the excitation propagation in the myocardium is considered a key cause for reentry tachycardia. Paradoxically, this is one of the frequent side effects of heart arrhythmia with chemically defined single substances.

▸ **Indications.** Motherwort is used in traditional folk medicine as a remedy for various nerve and heart disorders. Weiss confirmed its efficacy especially for **vegetative functional heart symptoms**. It seems to be primarily a sedative like valerian but needs to be used for several months.

Yellow Jessamine (Gelsemium sempervirens)

This vine originates from Mexico and Guatemala. Its rootstock, **Gelsemii rhizoma**, provides a 10%, light brown, bitter-tasting tincture.

▸ **Pharmacology.** Yellow jessamine contains the indol alkaloids gersemin and sempervirin.

Yellow jessamine also lowers the excitability of the sympathetic and parasympathec nervous systems and calms hypertonic vascular systems. Its action is **cardiosedative**. Unlike Scotch broom, yellow jessamine does not have a specific effect on the cardiac conduction system (CCS).

▸ **Indications.** The Commission E compiled a negative monograph for yellow jessamine because of its narrow therapeutic application and numerous cases of toxicopathy, including deaths.

Despite that, yellow jessamine, best taken as a tincture, has been proven in practice for calming the heart, especially for **extrasystoles** and **functional heart disorders**. However, it should always be prescribed and monitored by a physician.

Preparation	

- **Tincture**
  Take 20–30 drops 2–4 × a day.

Proven Prescriptions

Prescriptions	

Rx
Tinct. Gelsemii 10.0 (yellow jessamine tincture)
Tinct. Valerian. aeth. ad 30.0 (ethereal valerian tincture)
D.S.
Take 20–30 drops 3 × a day.

Prescriptions	

Rx
Tinct. Gelsemii 10.0 (yellow jessamine tincture)
Extr. Adonidis fluid. 10.0 (pheasant's eye fluid extract)
Tinct. Valerian. aeth. ad 30.0 (ethereal valerian tincture)
D.S.
Take 20–40 drops 3 × a day.

Prescriptions	

Rx
Tinct. Gelsemii 12.0 0 (yellow jessamine tincture)
Extr. Crataegi fluid. ad 30.0 (hawthorn fluid extract)
D.S.
Take 20 drops 3 × a day.

Bibliography

Ritter M, Melichar K, Strahler S, et al. Cardiac and electrophysiological effects of primary and refined extracts from Leonurus cardiaca L. (Ph.Eur.). Planta Med. 2010; 76(6): 572–582

Wichtl M, Ed. Teedrogen und Phytopharmaka. 5. Auflage. Stuttgart: Wissenschaftliche Verlagsgesellschaft; 2008

4.3 Functional Heart Disorders

This chapter presents a summary of the important reasons why phytotherapy and its remedies are an indispensable part of modern pharmacotherapy in the realm of cardiology.

4.3.1 The "Nervous" Heart

Without a doubt, modern medicine in the 21st century should recognize that a delineation of organic and functional disorders, for example of the heart, does not make sense. Representatives of a mechanistic philosophy should be especially cognizant of the fact that a healthy organ is a functioning organ. For example, an engine that allows a car to be driven but constantly sputters would not be acceptable to its owner and would quickly be taken to an auto repair shop. This book, however, is based on the thinking that the human organism neither corresponds to mechanistic principles nor does it follow mechanistic functions. In addition to the purely physical level, the human organism also operates on a living, feeling plane, and is conscious of itsself. When one takes this into consideration, it becomes obvious that impaired function is already organic in nature, and in many cases, is a precursor to manifest organic disease. Given the significance of prevention, functional organ disorders should be taken seriously and therapy—ideally, causal therapy—should be provided.

Another important aspect relates to the fact that humans place a high value on the impact of a disturbed state of mind on their health and sense of well-being. Frequently, this impact is subjectively rated as higher than organically manifested findings. This state can also be described as latent disease. Traditional medicine called this the "nervous" heart. Paroxysmal, supraventricular tachycardia, benign extrasystoles ("chaotic heart" or allodromy), functional angine pectoris without demonstrable findings relating to the coronary arteries—they all can create the emotional symptom of fear, even fear of death, in addition to symptoms related to the organ. Rather than immediately resorting to remedies that interfere with the function of important organ systems—for example, beta-blockers—choosing remedies that reestablish the body's own regulating abilities in a way that enable it to deal with disturbed function must be, in terms of a truly humane therapy, the first choice for every practitioner.

Plants for Treatment

The individual sections of this chapter contain multiple references to the phytotherapeutic treatment options for functional heart disorders. The relevant medicinal plants are described in the chapters that correspond to their leading symptom—heart failure and angina pectoris (see Section 4.1.2 (p. 147)), congestive Heart Failure (p. 147), arrhythmia (see Section 4.2.1, Benign Cardiac Arrhythmia (p. 163)), and circulatory system dysregulation (see Chapter 4.4, Circulatory System Dysregulation (p. 167)). The sample prescriptions in those chapters also encompass more complex symptoms.

Special Treatments

Another treatment option is the **external application of heart salves and heart ointments**, which frequently contain essential oils. In the authors' experience, they often work well and are always helpful as an adjuvant to other treatments. They are especially applicable for functional heart disorders with **angina pectoris symptoms** and should be applied by the patient in the morning and evening.

Preparation

Rosemary Composite Ointment (Ungt. Rosmarini comp. according to the German Pharmacopoeia DAB)

Ungt. Rosmarini comp.:

16 parts pig lard, 8 parts mutton fat, 2 parts yellow bee wax, 2 parts mace (Myristica fragrans) balm (produced from mace by hot squeezing) are melted together and—after slight cooling—mixed with 1 part each of rosemary oil and juniper berry oil.

Bibliography

Weidinger G. Waarenlexikon der chemischen Industrie und der Pharmacie. 1. ed, Verlag H. Haessel. Leipzig, 1868, 548

4.4 Circulatory System Dysregulation

The term "circulatory system dysregulation" describes all changes that present as functional disturbances of the life essential circulation regulatory system. Much too often, circulation is equated with blood pressure. Blood pressure is an important symptomatic expression of circulation, but the two are not identical. Circulation refers to blood flow characteristics, the distribution of arterial and venous blood in the entire organism, including the organs involved, and the regulation of substance transport and exchange.

However, the primary role of the circulatory system is to be a "location" of a subtle balance that is of utmost importance for the health and sense of well-being of human beings. Much too little attention is still being paid to the mental and emotional influence on the circulatory system because it cannot be treated by selective *in vitro* pharmacology.

Clinical practitioners know that blood pressure that gradually rises to extreme values does not have to present with any subjective symptoms and may not be discovered until an apoplectic insult occurs. On the other hand, labile hypertension (prehypertension) with erratic and sudden rises in blood pressure caused by endocrine disorders (pheochromocytoma) immensely impacts how a person feels. The same applies to hypotension. Many people suffering from low blood pressure actually can have completely normal blood pressure but suffer from all the symptoms of hypotension. On the other hand, patients with constitutional hypotension—whose blood pressure rarely rises above 100 mmHg—can enjoy perfect health and full vitality. Readers of the following sections are invited to always remember that symptoms associated with high or low blood pressure are but one aspect of a more comprehensive circulatory system dysregulation.

4.4.1 Arterial Hypertension

Medicinal Plants
Indian Snakeroot, Rauwolfia serpentina
Indian Snakeroot root, Rauwolfia radix
Mistletoe, Viscum album
Mistletoe herb, Visci herba
Olive, Olea europaea
Olive leaf, Oleae folium

Most cases of hypertension are considered idiopathic. This surprising fact indicates that, as a rule, no demonstrable causes can be found. Endocrine and renal causes are found in only a few cases.

Since hypertension is a significant contributor to the development of vascular sclerosis, treating hypertension is also a preventive measure.

Nowadays, early diagnosis and preventive treatment are considered standard treatment for hypertension.

The plethora of effective synthetic antihypertensive drugs raises the question if phytotherapy reaches its limits with this indication. This is certainly true for fixed and malignant types of hypertension. However, especially with labile hypertension, which presents with obvious functional and emotional components, phytotherpeutics that regulate and normalize blood pressure rather than symptomatically lower blood pressure can be helpful. Few drugs are available that are able to accomplish that. The primary remedy is **Indian snakeroot** (Rauwolfia serpentina). Other options are garlic (p. 154), which is discussed extensively earlier in this book, and, with some limitations, **mistletoe** and **olive**.

Plants for Treatment

Indian Snakeroot (Rauwolfia serpentina)

Indian snakeroot is a member of the Apocynaceae or dogbane family that also includes strophanthus, oleander, and periwinkle along with other valuable medicinal plants.

This ancient Indian medicinal plant primarily grows on the slopes of the Himalayas. In addition to Indian snakeroot (Rauwolfia serpentina) (▶ Fig. 4.13) there are a number of other types of Rauwolfia that largely have the same effects. Commercially suitable types of Rauwolfia grow in the tropical areas of the Congo. Indian snakeroot is extensively cultivated in India to better meet the demand for this plant.

Medicinal applications use the **Indian snakeroot root** (Rauwolfiae radix).

▶ **Note.** The name Rauwolfia refers to the German physician Leonhard Rauwolf (1535–1596) from Augsburg. He traveled to Asia in the middle of the 16th century and subsequently wrote a widely renowned book about herbs. The book, however, did not describe the Rauwolfia plant itself. It was

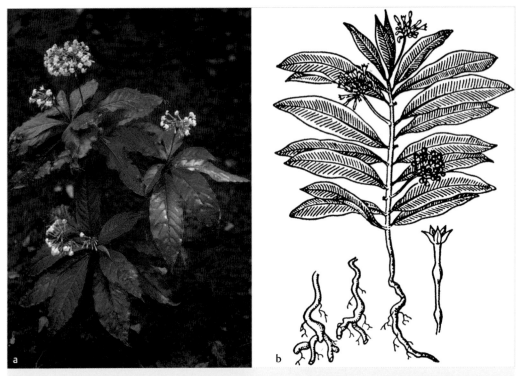

Fig. 4.13 a and b Indian Snakeroot, Rauwolfia serpentina. Photo: Dr. Roland Spohn, Engen.

discovered a century later by a French botanist and named after Rauwolf to honor him for his travels, which greatly benefited botany.

Indian snakeroot was introduced to clinical use by the Indian physician Vakil in 1940 after Chopra et al. had discovered the blood pressure-lowering action of Rauwolfia in animal experiments. Vakil reported that Rauwolfia was already mentioned in old Hindu texts around 1000 BC and referred to by its Sanskrit name *sarpagandha* around 200 AD.

Reports describing the application of Indian snakeroot for various diseases go back several hundred years. As with many plants used in folk medicine, the indications for Indian snakeroot varied widely. It was indicated as a remedy for snake and insect bites, headaches, agitation and anxiety, fever, and abdominal symptoms. A review of indication areas for this remedy makes it clear that nervous system conditions play a predominant role. Indian snakeroot seems to have been primarily used as a **universal tranquilizer.**

▶ **Pharmacology.** Indian snakeroot contains at minimum of 1% alkaloids, calculated as reserpine in the dried drug. Other known alkaloids include rescinamine, deserpidine, serpentine, and raubasin.

The action of reserpine and other alkaloids contained in Indian snakeroot is sympatholytic via depletion of catecholamine by sequestering and inhibiting reabsorption of noradrenalin in the vesicles of noradrenergic nerve endings. This provides the **blood pressure-lowering** and simultaneous **sedative** effects. The Indian snakeroot constituent ajmalin is known to have **antiarrhythmic effects** via membrane stabilization. The resorption rate of reserpine is 40% and its blood pressure-lowering action takes time to develop.

Nowadays, literature about snakeroot is too extensive even for experts to keep up with. It has been studied chemically, pharmacologically, and clinically, many times and very precisely, especially in the United States and in the United Kingdom.

▶ **Indications.** Indian snakeroot positively affects primarily the **subjective symptoms** of hypertension, such a headache, vertigo, heart anxiety, and general restlessness.

Snakeroot does not have immediate effects. Its effect develops gradually, and it often takes 2 to 3 weeks to notice them. However, the effects persist after the remedy is stopped, sometimes for several weeks.

The Commission E listed the following indications for snakeroot: **mild, essential hypertension** (borderline hypertension), especially with increased tonus of the sympathetic nervous system and sinus tachycardia, anxiety and tension, and psychomotor agitation.

Side effects of snakeroot include nasal congestion, fatigue, sexual arousal disorders, and depressive states. Snakeroot can also significantly impact reaction capacity. Interactions with other drugs include reciprocal potentiation with neuroleptics and barbiturates, pronounced bradycardia in combination with digitalis glycosides and antagonism to (lowering the effects of) levodopa (L-dopa). Other contraindications, also due to its interactions with other drugs are depression, pheochromocytoma, gastric ulcers, pregnancy, and lactation.

For a long time, snakeroot was one of the most widely used antihypertension drugs. It was successively pushed into the background by the isolation of the snakeroot alkaloid reserpine and by the discovery of numerous new synthetic antihypertensive drugs (α-methyldopa, nifedipine, ACE inhibitors, ganglionic blockers). More recently, a change in thinking is starting to take place, bolstered by the fact that many synthetic antihypertension drugs have significant negative effects that impact how hypertension patients feel. It was shown that a whole extract of snakeroot with a standardized alkaloid content is as effective as the isolated reserpine, but with significantly higher tolerability. It is too early to talk about a snakeroot renaissance for hypertension treatment, but it should be increasingly viewed as an alternative for the treatment of hypertension.

However, due to increasingly strict rules for testing and approval of drugs and the availability of highly efficacious synthetic antihypertension drugs, finished pharmaceuticalwhole extract products of Indian snakeroot are no longer available. The only options are to prescribe the tincture, possibly combined with other blood pressure-lowering plant remedies, or to use homeopathic preparations or combination remedies that contain the tincture.

Weiss summarized the **clinical significance of Indian snakeroot** for essential (idiopathic) hypertension as follows:

- Snakeroot is the **mildest of all hypotensive remedies** and one of the most useful. Its advantages include its simple peroral application and a desired sedative effect. This almost makes snakeroot a "causal therapeutic" because the "tension" exhibited by hypertension patients is obvious.
- Snakeroot suffices as the only remedy for mild and moderate cases of **essential hypertension**. It needs to be taken from 2–3 months to 1 year or an average of 6 months.
- Treatment starts with a low dosage that is gradually increased until blood pressure drops or undesirable symptoms occur. If side effects are too severe, the dosage is reduced. It rarely needs to be discontinued altogether. When sufficient lowering of blood pressure has been reached, the patient is stabilized on that dosage for a longer period.
- Snakeroot is either used as a **whole extract** or as the pure reserpine alkaloid. Their effects on patients is the same. From a phypotherapeutic perspective, whole extracts featuring a defined alkaloid content is preferred.
- Snakeroot cannot be expected to cure hypertension. However, in a significant percentage of patients, it positively and sufficiently impacts the subjective manifestations of hypertension and reduces its implications, especially for the vascular system.

Preparation ☞

- Tincture

Mistletoe (Viscum album)

Mistletoe is a spheroid shrub (▶ Fig. 4.14) in the Loranthaceae family and grows on deciduous and coniferous trees.

Mistletoe stems are dichotomously forked in a manner otherwise primarily seen in "lower" plant species such as algae. Its yellowish-green flowers are completely inconspicuous. Its white berries, however, are more noticeable and contain a sticky, mucilaginous mass. Its leaves are opposite, yellowish green, and perennial.

Medicinal applications use the **whole mistletoe herb** (fresh or dried younger branches with flowers and fruits, Visci herba).

▶ **Pharmacology.** Many constituents of mistletoe have been identified, including toxic polypeptides (viscotoxins), lectins, flavonoids, biogenic amines, phenylpropane derivatives, and lignans. Until now, none of these constituents was identified as being responsible for the blood pressure-lowering effect traditionally attributed to mistletoe.

▶ **Research.** According to Wagner and Wiesenuer, studies by Sih et al. have shown that the only potential constituents for lowering blood pressure are flavone compounds and lignan or phenylpropane compounds. This is because the lignan pinoresinol, a related compound, has blood pressure-lowering effects.

▶ **Indications.** There are no newer, controlled studies demonstrating long-term efficacy for a larger patient cohort. Therefore, the decision criterion for the use of mistletoe is found in the practitical experience of traditional medicine, which has made use of mistletoe as a blood pressure regulator with mild blood pressure-lowering effects.

Weiss characterized mistletoe as a typical **mild** (**"mite"**) **phytotherapeutic** without objective immediate effect and minor blood pressure-lowering effects compared to snakeroot. However, its beneficial effects on subjective symptoms like headaches, dizziness, reduced stamina, irritability, and other symptoms associated with high

blood pressure make it a proven remedy in practice, especially because it has no known negative side effects. Minor to moderately high blood pressure values decrease in the course of treatment or only occur sporadically during increased physical exertion or emotional stress. As a mild therapeutic, Weiss viewed mistletoe as a remedy that can be used for **long-term treatment or regimens.**

Preparation

- **Maceration**

Prescriptions

Rx
Viscum alb. herb. conc. 100.0 (mistletoe herb concoction)
M. f.
Add 250 mL of cold water to 2–4 teaspoons. Soak overnight.
D.S.
Drink 1 cup each in the morning on an empty stomach and in the evening.

- **"Blood Pressure Tea" according to R.F. Weiss**
  According to Weiss, this "blood pressure tea" has been a proven remedy for decades. It contains equal parts of mistletoe formulated as follows for mild blood pressure lowering, hawthorn to increase coronary circulation, and lemon balm as a cardiac sedative:

Prescriptions

Rx
Visci albi herb. (mistletoe herb)
Crataegi fol. et flos (hawthorn leaves and flowers)
Melissae fol. āā ad 100.0 (lemon balm leaves)
M. f.
Add 1 cup of hot water to 2 teaspoons of the blend. Steep covered for 5–10 minutes, then strain.
D.S.
Drink 1 cup each warm in the morning and evening in small sips. May be sweetened with honey.

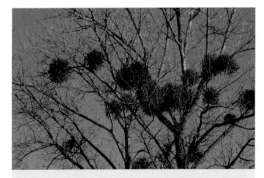

Fig. 4.14 Mistletoe, Viscum album. Photo: Dr. Roland Spohn, Engen.

Olive (Olea europaea)

The olive tree is one of the most important plants in the Mediterranean. It can reach a very old age. Its black-blue fruit, called olives, provide the popular olive oil. Its leaves are evergreen, leathery, and covered in scaly hairs on the underside.

Medicinal applications use the **olive leaves** (Oleae folium). They are recommended as a blood pressure-lowering remedy. The French phytotherapist Henri Leclerc (1870–1955) reported about this characteristic of olive leaves in the early part of the 20th century.

▶ **Pharmacology.** The active principle of olive leaves is presumed to be the secoiridoid glycoside oleuropein. According to studies by Petkov and Manolov, oleuropin has hypotensive, antiarrhythmic and coronary dilating effects. Mild calcium antagonistic effects have also been found.

▶ **Indications.** Weiss considered the blood pressure-lowering effects of olive leaves to be weaker than those of mistletoe and also referred to gastric distress due to local irritation as an unpleasant side effect.

▶ **Therapy Recommendation.** Treatment should use olive leave extract preparations, exclusively.

Bibliography

Chopra RN, Gupta JC, Mukherjee SN. The pharmacological action of an alkaloid obtained from Rauwolfia serpentina Benth. A preliminary note. Indian J Med Res. 1933; 21:261–271

Leclerc H. Précis de phytothérapie. Essais de thérapeutique par les plantes françaises. Issy-les-Moulineaux: Elsevier Masson; 2000

Petkov V, Manolov P. Pharmacological analysis of the iridoid oleuropein. Arzneimittelforschung. 1972; 22(9):1476–1486

Rauwald HW, Brehm O, Odenthal KP. Evaluation of the calcium antagonistic activity of Peucedanum ostruthium and Olea europaea constituents. Pharmaceutical and Pharmacological Letters. 1991; 1:78–81

Sih CJ, Ravikumar PR, Huang FC, Buckner C, Whitlock H, Jr. Isolation and synthesis of pinoresinol diglucoside, a major antihypertensive principle of Tu-Chung (Eucommia ulmoides Oliver). J Am Chem Soc. 1976; 98:5412–5413

Vakil RJ. Rauwolfia serpentina in the treatment of high blood pressure. Lancet. 1954; 267(6841):726–727

Wagner H, Wiesenauer M. Phytotherapie. Phytopharmaka und pflanzliche Homöopathika. 2nd ed. Stuttgart: Wissenschaftliche Verlagsgesellschaft; 2003

Wichtl M, Ed. Teedrogen und Phytopharmaka. 5th ed. Stuttgart: Wissenschaftliche Verlagsgesellschaft; 2008

4.4.2 Arterial Hypotension

Medicinal Plants

Rosemary, Rosmarinus officinalis
Rosemary leaves, Rosmarini folium
Motherwort, Leonurus cardiaca
Motherwort herb, Leonuri cardiacae herba
Camphor, Cinnamomum camphora
Camphor (steam distillate), Camphora

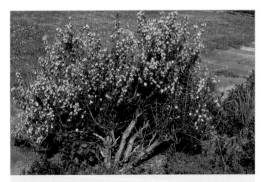

Fig. 4.15 Rosemary, Rosmarinus officinalis. Photo: Dr. Roland Spohn, Engen.

Hypotension, or low blood pressure, is more difficult to treat than high blood pressure. It is more frequently idiopathic than in hypertension, and organic causes for low blood pressure are extremely rare, for example, endocrine disorders such as adrenal insufficiency.

Constitutional hypotension is considered a domain of physical therapy. There are practically no synthetic drugs that produce results comparable to those of antihypertension drugs. Some of these include catecholamine derivatives and vasoconstrictive drugs. With the exception of dihydroergotamine derivatives, the many remedies on the market have shown little usefulness in practice and are not popular with patients. Truly effective synthetic antihypotension drugs are primarily used in shock situations in intensive and emergency care.

Phytotherapy offers two types of action for hypotension: **cardiosedatives** for hypotonic dysregulation, primarily characterized by functional heart symptoms and tachycardia, and **cardiotonics** for hypotensive dysregulation in a narrower sense, characterized by rapid fatigability and orthostasis. Typical cardiosedatives include Scotch broom (p. 163) and motherwort (p. 173). Cardiotonics include pheasant's eye (p. 149), lily-of-the-valley (p. 149), and yellow jessamine (p. 165). Simple combinations that are easy to formulate have also proven to be useful. Some examples are described in the sections on digital glycosides and strophanthin, see Congestive Heart Failure (p. 147).

Remedies specific to hypotensive dysregulation include rosemary, motherwort, and camphor.

Plants for Treatment

Rosemary (Rosmarinus officinalis)

Rosemary is a member of the Lamiaceae family that originates from the Mediterranean region.

This subshrub has small leaves that are curled at the margin (► Fig. 4.15) and exudes an intense, camphor-like fragrance. Its flowers are a light lavender color.

Rosemary grows widely in dry heaths or macchie together with other highly fragrant plants that we also highly value as medicinal plants, for example, sage, thyme, and lavender.

Medicinal applications use the **rosemary leaves,** gathered while flowering (Rosmarini folium, in the past also called *folia anthos*).

► **Pharmacology.** Rosemary leaves contain a minimum of 1.2% volatile oil (Oleum Rosmarini) along with tannins, bitters, and resins. Its main active constituent is volatile oil, which contains rosemary camphor and 1,8-cineol, borneol, and α-pinene. The action of rosemary camphor is analogous to the effects of camphor derived from the camphor tree (Cinnamomum camphora).

► **Indications.** Rosemary is a general circulation and nervous system tonic, especially for the vascular nervous system. This is why it is especially recommended for all **chronic weakness conditions of the circulatory system** with symptoms of hypotension. Rosemary is especially efficacious for asthenic, pale young people with little physical stamina and who do not exhibit organic circulatory system disorders. Rosemary is also a suitable remedy for older people in a weaked state (possibly postinfection).

► **Research.** A randomized, placebo-controlled, double-blind study documented the efficacy of

Preparations

- **Tea**
  Add 1 cup of hot water to 1 teaspoon of the finely chopped drug. Steep covered for 3 minutes, then strain.
  Drink 1 cup warm in the morning and midday.
- **Tincture (1:5)**
  Add 5 drops to a small amount of warm water.
  Drink 15 minutes before meals 3 × a day.
- **Infusion for Baths**
  - **Full bath or sitz bath**
  - Add 1 L of hot water to 50 g of the drug. Steep covered for 30 minutes, then strain, and add to the bath water for full baths or sitz baths.
- **Foot Bath**
  Rosemary footbaths have been proven and are easier to use than the full bath recommended by Weiss. Rosemary baths are tonic and stimulating. They could interfere with sleep and should therefore be taken in the morning, shortly after rising. Bath duration should be 10 minutes in water at a temperature of 34–36 °C, followed by 1 hour of rest, if possible.
  Weekend regimens with rosemary baths taken every Saturday and Sunday morning have been proven effective for people with a tendency toward hypotension who are outside their homes during the workweek.
- **Rosemary Spirit**
  Rosemary spirit is primarily indicated for functional heart symptoms as an external rub applied in the area of the heart.
- **Rosemary Ointment** (Ungt. Rosmarini comp., according to the German Pharmacopoeia, DAB)
  This ointment is listed in the German Pharmacopoeia (DAB) for external application in the area of the heart in case of functional heart symptoms.
  Ungt. Rosmarini comp.:
  16 parts pig lard, 8 parts mutton fat, 2 parts yellow bee wax, 2 parts mace (Myristica fragrans) balm (produced from mace by hot squeezing) are melted together and—after slight cooling—mixed with 1 part each of rosemary oil and juniper berry oil.

rosemary leaves in 40 patients diagnosed with arterial hypotension. The patients treated with a placebo did not show any changes in blood pressure. The systolic blood pressure of patients who received rosemary rose by 20–40 mmHg while their diastolic blood pressure remained nearly unchanged (Scarlat and Tamas).

Motherwort (Leonurus cardiaca)

Motherwort is a member of the Lamiaceae family. It is easily recognizable by its tall, stiff growth, and large leaves with five laciniate lobes. Its flowers are small, inconspicuous and pale red, and crowded into the leaf axils. In Germany, motherwort frequently grows in inhospitable locations near buildings, along the edges of village streets, and along fences.

Medicinal applications use the **motherwort herb** (above-ground parts of the whole plant, gathered during flowering season; Leonuri cardiacae herba).

▶ **Pharmacology.** This drug contains alkaloids, for example stachydrine and bitter glycosides, in addition to other constituents.

In 2010, Ritter et al. published a detailed study of motherwort's pharmacology. It involved the use of a bioassay-guided extract fractionation procedure, resulting in the development of a cardioactive Leonurus cardiaca refined extract (LCRE) from the aqueous Soxhlet extraction of Leonurus cardiaca. Intracoronary application of this special extract in isolated rabbit hearts perfused according to the Langendorff technique prolonged the PQ-interval and increased both the basic cycle length and the activation recovery interval. In concurrent voltage clamp experiments, LCRE exerted a calcium antagonistic activity by I(Ca.L) blockade, reduced the repolarizing current I(K.r), and prolonged the action potential (AP) duration. LCRE displayed only weak effects on the amplitude and voltage dependence of the I(f) amplitude of the adult guinea pig sinus node; and it significantly prolonged the activation time constant of I(f). I(Na) was not affected by the application of LCRE. This study shows a significant effect for the special LCRE extract used on a number of electrophysiological targets, especially I(Ca.L), I(K.r), und I(f), on the organ, and on the cellular level.

▶ **Indications.** Motherwort is used in traditional folk medicine as a remedy for various nerve and heart disorders. Weiss confirmed its efficacy especially for **vegetative functional heart symptoms**. It seems to be primarily a sedative like valerian but needs to be used for several months.

Preparation

- **Tea**
  Add 1 cup of hot water to 2 teaspoons of motherwort herb. Steep covered for 5 minutes, then strain.
  Drink 1 cup each in the morning and in the evening.

- **Combination with Lily-of-the-Valley and the Sedative Effects of Lemon Balm**

Prescriptions

Rx
Leonur. card. herb. (motherwort herb)
Convallar. herb. (lily-of-the-valley herb)
Melissae fol. āā ad 100.0 (lemon balm leaves)
M. f. spec.
Infusion of 2 teaspoons in 1 cup of water.
D.S.
Drink 1 cup each in the morning and in the evening regularly for several weeks.

Camphor (Cinnamomum camphora)

The camphor tree originates from the mountain forests of China, Taiwan, and the southern islands of the Japanese archipelago. In those regions, it can grow to a height of 20 m, sometimes to 50 m. Its preferred growth medium is mixed sand and loam.

The gnarled, branched tree has elongated to elliptical leaves that are up to 11 cm long and feature three veins. The leaf surface is shiny and the underside is bluish green. Camphor tree flowers are greenish yellow and its fruit is purple black.

Camphor is derived through steam distillation of the chipped wood. The camphor crystallizes from the raw oil and is purified through centrifugation and supplimation. For some time now, camphor has also been distilled from the camphor tree leaves.

▶ **Note.** Camphor has been used since ancient times. It can also be found depicted in drawings from the Middle Ages, for example, by Hildegard von Bingen. In modern medicine, it was used as a central analeptic (central nervous system stimulant). Camphor injections were a typical remedy for emergency and acute treatment of collapse and syncope (unconsciousness).

▶ **Pharmacology.** Camphor contains (1R,4R)-2-bornanone, at least half of which is present as (1R)-isomeres. R-(+)-camphor is a bicyclic monoterpene. Natural camphor also contains traces of cineol, borneol, eugenol, and other monoterpenes.

Camphor is largely metabolized by the organism, conjugated with glucuronic acid and excreted via the kidneys. Only a small amount of camphor is excreted via exhalation. Its rapid metabolization explains camphor's short-term effects.

Camphor stimulates the respiratory and vasomotor centers and therefore has a **tonic effect on the circulatory system** as well as **bronchospasmolytic** effects. Camphor's analeptic action is minor and requires almost toxic dosage levels to be effective. External applications of camphor produce **hyperemic effects** and inhalations of camphor are a bronchial secrolytic.

▶ **Indications.** The primary indications for oral administration of camphor are **circulatory system disorders with hypotension**. Camphor is also used externally as an ointment to treat **chest tightness (heart anxiety)** in the area of the heart. Camphor should only be applied to intact skin as it can cause redness, irritation, and painful inflammation in higher concentrations.

The Commission E monograph for camphor lists the following indications: muscular rheumatism, cardiac symptoms (external applications) and hypotonic circulatory regulation disorders (internal application).

> ## Caution
>
> The internal use of camphor as a respiratory analeptic is obsolete.
>
> The camphor content of remedies used with infants and young children should not exceed a maximum of 5%, if it is used at all, due to its pronounced irritation potential. Under no circumstances should camphor be applied to the face, especially not near the nose, as this can lead to a closure of the glottis and depressed respiration and, worst case, to suffocation (Kratschmer reflex).

▶ **Research.** A randomized, placebo-controlled, double-blind study documents a significantly stronger effect of the camphor-containing combination remedy on low blood pressure (Schandry et al.). This provides evidence-based confirmation of the decades of positive experience of using this remedy, which also has acute effects.

> ## Preparations
>
> * **Ointments and Liniments**
>   They contain 10–20, up to a maximum of 25% camphor.
>   Apply externally several times a day.
> * **Camphor Spirit** (Spiritus camphoratus, in accordance with the German Pharmacopoeia DAB 10)
>   This spirit is prepared using 9.5–10.5% camphor and is also suitable for external applications (see caution on this page above for infants and young children).
>   Apply externally several times a day.

Bibliography

Czygan I, Czygan FC. Rosmarin-Rosmarinus officinalis L. Portrait einer Arzneipflanze. Z Phytother. 1997; 18(3):182–186

Ritter M, Melichar K, Strahler S, et al. Cardiac and electrophysiological effects of primary and refined extracts from Leonurus cardiaca L. (Ph.Eur.). Planta Med. 2010; 76(6): 572–582

Scarlat MA, Tamas M. Vorläufige Ergebnisse einer klinischen Studie über die Wirkung von Rosmarini folium pulvis 2 × 0,5 g/d zur Behandlung arterieller Hypotonie. Z Phytother. 2006; 27(3): 120–121

Schandry R, Nussbaumer J. Hahnenkamp SDie Wirkung eines campherhaltigen Phytopharmakons auf den Ruheblutdruck und die kognitive Leistung bei essenzieller Hypotonie. Z Phytother. 2008; 29 Suppl 1:14

4.5 Venous System Disorders

4.5.1 Chronic Venous Insufficiency

Medicinal Plants

Horse Chestnut, Aesculus hippocastanum
Horse Chestnut seeds, Hippocastani semen
Sweet Clover, Melilotus officinalis
Sweet Clover herb, Meliloti herba
Common Grape Vine, Vitis vinifera
Common Grape leaves, Vitis viniferae folium

Vascular system disorders are characterized by thrombotic and inflammatory processes: **thrombophlebitis** and **varicosities** (varicose veins), based primarily on constitutional factors and weak connective tissue. Therapy is dominated, on the one hand, by anticoagulants such as dicumarol and heparin, and, on the other hand, by physical therapy and vascular surgery.

The most important application area for phytotherapeutics is **chronic venous insufficiency**, which most frequently occurs in conjunction with varicose veins. This disorder is very prevalent in industrialized countries. It is almost always preceded by deep vein thrombosis, which may go unnoticed. This causes changes in the venous walls, especially to destruction of venous valves, and creates the typical set of symptoms indicative of stasis, such as local edema that occurs especially in situations of static pressure (sitting, standing), leg cramps in the calf area, pain, and fatigued, heavy, and itchy legs. In the late stages of this disorder, chronic venous ulcers of the lower leg are a sign of a perfusion disorder.

Since the underlying connective tissue disorder (weakness) is not treatable, primary therapy consists of support and compression measures. Frequently, varicose veins are sclerotized or surgically removed. Before the decision to undergo such invasive measures, however, this complex set of symptoms can be very successfully treated with medicinal plant remedies. The primary remedy is **horse chestnut**, which is supported by voluminous clinical literature, followed by **sweet clover**.

Plants for Treatment

Horse Chestnut (Aesculus hippocastanum)

The horse chestnut tree (▶ Fig. 4.16) provides a valuable remedy, especially for venous disorders, in its usually shiny-smooth seeds called **chestnuts** (Hippocastani semen). The seeds have to be processed in a certain manner to provide usable horse chestnut preparations.

▶ **Note.** Horse chestnuts need to be differentiated from the sweet chestnut (Castanea vesca), which provide the edible fruit (marron) and are not used medicinally.

▶ **Pharmacology.** Horse chestnuts contain 3–10% of an acidic, complex triterpene saponin mixture, calculated as anhydrous aescin based on a drug dehydrated at 100–105 °C. They also contain purine derivatives and flavonoids.

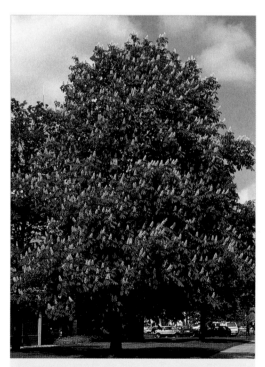

Fig. 4.16 Horse Chestnut, Aesculus hippocastanum. Photo: Dr. Roland Spohn, Engen.

Aescin is the primary active constituent of horse chestnut. Like all saponins, it has strong **hemolytic** effects, but these do not play a role in clinical applications. Horse chestnuts contain two different types of aescin, α-aescin and β-aescin: β-aescin is easily water-soluble and is resorbed at a rate of 5%, whereas α-aescin has about twice the rate of resorption. The elimination half-life of α-aescin is longer because its plasma albumin bond is higher than for β-aescin.

Aescin has a positive effect on the capillary permeability of venous walls that is **protective against edema** and **anti-exudative**. This effect is likely not due to a sealing effect on the vessel walls, but on protection of venous walls by the endothelium. This action is considered nonspecific. Animal experiments of α-aescin have also shown **vasoactive** effects on veins and arteries. It initially causes a transient widening followed by the constriction (toning) of vessel walls. **Natriuretic** effects are also ascribed to aescin.

▶ **Indications.** Objectifying the therapeutic effects and efficacy of horse chestnut for **chronic venous insufficiency** is not easy. There is no question that standardized horse chestnut preparations provide effective, symptomatic treatment (Fintelmann; Pittler and Ernst). They simultaneously complement and are an important aspect of phlebological therapeutic concepts.

The Commission E monograph for horse chestnut lists the following indications: chronic venous insufficiency (pain and sensation of heaviness in the legs, cramps in the calves, pruritis, and swelling of the legs).

Clinical studies document that horse chestnut can also be used as a preventive for travel on long-distance flights.

▶ **Research.** In 1994, Marshall and Loew summarized the measures undertaken to prove the efficacy of **vein pharmaceuticals**. A finished pharmaceutical whole extract product standardized for aescin was shown in two crossover double-blind studies to achieve superiority in improving subjective symptoms in outpatients compared to placebo (Friederich et al.; Neiss and Böhm).

To counter the objections that these studies only examined subjective test variables, in 1981, Pauschinger et al. conducted a placebo-controlled and double-blind study in which they tested the behavior of filtration coefficients using venous-occlusion plethysmography in reference to the same study drug. They showed a statistically significant **lowering** of the **capillary filtration coefficient** compared to placebo. In 1986, Bisler et al. conducted a study using the same criteria with venous insufficiency patients. They reached the same conclusions as Pauschinger et al.

In 1990, in a randomized, placebo-controlled, crossover double-blind study, Steiner examined changes in leg volume in venous insufficiency patients. He employed water displacement plethysmometry. Patients first received a placebo and showed no changes. When given the study drug (Venostatin), patients exhibited substantial **reductions in leg volume**. A second group that initially received the study drug responded with immediate substantial reductions in leg volume that returned to the levels measured at the beginning of the study during the placebo period. These differences were statistically significant.

In order to show that the measured changes in leg volume resulted only from changes in filtration and not from other interference factors such as blood pooling, Rudofsky et al., in 1986, studied leg volume changes during the course of therapy under normal conditions and with reduced fixed leg volume. The resulting data of the two experiments did not deviate from each other, which means that leg volume measurements are based exclusively on changes in tissue edema volume. These results were confirmed in further studies (Diehm et al.; Lohr et al.).

In 1987, Marshall and Dormandy conducted another interesting study based on the observation that during **long-distance flights**, the lower extremities usually develop significant swelling based on a lack of use of the calf muscle pump. A randomized, double-blind study that measured leg volume during a long-distance flight showed that horse chestnut extract significantly reduced leg swelling compared to placebo. Considering the discussions about the complications of thrombosis and embolism resulting in acute deaths in conjunction with long-distance flights, this indication for horse chestnut should be publicized more.

▶ **Therapy Recommendation.** Horse chestnut seeds should be used as extract preparations standardized for aescin content.

▶ **Note.** A pure aescin product has been available commercially for a long time in various preparations. Its indications are limited to antiphlogistic effects for traumatic swelling.

Sweet Clover (Melilotus officinalis)

Sweet clover (Melilotus officinalis, derived from the Latin *mel* = honey, *lotos* = clover) is a common plant along the edges of forests and meadows in Germany (▶ Fig. 4.17). It is a member of the Leguminosae family. Its small, yellow flowers exude a pleasant, sweet fragrance reminiscent of honey. When dried, the plant develops a typical coumarin odor, similar to woodruff or sweet vernal grass (Anthoxanthum odoratum), which is a main constituent in hay flower.

Medicinal applications use the **sweet clover herb** (dried or fresh leaves and flowering branches, **Meliloti herba**).

▶ **Note.** In the early 20th century, dairy farming areas of the US state of Wisconsin were plagued by a mysterious disease, which led to a high number of cattle deaths by internal bleeding. After several years of research to find the potential pathogenic bacterium had failed, the British-Canadian veterinarian Frank W. Schofield was able, in 1922, to identify the anticoagulant effect of large amounts of sweet clover in the cows' diet as the cause of the disease. Subsequent analysis led to the discovery of coumarins contained in sweet clover. When sweet clover decomposes (spoils), these coumarins, which are not anticoagulants in their original state, degrade into the anticoagulant dicumarol.

▶ **Pharmacology.** The sweet clover drug contains 5,6-benzo-α-pyron (coumarin). Other active substances include 3,4-dihydrocoumarin (melilotin), o-coumaric acid, melilotoside, and flavonoids.

Sweet clover has anti-exudative effects on inflamed edema and venous stasis edema by increasing venous return flow and improving lymph kinetics. It has also been shown to accelerate would healing in animal experiments.

There are few pharmacologic studies of sweet clover.

▶ **Indications.** Sweet clover is primarily used to treat symptoms of **chronic venous insufficiency**. It also provides supportive treatment for **thrombophlebitis** and **postthrombotic syndrome**. Sweet clover is also indicated for **lymph stasis**.

The Commission E monograph for sweet clover lists numerous indications: chronic venous insufficiency, supportive internal use for treatment of thrombophlebitis, hemorrhoids, lymphatic congestion, and postthrombotic syndromes. It also indicates external use for contusions, sprains, and superficial effusions of blood (hematomas).

> ### Preparations
>
> - **Tea**
>   Add 1 cup of simmering water to 1–2 teaspoons of the finely chopped drug. Steep covered for 10 minutes, then strain.
>   Drink 1 cup 2–3 × a day.
> - **Cataplasm**
>   Moisten the drug thoroughly with an equal amount of simmering water, allow to cool, and use externally.

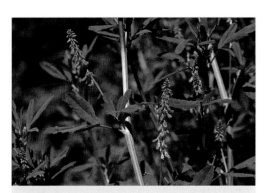

Fig. 4.17 Sweet Clover, Melilotus officinalis. Photo: Dr. Roland Spohn, Engen.

Common Grape Vine (Vitis vinifera)

Grape vines have been used as a traditional medicinal plant going back to antiquity and are being rediscovered as a modern medicinal. Most everyone is probably familiar with wine grape plants. They were cultivated from the wild plant, which is actually a climbing vine. The common grape vine still grows in the wild and can climb and cover trees up to 30 m in height and form trunks up to 0.5 m thick (Pelikan). In Germany, they are frequently found growing on the walls of houses, where they can cover large areas. Its berries are much smaller than wine grapes but can become quite sweet in areas with sufficient sun.

Medicinal applications use the **red leaves** (Vitis viniferae folium) of specific types of grapes known for the intense red color of their leaves and berries. Their use as a source drug to treat vein disorders has a long history, especially in the old wine country of France (Schneider).

▶ **Pharmacology.** The most important constituents of grape vines include tannins, anthocyanins that lend color, flavonoids (for example, quercetin, rutin, and kaempferol), polyphenols, and organic acids. Its whole extract exhibits antiedematous, anti-inflammatory and capillary healing, and antioxidant properties. It also inhibits thrombocyte aggregation.

The common grape vine's effect on the venous system is described as acting on the endothelium by preventing the opening of the venular endothelium barrier and thereby preventing extravasation (Nees et al.).

▶ **Indications.** The common grape vine is indicated for **chronic venous insufficiency** presenting with symptoms of heavy legs, swelling (edema), pain, and a feeling of pressure. Its positive clinical efficacy for this indication was confirmed by an observational study (Schaefer et al.). The study emphasized that this remedy was also well tolerated and there were no indications of stomach irritation.

▶ **Therapy Recommendation.** Treatment should exclusively make use of finished pharmaceutical products.

Bibliography

Bisler H, Pfeifer R, Klüken N, Pauschinger P. Wirkung von Rosskastaniensamenextrakt auf die transkapilläre Filtration bei chronischer venöser Insuffizienz [Effects of horse-chestnut seed extract on transcapillary filtration in chronic venous insufficiency]. Dtsch Med Wochenschr. 1986; 111(35):1321–1329

Diehm C, Vollbrecht D, Hübsch-Müller C, Müller-Bühl U. Clinical efficacy of edema protection in patients with venous edema due to chronic venous insufficiency. Phlebologie. 1989; 89:712–715

Emter M. Adäquate Therapie in der Phlebologie unter besonderer Berücksichtigung pflanzlicher Venenpräparate. In: Loew D, Blume H, Dingermann T, ed Phytopharmaka. Vol V. Darmstadt: Steinkopff; 1999: 119–126

Fintelmann V. Moderne Pharmakotherapie mit Phyto-therapeutika. Die Wirksamkeit von pflanzlichen Arzneimitteln am Beispiel von Rosskastanienextrakt. Natur- und Gan-zheitsmedizin. 1991; 4: 636–638

Friederich HC, Vogelsberg H, Neiss A. Ein Beitrag zur Bewertung von intern virksamen Venenpharmaka [Evaluation of internally effective venous drugs]. Z Hautkr. 1978; 53(11):369–374

Loew D, Schrödter A. Pharmakokinetik und Äquivalenz von Zubereitungen aus Hippocasti semen. In: Loew D, Blume H, Dingermann T, ed Phytopharmaka. Vol V. Darmstadt: Steinkopff; 1999: 135–143

Lohr E, Garanin G, Jesau P, Fischer H. Ödempräventive Therapie bei chronischer Veneninsuffizienz mit Ödemneigung. Munch Med Wochenschr. 1986; 128:579–581

Marshall M, Dormandy JA. Oedema of long distant flights. Phlebology. 1987; 2:123–124

Marshall M, Loew D. Diagnostische Maßnahmen zum Nachweis der Wirksamkeit von Venenpharmaka. Phlebology. 1994; 23:85–89

Nees S, Weiss DR, Reichenbach-Klinke E, et al. Protective effects of flavonoids contained in the red vine leaf on venular endothelium against the attack of activated blood components in vitro. Arzneimittelforschung. 2003; 53(5):330–341

Neiss A, Böhm C. Zum Wirksamkeitsnachweis von Ross-kastaniensamenextrakt beim varikösen Symptomkomplex. Munch Med Wochenschr. 1976; 118:213–216

Pauschinger P, Wörz E, Zwerger E. Die Messung des Filtrationskoeffizienten am menschlichen Unterschenkel und seine pharmakologische Beeinflussung. Med Welt. 1981; 32: 1954–1956

Pelikan W. Heilpflanzenkunde. Vol. 2. Dornach: Philosophisch-Anthroposophischer Verlag am Goetheaneum; 1962:112–119

Pittler MH, Ernst E. Rosskastanien-Extrakt zur Behandlung der chronisch-venösen Insuffizienz. Ein systematischer Review. In: Loew D, Blume H, Dingermann T, ed Phytopharmaka. Vol V. Darmstadt: Steinkopff; 1999: 127–134

Rudofsky G, Neiss A, Otto K, Seibel K. Ödemprotektive Wirkung und klinische Wirksamkeit von Rosskastanienextrakt im Doppelblindversuch. Phlebol Proktol. 1986; 15(2):47–54

Schaefer E, Peil H, Ambrosetti L, Petrini O. Oedema protective properties of the red vine leaf extract AS 195 (Folia vitis viniferae) in the treatment of chronic venous insufficiency. A 6-week observational clinical trial. Arzneimittelforschung. 2003; 53(4):243–246

Schneider E. Rotes Weinlaub—Geschichte der Verwendung. Z Phytother. 2007; 28(5):250–258

Schofield FS. Canadian Vet Rec. 1922; 3:74

Schofield FS. Jour Amer Vet Assoc. 1924; 64:553

Shats D, Bommer S, Degenring FH. Aesculaforce bei chronisch venöser Insuffizienz. Doppelblindstudie zum Nachweis der Wirksamkeit und Verträglichkeit eines Phyto-therapeutikums. Schweiz Zeitschrift Ganzheitsmedizin. 1997; 9(2):86–91

Steiner M. Untersuchungen zur ödemvermindernden und ödemprotektiven Wirkung von Rosskastaniensamenextrakt. Phlebol Proktol. 1990; 19:239–242

Questions

1. What makes hawthorn a "comprehensive" medicinal plant?
2. What does "cardioprotective" mean?
3. What dosage of hawthorn would you use for congestive heart failure NYHA II/III?
4. Is hawthorn tea an appropriate treatment for congestive heart failure?
5. What is the effective method of use for arnica with angina pectoris?
6. Are there heart glycoside alternatives for digitalis?
7. Which medicinal plants have evidence-based proof of efficacy for prevention and curative treatment of arteriosclerotic vascular disease?
8. Name plants used to treat hypotension.

Answers (p. 422) for Chapter 4

5 Respiratory Disorders

Medicinal plants have played an important role in the treatment of respiratory disorders from time immemorial. Today, cough remedies such as teas, tinctures, and syrups are some of the most widely used medicines overall. Of the astoundingly large number of plants suitable for the treatment of respiratory disorders, this chapter presents a selection of medicinal plants that have been shown to be especially effective from a modern perspective.

Respiratory disorders are extremely common and have a profound economic impact. Most of these disorders are acute and chronic infections with bacterial, viral, or toxic causes. Much too often, these indications are treated with antibiotics. Specific phytopharmaceuticals are very much underutilized. This is especially true for **viral infections**, which include all manifestations of the "common" cold. These are hardly ever recognized as diseases anymore even though their impact on well-being and stamina can cause a substantial loss of working hours.

Bronchial asthma represents another important segment of respiratory disorders. While this disorder can be effectively treated with synthetic drugs, it nevertheless frequently represents an eminently chronic and lifelong disorder that is largely incurable. Other respiratory disorders that are being diagnosed more frequently again are pulmonary tuberculosis and lung cancer. These are not discussed here because there are no phytotherapeutic treatment options available for these indications.

Respiratory disorders are divided into "upper" and "lower," with the larynx forming the dividing line (Riechelmann and Klimek). This approach makes sense for specialization in the areas of ear, nose and throat or pulmonology. It makes little sense for the use of phytopharmaceuticals. Phytopharmaceuticals are primarily symptom oriented. This determines their categorization and differentiated therapeutic use.

As was already mentioned, the number of medicinal plants suitable for treatment of respiratory disorders is substantial. However, their therapeutic efficacy varies widely.

This chapter focuses on a detailed discussion of medicinal plants or drugs that are emphasized for treatment and for which modern experimental and/or clinical verification procedures are available.

Plant-based respiratory therapeutics are largely classified as category 2 and 3 in the therapeutic categories for phytotherapeutics developed by the authors (▶ Table 1.3). They are prescribed as alternatives to synthetics or as adjuvants.

These remedies are frequently used for **self-medication**. This therapy segment continues to grow since health insurance programs, worldwide, generally do not cover nonprescription medications.

Medicinal Plants

Acute and Chronic Respiratory Infections
Marshmallow, Althaea officinalis
Coltsfoot, Tussilago farfara
Hollyhock, Althaea rosea
Mallow, Malva sylvestris
Mullein, Verbascum densiflorum
Narrowleaf Plantain, Plantago lanceolata
Iceland Moss, Cetraria islandica
Irish Moss (Carrageen), Chondrus crispus
Usnea, Usnea barbata
Cowslip/Oxlip Primrose, Primula veris/elatior
Sweet Violet, Viola odorata
Pimpinella, Pimpinella saxifraga
Anise, Pimpinella anisum
Soapwort, Saponaria officinalis
Lungwort, Pulmonaria officinalis
Elecampane, Inula helenium
Thyme, Thymus vulgaris
Wild Thyme, Thymus serpyllum
Roundleaf Sundew, Drosera rotundifolia
Ivy, Hedera helix
African Geranium, Pelargonium sidoides DC.
Nasturtium, Tropaeolum majus
Horseradish, Armoracia rusticana

Sinusitis
Fixed combination of gentian root, primrose flowers (Primula veris), garden sorrel (Rumex acetosa), European elderberry flowers (Sambucus nigra), and verbena (Verbena officinalis).
African Geranium, Pelargonium sidoides DC.

Asthmatic Bronchitis
Bishop's weed, Ammi visnaga
Thyme, Thymus vulgaris
Roundleaf Sundew, Drosera rotundifolia
Ivy, Hedera helix
Onion, Allium cepa

Flu and Colds
Echinacea, Echinacea purpurea/pallida, Echinacea angustifolia
Wormwood, Artemisia absinthium
European Elderberry, Sambucus nigra
Linden flower, Tilia cordata/platyphyllos
Jaborandi, Pilocarpus pennatifolius
Lemon, Citrus limon
Dog Rose, Rosa canina
Sea Buckthorn, Hippophae rhamnoides
Black Currant, Ribes nigrum

5.1 Acute and Chronic Respiratory Infections

Medicinal Plants

Demulcents
Marshmallow, Althaea officinalis
Marshmallow root and leaves, Althaeae radix et folium
Coltsfoot, Tussilago farfara
Coltsfoot leaves, Farfarae folium
Hollyhock, Althaea rosea
Hollyhock flowers, Malvae arboreae flos
Mallow, Malva sylvestris
Mallow flowers, Malvae flos et folium
Mullein, Verbascum densiflorum
Mullein flowers, Verbasci flos
Narrowleaf Plantain, Plantago lanceolata
Narrowleaf Plaintain herb, Plantaginis lanceolatae herba
Iceland Moss, Cetraria islandica
Iceland Moss, Lichen islandicus
Irish Moss (Carrageen), Chondrus crispus
Irish Moss, Fucus irlandicus
Usnea, Usnea barbata
Usnea

Expectorants
Cowslip/Oxlip Primrose, Primula veris/elatior
Primrose root, Primulae radix
Sweet Violet, Viola odorata
Sweet Violet root, Violae odoratae radix
Pimpinella, Pimpinella saxifraga
Pimpinella root, Pimpinellae radix
Anise, Pimpinella anisum
Anise seeds (fruit), Anisi fructus
Soapwort, Saponaria officinalis

Soapwort root, Saponariae rubrae radix
Lungwort, Pulmonaria officinalis/maculosa
Lungwort herb, Pulmonariae herba
Elecampane, Inula helenium
Elecampane root, Helenii radix

Cough Medicine (Antitussives)
Thyme, Thymus vulgaris
Thyme herb, Thymi herba
Wild Thyme, Thymus serpyllum
Wild Thyme herb, Serpylli herba
Roundleaf Sundew, Drosera rotundifolia
Roundleaf Sundew herb, Droserae herba
Ivy, Hedera helix
Ivy leaves, Hederae helicis folium
African Geranium, Pelargonium sidoides DC.
African Geranium root, Pelargonii sidoidi radix

These typically bacterial and mostly acute respiratory infections are a primary indication for antibiotics. This unambiguous statement is called into question by the fact that bacterial infections are difficult to verify specifically. In most cases, the criteria for correct diagnosis are the experience of the practitioner and the severity of the disease. In the past, antibiotics were prescribed much too frequently, and this has led to increasing antibiotic resistance. Treatment decisions for these diseases should take under consideration whether it makes sense to support the body's significant self-healing processes by providing **supportive therapy,** for example, phytopharmaceuticals, or if a prescription for synthetics is unavoidable. The following discussion differentiates between sinus infections, throat and bronchial infections and colds (catarrh).

5.1.1 Bronchial Infections

Chronic infections are one of the domains for phytopharmaceuticals and their excellent tolerability allows for long-term use. Prevention in cases of proven susceptibility to infections is another area where herbal medicines are especially suitable.

The following delineation of remedies has been proven in practice: mucolytic **demulcents, expectorants**, and cough-quieting **antitussives**. Plant medicines exhibiting these actions can also be combined and many of them are already a "natural" combination. This delineation into main active principles is used here because it helps with understanding these plants and putting them to their best use.

Plants for Treatment: Demulcents

Demulcents are especially suitable for treating **acute respiratory infections**. They calm irritated mucosa and provide relief from symptoms of the disorder. Prescribing a cough remedy from the group of saponin drugs for acute catarrh (cold) is not indicated. These remedies should be reserved at the earliest for subacute stages and are primarily indicated for chronic bronchitis, when the goal is to "loosen" the cough.

Chronic bronchial catarrh can present with stages of increased irritability that require the use of demulcents. However, the indications outlined above should be used as a guideline for prescribing demulcents.

For the use of demulcents for disorders of the oral and pharyngeal mucosa, see Chapter 3.1.

Marshmallow (Althaea officinalis)

Marshmallow is a member of the mallow family with large reddish-white flowers. It grows to a height of more than 1 m and its leaves have three to five lobes and are velvety and tomentose on both sides (▶ Fig. 5.1).

In Germany, marshmallow grows wild. It prefers saline meadows such as the ones that can be found in the Northern Lowland. The supply does not meet the demand for this plant and the plants used medicinally are exclusively derived from cultivation. In North America, marshmallow has been introduced and has naturalized in many US Eastern and Midwestern states.

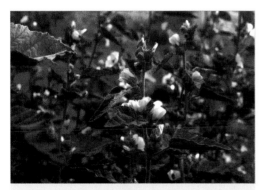

Fig. 5.1 Marshmallow, Althaea officinalis. Photo: Thieme Verlagsgruppe, Stuttgart.

Medicinal applications use the **marshmallow root** (Althaeae radix) and **leaves** (Althaeae folium). However, the leaves are less efficacious than the drug made from the root.

▶ **Pharmacology.** The drug contains a minimum of 35% mucilage, 38% starch, and 10% each of pectin and sucrose.

▶ **Indications.** The Commission E monograph for marshmallow lists the following indication, among others: **dry, irritated cough**.

Preparations

Marshmallow decoctions should only contain mucilage and not the starch that is soluble in hot water. Therefore, the German Pharmacopoeia (DAB) calls for marshmallow decoctions to be cold water preparations, counter to its name. However, if marshmallow tea is to be used for gargling, it is helpful to dissolve some of the starch into the solution.

- **Cough Tea**
  Add 1 cup of cold water to 1 tablespoon of marshmallow leaves or 1 teaspoon of marshmallow root. Soak for 1–2 hours while stirring frequently. Strain and gently heat to a lukewarm temperature. Drink 1 cup several times a day. Tea prepared from marshmallow root can also be used for gargling.
- **Syrup**
  This preparation is very suitable for adding to cough mixtures.
- **"Chest Liquor"** (Liquor pectoralis, according to the German Prescription Formulas, DRF)
  In this preparation, anisated solution of ammonia (Liquor Ammonii anisati) increases the action of the marshmallow syrup.

Prescriptions

Rx
Sir. Althaeae 30.0 (marshmallow syrup)
Liqu. Ammon. anisat. 5.0 (anisated solution of ammonia)
Aqu. dest. ad 200.0 (distilled water)
D.S.
Take 1 tablespoon every 2 hours. Shake before use.

Preparations

- **Marshmallow Maceration** (Maceratio Althaeae, according to the German Prescription Formulas, DRF)
  Take 1 tablespoon every 2 hours.
- **Marshmallow Syrup with Fennel Honey and Narrowleaf Plantain Syrup**

Prescriptions

Rx
Sir. Althaeae (marshmallow syrup)
Sir. Plantaginis lanc. (narrowleaf plantain syrup)
Mel. Foeniculi āā ad 100.0 (fennel honey)
D.S.
Take 1 teaspoon every 2 hours

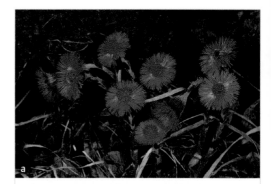

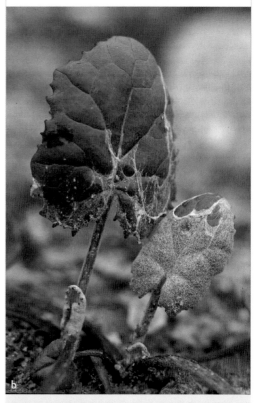

Fig. 5.2 a and b Coltsfoot, Tussilago farfara. Photos: Dr. Roland Spohn, Engen.

Coltsfoot (Tussilago farfara)

The yellow flower heads of coltsfoot can be seen sprouting from the earth in the spring, around the time of snowmelt. This plant is very common everywhere in Germany. This plant loves loamy clay soil. Its leaves are angled, heart shaped and their underside is tomentose with white hair (▶ Fig. 5.2). The leaves are similar to butterbur (Petasites hybridus), only much smaller.

Medicinal applications use the **coltsfoot leaves** (Farfarae folium).

▶ **Pharmacology.** In addition to mucilage, coltsfoot contains a bitter substance and a tannin. The tonic effects caused by coltsfoot's bitter constituent complement its expectorant action.

Coltsfoot is one of the drugs that contain pyrrolizidine alkaloids. The basic issue of toxicology assessment was discussed in the introduction of this book, see side effects (p. 15). Its pyrrolizidine alkaloid content does not negate coltsfoot's value as a cough remedy.

Caution ⚠

According to the Commission E monograph, the maximum daily dose of 1 µg of toxic pyrrolizidine alkaloids with 1,2-unsaturated necin structure must not be exceeded. The responsibility for the concentration of pyrrolizidine alkaloids rests with the pharmacist.

▶ **Indications.** Coltsfoot is an ideal remedy for **chronic bronchitis**. It can be found as an constituent in many cough teas and is a proven cough remedy.

Weiss viewed coltsfoot to be especially suitable for treatment of chronic obstructive pulmonary disease (COPD) and silicosis.

The Commission E monograph for coltsfoot lists the following indications: acute catarrh of the respiratory tract with cough and hoarseness.

- **Infusion**
  Add 1 up of hot water to 1– 2 teaspoons of the drug. Steep covered for 10 minutes, then strain.
  Drink hot several times a day.

▶ **Therapy Recommendations.** Weiss recommended to patients with COPD and silicosis to drink a cup of hot coltsfoot tea before breakfast, ideally before getting out of bed in the morning. The tea can be sweetened with a teaspoon of honey and provides great relief to patients. It can be prepared in the evening and kept in a thermos on the night table overnight. A cup of coltsfoot tea is also indicated before bed, possibly together with an antispasmodic, for example Bishop's weed (p. 202).

As a rule, coltsfoot should only be prescribed for a limited duration of about 2–3 weeks. With cases of advanced pulmonary emphysema or silicosis, coltsfoot may be taken for longer periods if prescribed by and under the professional responsibility of a medical practitioner; this applies especially to the method of morning use as described above.

Hollyhock (Althaea rosea)

Hollyhock (▶ Fig. 5.3), a common decorative plant in the garden, is similar to marshmallow in its effects.

Medicinal applications use the hollyhock flowers (Althaeae flos), also referred to as black hollyhock. The flowers of this plant may be white to dark red, including pink, yellow, and orange. Its

main constituents are mucilage, tannins, and the blue pigment althaein.

The beautiful, large, dark red flowers also make a fairly attractive drug. They are frequently added to cough teas not so much because of their effects, but as a decorative drug.

Mallow (Malva sylvestris)

Mallow can be found all over Germany. Unlike marshmallow, medicinal applications of mallow use the **mallow flowers** (Malvae flos) and **leaves** (Malvae folium).

Internal use of mallow is much less prevalent than that of marshmallow.

- **Tea**
  Add 1 tablespoon of finely chopped flowers or 2 tablespoons of finely chopped leaves to 1 cup of cold water. Bring to a brief boil. Steep covered for 10 minutes, then strain.
  Use liquid to gargle several times a day.

Mullein (Verbascum densiflorum)

Dense-flowered mullein (Verbascum densiflorum) (▶ Fig. 5.4) and the very similar orange mullein (Verbascum phlomoides) both have a well-deserved special reputation as a cough remedy. In Germany, both plants and several other types of mullein grace many rocky areas and dry slopes from the mountains to the lowland areas. A proud and commanding presence, mullein can grow up

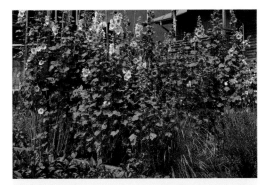

Fig. 5.3 Hollyhock, Althaea rosea. Photos: Dr. Roland Spohn, Engen.

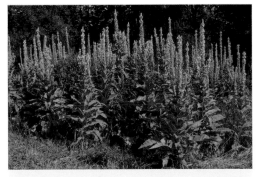

Fig. 5.4 Mullein, Verbascum densiflorum. Photos: Dr. Roland Spohn, Engen.

to a height of 1 m or more. Its brilliantly yellow flowers can be seen from afar. Its stem and leaves are densely covered in woolly hair (pilose).

Mullein is a biannual, like foxglove. In the first year, it grows a rosette of basal leaves and in the second year, a stiff, upright flower stem rises up from this base.

Medicinal applications use the **mullein flowers** (Verbasci flos).

▶ **Pharmacology.** Mullein flowers contain plentiful amounts of mucilage as well as acidic saponin and a small amount of volatile oil. Mullein is not a purely mucilaginous plant but represents a transition to expectorants containing saponin. This combination makes mullein special and is the reason for its positive therapeutic effect.

▶ **Indications.** Mullein flowers are both demulcents and expectorants. This drug is primarily prescribed for **subacute catarrh** and **chronic bronchitis** with still significant mucosa irritation. It is also an constituent in the officinal cough tea mixtures (Species pectorales).

The Commission E monograph for mullein lists the indication catarrhs of the respiratory tract.

Preparation

- **Tea**
  Add 1 cup of boiling water to 1 tablespoon of the finely chopped drug. Steep covered for 10–15, then strain.
  Drink 1 cup several times a day.

Narrowleaf Plantain (Plantago lanceolata)

Narrowleaf plantain is one of the most common plants in Germany. It grows in arid meadows, along the edges of paths, and in agricultural fields. Its flower stem arises from a basal rosette of narrow, pointed leaves. It bears a claviform flower spike of long, graceful stamens.

Medicinal applications use the **narrowleaf plantain herb** (dried above-ground parts of the plant, harvested during flowering season; Plantaginis lanceolatae herba).

▶ **Note.** Narrowleaf plantain should not be confused with the even more common broadleaf plantain (Plantago major), which grows in paths and in

inhospitable locations, in Germany. Broadleaf plantain is also traditionally collected as a folk remedy and used in the same manner as narrowleaf plantain. However, narrowleaf plantain is a far better remedy, at least for coughs. Broadleaf plantain is used more as an external remedy for wounds and areas of infected skin.

▶ **Pharmacology.** The narrowleaf plantain drug contains primarily mucilage along with iridoid glycosides such as aucubin and catalpol, plus phenylethanoids (for example, acteoside), tannins, and substantial amounts of silicic acid. Narrowleaf plantain is not a pure demulcent but is positioned between demulcents and silicic acid drugs.

▶ **Research.** In 1999, Paper and Marchesan compiled an overview of the pharmacology data for narrowleaf plantain. As is typical for medicinal plants, it showed an entire profile of effects, especially antibacterial, anti-inflammatory and antitussive actions. These actions were also demonstrated for the active constituents such as the iridoid glycosides aucubin and catalpol and the phenylethanoid acteoside. The iridoid glycosides were also shown to have spasmolytic and antiviral effects.

An observational study followed patients who presented with nonspecific respiratory disorders dominated by acute infections, acute bronchitis, and dry cough following acute respiratory infections (Kraft). The average prescribed dosage was 1 tablespoon of narrowleaf plantain syrup 3 times a day. Symptoms decreased by 58% compared to symptom severity measured at the beginning of the study, after 3 to 14 days of therapy, regardless of diagnosis. Cough intensity and frequency decreased by 67 or 65%, respectively. Two-thirds of patients experienced noticeable effects within 3 days. One notable result was the especially pronounced effect on dry cough symptoms.

▶ **Indications.** The indication of catarrh of the respiratory tract listed in the Commission E monograph for narrowleaf plantain does not do justice to the special characteristics of this plant. This drug offers a comprehensive spectrum of therapeutic options and is the remedy of choice for **acute respiratory tract disorders** in children and adults. This is confirmed by the results of the extensive observational study on narrowleaf plantain described by (Wegener 1999).

Narrowleaf plantain is likely less of a cough inhibitor and more of a **topical anti-inflammatory**.

Experience to date has shown that narrowleaf plantain does not suppress the cough center in the brain. It therefore does not inhibit the necessary elimination of bronchial secretions.

Preparations

- **Pressed Juice**
  Prepare a pressed juice from the fresh drug. Boil the raw juice with equal parts of honey for about 20 minutes.
  Take 1–2 tablespoons 3 × a day.
  The juice will keep for some time in a tightly closed container.
- **Syrup**
  Take 1 tablespoon 3 × a day.

▶ **Therapy Recommendation.** Therapy should primarily make use of defined finished pharmaceutical manufactured products.

Iceland Moss (Cetraria islandica)

This lichen (p. 61) was introduced earlier in the book in the section about treating chronic gastric disorders. It is discussed here because of its mucilage content.

The active constituents of Iceland moss are mucilage and bitters. Since bitters have a tonic effect, the Iceland moss drug is used as a remedy for **chronic bronchial catarrh** with **recurring bouts of acute irritation**. This drug is especially indicated for older or asthenic people or for people who have been weakened by a long-lasting cough for whom the simultaneous tonic effect of bitters is desired. Iceland moss also stimulates gastric juice secretion as well as the autonomic nervous system.

Preparation

- **Tea**
  Add 1 cup of boiling water to 1–2 teaspoons of the finely chopped drug. Steep covered for 10 minutes, then strain.
  Drink 2–3 cups a day for several months.

Irish Moss (Carrageen, Chondrus crispus)

Irish moss is the dried thallus of the red algae Chondrus crispus, which grows in the Atlantic Ocean. It should not be confused with Iceland moss.

The drug derived from Irish moss is referred to as **carrageen**–sometimes still referred to in Germany by the long outdated synonym **Fucus irlandicus**. It contains substantial amounts of mucilage as well as proteins, iodide, and bromide. For this reason, it is recommended as an **abirritant** for coughs. However, it is much less significant than Iceland moss and is rarely used in Germany.

▶ **Note.** In some Asian countries, Irish moss is used as a foodstuff.

Usnea (Usnea barbata)

Usnea (p. 62) is a lichen that grows in mountainous forests in Germany. It contains bitter lichen acids such as usnic acid. **Bacteriostatic** effects have been attributed to usnic acid.

Expectorants

Expectorants decrease the viscosity of thick bronchial secretions and promote the ejection of mucus by coughing.

The mucolytic and secretolytic action of expectorants is primarily promoted by saponins. The secretolytic effect is also due to certain volatile oils. Decreasing mucus viscosity and increasing the water content of bronchial secretions are important prerequisites for sufficient expectoration. The secretion motoricity (mucociliary clearance) promoting effect depends on the cilia of the bronchial epithelium. The mucociliary clearance speed required for transporting mucus is 4–20 mm/min. Saponin and volatile oil containing drugs also play a key role in phytotherapeutic expectorants.

▶ **Note.** In the past, ipecac (Cephaelis ipecacuanha) was considered the most important phytotherapeutic expectorant. It originates from South America and its main active constituents are alkaloids, for example, emetine. This drug is no longer recommended for phytotherapy but is still considered significant in homeopathy.

Primrose (Cowslip, Oxlip) (Primula veris, Primula elatior)

Oxlip primrose (Primula elatior) is more common in the western part of Germany and is a beautiful yellow spring flower found in mountain forests. Its calyx is narrow and funnel-shaped and the corona is diffuse and flat. **Cowslip** primrose (Primula veris)

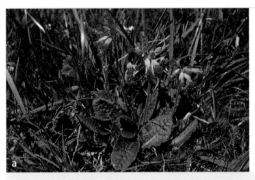
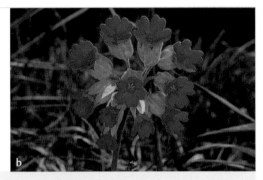

Fig. 5.5 a and b Cowslip primrose, Primula veris. Photos: Dr. Roland Spohn, Engen.

can be found in damp meadows, especially in the eastern parts of Germany. It is found only scattered in northwest Germany, but always in clusters. Its bulging calyx has short, wide teeth (dentate). Its corona leaves are bell-shaped (▶ Fig. 5.5). In recent decades, this plant has also been found more frequently in the alpine foothills of southern Germany as well as in Austria and Switzerland. Cowslip primrose has also been introduced in the northeastern regions of North America.

Medicinal applications use the **primrose root** (Primulae radix).

▶ **Pharmacology.** The primrose root drug contains 5–10% triperpene saponins along with the salicylic acid glycosides primulaverin and primverin as well as flavonoids. The salicylic acid derivatives content makes it likely that this drug has additional antiphlogistic actions.

The expectorant action of saponins is thought to be primarily due to irritation of the gastric mucosa, which triggers parasympathetic reflexes.

▶ **Note.** In Germany, native primroses represent highly valuable saponin drugs and can take the place of the North American senega snakeroot (Polygala senega), which is a saponin drug not native to Germany. The senega snakeroot drug (Senegae radix) is similar to the native German cowslip primrose in its saponin and salicylic acid compounds. Senega snakeroot does not seem to have a distinct advantage over cowslip primrose.

▶ **Indications.** As an expectorant with primarily saponin-derived effects, cowslip and oxlip primrose are primarily indicated for all types of **chronic bronchitis**, especially for simple, protracted cough

with insufficient ejection of mucus. For this reason, it is contained in many finished pharmaceutical products and is frequently combined with other expectorants such as thyme and volatile oil drugs.

The Commission E monograph for primrose lists the indication catarrh of the respiratory tract.

Preparations

- **Tea**
  Add ¼ teaspoon of the finely chopped drug to 1 cup of cold water. Cover, heat to a simmer, and allow to steep for 5 minutes, then strain.
  Drink 1 cup sweetened with a bit of honey every 2–3 hours.

- **Combination with Other Expectorants**

Prescriptions

Rx
Primulae rad. 20.0 (cowslip and/or oxlip primrose root)
Anisi fruct. (anise seeds)
Foeniculi fruct. (fennel seeds)
Farfarae fol. āā ad 50.0 (coltsfoot leaves)
M. f. spec.
Add 1 cup of boiling water to 2 teaspoons of the blend. Steep covered for 10 minutes, then strain.
D.S.
Drink 1 cup several times a day.

- **Primrose Decoction** (Decoctum Primulae, according to the German Prescription Formulas, DRF)

Prescriptions

Rx
Decoct. Primul. rad. 6.0/180.0 (cowslip and/or oxlip primrose decoction)
Elixir e Succo Liquiritiae ad 200.0 (licorice elixir and juice) [DAB6, 1926]
D.S.
Take 1 tablespoon every 2 hours.
Licorice Juice (Succo Liquiritiae) as per Johann Carl Leuchs. Allgemeins Warenlexikon oder vollständige Warenkunde, Vol. 2 (N-Z), 2. Auflage, Nürnberg, Verlag C. Leuchs & Comp. 1836, p. 417:
Licorice juice, contrary to its name, is not a liquid, but refers to the totality of all hot-water soluble components of licorice (Glycyrrhiza glabra) root, which have been solidified into a solid mass. This is achieved by first cooking the crushed raw drug and—after filtration—cooking it again until most of the water is gone and an extract with the consistency of dough remains. This "dough" is formed into elongated cylindrical shapes of 20 cm in length and 4 cm in circumference. These are subsequently wrapped with laurel (Laurus nobilis) leaves. In this form, licorice juice is suitable for long-term storage and soon becomes completely hard. When broken, the fragments look like splintered obsidian. Licorice juice of good quality is completely soluble in water.
By redissolving licorice juice in water at room temperature, filtrating, and subsequent resolidifying as described above, purified licorice juice is obtained.
Elixir e Succo Liquiritiae (licorice juice elixir) [DAB6, 1926]:
40 parts purified licorice juice, 120 parts water, 6 parts ammonia water (10% NH_3 in H_2O), 1 part anise essential oil, 1 part fennel essential oil, 32 parts alcohol.
The purified licorice juice is dissolved in the water and mixed with the ammonia water. The resulting mixture is allowed to settle for 36 hours. Subsequently, the essential oils are dissolved in the alcohol. This solution is then added to the first mixture and stirred intensively. The combination of all parts is allowed to settle for 1 week. The supernatant is then decanted, and the rest is filtered to remove all solid parts. It is important to take care that the temperature of the liquid is always close to room temperature and never falls below 15 °C during the whole process. Otherwise, the anise essential oil constituents will separate from the liquid, crystallize on the surface, and must be removed in the filtration step. It is best, however, not to allow the crystallization to occur during the process.

Prescriptions

Rx
Decoct. Primul. rad. 5.0/150.0 (cowslip and/or oxlip primrose decoction)
Liqu. Ammon. anisat. 10.0 (anisated solution of ammonia)
Sir. Althaeae ad 180.0 (marshmallow syrup)
D.S.
Take 1 tablespoon 3 × a day.

- **Tincture**
  Take 20 drops 4 × a day.
- **Fluid Extract**
  Take 20 drops several times a day.

The extract has a stronger effect and is highly recommended.

- **Combination with other cough remedies**

Prescriptions

Rx
Ol. Anisi 2.0 (anise essential oil)
Extr. Primul. fluid. (cowslip and/or oxlip primrose fluid extract)
Tinct. Pimpinellae āā 20.0 (pimpinella tincture)
Pimpinella tincture is made from 1 part of powdered Pimpinella saxifraga root via maceration in 5 parts of diluted alcohol (60%).
D.S.
Take 10 drops 3 × a day.

Prescriptions

Rx
Extr. Primul. fluid. (cowslip and/or oxlip primrose fluid extract)
Extr. Thymi fluid. āā 20.0 (thyme fluid extract)
D.S.
Take 20 drops 3 × a day.

Sweet Violet (Viola odorata)

Sweet violet is known as a beautiful spring flower in Germany. It frequently grows in large clusters in shaded deciduous forests and in undergrowth shrubbery.

Medicinal applications primarily use the **sweet violet root** (Violae odoratae radix).

▶ **Pharmacology.** Sweet violet contains saponins, an anthocyanin (violanin), and small amounts of an alkaloid (violin) that has emetine-like effects. Because of this alkaloid, sweet violet has also been referred to as "German ipecac," but sweet violet's effect does not nearly come close to this plant. Sweet violet's most important constituent is its **saponin** content.

▶ **Note.** Iridin and its aglycone irigenin are found together in the roots of several iris types (Iris florentina, Iris germanica, Iris pallida) and in leopard lily (Belamcanda chinensis, syn. Iris domestica). It is mention in this context because the rootstock of Iris florentina is referred to as "violet root" in German pharmacies. They must not be confused with the true violet mentioned here.

▶ **Indications.** The indications for sweet violet are the same as for cowslip and oxlip primrose, but its effect is significantly weaker. It can be considered a useful expectorant. The authors prescribe it for **chronic bronchitis**.

Prescriptions

Tea with Marshmallow
Rx
Decoct. Violae odoratae rad. 3.0/150.0 (sweet violet decoction)
Sir. Althaeae ad 180.0 (marshmallow syrup)
D.S.
Take 1 tablespoon 4 × a day.

▶ **Therapy Recommendations.** Sweet violet works best if prescribed as part of a tea blend formulation.

Prescriptions for sweet violet should always specify "odoratae" to prevent it from being confused with heart's ease (Viola tricolor).

Pimpinella (Pimpinella saxifraga, Pimpinella nigra)

Pimpinella grows wild throughout Germany in arid, grassy forests, dry meadows, and on dry slopes. In North America, this plant has been introduced in the Northeast and in some areas of the Northwest. It is a member of the Apiaceae family. Its leaves are pinnatepartite and its flowers are whitish and inconspicuous (▶ Fig. 5.6).

Medicinal applications use the **pimpinella root** (Pimpinellae radix).

The more robust pimpinella variety, Pimpinella nigra, is collected more frequently than the main variety Pimpinella saxifraga.

▶ **Note.** Pimpinella saxifrage is often confused with salad burnet (Sanguisorba minor), which has remotely similar pinnatepartite leaves, but has very different reddish flowers that are clustered into flower heads. Salad burnet is a member of the rose family. It is often planted in gardens and its leaves are used as a cooking spice and salad constituent.

▶ **Pharmacology.** Pimpinella contains saponins and a minimum of 0.4% volatile oil. It is not yet well known as an expectorant.

▶ **Indications.** Pimpinella's efficacy is not very pronounced, but well documented enough to be recommended for **colds**.

The Commission E monograph for pimpinella lists the indication catarrh of the upper respiratory tract.

Preparations

- **Tincture**
  This is especially well suited for combining with different cough remedies.
- **Tea**
  Add 1 cup of cold water to 2 tablespoons of the finely chopped drug. Bring to a brief boil, then strain.
  Drink 1 cup several times a day sweetened with a small amount of honey.

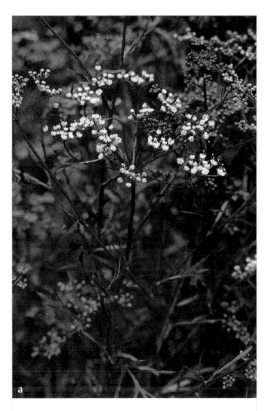

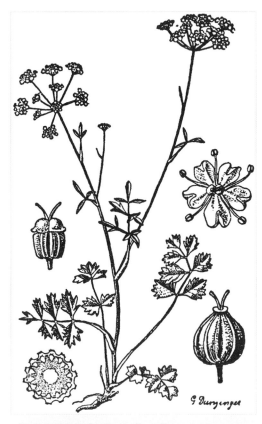

Fig. 5.6 Pimpinella, Pimpinella saxifraga.

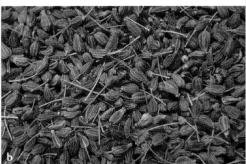

Fig. 5.7 a and b Anise, Pimpinella anisum. Photos: Dr. Roland Spohn, Engen.

Anise (Pimpinella anisum)

With regards to its volatile oil content, pimpinella (Pimpinella saxifraga) is similar to anise (Pimpinella anisum), its close relative (▶ Fig. 5.7). As a carminative, anise's expectorant action supersedes that of caraway (p. 73) and fennel, which are also carminatives with expectorant characteristics.

Medicinal applications use the **anise seeds** (Anisi fructus).

▶ **Indications.** Anise is a mild, sedating, and pleasant tasting cough remedy. It has been mentioned several times in prescription formulas in this book as anisated solution of ammonia (Liquor Ammonii anisati).

The Commission E monograph for anise lists the indication catarrh of the respiratory tracts.

Preparations

- **Anisated Solution of Ammonia** (Liquor Ammonii anisati)
  Adults take 15 drops and children take 5 drops in tea or sugar water 3–4 × a day for dry bronchitis and tracheobronchitis. Its pleasant taste also makes this remedy a suitable single remedy for children.
- **Tea**
  Add 1 cup of boiling water to 1 heaping teaspoon of the crushed or coarsely powdered drug. Steep covered for 10–15 minutes, then strain. Drink 1 cup several times a day.
- **Anise Seed Essential Oil**
  Take 3 drops on one sugar cube several times a day.

Caution

- This is anise (Pimpinella anisum) oil, not star anis (Illicium verum) oil. These are two completely different plants that must not be confused with one another!

- **Combination with Pimpinella**

Prescriptions

Rx
Ol. Anisi 0.2(–0.4) (anise seed essential oil)
Tinct. Pimpinellae 30.0 (pimpinella tincture)
D.S.
Take 10–30 drops 4 × a day.

Soapwort (Saponaria officinalis)

Soapwort grows wild along the edges of streams and in hedges and is also cultivated, in Germany. Its leaves are opposite, and its flowers are reddish to a light-fleshy color.

Medicinal applications use the soapwort root (**Saponariae rubrae radix**). This root is different from the drug Saponariae albae radix, which is derived from its close relative, white soapwort (Gypsophila panniculata), which does not have medicinal significance today.

▶ **Pharmacology.** The soapwort drug contains saponins, tannins, and starch. Soapwort is a typical representative of saponin plants with expectorant action.

▶ **Indications.** The indication for soapwort is **chronic bronchitis**, which is also listed as an indication in the Commission E monograph for soapwort.

▶ **Note.** Soapwort was the most frequently used native cough remedy in Germany for many years. It has now been surpassed by cowslip and oxlip primrose and by sweet violet.

Preparation

- **Tea**
  Add ½ a teaspoon of the drug, chopped medium fine, to 1 cup of water. Bring to a boil and strain.
  Drink 1 cup warm and sweetened with a little honey several times a day.

Lungwort (Pulmonaria officinalis, Pulmonaria maculosa)

Its name indicates that lungwort has been used as a traditional folk remedy for respiratory tract disorders for a long time.

Lungwort is part of the spring flora in the deciduous forests of Germany. Its flowers initially bloom red, but then increasingly turn violet blue. Its basal leaves are wide and heart shaped at the base. The conspicuous large white spots on its ovate leaves make the plant easy to recognize even after the flowers have disappeared (▶ Fig. 5.8). The entire herb is covered in prickly hairs (aculeate).

Medicinal applications exclusively use the **lungwort herb** (dried above-ground parts, Pulmonariae herba)

▶ **Pharmacology.** Lungwort's saponin content is not substantial and is not homogenous. However, its silicic acid content of 3% and tannin content of

6–10% is substantial. For this reason, lungwort cannot really be referred to as a saponin-based expectorant, but instead represents a transition to silicic acid drugs. Its low saponin content determines its weak expectorant effects.

▶ **Indications.** Lungwort is no longer considered a significant expectorant. However, since there are no risks associated with prescribing it, prescription formulas that combine lungwort with typical saponin drugs are definitely justified.

The Commission E issued a negative monograph for lungwort because its efficacy is not sufficiently proven.

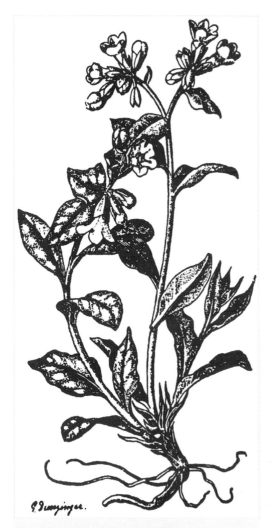

Fig. 5.8 Lungwort, Pulmonaria officinalis.

Elecampane (Inula helenium)

This stiff and erect plant with beautiful large yellow flowers can grow to a height of more than 1.5 m and is a member of the Asteraceae family (▶ Fig. 5.9). Elecampane originates from Asia but has been cultivated in gardens for quite a while from which it has spread and naturalized. In Germany, it grows along roads, hedges, and riverbanks, and gives the impression of being a native plant.

Medicinal applications use the large main **elecampane root** (Helenii radix, also referred to as Enulae radix or Inulae radix), which is sourced from cultivated plants.

▶ **Pharmacology.** The elecampane drug contains 1–3% of a volatile oil, bitters, and substantial amounts of inulin. Elecampane has expectorant effects and is a popular component of many finished pharmaceutical products, for example, cough syrups, lozenges, and pills.

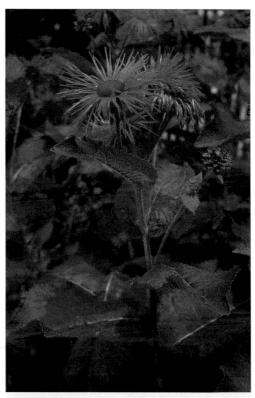

Fig. 5.9 Elecampane, Inula helenium. Photo: Dr. Roland Spohn, Engen.

▶ **Note.** Inulin is a starch-like carbohydrate that tastes slightly sweet. It is used as a sugar substitute for diabetics and is also contained in some foods for diabetics. It is also increasingly being added to foods as a **prebiotic.** Elecampane's water-soluble fiber is thought to be especially supportive for the intestinal flora.

▶ **Indications.** Elecampane is a remedy for **chronic cough** that impacts overall well-being, including appetite. It is indicated for **protracted bronchial catarrh, COPD,** and also for chronic **cough in seniors.** For this indication, elecampane is similar to coltsfoot.

The Commission E issued a negative monograph for elecampane because its efficacy for the indications it is used for in practice has not been sufficiently documented and the risk of potential allergic reaction based on the drug's sesquiterpene lactone content was not considered acceptable.

Preparation 👉
• Tea

The following prescription formula is recommended:

Prescriptions 🔍
Rx Helenii rad. (elecampane root) Primulae rad. (cowslip primrose and/or oxlip primrose root) Farfarae fol. āā ad 100.0 (coltsfoot leaves) M. f. spec. Add 1 cup of hot water to 2 teaspoons of the blend. Boil for 5 minutes, and steep covered for 15 minutes, then strain. D.S. Drink 1 cup 3 × a day.

Antitussives

Antitussives are especially suitable for treating **spasmodic cough** (dry cough). This type of cough is often found in adults in conjunction with viral infections that dry out mucus membranes.

Whooping cough represents a special case. This childhood disease is occurring in an atypical form more frequently in adults as a chronic spasmodic cough. Frequently, it is not diagnosed or even misdiagnosed as asthmatic bronchitis. Serologic proof for whooping cough can provide quick clarification. Whooping cough is an unambiguous indication for the medicinal plants discussed in this chapter, especially for thyme.

▶ **Note.** The indication "dry cough" requires **abundant consumption of fluids** in addition to the prescribed remedy.

Thyme (Thymus vulgaris)

Thyme is a member of the Lamiaceae family. Its stems are branching, erect and shrub-like at the bottom (▶ Fig. 5.10). Its flowers are small and reddish to red. The entire plant exudes an intensive, pleasantly volatile fragrance.

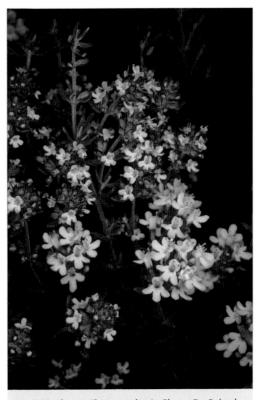

Fig. 5.10 Thyme, Thymus vulgaris. Photo: Dr. Roland Spohn, Engen.

Thyme grows in large quantities in macchie (shrub heaths) in the mountains in southern France, Spain, and Italy. It has also been introduced and naturalized in some areas of in the northeastern United States. Thyme planted in a garden (garden thyme) is more of a spice. For medicinal purposes, wild harvested thyme from the Mediterranean should be used. It grows taller than garden thyme, has a much more intense fragrance, and contains substantially more volatile oil.

Medicinal applications use the **thyme herb** (stripped and dried leaves and flowers, Thymi herba).

▶ **Note.** Thyme was listed in the capitularies of Charlemagne, King of the Franks, in the late 8th century. This collection of civil ordinances of the Carolingian Empire contains detailed instructions for the types of medicinal plants of value to the population that were to be planted in cloister gardens.

▶ **Pharmacology.** Thyme contains a multitude of constituents. The most important of these is its volatile oil content of a minimum of 1.2%, including at least 0.5% thymol. In addition, thyme contains tannins, saponins, and bitters.

Thyme is as complex in its actions as its diversity of constituents would suggest. Its action is dominated by the **volatile thyme oil** with its **secretolytic, secretomotor, broncholytic,** and mildly disinfecting (antibacterial) effects.

Thyme oil taken orally is largely excreted via the pulmonary alveoli of the lungs. This places thyme oil's concentrated effect right where it is needed. Its **spasmolytic** effects on the bronchioles are particularly important. Thyme baths enable the inhalation of the thyme oil rising from the bath water.

▶ **Indications.** Thyme's expectorant action with spasmolysant effects determines its indications. Thyme can be helpful with **spasmodic acute or chronic coughs**. Its spasmolytic action can even help with **emphysema** and asthma, even if thyme is used as an adjuvant to other therapies for these conditions. Thyme has a large spectrum of indications. Its significance for the trachea and bronchia is analogous to that of peppermint for the gastrointestinal system.

The Commission E monograph for thyme lists symptoms of bronchitis and whooping cough as well as catarrh of the upper respiratory tract.

Preparations

- **Tea**
  Add 1 cup of hot water to 2 teaspoons of the finely chopped drug. Steep covered for 5 minutes, then strain.
  Drink 1 cup several times a day.
- **Tincture**
  Take 5–10 drops in a small amount of water or on 1 sugar cube several times a day.
- **Fluid Extract**
  Take ½ teaspoon diluted in a small amount of water several times a day.

▶ **Therapy Recommendations.** Thyme can also be prescribed in high dosages. Frequently this is needed to accomplish the therapeutic goal.

For clearly identified indications, prescribing one of the standardized, finished pharmaceutical products is recommended.

Wild Thyme (Thymus serpyllum)

This close relative of thyme (Thymus vulgaris) is native to Germany and grows on arid slopes, in sandy pine forests, and in sunny, rocky areas. In midsummer, this herb, with its aromatic fragrance and its clusters of reddish-violet flowers, is hard to miss (▶ Fig. 5.11). Wild thyme often grows together with heather.

Medicinal applications use the **wild thyme herb** (dried, flowering above-ground parts Serpylli herba).

The constituents of wild thyme are similar to those of thyme. However, its volatile oil content is lower, and the oil is not as valuable as the thyme oil from Thymus vulgaris. Wild thyme is less significant as a cough and whooping cough remedy, but it is very well suited for **herb baths and herb pillows**.

Roundleaf Sundew (Drosera rotundifolia)

Roundleaf sundew is known as a carnivorous (insect-digesting) plant. In Germany, it grows in bogs, especially the peat moss bogs of hill moors. Its basal rosette hugs the ground. In late summer, a stem bearing small white flower rises from its center to a height of 5–15 cm (▶ Fig. 5.12).

Roundleaf sundew leaves feature a peculiar corona of glandular hairs. These hairs exude a sticky

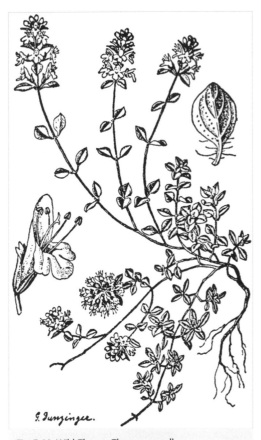

Fig. 5.11 Wild Thyme, Thymus serpyllum.

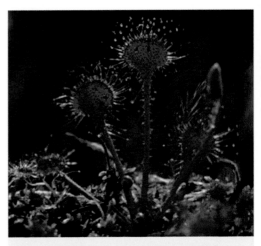

Fig. 5.12 Roundleaf Sundew, Drosera rotundifolia. Photo: Naturfoto Franke Heckler, Panten-Hammer.

▶ **Pharmacology.** The roundleaf sundew herb contains 0.14–0.22% naphthoquinone derivatives, calculated as juglone and based on the anhydrous drug. Finished pharmaceutical products have been shown to contain very little naphthoquinone, which may be due to extended storage. Other constituents of the roundleaf sundew herb include flavonoids, anthocyanin glycosides, and ellagic acid.

Roundleaf sundew's significant **spasmolytic, antiphlogistic** and **antibacterial** actions make it a cough suppressant. Its spasmolytic action is dosage dependent. Consumption of roundleaf sundew turns urine a dark color.

▶ **Research.** Roundleaf sundew's spasmolytic effects have been relatively extensively studied experimentally on the ileum and on isolated guinea pig trachea strips. Alcoholic extractions were shown to be much more effective than aqueous extractions. A hot water extract showed significant antibacterial effects for roundleaf sundew on two different strains of *Staphylococcus aureus* und *Escherichia coli*. The study also showed anti-inflammatory effects based on inhibition of human neutrophil elastase (Krenn and Kartnig).

▶ **Indications.** The Commission E indications for roundleaf sundew are coughing fits (spasmodic cough) and dry cough.

Roundleaf sundew also works well for whooping cough (p. 338). A proven remedy is the combination of thyme with a small addition of roundleaf sundew.

glandular substance that sparkles in the sunlight like a precious stone. When an insect lands on the leaf, it is first held captive by the adhesive power of the glandular hairs. Soon, the more distant hairs start to bend toward the insect. This initiates the excretion of an enzymatic substance that breaks down the insect's protein substances and allows them to be absorbed by the plant. This process is similar to the action of gastric juices in the stomach. The roundleaf sundew plant requires this additional source of proteins to survive in its very barren, protein-deficient peat moss soil and peat moss (sphagnum) growth habitat. In Germany, roundleaf sundew has been placed under strict protected status and medicinal plants are now sourced from other sundew varieties, primarily from East Africa. In North America, roundleaf sundew is abundant.

Medicinal applications use the roundleaf **sundew herb** (above-ground parts of the plant, Droserae herba).

▶ **Therapy Recommendations.** Finished pharmaceutical products are clearly the most reliable remedy.

Roundleaf sundew must be taken in small amounts. The average daily dose is 3 g.

Ivy (Hedera helix)

Ivy is a very old cult and medicinal plant. It has been written about as far back as Roman times. In Germany, ivy grows in damp forests. It is a climbing plant and a member of the special group of root climbers (plants that use adventitious roots to cling to surfaces). In the past, ivy was thought to be a parasite, but that has been proven not to be the case. Ivy uses the plants it climbs as a surface to which to attach itself. However, it can choke a tree it entwines of nutrients, water, and sunlight, and cause it to die.

Medicinal applications use the **dried ivy leaves** (Hederae helicis folium).

▶ **Pharmacology.** The most important constituents of ivy are triterpene saponins, flavone glycosides, and phenol carbon acids. Its effects are primarily **spasmolytic**. Ivy is also **secretolytic** and a **mild sedative**. Using these mechanisms, ivy can calm whooping cough by reducing the number of coughing fits and especially by reducing spasmodic coughing. One of ivy's interesting therapeutic actions is attributed to the saponin α-hederin. It inhibits the downregulation of $β_2$-receptors caused by over irritation of the bronchial mucosa in bronchial muscle cells and lung epithelium. This causes bronchial dilation and increased production of surfactants, which enhances secretion.

▶ **Indications.** Ivy is used therapeutically in some specialized preparations as a **whooping cough remedy** and for treatment of **spastic inflammatory respiratory disorders**, including dry cough.

The Commission E monograph for ivy lists the indications catarrhs of the respiratory passages and symptomatic treatment of chronic inflammatory bronchial conditions.

▶ **Therapy Recommendation.** Liquid ivy leaf extract solutions can also be used for inhalation. This application is also suitable for children.

▶ **Research.** Rudkowski and Latos describe a 3-week course of inhalation treatment using 20 drops of a Hedera helix preparation diluted in water at a 1:5 ratio. This solution was inhaled 3 times a day using an ultrasonic vaporizer.

African Geranium (Pelargonium sidoides DC)

African geranium is found in its native habitat in South Africa near the coast at elevations of up to 2,000 m. This plant has narrow deep-red flowers and large heart-shaped leaves. The leaves are densely covered in hair and feel soft and velvety to the touch. Their tips are rounded and have a finely ribbed margin (Kolodziej and Kayser).

The African geranium is part of the large Geraniacea family. This family includes many types, which are used as decorative plants nowadays. These decorative plants are called geraniums, but modern botany classifies them as the genus Pelargonium, the most prominent ornamental variety is Pelargonium × hortorum.

Medicinal applications use the dried **African geranium root** (Pelargonii sidoidi radix).

▶ **Note.** The Zulu name "umckaloabo" for African geranium in its native habitat means "severe cough." This drug was imported to England at the end of the 19th century as a tuberculosis remedy. However, it did not establish itself for this indication long term. When tuberculosis ceased to be a public health concern in West Germany in the mid-20th century, the use of Pelargonii sidoidi radix preparations shifted to less severe pulmonary infections for which it proved to be much more successful.

▶ **Pharmacology.** The important constituents of African geranium are coumarins, gallic acid, and tannins.

▶ **Research.** Various experimental studies of the drug and its isolated constituents have shown **antibacterial**, **antiviral**, and **immune-modulating characteristics** (Kolodziej and Kayser). Especially the coumarins contained in the drug, for example, exhibit pronounced inhibitory effects against gram-positive and gram-negative bacteria that occur frequently with respiratory infections. The drug also showed immune-modulating effects on several components of the immune system, for example, macrophages, interferon, and tumor necrosis factor alpha. This effect is primarily attributed to gallic acids.

Other studies also show an **increase in the phagocytosing ability** of human peripheral blood phagocytes (PBP). The study conducted by Conrad et al., in 2008, showed that the absolute number of PBPs was increased by a maximum of 56%. The application of EPs 7630 also led to a concentration-dependent and significant increase in the number of burst-active PBPs. The study also showed a significant increase in the intracellular killing of yeast cells as test organisms. The study did not show which active constituents are responsible for this effect.

▶ **Indications.** African geranium is used for nonspecific infections of the entire respiratory tract, with emphasis on acute or **acute exacerbating chronic bronchitis, sinusitis, and nonpyogenic tonsillitis.**

There is no Commission E monograph for this drug.

▶ **Research.** Older clinical studies (Haidvogel et al.; Heil and Reitermann) have been augmented by numerous modern, evidence-based studies. Following are the results of two of these studies:

A randomized, double-blind, placebo-controlled study of 124 patients with acute bronchitis showed that EPs 7630 was significantly superior to placebo in symptom improvement (p < 0.001). In the verum group, remissions within 4 days occurred 69% of the time and in the placebo group 33% of the time. Tolerability was equally good in both groups (Chuchalin et al.).

These results were comprehensibly confirmed by another randomized, double-blind, placebo-controlled study of 217 patients with acute bronchitis. One interesting aspect of this study was the difference in thr effects on symptoms: The differences between the verum group and the placebo group were most pronounced for the symptoms of cough, rales, weakness, fatigue, expectoration, hoarseness and headaches, in that order. The impact on symptoms of dyspnea, chest pain, limb pain, and fever were much less pronounced. Another significant result was patient satisfaction (84% for EPs 7630, 48% for placebo). Tolerability was very good (Matthys and Heger).

For some time, there was a discussion of **liver toxicity** and interactions with other coumarins or coumarin derivatives. However, this was not confirmed and has also been partially disproven experimentally (Loew and Koch). In 2015, Tisch published a current review of the use of phytopharmaceuticals for the treatment of respiratory tract disorders.

A controlled, randomized, three-armed, placebo-controlled, double-blind study showed significant recidivism prevention in patients susceptible to respiratory tract infections. The study tested two different dosages of a combination of nasturtium herb and horseradish root against placebo. A higher daily dose of 3 × 2 tablets was shown to be most effective and significantly superior to placebo. Tolerability was very good (Fintelmann et al.).

Proven Prescription Formulas for Cough Teas

Cough teas should be considered in addition to the finished pharmaceutical products recommended in this section. Tea provides abundant hydration, which is almost always appropriate. Its warmth stimulates the organism, and it can be formulated to contain different drugs that are adapted for the specific symptoms a patient is experiencing.

Tea for Acute Urge to Cough (Acute Tracheobronchitis)

Rx
Verbasci flos (mullein flowers)
Farfarae fol. (coltsfoot leaves)
Althaeae rad. (marshmallow root)
Anisi fruct. āā ad 100.0 (anise seeds)
M. f. spec.
Add 1 cup of hot water to 2 teaspoons of the blend. Steep for 20 minutes, then strain.
D.S.
Drink 1 cup hot several times a day, optionally sweetened with honey.

Tea for Spasmodic Cough, Whooping Cough, Asthma, Chronic Obstructive Pulmonary Disease (COPD)

Rx
Thymi herb. (thyme herb)
Droserae herb. (roundleaf sundew herb)
Eryngii plan. herb. (sea holly herb (p. 352))
Anisi fruct. āā ad 100.0 (anise seeds)
M. f. spec.
Add 1 cup of hot water to 1 teaspoon of the blend. Steep for 20 minutes, then strain.
D.S.
Drink 1 cup several times a day.

Tea to Stimulate Expectoration with Subacute or Chronic Bronchitis

Rx
Primulae rad. (cowslip or oxlip primrose root)
Thymi herb. (thyme herb)
Plantagin. lanc. herb. āā ad 100.0 (narrowleaf plantain herb)
M. f. spec.
Add 1 cup of hot water to 1 heaping teaspoon of the blend. Steep for 20 minutes, then strain.
D.S.
Drink 3 cups a day.

Tea for Chronic, Recurring Bronchitis and General Weakness

Rx
Helenii rad. (elecampane root)
Lichen island. (Icelandic lichen)
Farfarae fol. (coltsfoot leaves)
Pulmonariae herb. āā ad 100.0 (lungwort herb)
M. f. spec.
Add 1 cup of hot water to 1 teaspoon of the blend. Boil for 15 minutes, then strain.
D.S.
Drink 3 cups a day.

Special Treatments: Inhalation

The remedies discussed in this section for the treatment of respiratory tract disorders—with cough as their most frequent symptom—are primarily taken internally. Inhalation represents a transition from internal to external application. For manifest upper respiratory catarrh, inhalation should be used several times a day. In some cases, inhalation is the only treatment required: It loosens coughs, clears the head by improving sinus drainage and reduces secretion and the urge to cough. Inhalations are also suitable as an adjuvant for cough tea treatments.

- **Chamomile Decoction**
  German chamomile (p. 42) is the most suitable plant medicine for inhalations.
  Add boiling water to a handful of German chamomile in a pot. Patients should place a towel or cloth over their heads in such a way that it also covers the pot. Patients should inhale the vapors rising up from the pot, with their mouth slightly open. The vapors can also be inhaled through a funnel made from sturdy paper.
- **Chamomile Decoction with Other Medicinal Plants**
  It makes sense to add additional medicinal plants to the chamomile decoction to increase its effectiveness. Thyme (Thymi herba), wild thyme herb (Serpylli herba) and oregano[1] (Origani herba/Origanum vulgare, above-ground parts) are

---

[1] Oregano is a common kitchen herb. It has some medicinal properties but not enough to justify a chapter of its own in this book. It is however useful in tea combinations and should therefore not be omitted entirely.

the most suitable herbs for this application. They contain volatile oils that are vaporized by the hot water. This allows them to reach the respiratory tract.

Prescriptions

Rx
Matricariae flos (German chamomile flowers)
Thymi herb. (thyme herb)
Origan. herb. āā 50.0 (oregano herb)
D.S.
Add 500 mL of boiling water to 1 tablespoon of the blend. Inhale the vapors.

- **Decoction of Dwarf Pine Oil (Oleum Pini pumilionis) or Eucalyptus Oil (Oleum Eucalypti)**
  Add 5 drops of the essential oil to 10–20 mL of distilled water. Inhale slowly (for example, using an inhalation device).
  Eucalyptus oil is the volatile oil distilled from the fresh leaves of the **eucalyptus tree** (Eucalyptus globulus). Its main constituent (about 70%) is 1.8-cineol. It is considered a secretolytic and expectorant primarily for external use, similar to camphor oil and menthol. The eucalyptus tree originates from Australia. Today, it is frequently found in Italy, where it was first planted in large numbers to dry up swamp areas and is now a popular tree along streets. It is easily recognized by its sickle-shaped drooping leaves that are covered by a layer of wax.
- **Japanese Mint Oil Decoction**
  Place 3–5 drops at the bottom of a small bowl, add hot water, and inhale the rising healing vapors for 5–10 minutes (using the method described for chamomile decoction above).
  This method has been proven to provide rapid self-help, even for protracted, chronic coughs.
  This oil is high in free menthol, which provides antibacterial action, stimulates secretion, and mildly anesthetizes irritated and inflamed upper respiratory mucosa. The menthol-rich vapors of Japanese mint oil are best inhaled into the irritated and infected bronchia at the first signs of catarrh of the nose, pharynx, and larynx.
  The volatile oil contained in Japanese mint oil (Oleum Menthae japonicum) is derived from Japanese mint (Mentha arvensis var. piperascens), a close relative of peppermint (Mentha piperita).

Inunctions

- **Balms and Ointments Containing Volatile Oils**
  Japanese mint oil, eucalyptus oil, and other volatile oils contained in the plants presented in this chapter for treatment of respiratory tract disorders also have **percutaneous (transdermal) effects**. This treatment provides reflex action (reflection) and absorption, even if the absorbed amounts are rather small. The effects of transdermal application are primarily **secretolytic** and **antiphlogistic**. Some oils, such as thyme, eucalyptus or sage oil, are also **antibacterial**. Some oils also have spasmolytic effects.
  Chest balm and chest ointment inunctions provide rapid and reliable relief. They are typically applied to the skin in the area of the sternum and on the back, between the shoulder blades.
  All chest balms and chest ointments can also be used for **dry chest wraps**: After applying one of the balms or ointments, a linen cloth is placed on the chest and back and covered by a thick wool cloth or scarf. This treatment is applied once or twice a day.

Prescriptions

Rx
Ol. Thymi (thyme essential oil)
Ol. Rosmarin. (rosemary essential oil)
Ol. Eucalypt. āā 2.0 (eucalyptus essential oil)
Ol. Camphorat. ad 50.0 (camphor oil)
D.S.
Apply to chest and neck

Caution

The balms, ointments, creams, or gels should be applied in a very thin layer because they can cause skin irritations. Extreme caution is especially advised for treatment of infants and young children. Inunctions of balms, ointments, or creams, etc. should never be applied to the face or to the area of the nose. This is especially important to remember when treating young children!

5.2 Sinusitis

5.2.1 Combination Preparation Sinupret

This indication, which falls into the category of upper respiratory infections in a larger sense, is included here because of the combination remedy Sinupret. This remedy has a special significance among phytopharmaceuticals. Without a doubt, however, the demulcents (p. 183) described in this book can also be used for adjuvant and symptomatic treatment of nonpyogenic sinusitis.

Recently, there are also indications that African geranium (Pelargonium sidoides DC., EPs 7630) is efficacious for treatment of sinusitis that does not require antibiotics.

Plants for Treatment: The Fixed Combination Remedy Sinupret

It is commonly assumed that the efficacy of a combination remedy containing more than three constituents, for which the contribution of each to the overall efficacy has not been shown, would not be rationally explainable. The emphasis of the argument is on the additive effects of such combinations, especially with a view toward synthetic substances. Plants, however, are multisubstances, which are the sum of their constituents. Using fixed or individually formulated combinations is a tradition in phytotherapy. This was repeatedly pointed out by Weiss. The fact that useful combinations can be viewed as a new entity, i.e., as a single medicine, is easily overlooked. The analogy here is the overall sound of an orchestra, which is more than the sum of its individual sounds: It represents a "new unit."

One prominent example of a finished pharmaceutical product on the German market that functions in accordance with this principle is Sinupret, a fixed combination remedy that contains gentian root (Gentiana lutea), cowslip primrose flowers (Primula veris), garden sorrel (Rumex acetosa), European elderberry flowers (Sambucus nigra) and verbena (Verbena officinalis). Compelling examples of proof of its pharmacological efficacy and clinical effectiveness document the special significance of this preparation (review by März et al.).

▶ **Pharmacology.** A classic Percy and Boyd model showed **secretolytic effects** for Sinupret and its constituent drugs. This effect was significantly higher than in control groups (19% alcohol by volume or 0.9% sodium chloride). A phenol red test produced the same results.

Anti-inflammatory effects for Sinupret and its constituents were shown in comparison with phenylbutazone and placebo. This was primarily attributed to the garden sorrel herb (Rumicis herba). **Antiviral effects** against influenza A, parainfluenza virus type 1, and human respiratory syncytial virus (HRSV) were also shown. These different effects were primarily attributed to different components of the remedy.

▶ **Indications.** Sinupret drops have been available since 1933 and Sinupret tablets were introduced in 1997. Numerous open trials and experiential reports confirm the good efficacy and excellent tolerability of this remedy for sinus infections. In the meantime, randomized, placebo-controlled studies provide impressive documentation for the efficacy of this remedy.

Sinupret is the remedy of first choice for acute and chronic **sinus infections**.

▶ **Research.** In a randomized, placebo-controlled study, 160 patients received Sinupret in addition to basic antibiotics treatment and local nasal decongestant drops. Sinupret showed significant superiority compared to placebo with regards to objective resolution (complete cure) and improvement of subjective symptoms (Schapowal). Further studies confirmed these results. Two randomized, blind studies of uncomplicated tracheobronchitis showed Sinupret's therapeutic equivalence to N-acetylcysteine and pronounced superiority compared to a competitor (Tisch).

A multicentric, prospective, open study (application observation) of the extract derived from African geranium root (Pelargonium sidoides DC.) was published in 2008, whereby 80.9% of patients indicated symptom resolution or significant improvement of their symptoms within 4 weeks. EPs 7630 is viewed as an interesting therapeutic alternative for sinusitis that does not require antibiotics (Schapowal and Heger).

5.3 Bronchial Asthma

5.3.1 Interval Therapy using Phytopharmaceuticals

> **Medicinal Plants**
>
> **Bishop's weed, Ammi visnaga**
> Bishop's weed fruit, Ammeos visnagae fructus
> **Thyme, Thymus vulgaris**
> Thyme herb, Thymi herba
> **Roundleaf Sundew, Drosera rotundifolia**
> Roundleaf Sundew herb, Droserae herba
> **Ivy, Hedera helix**
> Ivy leaves, Hederae helicis folium
> **Onion, Allium cepa**
> Onion bulb, Allii cepae bulbus

Bronchial asthma is not a uniform disorder. One indicator is the differentiation between extrinsic asthma, which is caused by allergens, and intrinsic asthma, which is caused by psychological factors. Each asthma patient will present with individual variations of this primarily chronic disorder to the practitioner.

Conventional and established bronchial asthma treatment encompasses primarily symptomatic treatment using synthetic drugs, mainly topical glucocorticoids, β-sympathicomimetics and theophylline derivatives. Phytotherapeutics are not indicated for the treatment of acute asthma, asthma attacks, and status asthmaticus. However, phytotherapeutics are indicated for **interval therapy**. Several plants can be recommended for adjuvant therapy. When taken regularly, they can help to reduce the frequency and daily dose of necessary synthetic drugs, which can increase the tolerability of these drugs or reduce their undesirable effects. It can be stated without reservation that these phytotherapeutics are beneficial for asthma patients.

Of the small number of plants that are indicated for asthma therapy, Bishop's weed is the most important. Other medicinal plants that have been introduced in this book for treating spasmodic cough or dry cough, so-called antitussives (p. 194), can be used as adjuvant therapy. This also applies to expectorants (p. 187), which are medicinal plants with strong secrolytic effects. Tenacious mucus located in the bronchioles that is very difficult to expectorate is one of the main pathogenic factors of this disorder. **Onions** (Allium cepa) should also

be mentioned because newer studies have shown antiasthmatic effects for this plant.

> **Caution** ⚠
>
> Treatment of the differentiated symptoms presented by bronchial asthma requires experience in prescribing phytotherapeutics to avoid overestimating their effectiveness. Insufficient treatment can lead to severe and possibly life-threatening complications.

Plants for Treatment

Bishop's weed (Ammi visnaga)

Bishop's weed is a member of the Apiaceae family. With its upright growth of up to 1 m and its finely feathered leaves (▶ Fig. 5.13), it resembles Daucus carota. Its flowers are white and its fruit resembles caraway fruit (seeds). They are slightly longer than

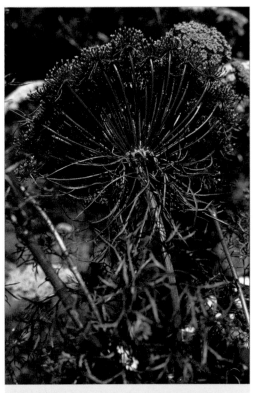

Fig. 5.13 Bishop's weed, Ammi visnaga. Photo: Dr. Roland Spohn, Engen.

they are wide and have ovate-oblong commissures. The entire plant exudes an aromatic fragrance, and its taste is spicy. Bishop's weed grows wild in the Mediterranean (primarily in Egypt).

Medicinal applications use the **bishop's weed fruit** (seeds, Ammeos visnagae fructus).

▶ **Note.** Bishop's weed is an ancient medicinal plant already known to ancient Egyptians and mentioned in the Ebers Papyrus (c.1550 BC). Ancient Egyptian folk medicine used this plant primarily for kidney stones because of its spasmolytic action. In 1946, the pharmacologist Anrep became aware of bishop's weed by coincidence while working in Egypt. In experimental studies, he discovered the plant's pronounced spasmolytic effects, especially on the bronchioles, but also on the coronary arteries and the ureter (Anrep et al.).

▶ **Pharmacology.** Bishop's weed's main constituents are furanochromones such as khellin and visnagin as well as pyranocoumarins, such as visnadin, samidin, and dihydrosamidin. It also contains flavonoids and a small amount of volatile oil.

Particularly khellin and visnadin have **spasmolytic** effects on the smooth vascular and bronchial muscles. Its **vasodilating effects** on coronary blood vessels can cause increased coronary and myocardial circulation. Mild positive inotropic effects have also been described for this plant.

No side effects or interactions with other drugs are known.

▶ **Note.** The synthetic khellin derivative **chromoglicic acid**, a new drug in the furanochromone group, was developed from bishop's weed. It appears as disodium chromoglicate in many finished pharmaceutical products available on the market. It is not a conventional asthma drug but does have antiallergic properties. This seems to make it especially suitable for the treatment of allergic types of bronchial asthma. It prevents the release of inflammatory mediators by stabilizing mast cell membranes. Chromoglicic acid is currently considered a prophylactic drug for the prevention of bronchial asthma exacerbation.

▶ **Indications.** The primary indications for bishop's weed are **mild stenocardia symptoms** and **spastic, asthmatic bronchial disorders**. However, bishop's weed is used exclusively for interval therapy. It is not suitable for treating asthma attacks.

Bishop's weed is also suitable for prevention of nighttime asthma attacks because its spasmolytic effects last a long time, about 6 hours on average. This differentiates bishop's weed from many other drugs in use.

Khellin accumulates in the organism and causes a cumulative effect, similar to digitalis. Three daily dosages of bishop's weed taken throughout the day are usually sufficient and one additional dosage at bedtime usually suffices to provide a restful night for asthmatics.

The Commission E issued a negative monograph for bishop's weed based on its risk assessment—which included isolated mentions of pseudoallergic reactions, cholestasis, and photosensitization—and because the efficacy of this plant was not sufficiently documented.

> **Preparation** ☞
>
> • Homeopathic Mother Tincture

Additional Therapy Options

Thyme (Thymus vulgaris), Roundleaf Sundew (Drosera rotundifolia), Ivy (Hedera helix)

Primarily thyme herb (p. 194) (Thymi herba), but also roundleaf sundew herb (p. 195) (Droserae herba) and ivy leaves (p. 197) (Hedera felicis folium), can be used as adjuvant treatment for bronchial asthma. This is due to their proven bronchial spasmolytic action. However, as mentioned above, they cannot replace synthetic antiasthmatic drugs under any circumstances. These spasmolytic remedies can be combined with typical expectorants and demulcents, depending on the symptoms of mucous congestion and impaired expectoration. This field is wide open for practitioners to formulate their own prescriptions.

Onion (Allium cepa)

Fresh onion juice has been used successfully in folk medicine to treat cough, bronchitis, and even asthma.

▶ **Pharmacology.** Studies by Dorsch et al. (1987; 1989) actually show antiasthmatic action for freshly prepared, lyophilized (freeze-dried) onion extract.

Thiosulfinates inhibit the following processes: anti-immunoglobulin-E (IgE)-induced release of histamine from peripheral granulocytes, leukotrine biosynthesis in prestimulated granulocytes by inhibiting 5-lipocygenase, and thromboxane-B_2-biosynthesis in platelet-rich human plasma and in pulmonary fibroblasts (Wagner et al. 1989). This makes these substances potent prostaglandin cascade inhibitors.

▶ **Indications.** The Commission E monograph for onion does not list bronchial asthma as an indication. It is confined to the indications lack of appetite and prevention of age-related vascular disorders.

This is likely because onion preparations that are suitable for clinical applications and for which the antiasthmatic component is sufficiently active are not yet available on the market. According to Wagner et al. (1989), the lack of chemical uniformity for homemade pressed onion juice means that the presence of sufficient amounts of the active constituents is not guaranteed.

Newer, primarily experimental results—combined with the experience of folk medicine—can open up the indication area of bronchial asthma for the onion. However, this requires comprehensive clinical application studies and, above all, the manufacture of an **onion extract that is standardized** for thiosulfinates.

▶ **Research.** Using whole body plethysmography of sensitized guinea pigs, Dorsch et al. (1989) showed that peroral treatment with lyophilized onion extract inhibits experimentally induced bronchial obstruction. In a human study, oral treatment with 2×100 mL ethanolic onion extract (= 400 g of onions) suppressed the immediate and delayed asthmatic reaction of a female patient to the inhalation of house dust mites (Dorsch et al. 1989).

5.4 Flu and Common Cold

Medicinal Plants

Immune-Modulating Phytotherapeutics
Echinacea, Echinacea purpurea/pallida/angustifolia
Echinacea herb and root, Echinaceae herba et radix
Wormwood, Artemisia absinthium
Wormwood herb, Absinthii herba

Diaphoretics
European Elderberry, Sambucus nigra
European elderberry flowers, Sambuci flos
Linden, Tilia cordata/platyphyllos
Linden flower, Tiliae flos
Jaborandi, Pilocarpus pennatifolius
Jaborandi leaves, Jaborandi folium

Plants that Contain Vitamin C
Lemon, Citrus limon
Lemon fruit, Citrus limonis fructus
Dog Rose, Rosa canina
Rosehip seed, Cynosbati semen
Sea Buckthorn, Hippophae rhamnoides
Sea Buckthorn fruit, Hippophae rhamnoides fructus
Black Currant, Ribes nigrum
Black currant fruit, Ribes nigrae fructus

5.4.1 Immune-Modulating Phytopharmaceuticals

Influenza (flu) and colds, like the ordinary rhinitis or laryngitis, are predominantly caused by viruses. Antibiotics and other chemotherapeutics are useless for treating these disorders. The commonly practiced use of antipyretics to reduce fever is also wrong and can lead to complications. As has been known for a long time, most human pathogenic viruses are not able to reproduce at high body temperatures. Therefore, fever constitutes causal treatment of viral infections.

Generally, influenza and colds nowadays are primarily treated only symptomatically. The actual treatment of the disease is left to the body's own defense systems. The body's natural nonspecific immune response is very important. For patients with increased susceptibility to infections who experience more than six—or in children, more than twelve—infections a year, therapies that strengthen or stimulate the immune system provide prevention as well as curative treatment in the early stages of infections. **Echinacea** is a plant that is especially suitable for this purpose.

We also know from folk medicine that influenza and colds can be successfully treated by inducing the organism to sweat. The most well-known and most suitable diaphoretics are elderberry and linden flower.

Plants for Treatment

Echinacea (Echinacea purpurea/pallida/angustifolia)

Echinacea (also known as coneflower) is possibly one of the most interesting medicinal plants. This shrub can grow to a height of 60–100 cm and starts to develop stems, leaves, and flowers shortly after its subterranean shoot sprouts. Its leaves are wide and ovate and more or less dentate and covered with bristly hair on both sides. The leaf surface is intensely green. Echinacea angustifolia has smaller, more linear, lancette-shaped leaves that are narrower at the base and divided by three veins. Echinacea flowers can be from purple to white. Echinacea purpurea flowers are the most vividly purple, hence its name.

Echinacea is a member of the Asteraceae family and originates from North America. Meanwhile, it can also be found in Europe as a common garden plant. Medicinal applications use the **fresh, aboveground parts of the Echinacea plant** (Echinaceae herba), harvested during flowering, and the **Echinacea root** (Echinaceae radix).

▶ **Note.** The Latin name *Echinacea* is derived from the Greek *echinos* (hedgehog) and refers to the appearance of the spiny seed head. Indigenous peoples of Nebraska and Missouri have known about Echinacea for a long time as a medicinal plant. It was brought to Europe and cultivated there at the end of the 19th century.

▶ **Pharmacology.** The main Echinacea constituents are polyene and polyyne compounds, volatile oil, resins, and heteropolysaccharides.

It is not yet fully understood if there are definitive differences in effects between the various preparations of Echinacea and the three types of Echinacea mentioned here. In a summary review, Wagner (1991) found no significant differences. At the time of this writing, the efficacy of the three types of Echinacea can be assumed to be comparable. Pressed juice of the above-ground parts of blooming Echinacea purpurea is the most well studied.

Echinacea is considered the most important immune-modulating phytotherapeutic. Given the great complexity and individuality of the human immune system, it is not surprising that very interesting experimental data about Echinacea's effect on the immune system but no exact description about how this plant impacts the human immune system is available. Most of what we know about this plant continues to come from clinical practical experience, supported by a large number of clinical trials and studies.

▶ **Research.** Bauer and Wagner provide a comprehensive review of the pharmacology of Echinacea. It delineates nonimmunologic and immunologic effects. The authors describe **anti-infective** and **antiphlogistic** effects on local tissue. The anti-infective effects are attributed to direct or indirect inhibition of the bacterial and tissue hyaluronic acid/hyaluronidase system. This explains the well-known ability of Echinacea to heal chronic, suppurating wounds or secondary skin infections. chinacea's antiphlogistic effect is attributed to polysaccharides and alkylamides.

Bauer and Wagner cite the following **immunogenic effects** of Echinacea: increase of properdin levels in guinea pigs, increased number of leucocytes in humans, increased number of granulocytes and rate of phagocytosis in mice and in humans exposed to radiation as well as increased phagocytosis (carbon clearance method). More recent studies also showed increases in T helper cells and in various cytokines, for example, interleukin-1, interleukin-6, and tumor necrosis factor (Ardjomand-Wodkart and Bauer). All of the above data can be summarized as an increasing natural nonspecific immune response.

▶ **Indications.** The main indications for Echinacea are **viral (influenza) infections** and **colds**. For other indications of Echinacea purpurea, see the chapters Wounds, Contusions, Distortions (p. 299), Kidney and Urinary Tract Disorders (p. 213) und Oncologic Disorders (p. 345).

The experience of the authors has shown that Echinacea can also be used as a preventive, for example, in cases of conspicuous and increased **susceptibility to infections**.

The Commission E monograph for Echinacea lists the following indications: for internal use, as a supportive treatment of chronic, recurring respiratory tract, and urinary tract infections. For external use to treat poor-healing surface wounds.

▶ **Research.** Numerous experiential reports to date as well as some proband and controlled studies confirm the indications listed above.

In 1994, Melchart et al. analyzed and evaluated 26 controlled studies in this context that also included the use of combination remedies containing Echinacea. Ardjomand-Wodkart and Bauer published a current review of the efficacy and medicinal safety data in 2014.

Preparation

- **Tincture**
  Adults can take 10 drops in a small amount of water several times a day. The dosage for children is lower at 5 drops 3 × a day.

▶ **Therapy Recommendations.** In cases of conspicuous susceptibility to infections, a dosage of 20–50 drops of echinacin in the morning for several months has been shown to be very effective. The Commission E recommends a shorter treatment duration.

There are no systemic or controlled studies of this indication and dosage. **Interval therapy** seems essential because the immunogenic effect of Echinacea almost certainly declines during long-term or continuous therapy. These statements are based entirely on practical experience.

Wormwood (Artemisia absinthium)

For more information about this plant, see wormwood (p. 111).

Wormwood generally **improves physical wellbeing** during influenza and colds. It is a potent tonic bitter that also provides a central stimulating effect.

Preparations

- **Tea**
  Add 1 cup of boiling water to 1–2 teaspoons of the finely chopped drug, ideally the fresh herb straight from the garden. Steep covered for 5 minutes, then strain.
  Drink 1 cup hot several times a day.
  Can be used as a tea regimen for 2–4 weeks in cases of postoperative and postinfection weakness with hypotonic symptoms.
- **Tincture**
  Take 20–30 drops in hot water several times a day.

5.4.2 Diaphorethics

European Elderberry (Sambucus nigra)

This shrub grows wild in European forests and along riverbanks and is also frequently planted in gardens and parks. Its small white flowers are clustered into umbrella-shaped inflorescences. Its berries are black and edible (▶ Fig. 5.14).

Medicinal applications use the **elderberry flowers** (Sambuci flos) and **berries** (Sambuci fructus). However, only the flowers are used as a diaphoretic and for increasing nonspecific immunity. The fruit is not suitable for this purpose. The fruit is a mild laxative and, in larger amounts, causes nausea and vomiting. Therefore, the Commission E monograph applies only to elderberry flowers. It lists colds as an indication.

▶ **Pharmacology.** The main constituents of European elderberry flowers are flavonoids,

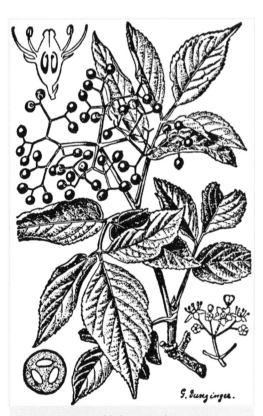

Fig. 5.14 European Elderberry, Sambucus nigra.

hydroxylphenyl carbon acid, phytosterines, and up to 0.2% volatile oils.

> **Preparation** ☞
>
> - **Tea**
>   Add 1 cup of boiling water to 2 teaspoons of the drug. Steep covered for 15 minutes, then strain.
>   To strengthen the immune system, drink 1 cup several times a day. To induce sweating for sweating regimens, drink approximately 500 mL.

▶ **Therapy Recommendation for Sweating Regimen.** The effects of sweating regimens are increased by a full hot bath following the consumption of the hot elderberry flower tea (see above). The bath should last long enough to induce pronounced sweating. Next, the patient should change over from the bath straight to a bed in which the patient is covered well in several blankets in order to continue sweating for at least 30 minutes. Then, patients need to thoroughly dry off the body. This step should be followed by another period of rest. Sweating regimens are best done in the evening. Please note that sweating regimens require the patient to have healthy and trained circulation to tolerate them well.

Littleleaf Linden (Tilia cordata), Bigleaf Linden (Tilia platyphyllos)

Linden trees are among the most well-known trees in Germany. **Bigleaf linden** is very rare nowadays. It can be recognized by its larger leaves with short hairs on the underside of the leaf. Its buds develop earlier than those of **littleleaf lindens** and it blooms about 8 to 14 days earlier. Littleleaf linden (▶ Fig. 5.15) has bare leaves that are sea green on the underside. It is frequently found in deciduous forests, but usually as an isolated, individual tree.

Medicinal applications use the **linden flowers** (Tiliae flos).

▶ **Pharmacology.** Linden flowers contain flavonoids, tannins, mucilage and small amounts of volatile oils (Czygan 1997). Like European elderberry flowers, linden flowers are a good diaphoretic.

Even if linden flowers do not cause bouts of sweating, they do achieve general strengthening of

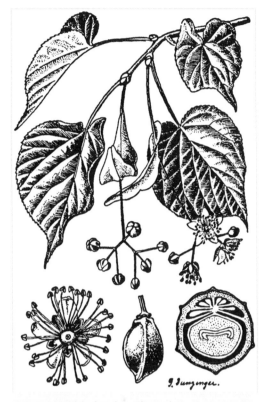

Fig. 5.15 Littleleaf Linden, Tilia cordata.

the immune system. The effects of both types of linden trees are about equally strong.

> **Preparation** ☞
>
> - **Tea**
>   Add 1 cup of hot water to 1 teaspoon of the drug. Steep covered for 10 minutes, then strain.
>   With influenza and colds, drink 1 cup several times a day slowly, in small sips, and as hot as can be tolerated.
>   Tea made from fresh linden flowers has a wonderfully aromatic fragrance and flavor, which is why children prefer it. It can be sweetened with honey.

Jaborandi (Pilocarpus pennatifolius)

The jaborandi shrub is a member of the Rutaceae family and grows almost exclusively in Brazil. It grows to a height of 1–3 m and has very little branching. Its upright, brownish-gray branches are covered in reddish-yellow hairs and the brittle bark is easy to peel. Its leaves are alternate and imparipinnate and are made up of two to five pairs of simple, opposite leaflets.

Medicinal applications use the **Jaborandi leaves** (Jaborandi folium).

▶ **Pharmacology.** The main constituent of jaborandi leaves is the alkaloid pilokarpin, which has been used as a synthetic single-constituent drug in medicine for a long time, for example in ophthalmology.

Jaborandi leaves are a "true" diaphoretic because they cause sweating directly, even without additional external application of heat.

The use of this drug requires considerable experience as a practitioner. A comprehensive overview can be found in the article by Scheerer (2000).

Caution ⚠
Jaborandi contains alkaloids and is therefore not suitable for use with children.

Preparation 👉
• **Tea** Add 1 cup of hot water to 1–2 teaspoons of the leaves. Do not boil! Steep for 5–10 minutes, then strain. Drink 1–2 cups and then spend some time in bed under plenty of covers in order to induce sweating.

5.4.3 Proven Prescriptions

Prescriptions
Diaphoretic Tea Blend Rx Sambuci flos (European elderberry flowers) Tiliae flos (linden flowers) Matricariae flos āā ad 100.0 (German chamomile flowers) M. f. spec. Add 250 mL of boiling water to 2–3 teaspoons of the blend. Steep for 10 minutes, then strain. D.S. Drink while hot in one sitting.

Prescriptions
Stronger Diaphoretic Tea Blend with Jaborandi Leaves Rx Jaborandi fol. 10.0 (Jaborandi leaves) Tiliae flos (linden flowers) Sambuci flos āā 20.0 (European elderberry flowers) M. f. spec. Add 1 cup of boiling water to 1 teaspoon of the blend. Steep for 10 minutes, then strain. D.S. Drink while hot.

5.4.4 Plants that Contain Vitamin C

Vitamins, especially vitamin C, strengthen the general immunity of the organism. Fever increases the body's use of vitamin C and it is now considered standard practice to administer plentiful amounts of vitamin C with any **acute infection**. The body should be satiated with vitamin C. Any excess will be excreted and toxicity is not a concern.

Lemon (Citrus limon)

The most well-known source of vitamin C is **lemon juice**. In addition to vitamin C, lemon juice also contains bioflavonoids (formerly called P-vitamins) such as citrin and hesperidin. This explains the traditional experience that the action of lemon juice is superior to vitamin C preparations for the treatment of scurvy.

However, lemon is not the only or necessarily the best source of vitamin C. A number of other fruits can also provide comparably high amounts of vitamin C. These include dog rose (rosehips), sea buckthorn, and black currants.

Dog Rose (Rosehip) (Rosa canina)

Rosehips, which are the fruit of the dog rose, are frequently processed into purees, preserves, and juice. Their red peel is high in vitamin C. Their medicinal name is **Cynosbati fructus** (from the Greek *kyon, kynos* for dog and *batos* for thorny bush). Their more fitting botanical name is Rosae pseudofructus. The red part of the rosehip fruit is the fleshy fruit receptacle (▶ Fig. 5.16).

Cutting open a rosehip reveals **rosehip seeds** (Cynosbati semen) that can also be used medicinally. They are a mild diuretic.

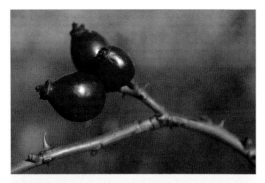

Fig. 5.16 Dog Rose (Rosehips), Rosa canina. Photo: Dr. Roland Spohn, Engen.

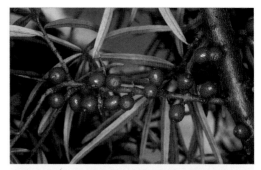

Fig. 5.17 Sea Buckthorn, Hippophae rhamnoides. Photo: Dr. Roland Spohn, Engen.

Preparation ☞

* **Tea**
  Add 1 cup of hot water to 2–5 g of the drug.
  Steep for 15–30 minutes, then strain.
  Drink 1 cup several times a day.
  Cold rosehip tea is good for quenching thirst caused by fever.

Sea Buckthorn (Hippophae rhamnoides)

Sea buckthorn grows wild primarily along rivers in the alpine foothills of Germany. It is also planted along beaches to fortify dunes. This many-branched shrub has lanceolate, silver-colored leaves and bright orange fruit (▶ Fig. 5.17).

Sea buckthorn fruit is high in vitamin C. It is processed into purees and juices, similar to rosehips. In Europe, sea buckthorn fruit became popular quickly because of its good taste, and it now has a considerable presence amount vitamin products.

Black Currant (Ribes nigrum)

Black currant is a fast-growing, deciduous shrub that can reach a height of 1–2 m. Its leaves are quite conspicuous. They can reach a width of up to 10 cm, are heart-shaped at the base, and have three to five lobes (▶ Fig. 5.18).

Black currants contain a considerable amount of vitamin C: 2000 mg/kg. They also contain potassium, rutin, and black pigment.

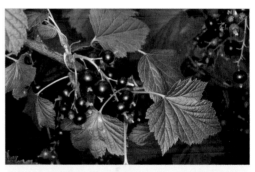

Fig. 5.18 Black Currant, Ribes nigrum. Photo: Dr. Roland Spohn, Engen.

Black currant juice is very well suited as a **hot beverage** during the early stages of influenza and colds. It can also be taken during convalescence (1 glass of juice midday and in the evening, with meals).

▶ **Note.** Red currents contain much less vitamin C and are not considered a medicinal remedy, but a good-tasting food.

▶ **Therapy Recommendation.** To preserve its vitamin content, black current juice should not be heated but diluted with hot water.

Ephedra (Ephedra sinica, Ephedra shennungiana)

Ephedra is a gymnosperm shrub resembling horsetail (▶ Fig. 5.19) and is related to the even more peculiar Welwitschia mirabilis, which is native to South Africa. Both are representatives of the

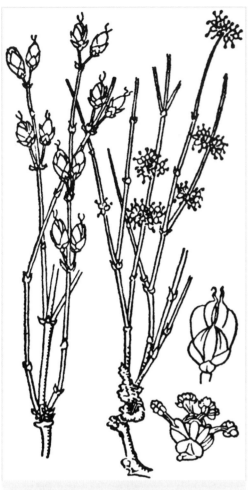

Fig. 5.19 Ephedra, Ephedra sinica.

gnetophyta division, a group of plants that have a unique place in the botanical system. They appear to be a relic from a long-forgotten period in the earth's history.

Ephedra species are found around the globe. It is possible that they are all subspecies of Ephedra sinica. Ephedra helvetica is rare and found on rocky outcroppings in the canton of Wallis in Switzerland. It is more common in Italy, Spain, and southern France. Ephedra distachia is found in Iran and India. It is an ancient medicinal plant that is mentioned in the Vedas (written in 1500–1000 BCE).

Research into ephedra began with Ephedra sinica, also known by its Chinese name *ma huang*.

This plant has been used since ancient times in Chinese medicine. It is said to have been used in China for treating asthmatic conditions for more than 5,000 years.

The discovery of ephedrine, one of the primary active constituents of Ephedra sinica, is closely connected with the pioneering lifework of the Japanese organic chemist and pharmacologist, Nagayoshi Nagai (1844–1929). Nagai was a major pioneer in scientific herbal medicine research and the first president of the Pharmaceutical Society of Japan, as of 1880. He first isolated ephedrine from Ephedra sinica in 1885 and recognized its pharmacological effect. In the mid-1920s, the German chemical company Merck developed synthetic ephedrine. Synthetic ephedrine differs from the natural, levorotary ephedrine alkaloid. The synthetic form is racemic, which means it is optically inactive because it consists of equal amounts of one levorotatory and one dextrorotatory isomer.

Practical experience has shown that the natural alkaloid as a constituent of ephedra has advantages over its synthetic form. The most important advantage is increased tolerability. It causes fewer heart symptoms, such as palpitations. Natural ephedrine, therefore, has not diminished in importance following the development of a synthetic form.

▶ **Pharmacology.** Ephedrine is derived from the amino acid phenylalanine. As an indirect sympathicomimetic, it stimulates the release of noradrenaline (norepinephrine) and causes **bronchodilation**.

The synthetic beta-sympathicomimetics commonly in use today are chemically derived from ephedrine or adrenaline (epinephrine).

Side effects to the pure compound include insomnia, motor unrest, irritability, headaches, nausea, vomiting, micturition problems, and tachycardia. Higher dosages can cause drastic increases in blood pressure and heart arrhythmia. Ephedrine dependence is also known to develop.

Contraindications to the pure compound include anxiety and restlessness, hypertension, narrow-angle glaucoma, cerebral circulation disorders, benign prostatic hyperplasia (BPH), prostate adenoma with residual urine retention, pheochromocytoma, and thyrotoxicosis. Interactions with other drugs can also occur, for example: Combining with heart glycosides or halothane can cause cardiac arrhythmia, combining with guanethidine can cause increases in sympathicomimetic effects, combining with MAO inhibitors can cause potentiation of sympathicomimetic effects, and combining with secale alkaloids or oxytocin can cause hypertension

▶ **Indications.** In the traditional Japanese system of Kampo medicine, the two ephedra combination preparations *kakkonto* [Pueraria lobata root 8.0 g, Ephedra sinica herb 4.0 g, jujube fruit (Ziziphus zizyphus) 4.0 g, cinnamon bark (Cinnamomum cassia) 3.0 g, peony root (Paeonia lactiflora) 3.0 g, licorice root (Glycyrrhiza uralensis) 2.0 g, dried ginger root (Zingiber officinale) 1.0 g] and *maoto* [Ephedra sinica herb 4.0–5.0 g, bitter apricot seed (Prunus armeniaca) 4.0–5.0 g, cinnamon bark (Cinnamomum cassia) 3.0–4.0 g, licorice root (Glycyrrhiza uralensis) 1.5–2.0 g] —the precise formulation varies by manufacturer—are some of the most frequently used cold remedies. Maoto is even named after the Japanese word for ephedra, which is *mao*.

⚠ Caution

In Western phytotherapy, ephedra preparations have also been used for interval therapy with bronchial asthma. However, given the side effects of ephedrine listed above, caution is advised regarding the long-term use of ephedra prescriptions that contain higher ephedrine concentrations than the Japanese prescriptions mentioned above.

Competition athletes should also note that drugs that contain ephedrine are on the doping list of the International Olympic Committee and the German Sports Federation.

Preparation

- Tinctures, Combined with Expectorants (according to Weiss)

Prescriptions

Rx
Tinct. Ephedrae benzoic. (ephedra benzoin tincture)
Tinct. Primulae (cowslip/oxlip primrose tincture)
Tinct. Pimpinellae āā 10.0 (pimpinella tincture)
D.S.
Take 20 drops 3 × a day.
Tinctura Ephedrae: 1 part Ephedra sinica herb is extracted and combined with 5 parts of dilluted alcohol (70 vol.%).
Tinct. Ephedrae benzoic.: 2 parts camphor, 4 parts bencoic acide, 183 parts dilluted alcohol (70 vol.%), 1 part anise essential oil, and 10 parts Tinctura Ephedrae are combined.

Bibliography

Anrep GV, Barsoum GS, Kenawy MR, Misrahy G. Ammi visnaga in the treatment of the anginal syndrome. Br Heart J. 1946; 8(4): 171–177

Ardjomand-Woelkart K, Bauer R. Echinacea. Eine Bestandsaufnahme der neueren Literatur. Z Phytother. 2014; 35(03):2–9

Bauer R, Wagner H. Echinacea-Monographie. Stuttgart: Wissenschaftliche Verlagsgesellschaft; 1989

Bauer R. Echinacea—Pharmazeutische Qualität und therapeutischer Wert. Z Phytother. 1997; 18(4):207–214

Chen KK, Schmidt CF. The action of ephedrine, an alkaloid from Ma Huang. Proc Soc Exp Biol Med. 1924; 21:351–354

Chuchalin AG, Berman B, Lehmacher W. Treatment of acute bronchitis in adults with a pelargonium sidoides preparation (EPs 7630): a randomized, double-blind, placebo-controlled trial. Explore (NY). 2005; 1(6):437–445

Conrad A, Bauer D, Hausmann C, Engels I, Frank U. Ein Extrakt aus Pelargonium sidoides (EPs® 7630) stimuliert die Phagozytose, den oxidativen Burst und die intrazelluläre Abtötung von Pathogenen in humanen peripheren Blutphagozyten. Z Phytother. 2008; 29 (1):15–18

Conrad A, Kolodziej H, Schulz V. Pelargonium-sidoides-Extrakt (EPs® 7630): Zulassung bestätigt Wirksamkeit und Verträglichkeit. Wien Med Wochenschr. 2007; 24:331–336

Czygan FC. Ätherische Öle und Duft. Universitas (Stuttg). 1987; 11: 1186–1199

Czygan FC. Linde (Tilia spec.)—Lindenblüten. Portrait einer Arzneipflanze. Z Phytother. 1997; 18(4):242–246

Dorsch W, Addmann-Grill B, Bayer T, et al. Zwiebelextrakte als Asthma-Therapeutika? Allergologie. 1987; 10:316–324

Dorsch W, Wagner H, Bayer T. Asthmaschutzwirkung von Zwiebelextrakten: Wirkprofil von Thiosulfinaten. Allergologie. 1989; 12(9):388–396

Fintelmann V, Schmitz G, Albrecht U, Schnitker J. Phytokombination geeignet zur Prophylaxe von Atemwegsinfekten. NaturaMed. 2013; 1:24–28

Frerichs G, Arends G, Zöring H, eds. Hagers Handbuch der Pharmazeutischen Praxis. Vol. 2., 2nd ed, Springer Verlag Berlin 1949, 450

Gaisbauer M, Zimmermann W, Schleich T. Die Veränderung immunologischer Parameter beim Menschen durch Echinacea pupurea Moench. Naturamed. 1986; 1:6–10

Geyer M, Mayer H, Pfandl A, Engelhard GM. Isländisches Moos – eine alte Heilpflanze aus heutiger Sicht. Pharm Ztg. 1986; 131: 2289–2301

Gstirner F. Prüfung und Verarbeitung von Arzneidrogen Vol. 2, Springer Verlag, Berlin 1955, 142

Haidvogel M, Schuster R, Heger M. Akute Bronchitis im Kindesalter—Multizenter-Studie zur Wirksamkeit und Verträglichkeit des Phytotherapeutikums Umckaloabo®. Z Phytother. 1996; 17:300–313

Heil C, Reitermann U. Atemwegs- und HNO-Infektionen Therapeutische Erfahrungen mit dem Phytotherapeutikum Umckaloabo®. Therapiewoche Pädiatrie. 1994; 7:523–525

Kolodziej H, Kayser O. Pelargonium sidoides DC. Neueste Erkenntnisse zum Verständnis des Phytotherapeutikums Umckaloabo®. Z Phytother. 1998; 19(3):141–151

Kraft K. Therapeutisches Profil eines Spitzwegerich-Fluidextraktes bei akuten respiratorischen Erkrankungen im Kindes- und Erwachsenenalter. In: Loew D, Rietbrock N, ed Phytopharmaka. Vol III. Darmstadt: Steinkopff; 1997: 199–209

Krenn L, Kartnig T. Sonnentau-Aktuelles über medizinisch genutzte Drosera-Arten. Z Phytother. 2005; 26(4):197–202

Loew D, Koch E. Cumarine: Differenzierte Risikobetrachtung mit dem Beispiel eines pflanzlichen Arzneimittels. Z Phytother. 2008; 29:28–36

Loew D, Rietbrock N, eds. Phytopharmaka. Vol. III. Erkrankungen der Atemwege. Darmstadt: Steinkopff; 1997: 81–215

März RW, Ismail C, Popp MA. Wirkprofil und Wirksamkeit eines pflanzlichen Kombinationspräparates zur Behandlung der Sinusitis. Wien Med Wochenschr. 1999; 149:202–208

Matthys H, Heger M. Treatment of acute bronchitis with a liquid herbal drug preparation from Pelargonium sidoides (EPs 7630): a randomised, double-blind, placebo-controlled, multicentre study. Curr Med Res Opin. 2007; 23(2):323–331

Melchart D, Linde K, Worku F, Bauer R, Wagner H. Immunmodulation mit Echinacea-haltigen Arzneimitteln. Forsch Komplementaermed. 1994; 1:27–36

Paper DH, Marchesan M. Portrait einer Arzneipflanze: Spitzwegerich (Plantago lanceolata L.). Z Phytother. 1999; 20:231–238

Reiter M, Brandt W. Erschlaffende Wirkungen auf die glatte Muskulatur von Trachea und Ileum des Meerschweinchens-Relaxant effects on tracheal and ileal smooth muscles of the guinea pig]. Arzneimittelforschung. 1985; 35(1):408–414

Riechelmann H. Klimek L Pathophysiologie und klinische Diagnostik entzündlicher Erkrankungen der oberen Luftwege. In: Loew D, Rietbrock N, ed Phytopharmaka. Vol. III. Darmstadt: Steinkopff; 1997: 111–134

Rudkowski Z, Latos T. Hedera helix: Wirksam bei Bronchitis im Kindesalter. Ärztl Prax. 1980; 80:2561–2562

Schapowal A, Heger M. EPs® 7630 Lösung (Umckaloabo®) bei Sinusitis. Z Phytother. 2007; 28(2):58–65

Scheerer J. Jaborandi—Pilocarpus microphyllus stapf ex wordleworth. Portrait einer Arzneipflanze. Z Phytother. 2000; 21:220–230

Schier W. Plantago lanceolata, P. major und P. media. Dtsch Apoth Ztg. 1990; 130:1457–1458

Schilcher H. Ätherische Öle—Wirkungen und Nebenwirkungen. Dtsch Apoth Ztg. 1984; 124:1433–1442

Schöneberger D. Einfluß der immunstimulierenden Wirkung von Preßsaft aus Herba Echinaceae pupureae auf Verlauf und Schweregrad von Erkältungskrankheiten (Ergebnisse einer Doppelblindstudie). Forum Immunologie. 1992; 2(8):18–22

Siegers CP. Mukolytika–Sekretolytika–Sekretomotorika. Therapeutischer Nutzen: Anspruch und Realität. Therapiewoche. 1994; 44(-7):414–418

Tisch M. Atemwegsinfekt-Mit Phytopharmaka gezielt behandeln. Phytokompass. 2015; 1:38–40

Wagner H, Bayer T, Dorsch W. Das antiasthmatische Wirkprinzip der Zwiebel (Allium cepa L.). Therapeutikon. 1989; 3(5):266–275

Wagner H, Wierer M, Bauer R. In vitro-Hemmung der Prostaglandin-Biosynthese durch etherische Öle und phenolische Verbindungen [In vitro inhibition of prostaglandin biosynthesis by essential oils and phenolic compounds]. Planta Med. 1986; 3(3):184–187

Wagner H, Wiesenauer M. Phytotherapie: Phytopharmaka und pflanzliche Homöopathika. 2nd ed. Stuttgart: Wissenschaftliche Verlagsgesellschaft; 2003

Wagner H. Pflanzliche Immunstimulanzien. Dtsch Apoth Ztg. 1991; 131:117–125

Wegener T. Anwendung von Spitzwegerichfluidextrakt (Broncho-Sern®) als Antitussivum mit antiinflammatorischen Eigenschaften bei akuten Erkrankungen des oberen Respirationstraktes. Abstracts 6. Phytotherapiekongress. Z Phytother. 1995; 16:22

Wegener T, Kraft K. Der Spitzwegerich (Plantago lanceolata L.): Reizlinderung bei Infektionen der oberen Atemwege. [Plantain (Plantago lanceolata L.): anti-inflammatory action in upper respiratory tract infections]. Wien Med Wochenschr. 1999; 149 (8–10):211–216

Weiss RF. Herbal Medicine. AB Arcanum, Gothenburg/Beaconsfield Publishers, Beaconsfield 1991

Questions

1. What are the three categories of phytotherapeutics for the treatment of respiratory infections?
2. Name a few typical demulcents.
3. Which important substance group primarily determines the effects of plant-derived (herbal) expectorants?
4. Which carnivorous plant constitutes a good antitussive?
5. Formulate a prescription for "cough tea."
6. Name some typical plant-derived (herbal) diaphoretics.

Answers (p. 422) for Chapter 5

6 Kidney, Urinary Tract, and Prostate Disorders

Phytotherapeutics have long been very popular in urology. "Flushing therapy" and its cleansing effect on the efferent urinary tract has been known for a long time.

In this chapter, you will learn more about the manifold indications for medicinal plants to treat disorders of the urogenital tract. These treatment options are not confined only to diuretic and aquaretic effects but also address prevention.

There are no specific phytotherapeutics for **nephritis** (parenchymal kidney disorders).

There are, however, many phytotherapeutic treatment options for **urinary tract disorders**, ranging from spasmolytic, antiphlogistic, and disinfecting phytotherapeutics to plant-based diuretics and aquaretics that are suitable for flushing therapy. However, the efficacy of herbal diuretics and aquaretics is not nearly comparable to that of modern synthetic diuretics. Herbal diuretics cause water diuresis by increasing the glomerular filtration rate and the creation of primary urine. This makes them very versatile for the treatment of **functional disorders** as well as for the **prevention of recurring urolithiasis**.

In addition to their aquaretic effects, these herbal remedies are also antidyscratic. They can be prescribed preventively and curatively to treat **metabolic disorders and deposition disorders**. This area was a primary application for herbal diuretics in the past and led to the concept of a "blood cleansing" effect. Even if such a concept no longer seems acceptable today, holistically oriented practitioners should especially revisit this field and develop different justifications for the treatment of deposition diseases, which are so prevalent today (see also Chapter 7 Rheumatic Disorders and Gout (p. 234)).

In the early stages of **benign prostatic hyperplasia** (BPH), phytotherapeutics are the treatment option of first choice. They are a category 1 plant medicine according to our classification system (see ▶ Table 1.3). While they do not inhibit the benign growth of prostate tissue, they are excellent for influencing the various subjective symptoms caused by it, such as micturition problems.

Medicinal Plants

Urinary Tract Infections
Uva-ursi, Arctostaphylos uva-ursi
Horseradish, Armoracia rusticana
Nasturtium, Tropaeolum majus
Cranberry, Vaccinium macrocarpon
Java Tea, Orthosiphon spicatus
Goldenrod, Solidago virgaurea
Rupturewort, Herniaria glabra and Herniaria hirsuta

Dysuria Symptoms
Juniper Berry, Juniperus communis
Parsley, Petroselinum crispum
Lovage, Levisticum officinale
Spiny Restharrow, Ononis spinosa
Couch Grass, Elymus repens
Horsetail, Equisetum arvense

Kidney and Urinary Tract Stones
Dandelion, Taraxacum officinale
Butterbur, Petasites hybridus
Goldenrod, Solidago virgaurea
Spiny Restharrow, Oonis spinosa
Java Tea, Orthosiphon spicatus

Bed-wetting
Gentian, Gentiana lutea
Sweet (Fragrant) Sumac, Rhus aromatica
St.-John's-wort, Hypericum perforatum

Irritable Bladder and Prostatopathy
Saw Palmetto, Serenoa repens
Pumpkin Seed, Cucurbita pepo

Benign Prostatic Hyperplasia (BPH)
Pumpkin Seed, Cucurbita pepo
Saw Palmetto, Serenoa repens
Stinging Nettle, Urtica dioica/urens
South African Star Grass, Hypoxis rooperi
Fireweed, Epilobium angustifolium

6.1 Urinary Tract Infections

6.1.1 Uncomplicated Acute and Subacute Cystitis

Medicinal Plants

Uva-ursi, Arctostaphylos uva-ursi
Uva-ursi leaves, Uva-ursi folium
Horseradish, Armoracia rusticana
Horseradish root, Armoraciae rusticanae radix
Garden Nasturtium, Monks Cress, Tropaeolum majus
Nasturtium herb, Tropaeoli maji herba
Cranberry, Vaccinium macrocarpon
Cranberry fruit, Vaccinii macrocarponi fructus
Java Tea, Orthosiphon spicatus
Java Tea leaves, Orthosiphonis folium
Goldenrod, Solidago virgaurea
Goldenrod herb, Solidaginis virgaureae herba
Rupturewort, Herniaria glabra
Rupturewort herb, Herniariae herba and Herniaria hirsuta

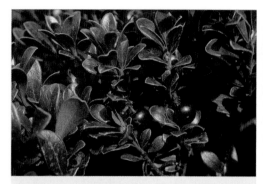

Fig. 6.1 Uva-ursi, Arctostaphylos uva-ursi. Photo: Dr. Roland Spohn, Engen.

Chronic urinary tract infections, often without symptoms or with few symptoms, are very common. These disorders mostly are no longer treated with chemotherapeutic or antibiotics, as was the recommendation in the early days of sulfa drugs and antibiotics. The recidivism rate is very high and there are increasing concerns about resistant bacteria.

Stammwitz points out that uncomplicated, acute cystitis, asymptomatic bacteriuria, and adjuvant therapy for long-term transurethral catheterization are important indications for the use of phytopharmaceuticals. **Uva-ursi** (Arctostaphylos uva-ursi) is featured as an effective representative of plants that are urine disinfecting. The following discussion will differentiate between plants with antibacterial, antiphlogistic, and spasmolytic effects.

Plants for Treatment

Uva-ursi (Arctostaphylos uva-ursi)

Uva-ursi—like cranberry and bilberry—is a member of the Ericaceae family. Its leaves are entire, leathery, evergreen and prominently veined (▶ Fig. 6.1). Its flowers are small and red, as are its stone fruit. This low-growing, ground-cover shrub

grows in coniferous forests, moors, and heaths. It is more common in northern Germany and less common in Bavaria. Uva-ursi grows wild in most of North America with the exception of the South and Southeast. It is also known as kinnikinnick or pinemat manzanita.

Medicinal applications use the **dried uva-ursi leaves** (Uva-ursi folium).

▶ **Pharmacology.** Uva-ursi leaves contain a minimum of 8% hydroquinone derivatives, calculated as anhydrous arbutin. They also contain flavonoids, tannins, organic acids, and triterpenes.

The main action of uva-ursi as a urine disinfectant is derived from arbutin. The action of this genuine constituent of the drug is indirect. Arbutin comes into contact with beta-glucosidase and hydrolyzes into the aglycone (hydroquinone) and glucose. Following resorption, it is bound to glucuronic and sulfuric acid and excreted via the urine. For optimal effectiveness, this process requires the urine to be alkaline. The hydroquinone released during this process constitutes the active disinfecting principle.

▶ **Research.** Experiments have shown that in healthy study participants, up to 70% of a given arbutin dose was excreted in the urine as conjugated hydroquinone within 24 hours. Measurable free hydroquinone levels were below 0.5% of the given arbutin dose (Stammwitz).

The **antibacterial action** of uva-ursi leaves was demonstrated in a comparison using the diffusion plate assay against a reference antibiotic (neomycin) (Stammwitz). It showed concentration-dependent growth inhibition of five strains of bacteria (*Escherichia coli*, Klebsiella pneumonia, Proteus vulgaris,

Pseudomonas aeruginosa, Staphylococcus aureus) and one yeast (Candida albicans).

▶ **Indications.** Uva-ursi is indicated for uncomplicated **acute and subacute urinary tract infections**, including **asymptomatic bacteriuria**.

The Commission E monograph for uva-ursi lists the indication inflammatory disorders of the efferent urinary tract.

Preparation 👉

- **Tea**
  Add 1 cup of cold water to 2 teaspoons of the drug. Soak for several hours, then heat briefly, and strain. Alternatively, add 1 cup of hot water to 2 teaspoons of the drug. Steep for 5 minutes, then strain.
  Drink 1 cup several times a day between meals.

▶ **Therapy Recommendations.** Uva-ursi treatment should be accompanied by increased fluid consumption.

The urine should be alkaline (pH 8) or should be alkalinized by the additional intake of sodium bicarbonate (baking soda).

Uva-ursi leaves contain a substantial amount of tannins. This can cause severe irritation of the gastric mucosa. Therefore, uva-ursi tea is primarily suitable for short-term use.

Horseradish (Armoracia rusticana)

Horseradish is a member of the mustard (Brassicaceae) family. It is known for its strong root growth. Its long horizontal runners and root sprouts prefer sandy moist soils. Once a plant has established itself, it is almost impossible to eradicate. It pushes up multiple heads bearing firm, green, juicy leaves that are up to 1.2 m long and long stemmed, fairly wide, undulate, and involute. Its large panicle features many loose flower racemes that contain many small, white flowers.

Medicinal applications use the **horseradish root** (Armoraciae rusticanae radix).

▶ **Pharmacology.** Horseradish root contains primarily mustard oil and mustard oil glycosides (isothiocyanates). Isothiocyanates give horseradish

its pungent odor and acrid taste. The mustard oil responsible for horseradish's action develops through fermentation of mustard oil glycosides. They are quickly absorbed in the small intestine, bind to glutathione, and are excreted as mercapturic acid via the kidneys.

Mustard oils are very volatile, and their stabilization presents a technical challenge.

▶ **Research.** The **antibacterial action** of horseradish root on gram-positive and gram-negative bacteria as well as yeasts was documented, and more recently confirmed and expanded to a wider spectrum of antibacterial actions (Conrad et al. 2008; 2013).

▶ **Indications.** In the author's practice, horseradish root has been shown again and again to be an **efficacious urine disinfectant**. It was frequently able to replace sulfa drugs or antibiotics.

The Commission E monograph for horseradish root lists its indication as a supportive therapy for infections of the urinary tract and restricts its indication in terms of efficacy compared to uva-ursi.

▶ **Research.** In view of the newer literature about a combination preparation containing horseradish root and nasturtium herb, this restriction by the Commission E is no longer justified. Two observational studies involving 1,649 adults (Goos et al. 2006) and 858 children (Goos et al. 2007) with acute urinary tract infections received either Angocin or an antibiotic. There were no differences in success rates.

A randomized, double-blind, placebo-controlled study examined the extent to which this herbal medicinal product reduces the recidivism rate of treated urinary tract infections. The difference compared to placebo after 3 months and even after 180 days was significant (Albrecht et al.).

▶ **Therapy Recommendations.** Mustard oils can cause irritation of gastric mucosa. Patients should be encouraged to drink plenty of fluids.

Since mustard oils are difficult to stabilize, finished pharmaceutical products should be used.

Garden Nasturtium, Monks Cress (Tropaeolum majus)

Garden nasturtium is an herbaceous annual plant that is very common in Germany and is also frequently found in gardens. Its stems are fleshy and its smooth, grayish-green alternate leaves are circular and attached at the bottom center of the leaf. Its beautiful flowers consist of a five-lobed calyx, with two petals forming a lower lip and three petals forming an upper lip. Its spur can grow to about 2.8 cm and is slightly curved and gradually acuminate. This species should not be confused with watercress or yellowcress (Nasturtium officinale), or its genus Nasturtium spec. which is a member of the Brassicaceae family, not of the Tropaeolaceae family.

Medicinal applications use the garden **nasturtium herb** (above-ground parts; Tropaeoli maji herba).

▶ **Pharmacology.** Garden nasturtium's main constituents are mustard oil glycosides.

▶ **Indications.** The indications for garden nasturtium are the same as for horseradish and uva-ursi.

The Commission E only issued a positive assessment of garden nasturtium's pharmacological properties because no single constituent garden nasturtium preparation is commercially available.

Preparation
• **Tincture (EB 6)**   Take 20–50 drops 3–5 × times a day in a small amount of water after meals.

Cranberry (Vaccinium macrocarpon)

The American cranberry is in the Ericaceae family and is related to bilberry (Vaccinium myrtillus) and lingonberry (Vaccinium vitis-idaea). It has increasingly found its way to Europe for the treatment of urinary tract infections; cranberries have been part of the standard treatment for these disorders in North America for quite some time. For this reason, many experimental, pharmacologic and evidence-based clinical studies are available for this plant (Nowack 2003).

Cranberry grows in natural or human-made acidic bogs in the northeastern region of North America. It is very similar to the European lingonberry, but the fruit of the cranberry is significantly larger. It is a low-growing and creeping shrub with long vines. Its flowers are said to be reminiscent of cranes (birds), which likely explains its name.

Medicinal applications use the **cranberry fruit** (Vaccinii macroparoni fructus) and sometimes the **leaves**.

▶ **Pharmacology.** Cranberry's action is primarily derived from proanthocyanidine, which are polyphenols in the flavanol group. These are primarily oligomers of catechin and epicatechin. Their **antibacterial** action is attributed to the inhibition of bacterial binding (adhesion) to the host tissue. For the highly uropathogenic *Escherichia coli*, this adhesion occurs through surface fimbriae expressing lectins.

▶ **Research.** The antibacterial action of cranberry has also been demonstrated in human volunteer studies (Nowack 2006).

Initial research has been conducted that expands the potential antibacterial action of cranberry to *Helicobacter pylori* and infections of the oral cavity with caries and periodontitis.

▶ **Indications.** Several evidence-based clinical studies document the specific efficacy of cranberry for **chronic urinary tract infections**. Studies by Avorn et al., Kontiokari et al., and Stothers examined and treated women only.

A randomized, placebo-controlled proband study examined the action of cranberry for **infections of the oral cavity** (Weiss et al.). After 6 weeks of treatment using mouth rinses containing either cranberry or placebo, the number of *Streptococcus mutans* bacteria and the total bacterial load in saliva was significantly lower in the cranberry group, compared to placebo.

Initial experimental studies of cranberry's effect on ***Helicobacter pylori*** showed that cranberry inhibits the adhesion of bacteria to gastric mucilage and gastric mucosa (Burger et al.).

These studies show the availability of established and potential antibacterial therapy options that provide sensible additions to European and traditional remedies.

Preparations
Cranberry preparations are currently only available as supplements.   • **Cranberry Capsules**

Supportive Plant Medicines (Aquaretics)

Java Tea (Orthosiphon spicatus, Orthosiphon stamineus, Orthosiphon aristatus, Koemis Koetjing)

Java tea is a member of the Lamiaceae family and grows wild on the Sunda Islands, Australia, southern China, the Indian subcontinent and Southeast Asia. This herb with its square stem not only resembles peppermint but also is related to it. Like peppermint, Java tea leaves are opposite across and lanceolate. Its flowers are spicate and light violet colored. A conspicuous feature is its long filaments that drape far beyond the flower. These have given the plant its Malaysian name, which is *koemis koetjin* and means cat's beard.

Java tea grows wild in large amounts on the Sunda Islands. However, this does not meet the increasing demand for this plant, which is now cultivated as a field crop.

Medicinal applications use the **Java tea leaves** (Orthosiphonis folium), similar to peppermint.

▶ **Note.** Java tea has played an important role among the Malaysian people for a very long time. Its healing power was discovered more recently for use in Western medicine. In Germany, it was first marketed as "Indian kidney tea."

▶ **Pharmacology.** Java tea leaves contain lipophilic flavones, for example, sinensetin, scutellarein tetramethyl ether, and eupatorin, along with volatile oil and approximately 3% potassium salts.

▶ **Indications.** Java tea has been officially adopted into the French, Indonesian, Dutch, and Swiss Pharmacopoeias. The plant seems to indeed have special efficacy for kidney disorders. It has been observed to promote the excretion not only of fluids, but also of nitrogen-containing substances and sodium chloride. Increased blood nitrogen levels as a diagnostic indicator for kidney failure decrease, at least to a certain degree. No damaging effects to the kidneys have been found even when this drug is given in large amounts. However, the studies regarding effects on the renal parenchyma are not yet reliable enough in terms of modern study techniques to base indications on these results. Yet, with its mild aquaretic and spasmolytic effects and the experimentally documented antiphlogistic effects, Java tea is very suitable overall for com-plementing urine disinfection remedies.

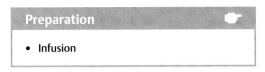

Preparation

• **Infusion**

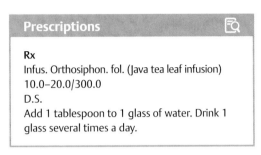

Prescriptions

Rx
Infus. Orthosiphon. fol. (Java tea leaf infusion)
10.0–20.0/300.0
D.S.
Add 1 tablespoon to 1 glass of water. Drink 1 glass several times a day.

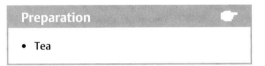

Preparation

• **Tea**

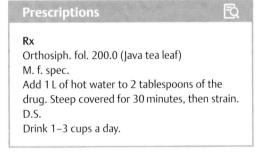

Prescriptions

Rx
Orthosiph. fol. 200.0 (Java tea leaf)
M. f. spec.
Add 1 L of hot water to 2 tablespoons of the drug. Steep covered for 30 minutes, then strain.
D.S.
Drink 1–3 cups a day.

Goldenrod (Solidago virgaurea)

Goldenrod grows in clusters on dry slopes, in pine forests, and in heath areas, in Germany. Its beautiful golden yellow flowers are grouped at the end of a stiff erect stem and glow from late summer into autumn (▶ Fig. 6.2).

Medicinal applications use the **goldenrod herb** (above-ground parts, Solidaginis virgaureae herba) collected and carefully dried during flowering. Solidago virgaurea, also sometimes called European goldenrod, is the only goldenrod native to Europe. In Germany, this type of goldenrod is referred to as "true goldenrod herb." Other common goldenrod species used medicinally are **Solidago canadensis** L. (Canadian goldenrod) and **Solidago serotina** (giant goldenrod, early Goldenrod, also known as

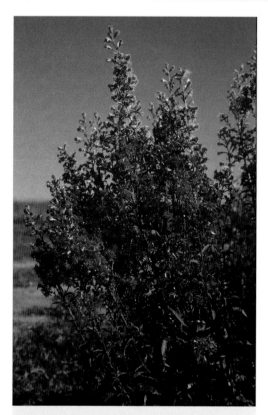

Fig. 6.2 Goldenrod, Solidago virgaurea. Photo: Dr. Roland Spohn, Engen.

S. gigantea Aiton) and their hybrids (see note directly below).

▶ **Note.** Two other types of goldenrod, **Solidago Canadensis L.** (Canadian goldenrod) and **Solidago serotina** (giant goldenrod, early goldenrod) are noticeable in late summer and autumn. Both of these North American species were originally imported as decorative plants. They are now naturalized in Europe and grow in large numbers along train tracks, riverbanks, and in inhospitable locations. Their flower panicles are much smaller and are located in large numbers at the end of the stems. This gives large clusters of goldenrod a remarkably yellow color that can be seen from afar.

The composition of constituents is markedly different in these three types of goldenrod. Scientific study results and experiential knowledge are based primarily on European goldenrod. However, the Commission E monograph for goldenrod treats the drugs derived from all three types equally. It remains to be seen if this can be maintained as

more detailed information about the differences is discovered (Bader).

▶ **Pharmacology.** Goldenrod herb contains flavonoids, tannins, saponins, diterpenes, volatile oil, caffeic acid derivatives, and phenyl glycosides.

Goldenrod's **antiphlogistic** and **diuretic** effects have been well studied in animal experiments. Studies have also shown **antimicrobial effects**, but these were not viewed as focus areas for goldenrod's pharmacological effect (Bader).

▶ **Research.** The isolated phenyl glycoside leiocarposide was shown to increase diuresis by 100% following intraperitoneal application (25 mg/kg body weight) in rats. By comparison, furosemide (6 mg/kg body weight) increased diuresis by 125%. Oral application showed less pronounced effects of 80% and 100% (Schilcher 1987).

▶ **Indications.** Its combination of **antiphlogistic**, **diuretic**, and **immune-modulating** effects makes goldenrod an ideal complement to drugs with direct antiseptic effects. Beyond its short-term use, it can be used as long-term "realignment" (transposition) therapy.

The Commission E monograph for goldenrod lists the indications irrigation therapy for inflammatory diseases of the lower urinary tract, urinary calculi, and kidney gravel, and as prophylaxis for urinary calculi and kidney gravel.

Based on the current state of knowledge about goldenrod, these indications seem to be on the conservative side. The observation made in the past that goldenrod can reverse albuminuria needs to be revisited in newer, more systematic studies. However, the indication "acute or subacute nephritis" that was referred to by Weiss may significantly overstate its—clearly present—anti-inflammatory activity.

Preparation

- **Tea**
  Add 1 cup of hot water to 2 teaspoons of the finely chopped drug. Steep covered for 10 minutes, then strain.
  Or add 2 teaspoons of the drug to 1 cup of cold water and bring to a brief boil, then strain.
  Drink 1 cup several times a day.
- **Infusion**

The efficacy of this infusion can be enhanced by adding parsley water (Aqua Petroselini).

Rupturewort (Herniaria glabra, Herniaria hirsuta)

This small, very inconspicuous plant is very common but is almost unknown. It grows on paths, in sandy fields, and in meadows. Rupturewort's prostrate stems grow to a length of 5–15 cm. Its small leaves are binate, and its small, greenish flowers are clustered in the leaf axils (▶ Fig. 6.3).

Rupturewort receives much too little attention as a medicinal plant. Medicinal applications use the **smooth rupturewort herb** (above-ground parts, Herniariae herba).

▶ **Pharmacology.** Rupturewort contains about 2% flavonol glycosides of quercetin and isorhamnetin along with triterpene saponins and coumarins.

▶ **Indications.** Rupturewort is primarily an **antispasmodic** for the urinary tract. As suggested by Weiss, we should advocate for a wider use of this medicinal plant.

The Commission E issued a negative monograph for rupturewort based on its assessment that its efficacy is not sufficiently documented.

▶ **Therapy Recommendations.** Rupturewort loses its efficacy during drying and needs to be used while fresh.

Rupturewort tea needs to be prepared by pouring hot water over the fresh herb. The tea must not

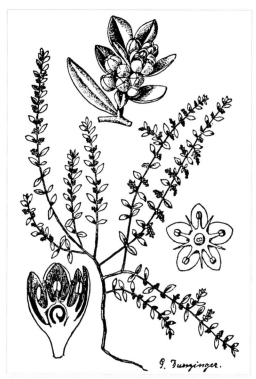

Fig. 6.3 Rupturewort, Herniaria glabra and Herniaria hirsuta.

be boiled because this causes essential components to be lost.

6.2 Dysuria Symptoms

6.2.1 Aquaretics and Antidyscratics

Medicinal plants used to treat dysuria symptoms were long referred to as diuretics. Schilcher (1987) deserves credit for having delineated the effects of these plants from the highly efficacious and precisely defined synthetic diuretics by referring to these plants as **aquaretics**. The term "water diuretics" is also frequently used because their action is said to be primarily water diuresis.

However, more recent research has shown that flavonoids contained in birch leaves and goldenrod, especially quercetin, inhibit metalloendopeptidase. Metalloendopeptidase catalyzes the degradation of atrial natriuretic peptides, which in turn influences **sodium-dependent diuresis** (Melzig and Major). This is another indicator for the special efficacy of medicinal plants compared to synthetic drugs that has been mentioned several times in this book: The action of medicinal plants interacts with the body's own regulation and control mechanisms and appears to realign imbalanced organism functions. Based on current understanding, and compared to synthetic diuretics, it does not appear justified to refer to the aquaretic effects of medicinal plants only as water diuresis. However, the effects of the medicinal plants described in this section are primarily aquaretic. They support flushing therapy and are suitable for treatment of all types of dysuria symptoms as well as for the prevention of urinary calculus and chronic urinary tract infections.

A true understanding of these drugs and their manifold recommendations in traditional phytotherapy requires full comprehension of the antidyscratic characteristics of these plants.

The traditional indications for these drugs were not targeted to the kidneys and efferent urinary tract. Instead, they were based on the perspective of "blood cleansing," which is why they were primarily prescribed for metabolic and deposition disorders ("rheumatism"). However, the concept of dyscrasia, which is based on the Hippocratic model of "humors," no longer fits into 21st century medicine.

One of the main functions of the kidneys is to excrete substances that the organism no longer needs and that would otherwise possibly be deposited or become endogenously toxic. Along these lines, the medicinal plants presented in this section are suitable for flushing therapy and should be more comprehensively indicated rather than be reduced to water diuresis.

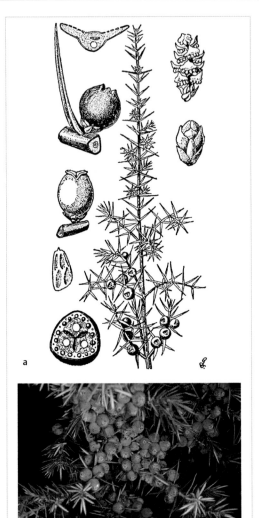

Fig. 6.4 a and b Juniper Berry, Juniperus communis. Photo: Dr. Roland Spohn, Engen.

Plants for Treatment

Juniper Berry (Juniperus communis)

Juniper berry is an evergreen conifer that grows wild in bogs and heaths in Germany, from lowlands to high mountains (▶ Fig. 6.4).

Medicinal applications use the blackish blue **juniper berries** (Juniperi fructus) that are actually the fleshy merged scales of ovulate cones, similar to those of the yew tree. They are also referred to as "cone berries." Consequently, the **juniper berry** drug is sometimes also referred to as "Juniperi pseudofructus."

▶ **Note.** Even though the English name for this drug refers to a berry, its Latin name is not Juniperi baccae (berry), but Juniperi fructus (fruit), or, what would be more botanically accurate, "Juniperi pseudofructus."

▶ **Pharmacology.** Juniper berries contain a minimum of 1% volatile oil, based on the dried drug. This volatile oil contains primarily terpene carbon hydrogens such as α-pinene and β-pinene, myrcenes, sabines, thujenes, limonenes, and sequiterpene hydrocarbons such as caryophyllene, cadines, elemenes, and terpene alcohols such as terpinen-4-ol. Juniper berries also contain flavone glycosides, tannins, sugar, and resinlike and waxlike substances.

Juniper berry's **aquaretic action** is primarily attributed to terpinen-4-ol. It increases blood flow through the kidneys, which increases glomerular filtration and increased the creation of primary urine.

▶ **Research.** Toxicological effects such as "kidney irritation" and "kidney damage" have been attributed to the essential oil (Juniperi aetheroleum) derived from the steam distillation of juniper berries. It has been stated that its aquaretic effect is achieved solely by damage to the glomeruli. However, Schilcher and Heil showed that there is no proof to date for any kidney damaging effects, or that this effect is derived from extreme excessive dosages given during certain animal experiments. According to the authors of that study, the most likely explanation is that earlier experiments used oil blends that were contaminated with turpentine oil, which is a close chemical relative, and that the known kidney damaging effects of turpentine oil were attributed to the juniper berry oil.

The clinical primary literature and newest studies do not show any kidney toxic effects for juniper berry oil, especially not at therapeutically appropriate dosages.

▶ **Indications.** In the authors' opinion, juniper berries are primarily indicated for the flushing therapy with **urinary tract infections** described at the beginning of this chapter. Juniper berries are not suitable for long-term therapy.

▶ **Note.** Juniper berry preparations or juniper berry oil are considered a prototype for plant-based diuretics. For this reason, it may be surprising that the main indications listed by Weiss for juniper berry are chronic arthrosis, chronic gout and the large group of rheumatic neuralgic muscle disorders, including tendinopathy and myogelosis. This makes sense against the backdrop of the overriding concept of antidyscratics. Juniper berry is also used for external indications.

Based on the supposedly kidney damaging effects, the Commission E monograph for juniper berry allows only for its use for dyspeptic symptoms. However, juniper berries are not viewed as a remedy of first choice for these symptoms.

> **Caution**
>
> Jupiter berries are contraindicated for chronic kidney failure (kidney insufficiency). Pregnancy is another contraindication for the juniper berry because of its potential abortive effects.

> **Preparation**
>
> - **Tea**
>   Add 1 cup of hot water to 1 teaspoon of the slightly crushed drug. Steep covered for 5 minutes, then strain.
>   Drink 1 cup 3 × a day.

Parsley (Petroselinum crispum)

The branched stems of this umbelliferous plant grow to a height of 1 m. Its leaves are multiple pinnatipartite and its flowers are inconspicuous and greenish yellow. Its fruit (seeds) resembles those of caraway.

Parsley is not only a popular herb in the kitchen but also an important medicinal plant that has been cultivated since ancient times. Its Latin name *petroselinum* is derived from *petra* = rock and *selinum* = selge. Selge refers to an umbelliferous plant native to the mountains of the Mediterranean.

Medicinal applications use the **parsley herb** and **parsley root** (fresh or dried plant sections, Petroselini herba et radix).

▶ **Pharmacology.** Parsley contains a volatile oil that includes apiol and myristicin, plus terpenes and flavonoids. The root also contains polyynes. Its active constituent is the volatile oil. Apiol, the main constituent of this oil, is toxic and has abortive effects. Nerve damage and extensive paralysis have been observed following abuse of this oil.

▶ **Indications.** Parsley is an excellent aquaretic. It is used when strong stimulation of urine excretion is needed, as is the case with disorders of the efferent urinary tract and kidney gravel.

The Commission E recommends parsley for flushing therapy of the efferent urinary tract in disorders of the same and in the prevention and treatment of kidney gravel.

Preparations

- **Tea**
  Add 1 cup of boiling water to 1–2 teaspoons of the finely chopped drug. Steep covered for 10–15 minutes, then strain.
  Drink 1 cup several times a day.
- **Parsley Water (Aqua Petroselini)**
  Suitable for composites, for example, it is contained in the "Mixtura diuretica" (according to the German Prescription Formulas, DRF).

Prescriptions

Rx
Liqu. Kalii acetici 30.0 (potassium acetate solution)
Aqu. Petroselini ad 200.0 (parsley water)
D.S.
Take 1 tablespoon 3 × a day.

Lovage (Levisticum officinale)

Lovage can grow up to a height of 2 m. Its upright growth is distinctive. Its leaves are bare, shiny, and single to bipinnatipartite. Its flowers are small and pale yellow and are gathered into umbels (▶ Fig. 6.5). The entire plant has a strong aromatic fragrance.

Lovage's origin is disputed. Some say it originates from southern Europe. Its wild origins are no longer known. It has been cultivated in herb gardens for centuries and is today cultivated in large amounts in some areas.

Medicinal applications use the **lovage root** (Levistici radix).

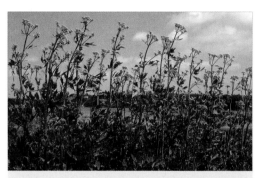

Fig. 6.5 Lovage, Levisticum officinale. Photo: Dr. Roland Spohn, Engen.

▶ **Pharmacology.** Lovage contains 0.4–1.7% volatile oil with its main constituent ligustilide and coumarin derivatives. The volatile oil has been shown to have spasmolytic effects on smooth muscles.

This drug is a main constituent in aquaretic tea blends, for example, Species Diuretica.

"Species Diuretica" are a group of diuretic tea prescriptions that are listed, for example, in the Austrian pharmacopoeia (ÖAB), where the following three species diuretica can be found. Note that only the Species dirureticae I is relevant to this section, as the others do not contain Levistici radix.

Preparations

Species diuretica I:
Levistici radix 25 g
Liquiritiae radix 25 g
Ononidis radix 25 g
Juniperi pseudofructus 25 g

Species diuretica II:
Solidagin. virgaur. herba 40 g
Orthosiphonis folium 30 g
Betulae folium 15 g
Equiseti herba 15 g

Species diuretica III:
Ononidis radix 40 g
Graminis rhizoma 40 g
Taraxaci radix 20 g

▶ **Indications. Lovage root** is used in flushing therapy with **inflammatory disorders of the efferent urinary tract** and as a preventive for **kidney gravel**.

- **Tea**
  Add 1 cup of boiling water to 1–2 teaspoons of the finely chopped drug. Steep covered for 10–15 minutes, then strain.
  Drink 1 cup warm several times a day before meals.

  Species diuretica I:
  Levistici radix 25 g
  Liquiritiae radix 25 g
  Ononidis radix 25 g
  Juniperi pseudofructus 25 g

Spiny Restharrow (Ononis spinosa)

This inconspicuous thorny subshrub belongs to the Fabaceae family and grows to a height of about 0.5 m. Its flowers are pale red, and its stalk bears one or two hairlike appendages (▶ Fig. 6.6). In Germany, spiny restharrow grows on dry slopes, along country roads and dirt paths, and in agricultural fields.

Medicinal applications use the **spiny restharrow root** (dried roots and rhizomes, Ononidis radix), harvested in autumn.

▶ **Pharmacology.** Spiny restharrow root contains isoflavonoids such as ononin, plus flavonoids, and small amounts of volatile oil.

Its aquaretic effect has been proven, but it is not very strong and is weaker than that of juniper berry and parsley. For this reason, spiny restharrow is primarily found in tea blends and combination remedies.

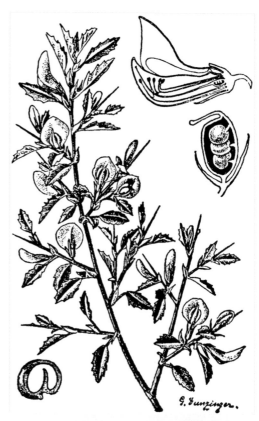

Fig. 6.6 Spiny Restharrow, Ononis spinosa.

- **Tea**
  Add 1 cup of boiling water to 1 teaspoon of the chopped drug. Steep covered for 30 minutes, then strain.
  Drink 1 cup several times a day.

Couch Grass (Elymus repens)

Couch grass is one of the most common and most pesky weeds in agricultural fields, in Germany. This enduring grass plant grows runners from a mostly subterranean root axis and its shoots can reach a height of 20–150 cm (▶ Fig. 6.7). Its stems and sheaths are smooth and bare, and its leaves are rough and covered in short hairs. Its long, straw-yellow rootstock contains hollow segments and provides good fodder for animals because of its high carbohydrate content.

Medicinal applications use the **couch grass rootstock** (rhizome, root and short stems; Graminis rhizoma). Couch grass derives its Latin name for its rootstock from the fact that it is the main representative of a group of healing grasses (**Gramineae or Poaceae**).

▶ **Pharmacology.** Couch grass rootstock contains volatile oil, saponins, mucilage, and polysaccharides. Its aquaretic effect is not pronounced.

▶ **Indications.** Couch grass rootstock is indicated in the context of flushing treatment for **inflammatory disorders of the efferent urinary tract** and **kidney**

223

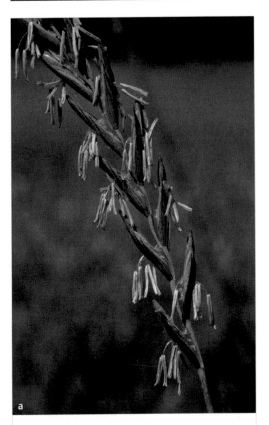

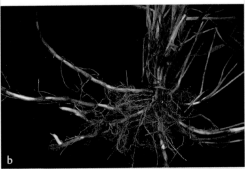

Fig. 6.7 a and b Couch Grass, Elymus repens. Photos: Dr. Roland Spohn, Engen.

gravel. This also reflects the recommendation of the Commission E monograph for this plant.

As a saponin-rich aquaretic, couch grass is found in many combination remedies.

▶ **Research.** An observational study of more than 300 patients confirmed the positive efficacy of a couch gross rootstock mono-preparation for

urinary tract infections and irritable bladder (Hautmann and Scheithe).

Horsetail (Equisetum arvense)

Horsetail is considered a noxious weed and prefers to grow in loamy soil. Its rhizome grows deep in the ground and is as thick as a pencil. In spring, in Germany, stems rise up from the roots and tubers that grow from the rootstock nodes to a height of about 20 cm. These stems bear brownish-yellow sporangium spikes (▶ Fig. 6.8). After these spike wilt, the plant grows light green leafy shoots that are rough, furrowed, and can reach heights of 10–50 cm. They bear the verticillate horsetail branches. Horsetail branch ash is high in silicic acid.

Medicinal application use the **horsetail herb** (fresh or dried, green, sterile stems; Equiseti herba).

▶ **Pharmacology.** This type of silica drug contains silicic acid in a mostly water-soluble colloidal form. This makes horsetail primarily a connective tissue remedy.

The application emphasis for horsetail is not its aquaretic effect, as had been widely assumed in the past, but on its **antidyscratic** and **humoral** effects. Horsetail's aquaretic effect is very limited: It is not based on silicic acid and the saponins usually required for aquaretic effects have not been found in horsetail (Veit).

▶ **Indications.** Horsetail is indicated for flushing therapy with **disorders of the efferent urinary tract** and **kidney gravel**.

Horsetail also **stimulates the metabolism** and this is a much more significant feature of horsetail than the aquaretic effect for which this drug is primarily known. Above all, it strengthens connective tissue. Since connective tissue also plays a role in rheumatic (arthritic) disorders, this explains horsetail's effect in this area.

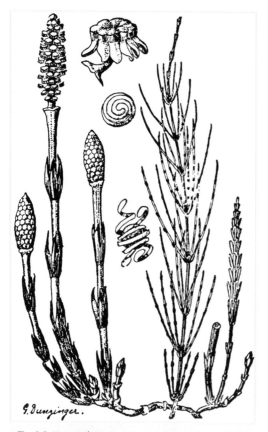

Fig. 6.8 Horsetail, Equisetum arvense.

Rx
Juniperi fruct. (juniper berry)
Ononidis rad. (spiny restharrow root)
Liquiritiae rad. āā ad 100.0 (licorice root)
M. f. spec.
Infusion of 1 cup of water and 2 teaspoons.
D.S.
Drink 3 cups a day.

Stronger Tea Blend
Rx
Juniperi fruct. (juniper berry)
Petroselini fruct. (parsley seeds)
Equiseti herb. (horsetail herb)
Ononidis rad. (spiny restharrow root)
Foeniculi fruct. (fennel seeds)
Menth. pip. fol. āā ad 200.0 (peppermint
leaves)
M. f. spec.
Add 1 cup of hot water to 1–2 teaspoons of the
blend. Steep covered for 20 minutes, then
strain.
D.S.
Drink 3 cups a day.

- **Tea**
  Add 1 cup of boiling water to 2 teaspoons of
  the chopped drug. Steep covered for
  15 minutes, then strain.
  Drink 1 cup several times a day.

Proven Tea Prescriptions

As a general rule, one or two aquaretics containing
volatile oils are combined with one or two aquaretics containing saponins. One or two other drugs
are added to improve taste and increase tolerability (reduce stomach irritation).

With Thyme as a Flavor Corrigent
Rx
Petroselini fruct. (parsley seeds)
Equiseti herb. (horsetail herb)
Thymi herb. āā ad 100.0 (thyme herb)
M. f. spec.
Add 1 cup of hot water to 2 teaspoons of the
blend. Steep covered for 20 minutes, then
strain.
D.S.
Drink 3 cups a day.

Squill is indicated for the treatment of cardiac edema or edema caused, for example, by obesity and some metabolic disorders. A good blend for this indication is the so-called Kreuser Tea recommended by Lichtwitz.

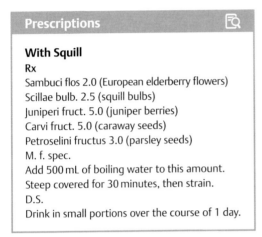

Prescriptions

With Squill
Rx
Sambuci flos 2.0 (European elderberry flowers)
Scillae bulb. 2.5 (squill bulbs)
Juniperi fruct. 5.0 (juniper berries)
Carvi fruct. 5.0 (caraway seeds)
Petroselini fructus 3.0 (parsley seeds)
M. f. spec.
Add 500 mL of boiling water to this amount.
Steep covered for 30 minutes, then strain.
D.S.
Drink in small portions over the course of 1 day.

6.3 Kidney Stones and Urinary Tract Stones

6.3.1 Flushing Therapy

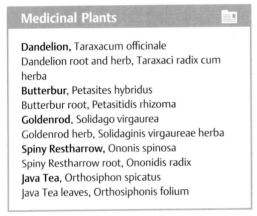

Medicinal Plants

Dandelion, Taraxacum officinale
Dandelion root and herb, Taraxaci radix cum herba
Butterbur, Petasites hybridus
Butterbur root, Petasitidis rhizoma
Goldenrod, Solidago virgaurea
Goldenrod herb, Solidaginis virgaureae herba
Spiny Restharrow, Ononis spinosa
Spiny Restharrow root, Ononidis radix
Java Tea, Orthosiphon spicatus
Java Tea leaves, Orthosiphonis folium

Phytotherapy has no direct role in dissolving stones that develop in the efferent urinary tract. This is primarily the domain of chemolysis. Phytotherapy can, however, be useful for flushing out small kidney and ureter calculi.

Plants for Treatment

The following plants are recommended in addition to the drugs that are suitable for flushing therapy.

Dandelion (Taraxacum officinale)

For more information about this plant, see Dandelion (p. 124).

Preparation

- **Tea**
  Add 500 mL of boiling water to 2 tablespoons of the drug. Steep for 10–15 minutes, then strain. Add warm water to make 1.5 L.
  Drink the entire amount within 15–20 minutes while it is still comfortably warm.

Butterbur (Petasites hybridus)

For more information about this plant, see Butterbur (p. 282).

Caution

Butterbur develops pyrrolizidine alkaloids with a 1.2-unsaturated necine structure. Therefore, its application is to be restricted to only a few days.

Goldenrod (Solidago virgaurea), Spiny Restharrow (Ononis spinosa), Java Tea (Orthosiphon spicatus, Orthosiphon stamineus, Orthosiphon aristatus)

These plants are described in detail earlier in this chapter. They are primarily used for the prevention of urolithiasis and for prophylactic treatment to prevent a relapse of this disorder. For information about prescriptions and finished pharmaceutical products, see (p. 216) and spiny restharrow (p. 223).

Proven Tea Prescription

The following prescription has been shown to be especially helpful for relapse prevention of urologic calculus disorders according to Weiss.

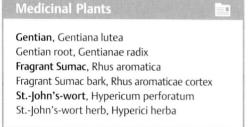

Prescriptions 📑

Rx
Taraxaci rad. c. herb. (dandelion root and herb)
Juniperi fruct. (juniper berries)
Petroselini fruct. (parsley seeds)
Herniariae herb. (rupturewort herb)
Anisi fruct. āā ad 200.0 (anise seeds)
M. f. spec.
Add 1 L of boiling water to 2 tablespoons of the blend. Steep for 20 minutes, then strain.
D.S.
Slowly drink the entire amount in small sips, once a day in the morning.

6.4 Functional Disorders

6.4.1 Bed-Wetting

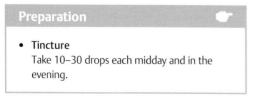

Medicinal Plants 📄

Gentian, Gentiana lutea
Gentian root, Gentianae radix
Fragrant Sumac, Rhus aromatica
Fragrant Sumac bark, Rhus aromaticae cortex
St.-John's-wort, Hypericum perforatum
St.-John's-wort herb, Hyperici herba

In the vast majority of cases, bed-wetting (nocturnal enuresis) is not a specific urinary tract disorder, but a functional disorder. Phytotherapeutic remedies often achieve good therapeutic results with this condition.

Plants for Treatment

Gentian (Gentiana lutea)

For more information about this plant, see Gentian (p. 54).

Gentian is one of the strong bitters that also achieves good results with children.

Preparation ☞

- **Tincture**
  Take 10–30 drops each midday and in the evening.

Fragrant Sumac (Rhus aromatica)

The bark of this shrub, **Rhus aromaticae cortex**, which is native to North America, is considered a specific remedy for enuresis.

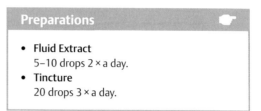

Preparations ☞

- **Fluid Extract**
  5–10 drops 2 × a day.
- **Tincture**
  20 drops 3 × a day.

St.-John's-wort (Hypericum perforatum)

For more information about this plant, see St.-John's-wort (p. 264).

This plant develops its effect via the nervous system.

6.4.2 Irritable Bladder and Prostatopathy

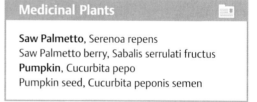

Medicinal Plants 📄

Saw Palmetto, Serenoa repens
Saw Palmetto berry, Sabalis serrulati fructus
Pumpkin, Cucurbita pepo
Pumpkin seed, Cucurbita peponis semen

Bladder disorders that are purely or primarily functional are less of clinical issue and more of an issue to be dealt with in the practice. The most important disorders are irritable bladder, which primarily occurs in women, and prostatopathy (also known as prostatodynia [painful prostate], chronic prostatitis, or chronic pelvic pain syndrome), and nonbacterial prostatitis, which is a frequent disorder in men.

Irritable bladder syndrome in women is a pathogenically complex problem and experience has shown that it is difficult to treat. It involves dysregulation of the interaction between the detrusor muscle of the bladder and the sphincter along with weakening of the bladder muscles, often in conjunction with general vegetative lability.

The symptoms of this disorder are similar to those of cystitis, but the urine is clear in most cases and the urinary sediment is normal. The most prominent symptom is micturition disorders, primarily increased and very agonizing urinary urgency. The individual amount of voided urine is small. Irritable bladder syndrome creates significant emotional and physical suffering and should be taken just as seriously as purely somatic cystitis.

In the same way, many men suffer from **prostate symptoms** that are mislabeled as "prostatitis" even though no signs of a true infection can be found in the prostate secretions. The symptoms of this disorder are also primarily characterized by micturition disorders and protracted discomfort in the pelvic region. Often, patients also suffer from carcinophobia.

Irritable bladder syndrome in women and prostatopathy in men are very similar pathogenically and in terms of symptoms. Therefore, they are frequently treated in the same way.

Plants for Treatment

Saw Palmetto (Serenoa repens, Sabal serrulata)

For more information about this plant, see Saw Palmetto (p. 229).

Pumpkin (Cucurbita pepo)

For more information about this plant, see Pumpkin (p. 229).

6.4.3 Benign Prostatic Hyperplasia (BPH)

> **Medicinal Plants**
>
> Pumpkin, Cucurbita pepo
> Pumpkin seeds, Cucurbitae peponis semen
> **Saw Palmetto**, Serenoa repens (Sabal serrulata)
> Saw Palmetto berry, Sabalis serrulatae fructus
> **Stinging Nettle**, Urtica dioica/urens
> Stinging Nettle root, Urticae radix
> **South African Star Grass**, Hypoxis rooperi
> South African Star Grass root, Hypoxis rooperi radix
> **Fireweed**, Epilobium angustifolium
> Fireweed root and herb, Epilobii radix et herba

In no other medical discipline does phytotherapy enjoy as much acceptance as in urology. One of the reasons is the indication area benign prostatic hyperplasia (BPH). It needs to be emphasized, however, that there is no medicinal plant remedy that can influence the cause of benign adenomatosis of the prostate. All phytotherapeutics used successfully with BPH treat the manifold symptoms of this disorder.

> **Definition**
>
> Alken divided the **symptoms of prostatic hyperplasia** into the following stages:
> - **Stage 1** (irritation stage): characterized by increased micturition frequency, pollakisuria, nocturia, and urinary hesitancy (delayed micturition stream).
> - **Stage 2** (urine retention): characterized by signs of beginning decompensation, small or larger amounts of urine retention, increased micturition frequency and pollakisuria.
> - **Stage 3** (urinary retention): characterized by complete decompensation of the bladder with constant dribbling of urine from an overfull bladder and kidney damage from urine backing up into the kidneys.

Stage 1 lists the main indications for phytotherapeutics, but they can also be applied for milder cases of stage 2. Sökeland and Sulke posit that phytotherapeutics represent a relatively economical treatment option for patients presenting with mild to moderate **micturition problems** caused by prostatic hyperplasia. Their main advantage is good tolerability, even for long-term treatment. The description of pharmacologic effects varies, for example, inhibition of prostaglandin synthesis, lowering of cholesterol levels, reduction of sex hormone binding globulin (SHBG); antiphlogistic, antiedematous and antiandrogenic effects, or inhibition of the 5-α-reductase or aromatase enzyme complex. All these statements rely, as a rule, on *in vitro* studies (Engelmann 1997; Sökeland and Sulke 1992).

The medicinal plants that can be used to treat the symptoms of benign prostatic hyperplasia are the same as those discussed for irritable bladder syndrome in women and prostatopathy in men. We can classify these remedies as "phyto-urologics."

Any efficacy assessment of phyto-urologics for treating BPH needs to consider that in its early stages, the symptoms of this disorder tend to improve spontaneously. This is why efficacy studies for this indication area should always be controlled and generally also be placebo controlled. On the other hand, there is no question that long, practical medical experience in the use of phytotherapeutics and the innumerable patients who have been treated with them already provide proof of efficacy. This applies especially to preparations derived from pumpkin seeds, saw palmetto extracts, stinging nettle, and also combinations with purple Echinacea.

Long-term phytotherapeutic therapy should be accompanied by regular checkups with a specialist to not miss the right point at which surgical treatment may become necessary.

The phytotherapeutics used to treat BPH have significantly fewer **undesirable effects** than those of hormone drugs and synthetic α-blockers (Popa). Cost of treatment is also substantially lower than for comparable synthetics, which can have a substantial economic impact given the prevalence of this condition and the fact that it always requires long-term treatment.

There are many effective finished pharmaceutical products available to treat BPH.

▶ **Note.** After the development and establishment of **transurethral resection** (of the prostate), it was believed for some time that prostatic hyperplasia should be resected as early as possible. This assessment, however, has been considered obsolete for some time. Transurethral prostate resection is now viewed as more of a measure at the end of the treatment process (Popa).

Plants for Treatment

Pumpkin (Cucurbita pepo)

There are many cultivated varieties of pumpkins as well as other squashes in the species Cucurpita pepo. Only one of these varieties, a special variety that originates from East Asia, is suitable for medicinal use (see p. 229).

Medicinal applications use the **pumpkin seed** (Cucurbitae peponis semen).

▶ **Pharmacology.** Pumpkin seeds contain primarily phytosterols in free and bound form. Their prototype is known as β-sitosterol. They also contain a minimum of 25 amino acids, including cucurbitin, gamma and beta tocopherol, as well as minerals, including selenium, plus fatty oil and protein.

The main ideas about the pharmacology of phyto-urologics were discussed in the introduction to this chapter. The action of phytosterols is mainly attributed to their influence on prostaglandin and prolactin metabolism. Constituents such as tocopherols and selenium can be assumed to have antiphlogistic and antioxidant effects.

Overall, the pharmacologic effects of these phytotherapeutics are much less well documented than their clinical effectiveness.

▶ **Research.** The medicinal use of pumpkin seeds is based on the observation that pumpkin seeds are a popular snack in many Balkan countries and that prostatic hyperplasia was less prevalent in these regions.

It made sense to apply this discovery therapeutically. In his studies, Schilcher (1986) discovered that the seeds of the precisely botanically verified source drug Cucurbita pepo L. convar. citrullinina I. Greb. var. styriaca. I. Greb. are sufficiently efficacious. This has been verified in many double-blind studies.

▶ **Indications.** The primary indications for pumpkin seeds are **stage 1** and mild forms of **stage 2** of BPH. Additional indications are functional-psychosomatic disorders such as **irritable bladder** and **prostatopathy**.

The Commission E monograph for pumpkin seeds lists the indications irritated bladder condition and micturition problems in stages 1 and 2 of BPH (according to Alken).

Tolerability of pumpkin seed preparations is very good, which contributes to high compliance.

▶ **Research.** An observational study using a German finished pharmaceutical product in 2,245 patients in stages 1 and 2 of BPH again confirmed the extensive experience regarding excellent efficacy and tolerability of pumpkin seeds. Undesirable effects were noted by only 22 patients (1%). Compliance was excellent, as could be expected (Schiebel-Schlosser and Friedrich).

Saw Palmetto (Serenoa repens, Sabal serrulata)

This true palm tree with its fan-shaped leaves and olive-size, dark red, berrylike fruit originates from the southern regions of North America. Today, it also grows wild in the Mediterranean regions of southern Spain, on the island of Mallorca, and especially in North Africa.

Medicinal applications use the **saw palmetto berry** (ripe, dried fruit; Sabalis serrulatae fructus).

▶ **Pharmacology.** Saw palmetto berries contain a fatty oil with phytosterols, polysaccharides, tannins, and sitosterol in glycoside bound form. Pharmacologically, the same considerations apply as for pumpkin.

The following effects have been demonstrated for saw palmetto berries: 5-α-reductase aromatase inhibition, influence on prostaglandin metabolism, inhibition of leukotriene B_4 and thromboxane B_2 synthesis, and other hormonal processes associated pathogenically with the development of BPH.

▶ **Indications.** Saw palmetto is indicated for micturition symptoms in stages 1 to 2 of BPH. This also reflects the indications issued by the Commission E.

▶ **Research.** A meta-analysis of all existing clinical studies of the treatment of benign prostatic hyperplasia with saw palmetto berry was conducted by Wilt et al. It congruently confirmed the therapeutic efficacy of saw palmetto berries with BPH according to the criteria of evidence-based medicine. Görne published a systematic review of saw palmetto berry (Sabalis serrulatae fructus).

A 6-month prospective study compared a pure saw palmetto berry extract with the selective α-receptor blocker tamsulosin for treating BPH. A third leg of the study compared a combination of the two drugs. This test of the "noninferiority" of saw palmetto berries resulted in uniform improvements in all three groups, without significant differences. The study did show differences in tolerability. Fifteen patients indicated undesirable effects. None of these were from the saw palmetto berry group. Twelve were from the tamsulosin group and three were from the combination group. The most frequently cited undesirable effect was ejaculation disorders (Hizli and Uygur).

These results once again point to the fact that a phytopharmaceutical can indeed be a remedy of first choice for prescriptions, in this case, for BPH.

Preparations
• **Tincture** Place 10 drops in a small amount of warm water and drink 3 × a day.
• **Percolate (1:3)** Take 20–30 drops 3 × a day.

▶ **Therapy Recommendations.** Treatment should primarily use standardized finished pharmaceutial saw palmetto berry preparations. A combination with stinging nettle makes sense.

Stinging Nettle (Urtica dioica, Urtica urens)

For more information about this plant, see Stinging Nettle (p. 237).

▶ **Indications.** Clinical experimental studies confirmed the beneficial effects of stinging nettles in **stages 1 and 2** of BPH with increased urine retention. These benefits are attributed to their phytosterol content. Stinging nettle roots are also strongly decongestive.

Since the pharmacological effects of stinging nettle differ from those of pumpkin seeds or saw palmetto berries, a combination of stinging nettle with one or the other of those two remedies seems to make sense.

▶ **Research.** A 1-year, double-blind study compared the 5-α-reductase inhibitor finasteride with a combination of saw palmetto berry extract and stinging nettle extract in patients in stages 1 and 2 of BPH (Sökeland and Albrecht). The results of the study showed therapeutic equivalence of both therapy principles (phytopharmaceutical/synthetic drug) for various measurements such as the International Prostate Symptom Score (I-PSS, Paris, 1993), maximum urinary flow per second and quality of life.

A randomized, double-blind study compared capsules containing a combination of 160 mg saw palmetto berries and 120 mg stinging nettle root with the selective α-receptor blocker tamsulosin. The study involved 140 men who were treated for 60 months. No difference in improvements of objective measurement parameters or statements about quality of life were shown between the two groups. Therefore, the efficacy of the phytopharmaceutical remedy was not inferior to the synthetic drug (Engelmann et al.).

Another randomized, double-blind, placebo-controlled, multicentric study showed significant superiority (p < 0.01) of a compound drug PRO 160/120 containing saw palmetto berries and stinging nettle compared to placebo during a 48-week treatment of 257 men with BPH (Lopatkin et al.).

A double-blind, placebo-controlled, long-term study also showed positive therapeutic effects for the same combination remedy (Metzker et al.).

South African Star Grass (Hypoxis rooperi)

South African star grass is native to South Africa. Its **root bulbs** (Hypoxis rooperi radix) contain high amounts of β-sitosterol. This compound is considered a chemically defined drug according to the German Pharmacopoeia (DAB 10) and not as a typical phytopharmaceutical. Its monograph was developed by the Commission B, but it should be included here because of its plant origin and beneficial effects. This is especially true as Hypoxis rooperi radix—and by extension the finished pharmaceutical product of this drug—contains not only β-sitosterol but also a vast variety of other phytosterols with similar pharmaceutical effects. The effectiveness of this blend of different phytosterols for the treatment of BPH is very well documented.

Fireweed (Chamaenerion angustifolium, Epilobium angustifolium)

This perennial plant is widespread in all regions of the Northern Hemisphere and likely originates from North America. It likes sunny locations and prefers to grow in open forest land. It is often one of the first plants to appear following the clearcutting of forests. Its root sprouts branch widely and help to build soil strength. The above-ground parts of the plant can grow to a height of 120 cm. Its leaves are small and lanceolate. They can be up to 20 cm long and exhibit pronounced reticulate venation on their underside. Its distinctive, large, racemiform flowers are reddish violet and bloom from June to August.

Medicinal applications use the **fireweed root** (Epilobii radix) as well as the **herb** (Epilobii herba), collected during flowering.

▶ **Pharmacology.** The main constituents of fireweed are tannins of the gallotannin type, plus numerous flavonoids that build on three aglycones: quercetin, kaempherol, and myrecetin.

▶ **Research.** Even though this plant has been known as a medicinal plant since ancient times—Theophrastus called it Oenothera—this plant never became one of the great medicinal herbs. Recent pharmacological studies, however, have provided indications for various effects (antiphlogistic, analgesic, antimicrobial, antiandrogenic, and proliferation inhibiting).

Its biologically significant content of peptidase (protease) seems to be of special interest in inhibiting the growth of prostate tissue (Lischka-Güntzel and Melzig). These authors view BPH as an important future indication for this plant because it could be a useful complement to drugs available today. However, there is no clinical proof of efficacy available.

Bibliography

Albrecht U, Goos KH, Schneider B. A randomised, double-blind, placebo-controlled trial of a herbal medicinal product containing Tropaeoli majoris herba (Nasturtium) and Armoraciae rusticanae radix (Horseradish) for the prophylactic treatment of patients with chronically recurrent lower urinary tract infections. Curr Med Res Opin. 2007; 23(10):2415–2422

Alken CE. Die grosse Prostata [The large prostate]. ZFA (Stuttgart). 1982; 58(27):1435–1439

Avorn J, Monane M, Gurwitz JH, Glynn RJ, Choodnovskiy I, Lipsitz LA. Reduction of bacteriuria and pyuria after ingestion of cranberry juice. JAMA. 1994; 271(10):751–754

Bader G. Die Goldrute. Inhaltsstoffe, Pharmakologie, Klinik und Anbau. Z Phytother. 1999; 20:196–200

Burger O, Ofek I, Tabak M, Weiss EI, Sharon N, Neeman I. A high molecular mass constituent of cranberry juice inhibits helicobacter pylori adhesion to human gastric mucus. FEMS Immunol Med Microbiol. 2000; 29(4):295–301

Conrad A, Biehler D, Nobis T, et al. Broad spectrum antibacterial activity of a mixture of isothiocyanates from nasturtium (Tropaeoli majoris herba) and horseradish (Armoraciae rusticanae radix). Drug Res (Stuttg). 2013; 63(2):65–68

Conrad A, Richter H, Bauer D, Nobis T, Engels I, Frank U. Breite antibakterielle Wirkung einer Mischung von Senfölen in vitro. Z Phytother. 2008; 29 Suppl 1:22–23

Engelmann U, Walther C, Bondarenko B, Funk P. Schläfke S. Efficacy and safety of a combination of sabal and urtica extract in lower urinary tract symptoms. A randomized, double-blind study versus tamsulosin. Arzneimittelforschung. 2006; 56(3):222–229

Engelmann U. Phytopharmaka und Synthetika bei der Behandlung der benignen Prostatahyperplasie. Z Phytother. 1997; 18(1):13–19

Fintelmann V. Unkomplizierte Infekte—Phytopharmaka Mittel der ersten Wahl. Ärztl Prax. 1992; 44:12–13

Goos KH, Albrecht U, Schneider B. Aktuelle Untersuchungen zur Wirksamkeit und Verträglichkeit eines pflanzlichen Arzneimittels mit Kapuzinerkressenkraut und Meerrettich bei akuter Sinusitis, akuter Bronchitis und akuter Blasenentztündung bei Kindern im Vergleich zu anderen Antibiotika [On-going investigations on efficacy and safety profile of a herbal drug containing nasturtium herb and horseradish root in acute sinusitis, acute bronchitis and acute urinary tract infection in children in comparison with other antibiotic treatments]. Arzneimittelforschung. 2007; 57(4):238–246

Goos KH, Albrecht U, Schneider B. Wirksamkeit und Verträglichkeit eines pflanzlichen Arzneimittels mit Kapuzinerkressenkraut und Meerrettich bei akuter Sinusitis, akuter Bronchitis und akuter Blasenentzündung im Vergleich zu anderen Therapien unter den Bedingungen der täglichen Praxis. Ergebnisse einer prospektiven Kohortenstudie. Arzneimittelforschung. 2006; 56(3):249–257

Görne RC. Systematischer Review zur Therapie von Symptomen der unteren Harnwege (LUTS) mit und ohne benigne Prostatahyperplasie (BPH) mit alkoholischen Extrakten von Sägepalmenfrüchten. Z Phytother. 2014; 35(03):111–118

Hautmann C, Scheithe K. Fluidextrakt aus Agropyron repens bei Harnwegsinfektionen oder Reizblase. Z Phytother. 2000; 21(5):252–255

Hizli F, Uygur MC. A prospective study of the efficacy of Serenoa repens, tamsulosin, and Serenoa repens plus tamsulosin treatment for patients with benign prostate hyperplasia. Int Urol Nephrol. 2007; 39(3):879–886

Kartnig T, Wegschaider O. Zur Kenntnis der Saponne aus Herniaria glabra[Saponins from Herniaria glabra]. Planta Med. 1972; 21(2):144–149

Kontiokari T, Sundqvist K, Nuutinen M, Pokka T, Koskela M, Uhari M. Randomised trial of cranberry-lingonberry juice and Lactobacillus GG drink for the prevention of urinary tract infections in women. BMJ. 2001; 322(7302):1571

Lichtwitz L. Die Praxis der Nierenkrankheiten. Berlin: Springer; 1934: 155

Lischka-Güntzel H, Melzig MF. Epilobium angustifolium L.—Porträt einer Arzneipflanze. Z Phytother. 2007; 28(4):201–206

Lopatkin N, Sivkov A, Walther C, et al. Long-term efficacy and safety of a combination of sabal and urtica extract for lower urinary tract symptoms—a placebo-controlled, double-blind, multicenter trial. World J Urol. 2005; 23(2):139–146

Melchior H, Schulze H, Seabert J, Sökeland J. Neue Perspektiven in der Behandlung der Prostatahyperplasie. Dtsch Aerzteblatt. 1994; 91:792–797

Melzig MF, Major H. Neue Aspekte zum Verständnis des Wirkungsmechanismus der aquaretischen Wirkung von Birkenblättern und Goldrutenkraut. Zeitschr f Phytotherapie. 2000; 21:193–196

Metzker H, Kieser M, Hölscher U. Wirksamkeit eines Sabal-Urtica-Kombinationspräparates bei der Behandlung der benignen Prostatahyperplasie (BPH). Urologe. 1996; 36:292–300

Nöske HD. Infektionsprophylaxe in der Prostata-Chirurgie. Natur- und Ganzheitsmedizin. 1989; 6:184–187

Nowack R. Cranberry als Phyto-Prophylaktikum bei bakteriellen Infektionen. Z Phytother. 2006; 27(4):163–171

Nowack R. Die amerikanische Cranberry (Vaccinium macrocarpon Aiton)—Porträt einer Arzneipflanze. Z Phytother. 2003; 24(1):40–46

Popa G. Phytotherapie der Prostata—die Rolle des praktisch tätigen Urologen. In: Loew D, Blume H, Dingermann T, ed Phytopharmaka. Vol V. Darmstadt: Steinkopff; 1999: 157–164

Rugendorff EW, Schneider HJ, Röhrborn CG. Ergebnisse einer randomisierten Doppelblindstudie über die Behandlung der benignen Prostatahyperplasie mit Prostagutt® vs. Beta-Sitosterin. Extr Urol. 1986; 9(2):115–118

Schiebel-Schlosser G, Friedrich M. Kürbissamen in der Phytotherapie der BPH. Eine Anwendungsbeobachtung. Zeitschr. f. Phytotherapie. 1998; 19:71–76

Schilcher H, Heil BM. Nierentoxizität von Wacholderbeerzubereitungen. Z Phytother. 1994; 15(4):205–213

Schilcher H. Cucurbita-Spezies—Kürbis-Arten. Z Phytother. 1986; 7:9–13

Schilcher H. Möglichkeiten und Grenzen der Phytotherapie am Beispiel pflanzlicher Urologika. Urologe. 1987; 27:368–370

Schilcher H. Pflanzliche Urologika. Dtsch Apoth Ztg. 1984; 124:2429–2436

Sökeland J, Albrecht J. Kombination aus Sabal- und Urticaextrakt vs. Finasterid bei BPH (Stad. I bis II nach Alken) (Stad. I bis II nach Aiken). Vergleich der therapeutischen Wirksamkeit in einer einjährigen Doppelblindstudie [Combination of Sabal and Urtica extract vs. finasteride in benign prostatic hyperplasia (Aiken stages I to II). Comparison of therapeutic effectiveness in a one year double-blind study]. Urologe. 1997; 36:327–333

Sökeland J, Sulke J. Harnwegsinfektionen. Dtsch Aerztebl. 1992; 89: 2319–2321

Sökeland J. Phytotherapeutika in der Behandlung des Prostatasyndroms. Z Phytother. 2004; 25(1):20–26

Stammwitz U. Pflanzliche Harnwegsdesinfizienzien – heute noch aktuell? Zeitschrift für Phytotherapie. 1998; 19:90–95

Stothers L. A randomized trial to evaluate cost effectiveness and cost effectiveness of naturopathic cranberry products as prophylaxis against urinary tract infection in women. Can J Urol. 2002; 9(3): 1558–1562

Veit M. Probleme bei der Bewertung pflanzlicher Diuretika. Z Phytother. 1994; 15:331–341

Wagner H, Eibl G, Lotter H, Guinea M. Evaluation of natural products as inhibitors of angiotensin I converting enzyme (ACE). Pharmaceutical and Pharmacological Letters. 1991; 1:15–18

Wegener T, Schmidt GP. Wacholderbeeröl—Aquaretikum. Biol Med Homotoxin J. 1995; 24:111–113

Weiss EI, Kozlovsky A, Steinberg D, et al. A high molecular mass cranberry constituent reduces mutans streptococci level in saliva and inhibits in vitro adhesion to hydroxyapatite. FEMS Microbiol Lett. 2004; 232(1):89–92

Weiss RF. Phytotherapie bei chronischen Blasen- und Nierenerkrankungen. Ärztez Naturheilverfahren. 1989; 30:956–960

Wilt TJ, Ishani A, Stark G, MacDonald R, Lau J, Mulrow C. Saw palmetto extracts for treatment of benign prostatic hyperplasia: a systematic review. JAMA. 1998; 280(18):1604–1609

Questions

1. Please explain what "aquaretic" means.
2. Are you familiar with any antibacterial medicinal plant remedies?
3. Are there contraindications for juniper berries? If yes, what are they?
4. Which mineral substance is found in unusually high concentrations in horsetail?
5. Formulate a prescription for an "aquaretic tea."
6. Which medicinal plants are suitable as a remedy of first choice for benign prostatic hyperplasia (BPH)?
7. According to recent studies, one medicinal plant has been shown to inhibit the growth of prostate tissue. What is the name of that plant?

Answers (p. 422) for Chapter 6.

7 Rheumatic Disorders and Gout

The preventive and curative effect of phytotherapeutics for metabolic and deposition disorders has been known for a long time, which earned them the reputation of "blood cleansers" early on. From a modern perspective, this point of view is no longer valid. However, it continues to illustrate the necessity for comprehensively intervening in metabolic processes to positively influence these difficult to treat disorders.

This chapter describes the therapeutic benefits of medicinal plant remedies with rheumatic disorders and gout that are even more suitable for holistic approaches toward healing than most synthetics.

Treatment success with chronic rheumatic disorders and gout is more difficult to assess than for most other areas of medicine. Improvements or worsening of symptoms associated with these disorders develop gradually over a period of months or years. Symptoms are ambiguous and, above all, subject to frequent changes. There are times when patients feel entirely or relatively well. Then their condition worsens again, and the causes cannot always be determined.

This is an important fact to keep in mind when assessing the effectiveness and prospects of success of medicinal plant therapy with this large and variable area of medicine. It is extraordinarily difficult to gauge whether improvements are spontaneous or the result of successful therapy. Frequently, this decision will be subjective. There are hardly any safe treatment methods that are certain to result in resounding success.

Medicinal plants used to treat chronic metabolic disorders are referred to as **antidyscratics**. This term needs to be comprehensively redefined because its meaning in the past—blood cleansing—no longer fits within the framework of modern medical thinking. Instead, it refers to providing a holistically oriented impact on complex metabolic processes and, above all, on the elimination of metabolites—also sometimes referred to as "waste." This process is central to our health. A wealth of prostaglandins and their derivatives point to the area of our metabolism involved in this process. These processes are also certain to be of key importance for our immunity.

Changes to joints only represent a partial view of much more comprehensive disease processes involved with rheumatic disorders. These processes primarily take place in the entire mesenchyme. Therefore, the disorders addressed here are also referred to as **collagenosis** or **connective tissue disorders**. The term "collagenosis" illustrates the primarily degenerative character of these disorders.

The focus of today's research is on arachidonic acid metabolism. Arachidonic acid is thought to play a key role in the development and symptoms of rheumatic disorders as the source material for the formation of leukotrienes and prostaglandins. The key enzymes involved are **lipoxygenase** and **cyclooxygenase**. Inhibition of these enzymes reduces inflammation in the joints and ameliorates the pain caused by inflammation. This has led to research into inhibitors of these enzymes as potential antirheumatic drugs.

In addition to more nonspecific antidyscratics like dandelion or stinging nettle, **devil's claw** (Harpagophytum procumbens) is of specific interest in this context. The iridoid glycosides it contains are viewed as lipoxygenase and cyclooxygenase enzyme inhibitors. Several very interesting study results for this plant are already available. Devil's claw may be the future antirheumatic medicinal plant remedy that can compete with synthetic drugs like nonsteroidal antirheumatic drugs. **Autumn crocus** (Colchicum autumnale) is a medicinal plant that is specific to the treatment of gout. Even with the availability of synthetic gout drugs, this plant remedy will remain valuable for the treatment of acute gout or for the prevention of gout flares.

This chapter also discusses several important plants that contain volatile oils and are successfully used as **external remedies** for symptomatic treatment of rheumatic disorders.

There are still more questions than answers about the etiology and pathogenesis of rheumatic disorders. For this reason, the answer to the question of which plants will be considered indispensable for the treatment of rheumatic disorders in the future remains open.

Medicinal Plants

Rheumatic Disorders

Dandelion, Taraxacum officinale
Stinging Nettle, Urtica dioica/urens
Birch, Betula pendula, Betula pubescens, Betula verrucosa
Woody Nightshade, Solanum dulcamara
Greater Burdock, Arctium lappa
Kidney Bean, Phaseolus vulgaris
Sand Sedge, Carex arenaria
Devil's Claw, Harpagophytum procumbens
Purple Willow, Salix purpurea
Comfrey, Symphytum officinale
Cayenne Pepper, Capsicum annuum, Capsicum frutescens
Hay Flower, Graminis flos
Calamus, Acorus calamus
Rosemary, Rosmarinus officinalis
Juniper Berry, Juniperus communis
Norway Spruce, Picea abies

Gout

Autumn Crocus, Colchicum autumnale
Olive Tree, Olea europaea

Willow bark, Salicis cortex
Comfrey, Symphytum officinale
Comfrey root, Symphyti radix
Grasses, Gramineae (Poaceae)
Hay Flower, Graminis flos
Rosemary, Rosmarinus officinalis
Rosemary leaves, Rosmarini folium
Calamus, Acorus calamus
Calamus rootstock, Calami rhizoma
Juniper, Juniperus communis
Juniper berry, Juniperi fructus
Stinging Nettle, Urtica dioica/urens
Stinging Nettle herb and leaves, Urticae herba et folium
Cayenne Pepper, Capsicum annuum, Capsicum fructescens
Cayenne Pepper fruit, Capsici fructus
Norway Spruce, Picea abies
Norway Spruce needle essential oil, Piceae abietis aetherolum

7.1 Rheumatic Disorders

Medicinal Plants

Dandelion, Taraxacum officinale
Dandelion herb and root, Taraxaci herba cum radix
Stinging Nettle, Urtica dioica/urens
Stinging Nettle herb and leaves, Urticae herba et folium
Birch, Betula pendula, Betula pubescens, Betula verrucosa
Birch leaves, Betulae folium
Woody Nightshade, Solanum dulcamara
Woody Nightshade stem, Dulcamarae stipites
Greater Burdock, Arctium lappa
Burdock root, Bardanae radix
Kidney Bean, Phaseolus vulgaris
Kidney Bean pods without seeds, Phaseoli fructus sine semine
Sand Sedge, Carex arenaria
Sand Sedge rootstock, Caricis rhizoma
Devil's Claw, Harpagophytum procumbens
Devil's Claw root, Harpagophyti radix
Willow, Salix purpurea/daphnoides

Modern rheumatology has developed extensive classifications and segmentations. What seems notable is that these pathogenically different disorders are subjected to largely similar therapies. This may be due to the perception that rheumatic disorders are largely caused by autoimmune processes. However, it also illustrates a severe lack of truly differential treatments. The following assumes that the cause of all rheumatic disorders is an **imbalance in the self-regulation** of metabolic processes, especially with a view toward elimination, that always leads to deposition disorders. This includes **gout (Arthritis urica)**, even though it requires a different therapy because it represents an imbalance of the uric acid metabolism.

7.1.1 Arthritis and Arthrosis

Arthritis and **arthrosis** are two poles of the same underlying disorder involving deposition, indurations, and loss of function. All inflammatory processes must first be examined for the presence of autoregulative self-healing processes. Suppressing these processes, for example, with immunosuppressives or antiphlogistics, can ameliorate the symptoms of pain associated with these disorders. However, it also compounds the actual disease process. Most valid therapy approaches for rheumatic inflammatory disorders are therefore primarily suited to treating acute symptoms but show very few satisfactory long-term results.

Given this situation, future studies need to examine the role of naturopathic therapies, including phytotherapy, in the overall treatment concept for rheumatic disorders. If the assumptions about these disorders are valid, one key task of phytotherapy would be to provide **basic therapy** for these disorders. We can now see antidyscratics in a new light, with a stronger justification for their use because we can better comprehend and assess humoral changes, especially with rheumatic disorders. The effects of antidyscratic remedies have always been seen as stimulation of all organs of excretion, not only the kidneys and the intestines but also all other large excretory glands, including the liver. Meanwhile, the aquaretic and choleretic effects of these remedies have been shown to be only part of their overall effect. A remarkably large number of antidyscratics also act on the digestion and could be referred to as antidyspeptics, as in the case of juniper berries, or as choleretics, as in the case of dandelion root and herb.

Antidyscratics encompass plants that have been described in previous sections of this book as aquaretics (p. 219) in a broad sense of the word. They also include some pure saponin drugs as well as plants whose constituents are not yet well studied.

Saponins is a term given to a group of nitrogen-rich glycosides. These plant components are converted by diluted acids into sugar and one or more organic compounds (aglycones). In most cases, they consist of only carbon, hydrogen and oxygen, and sometimes also nitrogen and sulfur. They are characterized by certain features. When agitated in aqueous solution, they create a soap-like foam. They emulsify oils and can dissolve red blood cells even when highly diluted. This hemolytic effect is used to detect saponins. Fish are killed by solutions containing minute amounts of saponins. Saponins are not absorbed or only absorbed in very small amounts through the intestinal wall, provided it is intact. However, they do promote absorption of many other compounds in the intestines.

The chemical makeup and effects of saponins vary widely. For example, saponins described for use as cough remedies are very different from those of antidyscratics; and even the latter are not a uniform group. Each saponin drug needs to be viewed as a specific drug and the task is to discover its specific area of application. Some of the saponins used in this area are more aquaretic, others are more antidyscratic or primarily dermotropic. At any rate, saponins and the drugs derived from them represent a very interesting area of phytopharmacology with highly significant practical applications that have not yet been sufficiently studied.

Devil's claw (Harpagophyti radix), based on current information, plays a special role in this context. Unlike traditional remedies that are endemic or common to Europe or North America such as stinging nettle, dandelion, and juniper, devil's claw originates from the tropical regions of Africa. It has very specific effects on the metabolic processes at the root of rheumatic disorders. On the other hand, it is worth noting that antidyscratic effects have also been ascribed to devil's claw. The primarily undesirable effects of devil's claw on the upper gastrointestinal tract may also be an indication that the efficacy of this plant is much more comprehensive than the pharmacologically defined effects currently attributed to it.

▶ **Therapy Recommendations.** Chronic disorders require **long-term treatment**. Antidyscratic plant remedies need to be taken consistently for longer periods of time to achieve treatment success. Interval treatment and varying remedies are useful strategies to stimulate the organism again and again. Expectations of achieving treatment success after only 4 weeks of taking a metabolic tea only lead to disappointment and to blaming treatment failure on the remedy rather than the method of treatment. Irritation therapy has taught us a gradual approach to crossing the body's stimulus threshold in small increments. Generally, strong responses should be avoided. Sometimes, it may be necessary to subject the organism to a strong stimulus at the beginning of treatment by using **remedies with acute effects** to motivate the organism into beginning to cooperate. Some medicinal plant remedies are excellent at achieving this effect. They can be given in intervals and impact the body at least as profoundly as fever cures. Schüllner and Mur published a good review of these topics.

Another important treatment consideration is that single medicinal plants usually cannot create sufficiently strong metabolic reactions. Usually, a **combination** of remedies is required. Purely metabolic effects need to be combined with a strong stimulation of excretion processes. Tolerability usually benefits from adding carminative drugs, similar to the formula for a purely laxative tea. A **metabolic antirheumatic tea** therefore should consist of:

- One or more antidyscratics
- One excretion remedy
- One carminative remedy

Remembering these clear categories provides orientation for the multitude of antidyscratic tea blends and for formulating suitable prescriptions.

Plants Used in Treatment: Internal Use

Dandelion (Taraxacum officinale)

For more information about this plant, see Dandelion (p. 124).

Medicinal applications use the chopped **dandelion root and dandelion herb** (entire plant gathered while flowering, Taraxaci radix cum herba).

▶ **Pharmacology.** The drug contains bitters such as lactucopicrin (taraxacin), triterpenoids, flavonoids, phenyl carboxylic acid, and phytosterols. Its bittering power is 600.

▶ **Indications.** Dandelion is one of our oldest medicinal plants and is mentioned in the context of many disorders.

The Commission E only lists dyspeptic complaints as an indication in its monograph for dandelion because no modern studies are available on dandelion's antidyscratic effects. However, dandelion holds substantial therapeutic potential for **rheumatic disorders,** and this is another important indication area for this plant.

Experimental studies have shown choleretic, aquaretic, antiphlogistic, and spasmolytic effects for dandelion. This drug increases gastric juice secretions and stimulates appetite. This documented comprehensive efficacy profile is expressed in dandelions **antidyscratic effects.**

Preparations

- **Tea**
  Add 1 glass of cold water to 1–2 teaspoons of the drug. Bring to a brief boil, remove from heat, and steep for about 10 minutes, then strain.
  Drink 1–2 cups in the morning and in the evening for several weeks.
- **Extract**
  The extract is contained in the following prescription formula.

Prescriptions

Rx
Extr. Taraxaci 30.0 (dandelion extract)
Aqu. Melissae ad 300.0 (lemon balm water)
D.S.
Take 1 tablespoon 3 × a day after meals.

Stinging Nettle (Urtica dioica/ Urtica urens)

This typical ruderal plant grows near human settlements, along garden fences, and in inhospitable areas, in Germany (▶ Fig. 7.1).

Antidyscratic preparations use fresh or dried **stinging nettle herb and leaves** (above-ground parts, Urticae herba et folium) collected during the flowering season.

▶ **Pharmacology.** The stinging nettle drug contains mineral salts, primarily calcium salt and potassium salt, and silicic acid. The hairs on its leaves contain biogenic amines such as histamines and serotonin. Unsaturated fatty acids and caffeoylquinic acids have also been identified.

Experimental studies have shown **mild aquaretic effects** attributed to the high potassium content of the drug. This effect requires a sufficient intake of fluids.

▶ **Indications.** Stinging nettle's comprehensive effect is **antidyscratic**.

The indications listed by the Commission E for stinging nettle are as irrigation therapy for inflammatory diseases of the lower urinary tract,

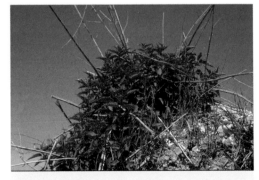

Fig. 7.1 Stinging Nettle, Urtica dioica. Photo: Dr. Roland Spohn, Engen.

prevention and treatment of kidney gravel, and as **supportive therapy for rheumatic ailments.**

For external applications, see Stinging Nettle (p. 247).

Preparations

- **Tea**
  Add 1 cup of hot water to 2 teaspoons of chopped stinging nettle leaves and/or herb. Steep for 10 minutes, then strain.
  Drink 1 cup several times a day, up to a total of 1 L a day.
- **Freshly Pressed Juice**
  Take 1 tablespoon 3 × a day.

Birch (Betula pendula, Betula pubescens, Betula verrucosa)

Birch trees are well known and require no description (▸ Fig. 7.2).

Medicinal applications use the fresh or dried **birch leaves** (Betulae folium).

▸ **Pharmacology.** Birch leaves contain a minimum of 1.5% flavonoids, computed as hyperoside, and based on the dried drug. They also contain saponins, tannins, and a volatile oil along with salicylates.

▸ **Research. Aqueous extracts** of birch leaves have been shown to be more efficacious than alcoholic extractions. They have been observed to produce increased urine excretion as well as increased electrolyte excretion (Schilcher).

▸ **Indications.** Their complex composition indicates that birch leaves are more of an antidyscratic than an aquaretic. They are suitable for general flushing therapy, but in our view, **rheumatic disorders** are a more important indication for birch leaves.

Preparation

- **Tea**
  Add 1 cup of hot water to 2 tablespoons of the drug, chopped medium fine. Steep covered for 10 minutes, then strain.
  Drink 1 cup warm several times a day, up to a total of 1 L per day.

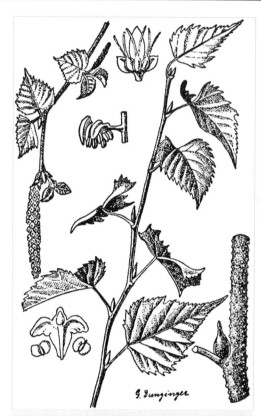

Fig. 7.2 Birch, Betula pendula, Betula pubescens, Betula verrucosa.

Woody Nightshade (Solanum dulcamara)

Woody nightshade grows in damp brush, along the edges of creeks and in alder fens. This climbing vine is native to Germany and is widely naturalized in North America. It is a member of the nightshade family and can climb up to 3 m on shrubs and trees. Its small, violet flowers have spots at the base of each lobe. Its leaves are heart shaped to ovoid and entire and its fruit are bright red (▸ Fig. 7.3).

Medicinal applications use the dried 2- to 3-year-old **stem tips** (Dulcamarae stipites) harvested in spring prior to leafing or late autumn after leaves have dropped.

▸ **Pharmacology.** Woody nightshade stem tips contain tannins, steroidal alkaloids, and saponins.

▸ **Indications.** This drug is considered one of the strongest antidyscratic remedies. It is not a

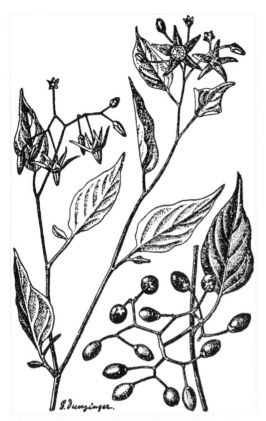

Fig. 7.3 Woody Nightshade, Solanum dulcamara.

significant diuretic. Its **metabolic transposition effect** is significantly stronger. This drug also has a slight, but distinctive narcotic effect.

> **Caution** ⚠
>
> Because of the potential for toxic damage (nightshade plant!), this drug should be dosed with restraint.

> **Preparations** ☞
>
> - **Tea**
>   Add 1 cup of water to 1–2 teaspoons of the drug. Bring to a brief boil, then strain.
>   Drink 1 cup in the morning and in the evening for longer periods.
> - **Extract**
>   The extract can be prescribed as follows.

> **Prescriptions**
>
> Rx
> Extr. Dulcamarae 5.0 (woody nightshade extract)
> Sirup. Juniperi ad 150.0 (juniper syrup)
> D.S.
> Take 1 teaspoon 3 × a day.

Greater Burdock (Arctium lappa, Lappa major)

This large member of the Asteraceae family is well known because of the distinct, uncinate involucral bracts of its flower and fruit receptacles. Greater burdock is common along paths, fences, and in forests, in Germany.

Medicinal applications use the **burdock rootstock** (fresh or dried underground parts, also referred to by the not very precise name of Bardanae radix. More recently, however, the synonym Arctii radix is used more frequently).

▶ **Note.** Common burdock (Arctium minus) and woolly burdock (Arctium tomentosum) are used in the same way as greater burdock (Arctium lappa). The rootstock is used for medicinal applications.

▶ **Pharmacology.** Greater burdock's main constituents include arctiin and its aglycon arctigenin, lappaoles, and caffeic acid; the rootstock contains inulin. Studies have shown anti-inflammatory, anti-oxidant, and antitumor effects along with an increased production of procollagen. Studies are also examining possible effects of inulin on metabolic disorders. In China, greater burdock is promoted as a food supplement (Baumgarten and Melzig). However, the significance of these partly well-studied pharmacologic effects is completely open as there are no clinical studies available at the time of this writing. Traditionally, greater burdock was used for dyspeptic symptoms, gout, rheumatic disorders, and skin disorders (psoriasis, slow-healing wounds). Today, greater burdock is used only in homeopathy and in Traditional Chinese Medicine (TCM).

Kidney Bean (Phaseolus vulgaris)

The unripe fruits of the kidney bean plant are known as the vegetable's "green beans." The vegetable's "white beans" consist of the ripe seeds of the same plant. The seed-free pods are yellowish white and look dried. They are a valuable medicinal remedy (▶ Fig. 7.4).

Medicinal applications use the **seed-free bean pods** (dried bean pods, ripe "beans" removed, Phaseoli fructus sine semine).

▶ **Pharmacology.** This drug contains phaseolin and structurally related phytoalexins as well as flavonoids. They have been shown experimentally and clinically to have a mild diuretic effect.

Dried kidney bean pods are a useful remedy as an aquaretic in a broader sense, with more antidyscratic characteristics. Their effects are not overly strong, but significant enough to justify their use, especially in antidyscratic tea formulations.

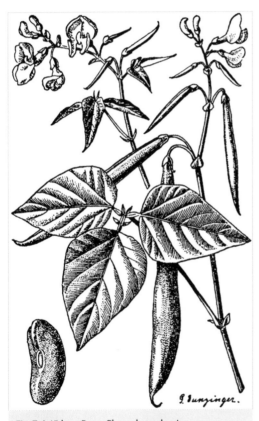

Fig. 7.4 Kidney Bean, Phaseolus vulgaris.

Preparation

- **Tea**
  Add 1 cup of boiling water to 1 tablespoon of the drug. Steep covered for about 10 minutes, then strain.
  Drink 1 cup of freshly prepared tea several times a day between meals.

Sand Sedge (Carex arenaria)

Sand Sedge is a common and characteristic plant in sandy fields and dry heaths. It can reach a length of several meters in areas that are too dry for most other plants to grow. Its underground rootstock can be traced by the linear, above-ground appearance of bushels of leaves (▶ Fig. 7.5). This plant typically appears in Germany on beaches and on the inland dunes of the North German lowlands, and in the coastal areas of North America.

Medicinal applications use the dried sand sedge **rootstock** (underground parts, Caricis rhizoma). Its aromatic scent is reminiscent of turpentine.

▶ **Pharmacology.** The drug contains silicic acid and saponins. However, its value as a saponin drug is not yet defined.

This plant is a much weaker antidyscratic than dandelion, stinging nettle, or birch. It is mostly used in combination with these plants.

Preparation

- **Tea**
  The **formulation** of this tea can be found in the section Proven Prescriptions (p. 244).

Devil's Claw (Harpagophytum procumbens)

This herblike plant is commonly found in southern Africa. It thrives in the red sand soils of the steppe regions in Namibia. After the first rains, young creeping stems grow from large tuberous roots. These stems grow along the ground and reach a length of 1–1.5 m. Bright red flowers grow from its leaf axils (▶ Fig. 7.6).

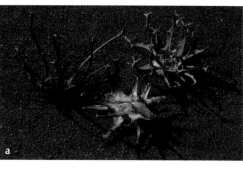

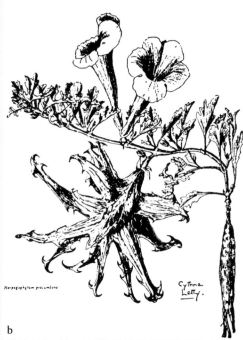

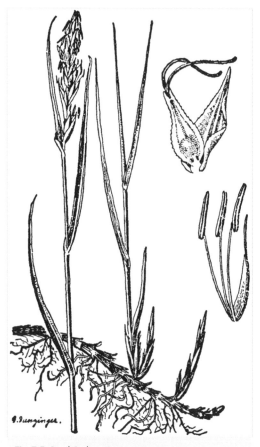

Fig. 7.5 Sand Sedge, Carex arenaria.

Its fruit turns woody and forms long, branched spines with hooks that gave the plant its name (Greek *harpagos* = grappling hook)

Medicinal applications of devil's claw use the secondary tubers (usually referred to as Harpagophyti radix, but they should more appropriately be called Harpagophyti tubera). These storage organs are up to 6 cm wide and up to 20 cm long. Several of them are often found on root branches in depths of up to 1 m. Secondary tubers are usually harvested by digging deep ditches and must be dried immediately because they quickly decay or become moldy.

▶ **Note.** The Aboriginal people of southern Africa have known about devil's claw for a long time and used decoctions of the dried roots as a tea for various ailments, especially for gastrointestinal and rheumatic disorders. The German farmer

b

Fig. 7.6 a and b Devil's claw, Harpagophytum procumbens. Photo: Dr. Roland Spohn, Engen.

Gottreich Hubertus Mehnert in (formerly) German Southwest Africa (modern-day Namibia) learned about its use and introduced it as a medicinal plant to Germany.

The German name *Teufelskralle* (devil's claw) was already in use at the time for a group of phyteuma plants belonging to the Campanulaceae family. Since these plants have no medicinal use, devil's claw became the commonly used name for Harpagophytum.

▶ **Pharmacology.** The main components of devil's claw are three iridoid glycosides: harpagoside, harpagide, and procumbide. It also contains a phytosterol mix, primarily β-sitosterin and stigmasterol, unsaturated fatty acids, triterpenes, flavonoids, and free acids (cinnamic acid, chlorogenic acid). This represents a comprehensive blend of active compounds (Wegener).

▶ **Research.** Even though this drug is used widely and is very popular, there is little pharmacologic evidence for its mode of action. Its constituents can have antiphlogistic and analgesic effects. However, its **analgesic effect** was weaker than aspirin in animal experimental studies (animal focal ray test) (Erdös et al.). Animal experimental studies also showed **antiphlogistic effects**, but studies by Lanhers et al. showed that these are certainly not attributable only to the plant's glycoside content.

Loew et al. (1996) demonstrated the impact of devil's claw on eicosanoid metabolism. Its inhibitory effect on 5-lipoxygenase is especially worth mentioning, but it is certainly not the only mechanism involved in its therapeutic efficacy. Sporer and Chubrasik point out that the type of extract used and its active iridoid glycoside content and stability, for example, when subjected to acidic gastric juices, decisively impacts the efficacy of devil's claw.

The pharmacology of devil's claw is a work in progress.

▶ **Indications.** The iridoid content of devil's claw, which has a bittering power of 6,000, and its antiphlogistic and analgesic effects makes this drug suitable for the indications appetite stimulation and **rheumatic disorders**. The focus here is on the latter.

The Commission E monograph for devil's claw lists the indications loss of appetite, dyspepsia, and supportive therapy of degenerative disorders of the locomotor system. The European Scientific Co-operative on Phytotherapy (ESCOP) also developed a monograph that is largely identical with the Commission E monograph but assumes a significantly lower dosage and longer application.

In the experience of the authors, this drug is an integral component of **complex therapy** for rheumatic disorders. Its significantly better tolerability compared to standard synthetic antirheumatic drugs should be emphasized. There are more effective remedies for lack of appetite—for example, bitters (p. 52) and this indication is not important for devil's claw.

Most studies show that the primary indication for prescribing devil's claw is **degenerative arthrosis** (Wegener).

▶ **Research.** Randomized placebo-controlled studies provide impressive evidence for this conclusion (Chrubasik and Ziegler 1996; Chrubasik et al. 1999; 2002). There appears to be an obvious connection between the type and galenics of the extract used. The assessment of analgesic efficacy varies widely.

Preparation

- **Tea**
  Add 2 cups of boiling water to 1 tablespoon of the finely chopped or coarsely powdered drug. Steep at room temperature for 8 hours, then strain.
  Drink warm in 3 portions shortly before meals.

▶ **Therapy Recommendation.** Preference should be given to unambiguously labeled, standardized, finished pharmaceutical products. Devil's claw tea is less significant therapeutically and is more suitable for prevention ("incipient arthrosis").

Willow (Salix purpurea, Salix daphnoides)

Like birch trees, willows are common and well-known trees and do not require a detailed description. Since ancient times, medicinal applications use the whole, chopped, or powdered dried **bark of young twigs** collected in spring (Salicis cortex).

▶ **Note.** In 1828, salicin was identified as the most important constituent of willow bark. In 1859, the German chemist Hermann Kolbe synthesized salicylic acid. In 1897, Felix Hoffmann synthesized acetylsalicylic acid (ASA), which became known as the antipyretic and analgesic drug aspirin that quickly spread across the globe. From that point forward, the use of willow bark extracts became obsolete. However, in the last third of the 20th century, a change of thinking occurred. Today, extract preparations standardized for salicin content are again used as efficacious phytopharmaceuticals, for example, to treat rheumatic disorders.

In 1984, the Commission E developed a monograph and, in 1991, willow bark was included in the German Pharmacopoeia (DAB 10). In 1997, the ESCOP also released a European monograph for willow bark.

▶ **Pharmacology.** The willow bark drug contains a minimum of 1% total salicin, determined as salicin, catechin tannins, caffeic acid derivatives, and flavonoids. Other characteristic constituents include salicortin, fragilin, and populin.

Salicin is a typical **prodrug**. It is nonactive and does not cause changes in the gastric mucosa. It is enzymatically catalyzed in the small intestine via hydrolysis and absorbed as saligenin. Saligenin is oxidized in the liver by cytochrome P450 into salicylic acid as the main active substance. It inhibits pain perception in the nociceptors by inhibiting cyclooxygenase (COX). Unlike the mobile acetyl groups in ASA, willow bark extract does not impact thromboxane B_2 synthesis or thrombocyte (platelet) aggregation.

Willow bark extract also has proven **antiphlogistic characteristics**.

▶ **Indications.** Willow bark is the most potent plant-based **analgesic**. Its additional antiphlogistic effect makes it a comprehensively efficacious remedy for rheumatic disorders.

The Commission E monograph and the ESCOP monograph list the indications fever, **rheumatic ailments**, and **headaches**. Numerous controlled studies and observational studies have confirmed these indications.

Willow bark extract should be given preference over nonsteroidal anti-inflammatory drugs (NSAIDS) or cyclooxygenase (COX2) inhibitors due to its positive benefit-risk quotient and significantly lower cost.

▶ **Research.** Studies showed the analgesic effect of willow bark extract to be significantly higher than with placebo. One study showed it to be equal to that of a modern COX2 inhibitor (Chrubasik 2000). The best results were achieved in adults with daily dosages of 240 mg salicin.

A randomized, double-blind, parallel group comparison study showed willow bark extract to provide the same pain relief as diclofenac for patients with hip joint and knee joint arthrosis. The study emphasized that willow bark extract was well tolerated (Lardos et al.).

▶ **Therapy Recommendation.** Only whole extract willow bark preparations standardized for salicin content should be prescribed.

Fixed Combination of Trembling Poplar, Goldenrod, and Ash Bark

The special finished pharmaceutical product Phytodolor tincture—a product of the world-famous German Bayer AG that is otherwise more known for synthetic drugs—is an alcoholic fresh plant extraction of trembling poplar bark and leaves (Populus tremula), European goldenrod herb (Solidago virgaurea) and common ash bark (Fraxinus excelsior). None of these plants has analgesic effects or can be characterized as a typical antirheumatic or antidyscratic, with the possible exception of goldenrod. However, the phytochemical composition and traditional use of Populus tremula are very similar to those of Salicis cortex.

▶ **Indications.** Excellent controlled and double-blind studies showed that Phytodolor was just as effective as, for example, the well-known nonsteroidal antirheumatic drug diclofenac for **painful disorders of the locomotor system.**

▶ **Research.** The following study results are emphasized to counter the frequent assertion that there are no plant-based analgesics that can compete with synthetic drugs. The authors have observed the excellent efficacy of Phytodolor in many clinical applications. A total of 25 clinical studies involving 1,124 patients demonstrate the efficacy and excellent tolerability of Phytodolor (Jorken and Okpanyi).

A review of all research results for Phytodolor was published in 2007 by Gundermann and Müller.

The following study is one example that illustrates the efficacy of Phytodolor. In this study, 43 patients received Phytodolor and 37 patients received diclofenac. Both groups of patients showed excellent results. Between 70 and 80% of target symptoms, which included resting pain, pressure pain, and motion pain, functional restrictions, and active and passive range of motion, were significantly improved or entirely abated.

Proven Prescriptions: Antirheumatic and Antidyscratic Teas

- Tea

Prescriptions

Rx
Urticae herb. (stinging nettle herb)
Dulcamar. stipit. (woody nightshade stem tips)
Caricis rhiz. (sand sedge rootstock)
Sennae fol. (senna leaves)
Foenicul. fruct. āā 20.0 (fennel seeds)
M. f. spec.
Add 500 mL of boiling water to 1–2 tablespoons of the blend. Steep covered for 10–15 minutes, then strain.
D.S.
Drink 1 cup each in the morning and in the evening.

Prescriptions

Rx
Taraxaci rad. c. herb. (dandelion root and herb)
Juniperi fruct. (juniper berries)
Sennae fol. (senna leaves)
Frangul. cort. (buckthorn bark)
Carvi fruct. āā 20.0 (caraway seeds)
M. f. spec.
Add 500 mL of boiling water to 1–2 tablespoons of the blend. Steep covered for 10–15 minutes, then strain.
D.S.
Drink 1 cup in the morning and one in the evening.

- Tea for **antidyscratic impact therapy** ("stoss therapy") with strong laxative effects; should only be prescribed for a few days as the initiation of long-term therapy.

Prescriptions

Rx
Taraxaci rad. c. herb. (dandelion root and herb)
Menth. pip. fol. āā 40.0 (peppermint leaves)
Foenicul. fruct. (fennel seeds)
Sennae fol. āā 20.0 (senna leaves)
M. f. spec.
Add 500 mL of boiling water to 1–2 tablespoons of the blend. Steep covered for 15 minutes, then strain.
D.S.
Drink half of the tea in the morning and the other half in the evening.

- Mixture

Prescriptions

Rx
Extr. Graminis (couch grass root extract)
Extr. Taraxaci (dandelion root extract)
Extr. Frangulae fluid. āā 10.0 (buckthorn bark fluid extract)
Aqu. Foeniculi (fennel water)
Aqu. Petroselini āā ad 150.0 (parsley water)
D.S.
Take 1 tablespoon 2–3 × a day for several weeks.

External Applications

Poultices (packs), inunctions, and baths have always played a significant role in the treatment of acute and chronic rheumatic disorders. Medicinal plants can be used for all three types of treatment. Comfrey and hay flower are primarily used for **poultices** and specific essential oil drugs are used for inunctions and baths.

Poultices

Comfrey (Symphytum officinale)

For a detailed description of this plant, see Comfrey (p. 294).

Poultices use **comfrey root and herb** (Symphyti radix, Symphyti herba).

▶ **Pharmacology.** Comfrey is a member of the Boraginaceae family and has been used medicinally since ancient times. In the past, it was used internally as well as externally. Its main applications were wound and bone healing (by promoting callus formation). Allantoin is considered to be the most important constituent of comfrey. It also contains mucilage as well as rosmarinic acid and other hydroxycinnamic acid derivatives such as caffeic acid and chlorogenic acid, which are important for the plant's pharmacodynamics. These constituents are said to be **anti-inflammatory** and **analgesic** (Koll et al.). There is no fundamental pharmacologic explanation for this action.

Internal use of comfrey extracts is considered obsolete since toxic and mutagenic effects of the pyrrolizidine alkaloids with a 1.2-unsaturated necine structure were demonstrated experimentally in comfrey.

Despite wide-ranging discussions, the Commission E decided to only approve **external use** up to a maximum pyrrolizidine alkaloid content of 10–100 µg a day in its comfrey monograph.

According to Brauchli J et al., alkaloids of Symphyti radix were present almost completely as N-oxides. Dermally absorbed pyrrolizidine-alkaloid-oxides are not or only to a small extent converted to the free alkaloids in the organism. This conversion, however, seems to be an essential step for the toxic action of pyrrolizidine alkaloid N-oxides, and the gut flora seems to play a major role in this process. This difference in the metabolism, together with the small degree of dermal absorption, makes it very likely that the occasional external use of Symphytum preparations should not be considered hazardous.

The currently available preparations all contain even lower dosages than the 10–100 µg per day recommended by the Commission E because they are derived from comfrey strains that are low in pyrrolizidine alkaloids or because pyrrolizidine alkaloids are removed to the point where they are no longer detectable. Therefore, even when comfrey preparations are applied to large areas of the body, the lower limit of 10 µg/day is not reached.

▶ **Indications.** The main indications for comfrey nowadays are **rheumatic muscle and joint disorders**, blunt trauma such as bruises, pulled muscles and sprains (Staiger 2007) and **slow-healing wounds** such as venous ulcers (see Chapter 9.3 Venous Ulcers (p. 294)).

▶ **Research.** Many controlled, evidence-based studies document the experiential data about the efficacy of comfrey for external applications. A double-blind, randomized, and placebo-controlled study in two study centers tested the efficacy of a commercial German comfrey extract ointment for **painful osteoarthritis of the knee**, whereby 220 patients received external applications of 6 g of the ointment (3×2 g a day) for 21 days. The study results showed significant superiority ($p < 0.001$) in pain reduction, improved mobility, and increased quality of life. Tolerability was very good (Grube et al.). A randomized, multicentric, double-blind, placebo-controlled parallel group comparison study tested the same product for the treatment of **ankle distortion**s (Koll et al.). Patients were treated $4 \times$ a day for 8 days. This study also showed very good results and highly significant superiority compared to placebo ($p < 0.0001$) for reduction of pain and edema as well as restoration of joint mobility. In Germany, an observation of application of the ointment according to the provisions of the Medicinal Products Act (§ 67 Section 6 Arzneimittelgesetz – AMG) confirmed these results in 163 patients (Tschaikin).

Staiger (2013)published a review of comfrey.

▶ **Therapy Recommendation.** Only defined finished pharmaceutical products should be prescribed.

Hay Flower (Graminis flos)

Hay flower is the flower of various grasses or Gramineae growing in meadows that are dried as hay. When these grasses are dried, a fermentation process takes place that creates a pleasing scent. When hay is stored in a barn, hay flowers and unripened seeds drop out and can be swept up from the barn floor at the end of the winter, after all the hay has been fed to the animals. Hay flower has been an important part of **Kneipp therapy** ever since Sebastian Kneipp, the Bavarian priest and one of the forefathers of naturopathic medicine, discovered their usefulness in the southern German Allgäu region. Kneipp only used hay flower as an addition to baths. Hay flower packs (poultices) used as moist hot compresses came into use later.

The characteristic scent of hay flower derives from **sweet vernal grass** (Anthoxanthum odoratum), one of the most common meadow grasses. It contains coumarin glycoside that is converted to coumarin when the grass wilts, similar to sweet woodruff (Galium odoratum, syn. Asperula odorata). This substance is similar to camphor in its effects and can be toxic when consumed in large amounts internally. External applications of coumarin increase hyperemia and skin stimulation.

▶ **Indications. Hay flower packs** provide excellent local energetic heat treatments for all rheumatic disorders.

They show outstanding effects for lumbago and similar **acute rheumatic muscle conditions**. For neuralgia, on the other hand, heat is only indicated when the condition has become chronic.

▶ **Research.** Fröhlich und Müller-Limmroth presented studies that used modern physics to confirm long-established experiential data about hay flower packs. Local increases in temperature caused by placing the hay flower pack directly on the skin provides analgesia and sedation. Axon reflexes increase blood circulation and tissue metabolism, decrease muscle tone, and increase connective tissue elasticity. During this process, active constituents are absorbed through the skin that can cause therapeutically useful local or generalized effects.

Preparation

- **Hay Flower Pack**
  Add about 2–3 finger's width of hay flowers to a flat linen sack. Place the sack into a pot and pour hot water over it. Cover the pot and let soak for 10 minutes. Carefully squeeze the pack until it is no longer dripping. Place it on the body area to be treated while it is still as hot as can be tolerated. Leave the pack in place for about 40 minutes. The temperature of the pack can be as hot as 42 °C (107.6 °F). The pack must be in close contact with the body and covered with a wool or flannel cloth to retain its heat.
  Use 1–2 × a day. The hay flower pack can be reused several times.

▶ **Therapy Recommendation.** Hay flower packs can be purchased ready-made in Germany. Making the packs using the drug (Graminis flos) however is much less expensive.

Inunctions

Inunctions are an important treatment component for rheumatic disorders. They are frequently used after heat treatments or massages. Inunctions are best applied to **warm muscles or joints**. At a minimum, inunctions should be applied early in the morning, while muscles or joints are still warm from being covered in bed.

Essential oils, for example, calamus oil, juniper oil, and rosemary oil in spirituous solution, which can be combined with alcoholic extractions of similar plants, are especially suitable for use in antirheumatic inunctions.

Rosemary (Rosmarinus officinalis)

For more information about this plant, see Rosemary (p. 172).

Preparation

- **Rosemary Oil**
  Apply to painful areas several times a day.

Calamus (Acorus calamus)

For more information about this plant, see Calamus (p. 59).

Preparation

- **Calamus Oil**
  Apply to painful areas several times a day.
- **Combination with Angelica Root**

Prescriptions

Rx
Ol. Calami 2.0 (calamus oil)
Spir. Angelicae Compos. ad 100.0 (spirit of angelica)
D.S.
Apply to painful areas several times a day.

Juniper Oil (Juniperus communis)

For more information about this plant, see Juniper (p. 220).

Preparation

- **Juniper Oil**
  Apply to painful areas several times a day.
- **Combination with Calamus**

Prescriptions

Rx
Ol. Juniperi 2.0 (juniper oil)
Spirit. Calami ad 100.0 (calamus spirit)
D.S.
Apply to painful areas several times a day.

Stinging Nettle (Urtica dioica, Urtica urens)

For more information about these plants, see Stinging Nettle (p. 237).

▶ **Indications.** This popular external application of stinging nettles makes use of the plants localized hyperemic effects and its ability to stimulate the cutaneous nervous system. It is used as a **supportive treatment** for neuralgia and rheumatic pain, especially resulting from degenerative and arthrotic disorders, for example, lumbago, sciatica, and tendinosis, and to treat distortions.

Preparation

- **Stinging Nettle Spirit**
  Carefully apply a few drops to painful areas of the body.

Cayenne Pepper (Paprika) (Capsicum annuum, Capsicum frutescens)

Capsicum varieties are members of the Solonaceae family. When used topically, they provide specific stimulation of peripheral nerve endings.

Medicinal applications use the **cayenne (paprika) fruit** (Capsici fructus).

▶ **Note.** No dosage-dependent neurotoxic effects were found even with long-term use of cayenne. This leads to the conclusion that these only occur as a result of overdosing (Loew 1997).

▶ **Pharmacology.** Cayenne fruit contains vanillylamide type acrid constituents, capsaicinoids such as capsaicin, dihydrocapsaicin, and other derivatives, plus flavonoids, carotenoids, and fatty oil.

For a long time the analgesic effect of cayenne was attributed to neurotoxicity. Newer studies have shown that cayenne and its active constituents interact with nerves in a specific way. This mechanism of action is based, on the one hand, on localized depolarization and nonspecific opening of voltage-gated sodium and calcium channels. This shifts the positive charge to the interior of the nerve cell. On the other hand, some cayenne constituents deplete certain neurotransmitters that are involved in processing pain information, for example, substance P, somatostatin and vasoactive polypeptides (Loew 1997; Nagy).

▶ **Indications.** The Commission E lists only external applications of cayenne ointments for painful muscle spasms in areas of the shoulder, arm, and spine of adults and school-age children.

During initial use, patients almost always experience localized burning pain that abates quickly and becomes less and less pronounced during the course of treatment.

▶ **Research.** Other indication areas documented by recent studies are diabetic polyneuropathy symptoms and postherpes neuralgia, which should be included here for the sake of completeness (Loew 1997).

▶ **Therapy Recommendation.** According to several studies, dosages should not exceed 0.075% for topical application. At this dosage, cayenne ointments can be used for up to 6 weeks. This differs from the information published by the Commission E, which limits the application to 2 days.

Baths

Rosemary (Rosmarinus officinalis)

For more information about this plant, see Rosemary (p. 172).

Preparation

- **Decoction for a Full Bath**
  Add 1 L of hot water to 50 g of the drug.
  Steep for 30 minutes, then strain, and add to bath water.

Norway Spruce (Picea abies)

This preparation refers to oil distilled from the needles and bark of spruce (Picea alba).

Preparation

- **Norway Spruce Essential Oil (Piceae abietis aetherolum)**
  For a full bath, add 5 g of the essential oil to bath water. Take 1 bath at least 3 × a week.

Hay Flower (Graminis flos)

For more information about this plant, see Hay Flower (p. 245).

Preparation

- **Decoction**
  Add 4–5 L of hot water to 500 g of hay flowers. Steep for approx. 3 minutes, then strain, and add to bath water.

7.2 Gout

As discussed in the introduction to this chapter, gout represents a special type of rheumatic disorder because it is a typical deposition disorder as well as a metabolic disorder. The clinical guiding (cardinal) symptom of gout is severe arthritis attacks, also called **gout flares**. The primary diagnosis is **hyperuricemia**. In three of four cases, this condition is caused by renal insufficiency in excreting uric acid. The remaining cases are caused by excess endogenous production of purines.

7.2.1 Acute Gout Flare

Despite the availability of modern synthetic pharmaceuticals such as allopurinol and benzbromarone, **autumn crocus** is still considered one of the best gout remedies, especially for treating acute gout flares.

Plants Used in Treatment

Autumn Crocus (Colchicum autumnale)

This beautiful plant grows in mountain meadows and derives its name from its late blooming period, which can be as late as October in Germany (▶ Fig. 7.7). The beautiful pink blossoms appear to emerge directly from the ground. Its fruit capsules migrate into the soil during the winter. This plant should not be confused with saffron crocus (Crocus sativus), which is also sometimes called autumn crocus.

Medicinal applications use the **dried autumn crocus seeds and flowers** harvested in the summer (Colchici semen and Colchici flos) or the chopped and **dried root tubers** collected later in the year and its preparations.

▶ **Pharmacology.** The main active constituent of autumn crocus is the alkaloid colchicine.

Autumn crocus or the pure colchicine alkaloid are not uricosuric but inhibit leucocyte phagocytosis and promote chemotaxis. They also inhibit prostaglandin release from macrophages and the induction of liposomal enzymes; thus the vicious circle of inflammation is interrupted in two locations.

Autumn crocus or colchicine is a **specific analgesic for gout flares**. It can be used ex juvantibus as a diagnostic tool for unconfirmed arthritis.

▶ **Indications.** The main indication for autumn crocus is **acute gout**.

▶ **Therapy Recommendations.** Autumn crocus should only be used as a finished pharmaceutical product that is standardized for colchicine content or as pure colchicine.

With acute gout flares, the dosage should be increased within a short time frame until the pain is relieved or until severe diarrhea occurs. The initial dosage is an amount corresponding to 1 mg of colchicine every 1–2 hours until pain relief is achieved. The maximum daily dose is 8 mg of colchicine and treatment should not exceed 3 days. A single dose of tincture equals 10–15 drops.

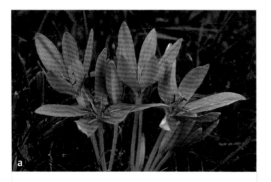

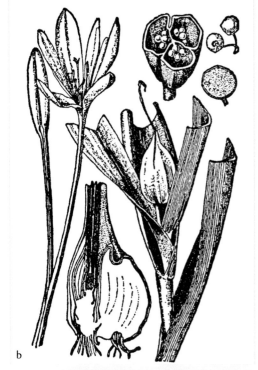

Fig. 7.7 a and b Autumn crocus, Colchicum autumnale. Photo: Dr. Roland Spohn, Engen.

Olive (Olea europaea)

Olive trees are some of the most important plants in the Mediterranean. They can reach a very old age. Olive oil is produced from its blackish-blue fruit, the olives. Its leaves are evergreen, leathery, and covered with scalelike hairs on the underside.

Medicinal applications use the **olive leaves** (Oleae folium). They are frequently used as a tea

for the treatment of gout, especially in Spanish folk medicine.

▶ **Pharmacology.** One important active principle for the treatment of gout is provided by oleuropein. Studies conducted by Flemmig et al. show that in an *in vitro* enzyme-kinetics experiment that this secoiridoid glycoside can significantly inhibit the enzyme xanthine oxidase (XO). This enzyme is closely associated with the development of gout. The specific effect of oleuropein was less pronounced than that of other isolated constituents of olive leaves studied in this experiment. However, the role of oleuropein in the efficacy of olive leaves for the treatment of gout can be considered significant. Other constituents of olive leaves, such as caffeic acid and luteolin, also seem to contribute to the efficacy of this drug for the treatment of gout. However, the flavone apigenin was shown to have the strongest specific enzyme inhibiting effect. Due to the low apigenin content in olive leaf extract, apigenin does not appear to contribute significantly to the efficacy of the extract against gout. However, the extract contains a high amount of apigenin-7-O-β-D-glucoside. This glycoside is inactive, but in the human body, it is transformed into the active apigenin aglycone. It follows that this aglycone plays an essential role in the activity of the olive leaf extract. Apigenin-7-O-β-D-glucoside, therefore, can be considered a prodrug for the indication of olive leaves for the treatment of gout.

▶ **Therapy Recommendation.** Olive leaves should only be used as extract preparations.

Bibliography

Baumgarten O, Melzig MF. Arctium lappa L. Z Phytother. 2014; 35 (06):298–304

Brauchli J, Lüthy J, Zweifel U, Schlatter C. Pyrrolizidine alkaloids from Symphytum officinale L. and their percutaneous absorption in rats. Experientia. 1982; 38(9):1085–1087

Chrubasik P. Weidenrindenextrakt. Dtsch Apoth Ztg. 2000; 140: 3825–3827

Chrubasik S, Eisenberg E, Balan E, Weinberger T, Luzzati R, Conradt C. Treatment of low back pain exacerbations with willow bark extract: a randomized double-blind study. Am J Med. 2000; 109 (1):9–14

Chrubasik S, Junck H, Breitschwerdt H, Conradt C, Zappe H. Effectiveness of Harpagophytum extract WS 1531 in the treatment of exacerbation of low back pain: a randomized, placebo-controlled, double-blind study. Eur J Anaesthesiol. 1999; 16(2):118–129

Chrubasik S, Thanner J, Künzel O, Conradt C, Black A, Pollak S. Comparison of outcome measures during treatment with the proprietary Harpagophytum extract doloteffin in patients with pain in the lower back, knee or hip. Phytomedicine. 2002; 9(3): 181–194

Chrubasik S, Ziegler R. Wirkstoffgehalt in Arzneimitteln aus Harpagophytum procumbens und klinische Wirksamkeit von Harpagophytum-Trockenextrakt. In: Loew D, Rietbrock N, ed Phytopharmaka. Vol II. Darmstadt: Steinkopff; 1996: 101–114

Erdös A, Fontaine R, Friehe H, Durand R, Pöppinghaus T. Beitrag zur Pharmakologie und Toxikologie verschiedener Extrakte, sowie des Harpagosids aus Harpagophytum procumbens DC [Contribution to the pharmacology and toxicology of different extracts as well as the harpagosid from Harpagophytum procumbens DC]. Planta Med. 1978; 34(1):97–108

Flemmig J, Kuchta K, Arnhold J, Rauwald HW. Olea europaea leaf (Ph.Eur.) extract as well as several of its isolated phenolics inhibit the gout-related enzyme xanthine oxidase. Phytomedicine. 2011; 18(7):561–566

Fröhlich HH, Müller-Limmroth W. Physikalische Untersuchungen zur thermotherapeutischen Wirkung des Kneippschen Heusacks. Munch Med Wochenschr. 1975; 117:443–448

Frohne D. Solanum dulcamara L. – Der Bittersüße Nachtschatten. Z Phytother. 1993; 14(6):337–342

Grube B, Grünwald J, Krug L, Staiger C. Efficacy of a comfrey root (Symphyti offic. radix) extract ointment in the treatment of patients with painful osteoarthritis of the knee: results of a double-blind, randomised, bicenter, placebo-controlled trial. Phytomedicine. 2007; 14(1):2–10

Gundermann KJ, Müller J. Phytodolor–effects and efficacy of a herbal medicine. Wien Med Wochenschr. 2007; 157(13–14): 343–347

Jorken S, Okpanyi SN. Pharmakologische Grundlagen pflanzlicher Antirheumatika. In: Loew D, Rietbrock N, eds. Phytopharmaka. Vol II. Darmstadt: Steinkopff; 1996: 115–126

Kaul R, Lagoni N. Weidenrinde – Renaissance eines Phytoanalgetikums. Dtsch Apoth Ztg. 1999; 139:3439–3446

Kienholz E. Behandlung von Arthrosen mit intracutanen Mistelinjektionen. Naturamed. 1990; 5:201–202

Koll R, Buhr M, Dieter R, et al. Wirksamkeit und Verträglichkeit von Beinwellwurzelextrakt (Extr. Rad. Symphyti) bei Sprunggelenksdistorsionen. Z Phytother. 2000; 21(3):127–134

Lanhers MC, Fleurentin J, Mortier F, Vinche A, Younos C. Anti-inflammatory and analgesic effects of an aqueous extract of Harpagophytum procumbens. Planta Med. 1992; 58(2):117–123

Lardos A, Schmidlin CB, Fischer M, et al. Wirksamkeit und Verträglichkeit eines wässrig ausgezogenen Weidenrindenextraktes bei Patienten mit Hüftund Kniearthrose. Zeitschrift für Phytotherapie. 2004; 25(6):275–281

Loew D, Schuster O, Möllerfeld J. Stabilität und biopharmazeutische Qualität. Voraussetzung für Bioverfügbarkeit und Wirksamkeit von Harpagophytum procumbens. In: Loew D, Rietbrock N, ed Phytopharmaka. Vol. II. Darmstadt: Steinkopff; 1996: 83–93

Loew D. Pharmakologie und klinische Anwendung von capsaicinhaltigen Zubereitungen. Zeitschrift für Phytotherapie. 1997; 18(6):332–340

Nagy JI. Capsaicin's action on the nervous system. Trends Neurosci. 1982; 5:362–365

Reuter HD. Phytotherapie bei Beschwerden am Bewegungsapparat. Naturamed. 1995; 10:13–20

Schilcher H. Möglichkeiten und Grenzen der Phytotherapie am Beispiel pflanzlicher Urologika. Urologe B. 1988; 28:90–95

Schmid B, Lüdtke R, Selbmann HK, et al. Wirksamkeit und Verträglichkeit eines standardisierten Weidenrindenextraktes bei Arthrose-Patienten. Randomisierte, placebo-kontrollierte Doppelblindstudie. Z Rheumatol. 2000; 59:1–7

Schüllner F, Mur E. Phytotherapie in der Rheumatologie. Zeitschrift für Phytotherapie. 2012; 33(4):158–167

Sporer F, Chrubasik S. Präparate aus der Teufelskralle (Harpagophytum procumbens). Untersuchungen zur pharmazeutischen Qualität. Z Phytother. 1999; 20(4):335–336

Staiger C. Beinwell – Stand der klinischen Forschung. Z Phytother. 2007; 28(3):110–114

Staiger C. Comfrey root: from tradition to modern clinical trials. Wien Med Wochenschr. 2013; 163(3–4):58–64

Tippler B, Syrovets T, Simmet T. Wirkung von Extrakten auf die Eicosanoidbiosynthese in Ionophor A 23187 – stimuliertem menschlichen Vollblut. In: Loew D, Rietbrock N, ed Phytopharmaka. Vol II. Darmstadt: Steinkopff; 1996: 95–100

Tschaikin M. Extrakt aus Symphytum officinale. Naturheilpraxis. 2004; 4:576–578

Wagner H, Fessler B, Knaus U, Wierer M. Zum Wirknachweis antiphlogistisch wirksamer Arzneidrogen. Z Phytother. 1987; 8 (5):135–140

Wagner H. Search for new plant constituents with potential antiphlogistic and antiallergic activity. Planta Med. 1989; 55 (3):235–241

Wegener T. Die Teufelskralle (Harpagophytum procumbens DC.) in der Therapie rheumatischer Erkrankungen. Z Phytother. 1998; 19:284–294

Wenzel P, Wegener T. Teufelskralle. Ein pflanzliches Antirheumatikum. Dtsch Apoth Ztg. 1995; 135:1131–1144

Questions

1. What are antidyscratics?
2. Which common plant native to Germany is a valuable antidyscratic and is especially suited for tea formulations?
3. Which parts of stinging nettle are used medicinally?
4. Which African plant constitutes an important antirheumatic remedy?
5. Which drug provides a potent plant-based analgesic?
6. Formulate an antidyscratic tea.
7. Which constituent of autumn crocus provides acute pain relief for gout flares?

Answers (p. 422) for Chapter 7.

8 Nervous System and Psychogenic Disorders

This chapter discusses medicinal plants that have been used for a long time to treat nervous system and psychogenic disorders. This includes St.-John's-wort, which is experiencing a veritable renaissance based on new research.

Phytotherapeutics provide gentle and holistic means of regulating the imbalanced organism on a mental and psychosomatic level. They have generally have few side effects and—with the exception of regulated substances like opium—carry no risk of addiction. They are also very suitable for long-term therapy, which is an important requirement for treatment of many psychogenic disorders.

The development of completely new **psychopharmaceuticals**—especially tranquilizers, but also neuroleptic drugs and tricyclic antidepressants—was considered a sensational breakthrough in modern pharmacotherapy. These drugs revolutionized the treatment of psychiatric disorders. It therefore comes as no surprise that traditional phytotherapeutics such as valerian, hops, and even powerful opium drugs were successively pushed into the background, belittled, or even dismissed as placebos. Since then, the euphoria about the effects of modern psychopharmaceuticals has been replaced by a more rational way of thinking about these drugs. Critical assessments in medical and lay literature have contributed toward this development. The "old" phytotherapeutics are experiencing a careful revival. This is partly supported by the fact that some of these remedies are now available as finished pharmaceutical products with much improved galenics, and their efficacy has been demonstrated in controlled trials (Schulz et al.).

One important disadvantage of modern synthetic psychopharmaceuticals is that they can lead to **habituation** and **dependence**, which can cause **addiction**. Suddenly stopping these drugs—for example tranquilizers—after long-term treatment can cause severe withdrawal symptoms, including psychotic episodes. Long-term use of psychopharmaceuticals is also associated with changes in personality. Some of these drugs are also sold as substitutes for illegal and nonprescription drugs on the street drug market. This is an especially important consideration in view of the current opioid epidemic in the United States.

Medicinal plant remedies are frequently observed to provide a **regulating** rather than displacing or narcotizing effect with nervous system and psychogenic disorders. These remedies help the body to rebalance itself and stimulate the body's self-healing power. With the exception of some very special personality structures, it is almost always possible to stop the use of phytotherapeutics—even those with deep psychic impacts in the long term—without causing withdrawal symptoms when the symptoms of the person being treated no longer require treatment. This represents a clear advantage compared to synthetic psychopharmaceuticals. However, medicinal plant remedies are almost never suitable for acute treatment and there are no real plant-based hypnotics or narcotics, with the exception of opium.

Deliberate nondogmatic practitioners can choose the synthetic and phytotherapeutic remedies most suitable for their patient's **individual situation**. Synthetics are likely to be more suitable for acute imbalances. Phytotherapeutics offer substantial advantages for long-term treatment. Synthetic psychopharmaceuticals are essential for premedication before surgical and diagnostic procedures. The same applies to the treatment of true psychosis. However, phytotherapeutics are the remedy of first choice for the large variety of states of anxiety and inner unrest, the increasingly frequent reactive depressive states or the many different types of dysautonomia.

Phytotherapeutics have also experienced a revolution. Modern **St.-John's-wort** preparations containing significantly higher dosages than in the past have shown such effective antidepressant and mood-lifting effects that they are considered today the remedy of first choice for **mild to moderate depression**. Their tolerability is excellent, and this makes them suitable for long-term therapy. They are not known to cause rebound phenomena when stopped abruptly. On the other hand, these remedies are known to cause clear interactions with some immunosuppressive and anti-AIDS drugs.

Neither synthetics nor phytotherapeutics can fill the large therapeutic gaps that still exist for treating **somatic disorders**. Some important medicinal plants have shown therapeutic value, for example, **ginkgo**. However, there are still no effective symptomatic or causal treatments available for many primarily degenerative disorders of the central nervous system, for example, multiple sclerosis (MS) or amyotrophic lateral sclerosis (ALS).

Medicinal Plants 📄

Nervous Unrest and Sleep Disorders
Valerian, Valeriana officinalis
Hops, Humulus lupulus
Lemon Balm, Melissa officinalis
Passionflower, Passiflora incarnata
Motherwort, Leonurus cardiaca
Lavender, Lavandula angustifolia
California Poppy, Eschscholtzia californica

Depressive Mood Disorders
St.-John's-wort, Hypericum perforatum
Indian Snakeroot, Rauwolfia serpentina
Kava, Piper methysticum

Psychophysical Exhaustion
Ginseng, Panax ginseng
Eleuthero, Eleutherococcus senticosus
Yerba Mate, Ilex paraguariensis
Kola Nut, Cola nitida
Calamus, Acorus calamus
Rosemary, Rosmarinus officinalis

Autonomic Dysregulation, Dysautonomia
Kava, Piper methysticum
Valerian, Valeriana officinalis
Lemon Balm, Melissa officinalis
Lavender, Lavandula angustifolia
Bugleweed, Lycopus virginicus/europaeus
Motherwort, Leonurus cardiaca
Rosemary, Rosmarinus officinalis

Degenerative Central Nervous System Disorders: Cognitive Brain Dysfunction
Ginkgo, Ginkgo biloba
Garlic, Allium sativum
Hawthorn, Crataegus laevigata/monogyna
Strophanthus kombe, Strophanthus kombe
Belladonna, Atropa belladonna
Henbane, Hyoscyamus niger
Jimsonweed, Datura stramonium

Vascular Headache, Neuralgia
Butterbur, Petasites hybridus
Peppermint, Mentha piperita
Yellow Jessamine, Gelsemium sempervirens

8.1 Nervous Unrest and Sleep Disorders

Medicinal Plants 📄

Valerian, Valeriana officinalis
Valerian root, Valerianae radix
Hops, Humulus lupulus
Hops glands and strobiles, Lupuli glandula et strobulus
Lemon Balm, Melissa officinalis
Lemon Balm leaves, Melissae folium
Passionflower, Passiflora incarnata
Passionflower herb, Passiflorae herba
Motherwort, Leonurus cardiaca
Motherwort herb, Leonuri cardiacae herba
Lavender, Lavandula angustifolia
Lavender flowers, Lavandulae flos
California Poppy, Eschscholtzia californica
California Poppy herb, Eschscholtziae herba

8.1.1 Limits and Possibilities of Phytopharmaceuticals

Nervous tension is not a scientifically recognized nosologic unit, but it is very prevalent in today's industrialized world. Its predominant symptoms are **states of restlessness and agitation**. Nowadays, these states tend to be expressed more and more frequently as aggression. They also exhibit an anxiety component, which in most cases signals a transition to depressive mood disorders. The primary cause of nervous tension is likely our hectic and arrhythmic lifestyle. We are no longer able to truly be at rest or—to use a term borrowed from our modern mechanistic world view—to "switch off." We seek to relax by watching television and do not notice how most of the content we consume actually increases tension.

The most typical sleep disorder is **difficulty falling asleep**. People suffering from this condition are exhausted and physically "dead tired," but they are so excited and tense and plagued by urgent thoughts that they become more and more awake and restless. This condition used to be referred to as neurasthenia. It basically involves overstimulation of the central nervous system. The central nervous system's physiologic task is to maintain alert consciousness: The body is physically tired, but the nervous system is too stimulated.

Perceptive practitioners will strive to help by prescribing a remedy or a combination of remedies. Good therapists will also help patients to become aware of the causes of nervousness, inner restlessness and sleep disorders and to find ways of resolving these causes or at least to mitigate their damaging effects. Modern medicine increasingly shows that long-standing functional imbalances or disorders frequently develop into somatic disorders that are difficult to treat. For this reason, a combination of helpful remedies and active participation by the individual patient are indicated to resolve the causes of this imbalance.

Nature offers a number of plants that can help to effectively treat restlessness and sleep disorders. Phytotherapy offers a multitude of options for treating nervous restlessness and sleep disorders and most of these remedies are pharmacologically, experimentally and clinically well documented.

Today's practitioners have access to **finished pharmaceutical products** of sufficiently high dosage whose quality and galenics conform to the monographs for these remedies. These remedies enrich and expand their therapeutic options and provide an important alternative to synthetic psychopharmaceuticals and hypnotics. The fact that these remedies do not force their effects on the organism but instead help the organism to activate its own self-regulation functions make these remedies of first choice for all treatments that are intended to be **long term**.

At the same time, **simple prescriptions** such as teas or tinctures and other recommended preparations are also useful. The act of preparing one's own sleep tea supports the efficacy of the tea. None of these therapies should be attempted without helping patients understand that they are responsible for resolving the causes at the root of their anxiety or sleep disorder. The role of medicines is to support a transition toward causal therapy.

Plants Used in Treatment

Valerian (Valeriana officinalis)

Valerian is a tall upright plant that can grow to a height of 1.5 m. Its leaves are opposite and pinnatisect (▶ Fig. 8.1) and its flowers are small, reddish white, and arranged in a polyanthus, umbel-like inflorescence.

Valerian is very common in Germany and grows wild in forests, along banks of streams, and in damp

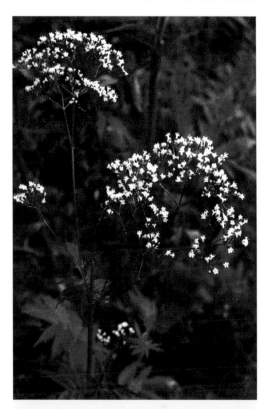

Fig. 8.1 Valerian, Valeriana officinalis. Photo: Thieme Verlagsgruppe, Stuttgart.

meadows. For medicinal use, valerian is cultivated, primarily in England, Belgium, and eastern Europe, and also, to some extent in Germany.

Medicinal applications use the **valerian root** (Valerianae radix).

▶ **Pharmacology.** The root drug contains 0.5–1% volatile oil with monoterpenes and sesquiterpenes (valerenic acid).

▶ **Research.** Valerian research conducted during the past decades illustrates the difficulty of modern pharmacology in dealing with phytotherapeutics, especially regarding active constituents. For example, the discovery of **valepotriates** by Thies and Funke led to the very one-sided conclusion that this constituent is responsible for valerian's action. This was shown to be not true at all in subsequent studies. These bicyclic monoterpenes are primarily found in South Asian and Mexican valerian and only in small amounts in the official version of the drug that is based on European valerian. They were also shown to be chemically very unstable. Valepotriates can only be detected in very carefully created preparations. They are not found at all in the types of preparations that are traditionally used.

Meanwhile, therapeutic effects have also been attributed to the valepotriate metabolite baldrinal. Without a doubt, the **volatile oil contained in valerian** constitutes another important active constituent. It contains several sesquiterpene compounds such as valeranone, valerenal, and valerenic acids. In animal experiments, these terpenes contained in valerian volatile oils have been shown to have a dampening effect on the central nervous system as well as spasmolytic and muscle relaxing effects. They also reduce motor activity (for example, Hendriks et al.). Riedel et al. also showed *in vitro* inhibition of the central neurotransmitter gamma-aminobutyric acid (GABA).

Valepotriates are considered to be sedative and tranquilizing and sometimes also stimulating. Those in the diene series were found to be more thymoleptic. Due to their epoxide structure, valepotriates have alkylating properties. However, according to Wagner and Jurcic, when administered orally, carcinogenic risk is not a concern because of the poor absorption rate and low bioavailability in the liver or in other organs. Wagner and Wiesenauer state that the research to date supports the conclusion that both the terpene compounds in valerian volatile oil and the valepotriates contribute to the overall efficacy of valerian.

More recent pharmacologic studies using different valerian root extracts in a mouse model showed no sedative effects, but significant **anxiolytic, antidepressant,** and **stress reducing effects** (Hattesohl et al.).

▶ **Indications.** Valerian is a useful sedative that has been used for a long time to treat nervous restlessness (anxiety). However, its significance was not recognized at first because the dosage used was often too low.

Based on medical experience as well as clinical and pharmacologic experimental studies, the main indications for valerian root and its preparations are **nervous agitation, nervous sleep disorders,** and **nervous heart symptoms.**

The Commission E monograph for valerian lists the indications restlessness and sleeping disorders based on nervous conditions.

▶ **Research.** A randomized, double-blind, placebo-controlled, parallel-design study showed for the first time that valerian can have acute effects with problems falling asleep and staying asleep (Dimpfel 2007). A newly developed method for determining periods of deep sleep showed that patients remained in deep sleep for longer periods and their sleep patterns began to normalize.

Combining valerian with hops increases the **sleep-promoting effects** of valerian. This was shown in a randomized, double-blind study by Koetter et al. It compared this combination with a single valerian root preparation and a placebo. The valerian root preparation in combination with hops was significantly superior to placebo. However, sleep latency (the time it takes to fall asleep) was significantly shorter for the combination preparation than for the single valerian root preparation (combination from 56 to 12 minutes = −44 minutes; single valerian root: from 46 to 24 minutes = −22 minutes; placebo: 64 to 70 minutes = +6 minutes).

Preparations

- **Tea**
  - ○ Method 1: Add 1 cup of hot water to 2 teaspoons of the chopped drug. Steep covered for 5 minutes, then strain.
  - ○ Method 2: Add 1 glass of cold water to 2 teaspoons of valerian root. Soak for 8–10 hours, then strain.
  - ○ Method 3: Macerated infusion: Add 1 cup of boiling water to 2 teaspoons of valerian root. Steep covered for 12 hours, then strain. For all the three methods drink 1–2 cups 30 minutes before bedtime.
  - ○ For Methods 2 and 3: In the morning, prepare the portion to be taken in the evening, and in the evening, prepare the portion to be taken the next morning on an empty stomach.
- **Combination with Valerian Tincture**
  Valerian tea can be fortified with 1 teaspoon of valerian tincture (see below) added to 1 cup of valerian tea.
- **Infusion**

Prescriptions

Rx
Infus. Valerian. rad. 15.0/150.0 (valerian root infusion)
Aqu. Menth. pip. ad 200.0 (peppermint water)
D.S.
Take 1 tablespoons 3 × a day.

Preparations

- **Tincture**
  1–2 teaspoons is considered a single dose. If this is not sufficiently effective, it can be repeated 2–3 × in short intervals.
- **Fluid Extract**
  Used more rarely, but recommended for some indications, especially for sedative mixtures.
- **Infusion for a Full Bath**
  Add 1 L of hot water to 100 g of the drug. Steep covered for 10 minutes, then strain, and add to bath water.
  Take a 20-minute bath 30–60 minutes before going to bed.

▶ **Therapy Recommendation.** Treatment success requires larger dosages of valerian, for example, 1–2 teaspoons of the tincture. Overdosing is rarely a concern.

Hop (Humulus lupulus)

This vine can be found growing wild in alder groves, along riverbanks, and in damp brush areas. The drug used for medicinal applications is derived exclusively from cultivation.

Hops are cultivated in almost all countries around the world, but primarily for bittering hops used in beer brewing. In Germany, hops are mostly cultivated in the southern regions. The largest and most well-known hops region is the Hallertau in Bavaria.

Hops are a valuable medicinal plant whose use was described in the Middle Ages. The special sedative and sleep-promoting effects of hops strobiles (Lupuli strobulus) and the lupulin glands (Lupuli glandulae) attached to the scales of the hops strobiles have been discovered more recently. These two medicinally used parts of hops are easily confused.

Hops strobiles (Lupuli strobulis) are the entire inflorescence with many individual fruits located behind large dry-skinned fruit scales. The arrangement of their scales resemble the familiar pattern of roof shingles (▶ Fig. 8.2).

All flower scales as well as the small flower bracteoles and the flower axis are copiously covered with small yellow **lupulin glands** (Lupuli glandulae). These can be separated by sifting freshly dried hops strobiles. They provide the medicinally active parts of the plant.

▶ **Note.** During the early Middle Ages, hops was considered diuretic, blood cleansing, and menstruation promoting. In the 8th century, the Assyrian Nestorian Yuhanna ibn Masawaih (c. 777–857, known in the West as "Mesue"), who was the personal physician to four caliphs in Baghdad, considered hop syrup a good remedy for gall fever and blood cleansing.

Paracelsus prescribed hops for digestive disorders. Hufeland valued hops as an aromatic bitter and nerve remedy. August Friedrich Hecker (1763–1811) was the first to describe the therapeutic use of the flower scales, attributing their tonic effect to the bittering compounds. He described the sedative effects on the nervous system but did not find any true narcotic effects.

▶ **Pharmacology.** The hops drug contains a minimum of 0.35% volatile oil, 15–30% resins (including humulone, lupulone and derivative compounds such as 2-methyl-3-butenol), tannins, bitter acids, and flavonoids.

Lupulin is not a pure constituent, but rather the drug isolated from the fruit scales, etc. It is identical to the hops glands. Whole hops strobiles are bulky and rustling and take up a lot of space. Lupulin, on the other hand, is a fine, yellow powder.

▶ **Research.** Gessner and Orzechowski write the following: "The bitter acids of hops are weakly hypnotic and also have mild sedative effects. In frogs, they initially cause paralysis of the hind limbs and later, of the fore limbs. At the same time, they decrease the excitability of striated muscles and motor nerve ends. No significant narcotic effects are seen in higher animals. The small amount of volatile oil contained in hops is likely to

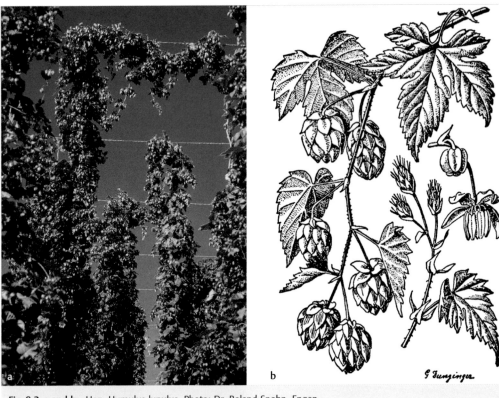

Fig. 8.2 a and b   Hop, Humulus lupulus. Photo: Dr. Roland Spohn, Engen.

play only a modest part in the overall effects of hops. Of the volatile oil constituents, humulene has central paralyzing effects presenting as deep anesthesia, following an initial state of primary agitation. The other constituents of hops play no role in the sedative effects of the drug."

In experiments on pigeons, Steidle found that the administration of a hops infusion caused mild sleepiness. Dogs developed diarrhea after receiving lupulin. Severe dyspnea along with increased respiratory rate was also observed. He discovered that the effects varied widely depending on the type of hops used. He also states that the efficacy of hops decreases rapidly during storage. He ascribes a limited role to the volatile oil contained in hops. In his opinion, the main active constituents responsible for the therapeutic effects of hops are its bitter acids. He expresses reservations about considering hops a narcotic substance or a narcotic recreational drug and considers it to be a substance that primarily influences autonomic functions. Steidle also ascribes antagonistic effects on nicotine to hops.

These results contradict the animal experiments conducted by Hänsel and Wagner (1965) in mice. They found no significant effects on motor activity in the exercise drum, locomotor activity in the exercise box, barbiturate potentiating effects, or tests using a rotating rod.

Hänsel and Schulz (1982; 1986) point out that the bitter compounds that determine the effects of hops are present in the freshly harvested drug but are present in a much lower concentration or not at all in extracts and finished pharmaceutical products. Even when hops are stored, their bitter compound content decreases by 50–70% within 6 months. The manufacture of extracts involves additional oxidative reactions. As a result, the type and amount of substances contained in extracts is largely unknown.

In earlier studies, Hänsel et al. (1982) showed that during storage of the drug, the bitter acids humulone and lupulone undergo a process of auto-oxidation and eliminate 2-methyl-3-buen-2-ol, a C-5 alcohol. The concentration of a C-5 alcohol depends on storage conditions and can be analyzed as a component of the volatile oil. Methylbutenol is chemically very similar to the closely related synthetic substance **methylpentynol**, which has been used as a sedative and hypnotic drug for some time. The methylbutenol content of hops continues to increase during storage and reaches its maximum after about 2 years at room temperature. This process is largely independent of the strain of hops. According to Hänsel et al. (1982), hops tea and bath preparations may contain relevant concentrations of methylbutenol. By comparison, hops extracts standardized for alpha acids contained relatively small amounts of this substance. Standardized sedative tablets contained only trace amounts, whereas standardized sedative bath preparations contained relatively high levels.

▶ **Indications.** Hops are a mild sedative that is not quite as potent as valerian. However, it has some special characteristics. It is considered especially sleep promoting. It is also said to have specific dampening effects on sexual arousal. It is therefore especially suitable for **sleep disorders**, especially **problems falling asleep** as well as for **sexual neurosis, nocturnal emissions**, and **premature ejaculation**. It is considered an anaphrodisiac for men.

The Commission E monograph for hops lists the indications restlessness and anxiety as well as sleep disturbances.

▶ **Note.** The effects of hops on sexual organs were first observed in young female hops pickers who experienced premature menstruation during hops harvests in the autumn (Verzele). This is thought to be due to significant amounts of plant metabolites with estrogen-like effects in hops, especially when it is freshly harvested (Milligan et al. 1999; 2000). This could explain the peculiar dampening effects of hops on sexual arousal in men, which is also thought to be a hormonal effect. Whether other hormonal effects besides estrogenic effects play a role in this process is still being discussed. Other authors contest any estrogenic effects.

Preparation

Hops is prescribed in different preparations, depending on the indication.

- **Extract in Combination with Valerian for General Nervous and Sleep Disorders**

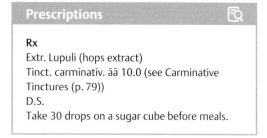

Prescriptions

Rx
Extr. Lupuli (hops extract)
Tinct. Valerian. āā 20.0 (valerian tincture)
D.S.
Take 30 drops in the evening before bedtime.

- **Extract in Combination with a Carminative for Nervous Stomach Disorders**

Prescriptions

Rx
Extr. Lupuli (hops extract)
Tinct. carminativ. āā 10.0 (see Carminative Tinctures (p. 79))
D.S.
Take 30 drops on a sugar cube before meals.

- **Combination of Hops and Valerian**
This tea contains equal parts of hops strobiles and valerian root and is the simplest prescription.
Add 1 cup of boiling water to 1 teaspoon of the chopped drug. Steep covered for 10 minutes, then strain. Drink 1 cup midday and in the evening.

Lemon Balm (Melissa officinalis)

For more information about this plant and its pharmacology, see Lemon Balm (p. 48).

▶ **Note.** Despite its Latin name, Carmelite water (Spiritus Melissae compositus) does not contain lemon balm. As specified by the German Pharmacopoeia (DAB), it contains citronella oil (Oleum Citronellae), which is also referred to as Oleum Melissae indicum. It is derived from Cymbopogon nardus (Cymbopogon winterianus, Andropogon nardus), a type of grass that is found in East India and is cultivated in Java, Sri Lanka, and Guatemala. Its scent is lemonlike and resembles lemon balm. Its main component is the essential oil derived from the herb.

The original formulation for Carmelite water, which was mentioned as a calming remedy as far back as the Middle Ages, specifies a distillate of true lemon balm and other herbs.

More information about the antidyspeptic and carminative effects of lemon balm can be found in Section 3.2.1 Acute Gastritis.

▶ **Indications.** Lemon balm is calming, antispasmodic, and carminative. It can be described as a nervine with a carminative element. Its main indications include **nervous heart disorders**, **nervous stomach disorders**, and **difficulties falling asleep** that are primarily caused by uncomfortable and anxious heart sensations.

The Commission E monograph for lemon balm lists the indications nervous sleeping disorders and functional gastrointestinal complaints. Its use for nervous sleeping disorders requires a sufficient amount of volatile oil.

Preparations

- **Tea**
  Add 1 cup of hot water to 2–3 teaspoons of the drug. Steep covered for 15 minutes, then strain.
  Drink 1 cup in the morning and especially in the evening before bedtime. The tea can be sweetened with a little honey.
  Lemon balm tea has a pleasant fragrance and taste, which make it a popular beverage. It is important to take sufficient dosages.
- **Combination with Peppermint Leaves**
  Nervous stomach disorders benefit from a combination of equal parts of lemon balm and peppermint.
- **Lemon Balm Water (Aqua Melissae)**
  Take 1 tablespoon 3–4 × a day.
- **Lemon Balm Spirit (Spiritus Melissae)**
  Take 1 teaspoon 3–4 × a day in a glass of sugar water. As a mild soporific, 1 teaspoon of this remedy can be taken after dinner and before bedtime.
  Lemon balm spirit can also be applied to the temples before bedtime.
- **Infusion for a Full Bath**
  Add hot water to 10 g of the drug. Steep covered for 5 minutes, then strain, and add to the bath water.

Additional Therapy Options

Passionflower (Passiflora incarnata)

Passionflower (▶ Fig. 8.3) is thought to originate on the South American continent and has a long history of medicinal use there, primarily for promoting sleep and for treating anxiety.

Passionflower is a recent arrival in Europe and initially was primarily valued as a decorative garden plant. As a climbing vine, it is planted on the walls of houses and on porches. Its fruit is known as maypop.

The medicinal use of passionflower has been described in detail since the 16th century. As a modern remedy, it has been used in North America since the 19th century but did not become an official medicinal remedy in Europe until the mid-20th century (Anagnostou and Staiger).

Medicinal applications use the **passionflower herb** (Passiflorae herba).

▶ **Pharmacology.** The drug contains flavonoids, primarily as glycosyles of apigenin and luteolin, as well as γ-pyrone maltol, various mono, oligo, and polysaccharides, and traces of volatile oil.

Studies have provided evidence of the anxiolytic and sedative effects of passionflower (Appel et al.). Animal experiments involving rats support the conclusion that passionflower extract inhibits GABA reuptake by binding to GABA(A) receptors and simultaneously exerting antagonistic effects on GABA(B) receptors (Hoffmann et al.).

▶ **Research.** Studies have shown **sedative** and **anxiolytic** effects for passionflower. In rodents,

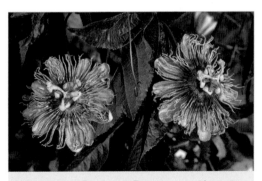

Fig. 8.3 Passionflower, Passiflora incarnata. Photo: Dr. Roland Spohn, Engen.

passionflower causes a dosage-dependent lengthening of barbiturate-induced sleep duration and a decrease in motor activity. However, some studies have also shown decreases in sleep duration. Anxiolytic effects were especially significant for the whole extract. The highest activity was seen with methanol extracts from passionflower leaves. Studies have also shown that a benzoflavone contained in passionflower can reduce symptoms of withdrawal with dependence on several psychotropic substances, including alcohol, nicotine, cannabis, or benzodiazepines (Krenn).

▶ **Indications.** For a long time, passionflower was thought to be a useful adjuvant remedy for other sedative or hypnotic drugs such as valerian or hops strobiles. Meanwhile, however, studies have also documented **anxiolytic effects** for passionflower as a single remedy.

The Commission E monograph for passionflower lists the indication **nervous restlessness**. The ESCOP monograph also lists problems falling asleep. In Switzerland and France, passionflower is also used for the indication of mild nervous heart symptoms.

▶ **Research.** An observational study of 190 patients using a **combination remedy** showed the expected effects, primarily shortening of the time to fall asleep and improved sleep quality (Staiger and Wegener).

Modern studies for single preparations are now also available. A randomized, controlled, double-blind study of 36 patients with anxiety disorders showed good anxiolytic effects for passionflower (Akhondzadeh et al.). Another study of 10 patients comparing passionflower with benzodiazepine showed passionflower to be superior because hardly any sedating and no muscle relaxing effects were observed (Ansseau).

Preparation

- **Tea**
  Add 1 cup of boiling water to 1 teaspoon of the chopped drug. Steep for 5 minutes, then strain.
  Drink 1 cup several times a day or 1–2 cups before bedtime.

Motherwort (Leonurus cardiaca)

Medicinal applications use the **motherwort herb** (Leonuri cardiacae herba).

▶ **Pharmacology.** Among other constituents, the drug contains betaines, like stachydrin, and labdane-type diterpenes.

Motherwort has a long tradition of use in central and eastern European phytotherapy for treating nervous restlessness. According to Kozo-Poljanskij, in Russia, in particular, it is viewed as an "equal substitute for valerian." In 1945, he wrote a booklet solely dedicated to the use of motherwort for treating anxiety disorders. The use of motherwort for this indication and its therapeutic similarity to valerian is less well known in western Europe. However, Weiss wrote about it in the second German edition of his *Lehrbuch der Phytotherapie.* European immigrants influenced the introduction of the drug to the US-American phytotherapy school of "eclectic medicine." In the classic standard, *The Eclectic Materia Medica,* Felter wrote in 1922 about motherwort "evidently having considerable control over the nervous system" and that it "has been advised in nervous debility with irritation and unrest."

This traditional indication has not been examined experimentally during the past decades. However, Rauwald et al. first published *in vitro* pharmacological data that seem to indicate motherwort's effects on $GABA_A$ receptors. The benzodiazepine binding sites do not seem to be involved in this process.

▶ **Indications.** In folk medicine, motherwort is used as a remedy for various nerve and heart disorders. Weiss confirmed this effect especially for **autonomic functional heart symptoms**. Like valerian, motherwort seems to have a predominantly calming effect, but needs to be taken for several months.

Lavender (Lavandula angustifolia, Lavandula officinalis)

Lavender is a member of the Lamiaceae family with small, blue flowers, and narrow leaves with rolled up edges. It grows wild in the Mediterranean on sunny mountain slopes in chalky soil, and it can reach a height of up to 1 m (▶ Fig. 8.4) in those areas. Lavender has been cultivated for centuries, especially because of its beautiful fragrance, which makes it suitable for use in cosmetics.

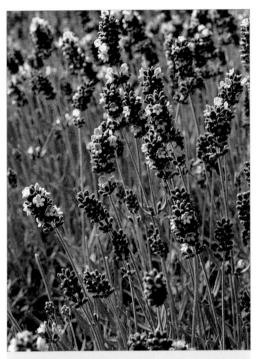

Fig. 8.4 Lavender, Lavandula angustifolia. Photo: Prof. Dr. Volker Fintelmann, Hamburg.

et al.). Several evidence-based studies of a whole lavender extract in humans showed anxiolytic effects for anxiety disorders of various causes. This assessment was primarily based on the Hamilton Anxiety Rating Scale (HAM-A). Two studies used a placebo as a control (Kaspar et al. 2010) and a third study chose the standard substance lorazepam (Woelk and Schläfke). Kaspar et al. (2010) compiled a review in 2010. It underscored that the new extract of lavender oil was reliably effective and well tolerated even during long-term use. Dyspeptic symptoms were cited as a rare adverse effect specific to the remedy because they were the exception in the placebo group and not at all seen in the lorazepam group. No sedation or rebound phenomena were observed. These clinical results were confirmed in a more recent animal experiment study (Kumar).

Preparation

- **Tea**
  Add 1 cup of hot water to 1–2 teaspoons of lavender flowers. Steep covered for 5 minutes, then strain.
  Drink 1–2 cups in the evening.

Medicinal applications use the **lavender flowers** (Lavandulae flos). They contain a minimum of 1.5% lavender oil (Oleum lavandulae) and about 12% lamiaceae tannins.

Lavender was considered a mild sedative and also used externally as a foot bath or oil dispersion bath. The Commission E issued a positive monograph for lavender with indications for external use in treating states of exhaustion.

Since 2010, a patented extract of lavender oil from lavender flowers with an entirely new efficacy profile has been introduced to the German market. Its efficacy and tolerability have been documented experimentally as well as in evidence-based clinical trials. This extract is significantly more effective than placebo and as effective as the reference substance lorazepam for anxiety disorders of various causes, especially generalized anxiety disorders (GAD). These studies also showed effective improvements for symptoms of depression that frequently accompany anxiety disorders (Kaspar and Dienel). The primary constituents in the extract are linalool, linalyl acetate, 1.8-Cineol, beta-ocimene, terpinen-4-ol, and camphor.

Animal experiments showed that linalool inhibits glutamate binding in the cerebral cortex (Elisabetsky

California Poppy (Eschscholtzia californica)

As indicated by its name, this plant belongs to the poppy family that also includes the opium poppy (Papaver somniferum). In Germany, the California poppy is known as a garden plant with beautiful orange flowers. In California, this flower grows abundantly in the wild.

Medicinal applications use the whole **California poppy herb** (Eschscholtziae herba).

▶ **Pharmacology.** Like opium poppy, California poppy contains several alkaloids that have **sedative** and **sleep-inducing** effects, primarily protopine, cryptopine, and chelidonine. These are isoquinoline alkaloids, a group that also includes papaverine and narcotin. Their narcotic effect is weaker than the phenanthrene alkaloids contained in morphine and codeine. In addition, California poppy also contains flavone glycosides (rutoside). California poppy's overall effect is mild and more **generally balancing** and not narcotic.

▶ **Indications.** Children also tolerate California poppy well. It is used to treat **sleep disorders** and for **bed-wetting**.

Preparation

- **Tea**
  Add 1 cup of hot water to 1 teaspoon of the drug. Steep for 5 minutes, then strain. Drink 1–2 cups warm in the evening.

Proven Prescriptions

The following "sleep teas" can frequently restore normal sleep patterns when used continuously for some time.

Nervine Tea (Species nervinae)

Teas that calm the nervous system can be easily created by combining the following drugs.

Prescriptions

Combination with Bitters for Atonic Conditions
Rx
Valerian. rad. (valerian root)
Melissae fol. (lemon balm leaves)
Lupuli strobul. āā ad 100.0 (hops strobiles)
M. f. spec.
Add 1 cup of hot water to 1–2 teaspoons of the blend. Steep 5 minutes, then strain.
D.S.
Drink 1–2 cups in the evening.

Prescriptions

Combination with Bitters for Atonic Conditions, with Peppermint to Calm the Stomach
Rx
Valerian. rad. (valerian root)
Melissae fol. (lemon balm leaves)
Menth. pip. fol. āā ad 100.0 (peppermint leaves)
M. f. spec.
Add 1 cup of hot water to 1–2 teaspoons of the blend. Steep 5 minutes, then strain.
D.S.
Drink 1–2 cups in the evening.

Prescriptions

Tea (according to Zimmermann) for Patients Who Dislike the Scent and Taste of Valerian
Rx
Angelicae rad. 20.0 (angelica root)
Rosmarini fol. 10.0 (rosemary leaves)
Melissae fol. 30.0 (lemon balm leaves)
Lavandulae flor. 10.0 (lavender flowers)
Lupuli strobul. 20.0 (hops strobiles)
Millefolii herb. 10.0 (yarrow herb)
M. f. spec.
Add 1 cup of hot water to 1–2 teaspoons of the blend. Steep 5 minutes, then strain.
D.S.
Drink 1–2 cups in the evening before bedtime.

Nervine Tincture (Tincturae nervinae)

The following combinations are all modifications of valerian tincture.

- **For nervous heart symptoms, also during menopause.**

Prescriptions

Rx
Tinct. Gelsemii (yellow jessamine tincture)
Tinct. Valerian. āā 10.0 (valerian tincture)
D.S.
Take 30 drops in a small amount of water 3–4 × a day.

Prescriptions

Rx
Tinct. Valerian. (valerian tincture)
Tinct. Convallariae āā 10.0 (lily-of-the-valley tincture)
D.S.
Take 20 drops 3–4 × a day.

- **Combinations of Valerian and Peppermint or Menthol**

These combinations are less intended for long-term use. However, they are calming and slightly stimulating remedies for conditions of "irritable weakness" that were referred to as neurasthenia in the past.

Prescriptions

Rx
Menthol. valerianic. 5.0
Tinct. Valerian. aeth. 10.0 (ethereal valerian tincture)
D.S.
Take 20 drops on a sugar cube.

Prescriptions

Rx
Mentholi 1.0 (menthol)
Ol. Menth. pip. 0.2 (peppermint essential oil)
Tinct. Valerian. aeth. ad 20.0 (ethereal valerian tincture)
D.S.
Take 5–10 drops for stimulation.

▶ **Therapy Recommendation.** Herb pillows are an old folk remedy already mentioned in Section 8.1.1.1.2 Hop (Humulus lupulus) (p. 255). They contain drug mixtures containing essential oils, for example, oregano (Origanum vulgare), thyme or lemon thyme (Thymus pulegioides). Lavender flowers, valerian root, and hops strobiles may also be added, all in about equal parts to make up a total amount of about 200–300 g.

These herb pillows are more than just suggestive remedies. They also have pharmacological effects by providing aromatherapy. Without a doubt, even very small entities can cause therapeutic effects, for example, endogenous hormones that are effective in nanogram amounts. There is also sufficient evidence now for the effects of homeopathically potentiated remedies.

Bibliography

Akhondzadeh S, Naghavi HR, Vazirian M, Shayeganpour A, Rashidi H, Khani M. Passionflower in the treatment of generalized anxiety: a pilot double-blind randomized controlled trial with oxazepam. J Clin Pharm Ther. 2001; 26(5):363–367

Anagnostou S, Staiger C. Passiflora—Jahrhundertealte Tradition und moderne Pharmazie. Z Phytother. 2006; 27(1):6–11

Anand CL. Effect of Avena sativa on cigarette smoking. Nature. 1971; 233(5320):496

Ansseau M. Evaluation des paramètres d'activité de gélules d'extrait sec de passiflore selon un modèle "en étoile." [Evaluation of activity parameters of passionflower dry extract capsules according to a "star" model].". J Pharm Belg. 2004; 59 (4):97–99

Appel K, Rose T, Fiebich B, Kammler T, Hoffmann C, Weiss G. Modulation of the γ-aminobutyric acid (GABA) system by Passiflora incarnata L. Phytother Res. 2011; 25(6):838–843

Bounthanh C, Bergmann C, Beck JP, Haag-Berrurier M, Anton R. Valepotriates, a new class of cytotoxic and antitumor agents. Planta Med. 1981; 41(1):21–28

Dimpfel B, Vonderheid-Guth B, Wedekind W. Das quantitative EEG als elektrischer Fingerprint von Phytopharmaka bei Ratte und Mensch. Zschr. f. Phytotherapie. 2001; 22(1):22–27

Dimpfel W. Akute Wirksamkeit eines Baldrianwurzel-Trockenextraktes auf die Schlaftiefe beim Menschen. Z Phytother. 2007; 28(1):7–16

Elisabetsky E, Marschner J, Souza DO. Effects of Linalool on glutamatergic system in the rat cerebral cortex. Neurochem Res. 1995; 20(4):461–465

Evans J. Opioid-Krise in den USA. Ein Drama mit vielen Akteuren. Pharmazeutische Ztg 2017. https://www.pharmazeutische-zeitung.de/ausgabe-502017/ein-drama-mit-vielen-akteuren/. Accessed July 18, 2019

Felter HW. The Eclectic Materia Medica, Pharmacology and Therapeutics. Cincinnati: John K Scudder; 1922: 251–252

Fintelmann V. Klinisch-ärztliche Bedeutung des Hopfens. Z Phytother. 1992; 13(5):165–168

Gessner O, Orzechowski G. Gift- und Arzneipflanzen von Mitteleuropa. 3rd ed. Heidelberg: Universitätsverlag Winter; 1974

Hänsel R, Schulz J. GABA und andere Aminosäuren in der Baldrianwurzel. Arch Pharm (Weinheim). 1981; 314:380–381

Hänsel R, Schulz J. Hopfen und Hopfenpräparate. Fragen zur pharmazeutischen Qualität. Dtsch Apoth Ztg. 1986; 126:2033–2037

Hänsel R, Schulz J. Valerensäuren und Valerenal als Leitstoffe des offizinellen Baldrians. Dtsch Apoth Ztg. 1982; 122:215–219

Hänsel R, Wagener HH. Versuche, sedativ-hypnotische Wirkstoffe im Hopfen nachzuweisen. Arzneimittelforschung. 1967; 17(1):79–81

Hänsel R, Wohlfahrt R, Schmidt H. Nachweis sedativ-hypnotischer Wirkstoffe im Hopfen. Planta Med. 1982; 45:224–228

Hänsel R, Wohlfart R, Coper H. Versuche, sedativ-hypnotische Wirkstoffe im Hopfen nachzuweisen, II. Z Naturforsch C. 1980; 35(11–12):1096–1097

Hänsel R. Pflanzliche Sedativa. Informierte Vermutung zum Verständnis ihrer Wirkweise. Erfahrungsheilkunde. 1989; 38: 327–332

Hattesohl M, Feistel B, Sievers H, Lehnfeld R, Winterhoff H. Pharmakologische Untersuchungen zu zentralnervösen Wirkungen von Zubereitungen aus Valeriana officinalis L. s. l. Z Phytother. 2008; 29 Suppl 1

Hendriks H, Bos R, Allersma DP, Malingré TM, Koster AS. Pharmacological screening of valerenal and some other components of essential oil of Valeriana officinalis. Planta Med. 1981; 42(1):62–68

Hoffmann C, Trompetter I, Weiß G. Wirkmechanismus der Passionsblume aufgeklärt. Z Phytother. 2014; 35(05):215–218

Hohmann-Jeddi C. USA—Lebenserwartung sinkt weiter. Pharmazeutische Ztg 2018. https://www.pharmazeutische-zeitung.de/lebenserwartung-sinkt-weiter/. Accessed July 18, 2019

Hölzl J. Inhaltsstoffe des Hopfens (Humulus lupulus L.). Z Phytother. 1992; 13(5):155–161

Kammerer E, Wegener T. Schlafstörungen und deren Behandlung. Stellenwert hochdosierter pflanzlicher Kombinationen. Naturamed. 1995; 10:2–8

Kaspar S, Anghelescu I, Dienel A. Efficacy of Silexan (WS 1265) in Patients with Restlessness and Sleep Disturbance. In: Annual Congress of the German Society for Psychiatry and Psychotherapy (DGPPN). Berlin, Germany, 2010

Kaspar S, Dienel A. Silexan (WS® 1265) vermindert begleitende depressive Symptome bei Patienten mit Angsterkrankungen. Z Phytother. 2013; 34(1): 58

Kasper S, Gastpar M, Müller WE, et al. Efficacy and safety of silexan, a new, orally administered lavender oil preparation, in subthreshold axiely disorders—evidence from clinical trials. Wien Med Wochenschr. 2010; 160:547–556

Kasper S, Gastpar M, Müller WE, et al. Silexan, an orally administered Lavandula oil preparation, is effective in the treatment of "subsyndromal" anxiety disorder: a randomized, double-blind, placebo-controlled trial. Int Clin Psychopharmacol. 2010; 25(5): 277–287

Koetter U, Schrader E, Käufeler R, Brattström A. A randomized, double-blind, placebo-controlled, prospective clinical study to demonstrate clinical efficacy of a fixed valerian hops extract combination (Ze 91019) in patients suffering from nonorganic-organic sleep disorder. Phytother Res. 2007; 21(9):847–851

Kozo-Poljanskij BM. Motherwort—the new pharmaceutical and technical crop from the Voronezh region. Voronezh 1945:1–10

Krenn L. Aktuelles über Passiflora incarnata. Zeitschrift für Phytotherapie. 2006; 27(1):47–50

Kumar V. Characterization of anxiolytic and neuropharmacological a-ctivities of Silexan. Wien Med Wochenschr. 2013; 163(3–4):89–94

Mair B. Passiflora incarnata L.—Passionsblume. Portrait einer Arzneipflanze. Z Phytother. 1995b; 16(2):115–126

Mair B. Passiflorae herba—pharmazeutische Qualität. Z Phytother. 1995 a; 16(2):90–99

Milligan SR, Kalita JC, Heyerick A, Rong H, De Cooman L, De Keukeleire D. Identification of a potent phytoestrogen in hops

(Humulus lupulus L.) and beer. J Clin Endocrinol Metab. 1999; 84(6):2249–2252

Milligan SR, Kalita JC, Pocock V, et al. The endocrine activities of 8-prenylnaringenin and related hop (Humulus lupulus L.) flavonoids. J Clin Endocrinol Metab. 2000; 85(12):4912–4915

Rauwald HW, Savtschenko A, Merten A, Rusch C, Appel K, Kuchta K. GABAA Receptor Binding Assays of Standardized Leonurus cardiaca and Leonurus japonicus Extracts as Well as Their Isolated Constituents. Planta Med. 2015; 81(12–13):1103–1110

Riedel E, Hänsel R, Ehrke G. Hemmung des gamma-Aminobutter-säureabbaus durch Valerensäurederivate [Inhibition of gamma-aminobutyric acid catabolism by valerenic acid derivatives]. Planta Med. 1982; 46(4):219–220

Schulz V, Hübner WD, Ploch M. Klinische Studien mit Psycho-Phytopharmaka. Z Phytother. 1997; 18(3):141–154

Sprecher E. Alte Drogen neu entdeckt. Dtsch Apoth Ztg. 1983; 123: 1337

Staiger C, Wegener T. Pflanzliche Dreierkombination bei Schlafstör-ungen und Unruhezuständen—Eine Anwendungsbeobachtung. Zeitschrift für Phytotherapie. 2006; 27(1):12–15

Steidle H. Naunyn Schmiedebergs Arch Pharmacol. 1993; 161:154

Thies PW. Funke S. Über die Wirkstoffe des Baldrians. Tetrahedron Lett. 1966; 11:1155–1170

Uhlmann B. Ein Land unter Drogen. Opioid-Krise in den USA. Süddeutsche Ztg 26.10.2017. https://www.sueddeutsche.de/gesundheit/suchtmedizin-ein-land-unter-drogen-1.3723553. Accessed July 18, 2019

Verzele M. 100 years of hop chemistry and its relevance to brewing. J Inst Brew. 1986; 92(1):32–48

Wagner H, Jurcic K. In vitro- und in vivo-Metabolismus von 14C-Didrovaltrat. Planta Med. 1980; 38(4):366–376

Wagner H, Sprinkmeyer L. Über die pharmakologische Wirkung von Melissengeist. Dtsch Apoth Ztg. 1973; 113:1159–1166

Wagner H, Wiesenauer M. Phytotherapie: Phytopharmaka und pfl-anzliche Homöopathika. 2nd ed. Stuttgart: Wissenschaftliche Verlagsgesellschaft; 2003

Weiss RF. Die Schafgarbe in der Phytotherapie. Z Phytother. 1982; 3 (2):295–296

Weiss RF. Lehrbuch der Phytotherapie. 2. ed Stuttgart. Hippokrates 1960;213

Woelk H, Schläfke S. A multi-center, double-blind, randomised study of the lavender oil preparation Silexan in comparison to Lorazepam for generalized anxiety disorder. Phytomedicine. 2010; 17(2):94–99

8.2 Depressive Mood Disorders

> ### Medicinal Plants
>
> **St.-John's-wort**, Hypericum perforatum
> St.-John's-wort herb, Hyperici herba
> **Indian Snakeroot**, Rauwolfia serpentina
> Indian Snakeroot root, Rauwolfiae radix
> **Kava**, Piper methysticum
> Kava rootstock, Piperis methystici rhizoma

Depression does not present a uniform clinical picture. One of the many more or less valid classifications differentiates between **somatogenic, endogenous, psychogenic,** or **reactive** depression. In the USA, endogenous depression is referred to as depression with unknown causes. Somatogenic depression occurs in conjunction with severe or chronic organ disorders.

The basic treatment concept involves prescription of antidepressants combined with psychotherapy and sociotherapy. The treatment focus for somatogenic depression is, of course, the underlying organ disorder. However, it also requires antidepressant treatment.

8.2.1 High Placebo Effect

Surprisingly, all placebo-controlled clinical studies (i.e., including those on synthetic antidepressants) show a high response rate of 50% to placebos. It is also worth knowing that 1 out of 5 depressed patients is resistant to typical synthetic antidepressants. Even though tricyclic antidepressants are frequently very effective, they are especially known to have adverse effects that should not be underestimated. Examples include rare, but serious cardiotoxicity. A significant number of patients with depression also reject synthetic antidepressants or take their prescribed medications very irregularly or not in high enough dosages. Against this backdrop and without questioning the usefulness and justification of modern synthetic antidepressives, plant-based alternatives such as **St.-John's-wort** (Hypericum perforatum), which has been used as a medicinal plant to treat depressive mood disorders for ages, are to be welcomed. Numerous recent studies have been published that document its effectiveness and reliable antidepressant effects and verify medical experience in this regard.

Depressive mood disorders are another area where medicinal plant remedies are better tolerated than synthetics. They are also much more easily and quickly discontinued when the symptoms of the depressive disorder have abated, and the patient has received sufficient therapy beyond that point.

Plants Used in Treatment

St.-John's-wort (Hypericum perforatum)

St.-John's-wort is a beautiful plant that grows, in Germany, on sunny slopes and in arid meadows, and is also found along the edges of pine forests. It starts to bloom around St. John's Day, near the summer solstice at the end of June, which gave it its name. Its bright yellow flowers make St.-John's-wort one of the most beautiful flowers in our flora (▶ Fig. 8.5). This plant features two curious characteristics that make it easy to recognize: When its leaves are held up to the light, one can see a number of translucent spots. They make the leaves seem perforated, hence its name "perforatum."

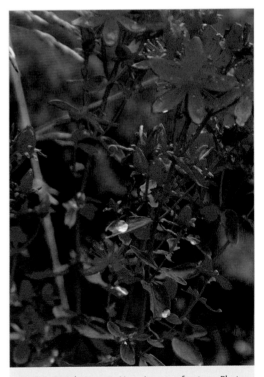

Fig. 8.5 St.-John's-wort, Hypericum perforatum. Photo: Prof. Dr. Volker Fintelmann, Hamburg.

These light spots in St.-John's-wort leaves are actually secretion glands that contain a translucent mixture of volatile oils and resin (Roth).

The second curious characteristic is its two-sided stem, which almost seems pressed flat. Stems are usually round or square. This two-sided stem is unique to Hypericum perforatum. All other varieties of St.-John's-wort, which grow in the wild, have four-sided stems.

Medicinal applications use the dried, **whole St.-John's-wort herb** (above-ground parts, Hyperici herba).

▶ **Note.** The stems of the square-stemmed St.-John's-wort variety Hypericum tetrapterum var. tetrapterum (syn. Hypericum quadrangulum) are winged on all four sides. This variety grows in damp meadows, is smaller than Hypericum perforatum, and is not used medicinally.

▶ **Pharmacology.** Upon close inspection, small black dots are visible on the sepals and on the leaves of the corolla of St.-John's-wort. When these dots are crushed, they produce a red substance that is also present in the other parts of the herb. This substance is hypericin, a photosensitizing compound that was previously considered to be the active constituent for the internal use of St.-John's-wort. The drug contains 0.1–0.3% total hypericin, which includes pseudohypericin, and protopseudohypericin. Its action resembles that of hematoporphyrin, an artificial metabolite of hemoglobin with antidepressant characteristics.

St.-John's-wort also contains 2–4% phloroglucinol derivatives, including hyperforin, flavonoids, and biflavonoids as well as tannins, pectin, and choline. Xanthones also seem to be important compounds (Hölzl). They are primarily found in gentian plants and have very strong monoaminoxidase (MAO)-inhibiting effects. *In vitro* tests showed that the xanthones contained in St.-John's-wort have similar effects.

▶ **Research.** The photosensitizing substance described above was discovered by observing cows. After eating large amounts of St.-John's-wort and lying in the sun for longer periods while digesting, cows developed skin inflammation and sunburn symptoms, sometimes including blisters. Humans can experience the same skin irritations following the internal use of St.-John's-wort if they spend too much time in the sun.

Five studies have examined the topic of **photosensitization** resulting from therapeutic dosages and from much higher dosages (up to 3600 mg/d) of St.-John's-wort extracts. All studies reached the same conclusion: Photosensitization at the daily dosages studied is very mild and occurs in very few study participants. Some participants even experienced decreased light sensitivity following maximum saturation. All reported cases add up to 1 case per 300,000 treated patients, and these cases only involved **mild skin reactions** (Schulz and Johne).

These results show that St.-John's-wort preparations should not continue to be stigmatized as being associated with increased photosensitivity. There are nearly 300 synthetic drugs available in the German medical market, which list, in part, much stronger photosensitizing characteristics, including several antidepressants (Schulz 2006). When prescribing St.-John's-wort preparations, patients should be made aware of the rare occurrence of increased photosensitivity without the consequence of limiting the profound usefulness of these remedies.

Many studies of the pharmacological effects of the constituents of St.-John's-wort have made a significant contribution toward understanding its therapeutic efficacy. However, questions remain for further study, which is also equally true for synthetic antidepressants. Depression is a complex "mental" set of symptoms that can be represented by somatically provable and measurable data. However, the infinite structure of emotional components that patients with depression experience is hard to describe directly. Animal experiments and studies of healthy subjects provide the following summarized results.

St.- John's-wort **inhibits the reuptake of the neurotransmitters** serotonin, noradrenalin, and dopamine. It also exerts a surprisingly strong inhibiting effect on the transmembrane proteins of nerve cells and the ion channels of GABA and NMDA receptors in cell membranes. No other antidepressant is known to have this type of effect. It is important to note that this represents a noncompetitive inhibition mechanism (Wonnemann et al.).

In healthy participants, St.-John's-wort also showed significant **effects on the central nervous system** compared to placebo based on electroencephalogram (EEG) measurements. After 8 days of treatment, the placebo group showed no changes compared with the initial examination. The verum group showed reproducible pharmacodynamic effects expressed primarily as higher levels of delta, theta, and alpha-1 waves (Trautmann-Sponsel).

Unlike tricyclic antidepressants, St.-John's-wort showed no adverse impact on autonomic functions. Instead, a tendency toward changes of autonomic functions (for example, vascular and sweat gland responses) indicated **more rapid dampening following sympathetic nervous system activation** (Mück-Weymann et al.).

These effects have been shown for whole extracts as well as for single constituents or groups of constituents. For a long time, hypericins were focused on as active constituents. However, newer research has shown special effects for the phloroglucinol derivative hyperforin. Other research showed strong efficacy for the flavonoid fractions and hyperoside (Butterweck et al.).

St.-John's-wort is another good example of the special characteristics of phytopharmaceuticals. Its comprehensive therapeutic efficacy is determined by a specific composition of constituents. This is what differentiates it from the frequently much more specific, but also more one-sided effects of synthetics. In addition, phytopharmaceuticals feature adjuvant constituents that are responsible for pharmacokinetics and pharmacodynamics, in this case, especially regarding tolerability.

Recently, **interactions** between St.-John's-wort preparations and other drugs have been documented, especially with the immunosuppressive cyclosporine, the HIV/AIDS drug indinavir, and other protease inhibitors as well as with oral contraceptives. Two studies have documented that concurrent use of the minipill and St.-John's-wort preparation does not cause the contraception protection of the minipill to be invalidated (Hall et al.; Pfrunder et al.; Schulz 2006).

However, since St.-John's-wort may tend to decrease the efficacy of these medications, their concurrent use needs to be carefully evaluated. Drug interaction with phytopharmaceuticals is an important topic in general and its relevance requires further study (Schulz 2004) (see Chapter 1.6 "Interactions (p. 17)").

▶ **Indications.** Clinical studies indicate mildly sedating, antidepressive, and anxiolytic effects for St.-John's-wort preparations. St.-John's-wort oil preparations (p. 301) for external use are antiphlogistic due to their high flavonoid content.

All available scientific research results, including medical experience, show that St.-John's-wort provides an important alternative for treating depressive disorders. Without a doubt, it is not suitable for treating endogenous depression. However, based on the experience of the authors, it is the remedy of first choice for **somatogenic and psychogenic depression**.

The Commission E monograph for St.-John's-wort lists the following indications: internal use for psychoautonomic disturbances, depressive moods, anxiety, and nervous unrest, and external use of oily preparations of St.-John's-wort for treatment and posttherapy of acute and contused injuries, myalgia, and first-degree burns.

St.-John's-wort's effects develop gradually. Experience has shown that it takes about 8 days to start working and 4 to 6 weeks before its full efficacy is reached. Those desiring quick effects associated with increased adverse effects should not take St.-John's-wort. If the goal, however, is satisfactory **long-term effects** without significant side effects, St.-John's-wort preparations should be given preference.

▶ **Research.** St.-John's-wort's **antidepressive** effect is documented by a multitude of modern clinical studies. Wagner and Wiesenauer cite 26 controlled clinical studies that were conducted and published prior to mid-1993. These studies compared St.-John's-wort to placebos as well as to synthetic antidepressants. Therapeutic efficacy was the same, but the rate of adverse effects was significantly lower for St.-John's-wort than for synthetics. Many participants experienced **increased cognitive performance** while taking St.-John's-wort. Since then, many other excellent studies have been conducted and published and some of these are cited here.

A randomized, double-blind comparative study compared St.-John's-wort (800 mg) to fluoxetine hydrochloride. The principal target criterion was the patient's global score on the Hamilton Rating Scale for Depression (Hamilton score). Other scaled questionnaires were also used. Treatment lasted 6 weeks. The efficacy of both medications was found to be statistically equivalent, and interestingly, so were the adverse drug reactions (ADRs). Of the 149 patients, 12 patients using St.-John's-wort indicated an ADR, leading to the withdrawal of 6 patients, whereas 17 patients using fluoxetine experienced an ADR, leading to the withdrawal of 8 patients (Schmidt et al.).

An open, multicenter trial of St.-John's-wort extract (900 mg/d) was conducted for 1 year with 313 patients. Of these patients, 251 concluded the study with complete data. This represents the first comprehensive **long-term study**, which is significant because treatment of depression frequently takes place over long periods of time. The Hamilton score showed highly significant improvements from 17.39 to 7.05 points ($p < 0.001$) after 1 year. This result was confirmed by additional scaled documentation. More than 80% of physicians and patients rated efficacy and tolerability as good to very good. ADRs seen in conjunction with St.-John's-wort were 2.2% (Hübner and Arnoldt).

A review of 8 clinical trials involving 629 patients confirmed the special **anxiolytic component** of St.-John's-wort (Friede and Wüstenberg).

A review by Schulz (1999) describes the special significance of St.-John's-wort for the treatment of depression. Another review by Reuter summarizes the pharmacology, toxicology, and clinical results.

A meta-analysis by Röder et al. also supports the efficacy and tolerability of St.-John's-wort for mild to moderate depression.

Comparative studies have also been published that compare St.-John's-wort preparations with standard synthetic medications such as setralin or, for example, citalopram, which has recently been identified as the lead serotonin reuptake inhibitors (SSRI) substance (Gastpar et al., Zeller and Gastpar). These studies proved therapeutic equivalence and led to **moderate depression** being recognized as an indication for special extracts. Tolerability for St.-John's-wort was significantly better.

In order to simplify long-term treatment, once-a-day dosages of 600–900 mg/d were also studied (Gastpar et al.; Kasper et al.). These studies also showed distinct proof of efficacy compared to placebo or to standard therapy. Increased dosages of, for example, 1200 mg/d showed no increase in efficacy.

> **Preparations**
>
> - **Tea**
>   Add 1 cup of hot water to 1–2 teaspoons of the finely chopped drug. Steep covered for 10 minutes, then strain.
>   Drink 1–2 cups in the morning and in the evening.
> - **Fluid Extract**
>   Take 5 drops 3 × a day, increase to up to 10 drops, for 3 weeks.

▶ **Therapy Recommendations.** The indications mild to moderate depression should only be treated with finished pharmaceutical products containing a daily dosage of 600–900 mg. Finished pharmaceutical extract products are especially suitable for also treating moderate depression. This indication is recognized for these remedies.

Traditional phytotherapeutic preparations can be used to treat mild types of mood swings, nervous restlessness, or generalized anxiety.

Indian Snakeroot (Rauwolfia serpentine)

This interesting plant-based phytopharmaceutical is primarily known as a blood pressure-lowering remedy and is discussed in detail in chapter 4 in that context (p. 167), which also mentions the fact that Indian snakeroot primarily effects the central nervous system.

The drug acts on the limbic system in the diencephalon. This is the same area acted on by drugs we refer to as **tranquilizers**. Low doses of Indian snakeroot lower the neural store of catecholamines and block the transport of noradrenaline and dopamine into the storage granules. This relaxes the peripheral vascular system and lowers blood pressure.

▶ **Indications.** When taken in dosages that are ten or more times as high as those for the treatment of hypertension, Indian snakeroot acts as a **neuroleptic** that can affect psychotic states of agitation with delusional and hallucinatory disorders. In the past, this effect was used for treating schizophrenia. Since then, Indian snakeroot treatment in this area has been replaced by phenothiazines and other types of drugs. Taken in high dosages, Indian snakeroot can produce **substantial adverse reactions**. The most important side effect is parkinsonism, as with all neuroleptics.

▶ **Note.** Low doses, often less than those used to treat hypertension, are sufficient to cause a **tranquilizing effect**. This relieves anxiety and tension, restores emotional balance, and provides a **regulating effect on the autonomic nervous system**. Most likely, the blood pressure-lowering effect of Indian snakeroot is a partial component of the remedy's more comprehensive tranquilizing effect. It is most effective in labile constitutional and essential types of hypertension where blood pressure rates and variations are substantially influenced by emotional factors.

Kava (Piper methysticum)

Kava (also known as kava kava) originates from the islands of the South Pacific Ocean and is a very common shrub in that region. It is a member of the pepper family (Piperaceae).

Traditionally, the islands' inhabitants chewed the root stock and prepared a beverage from it (kava, ava, yangona) that produced a dose-dependent state of relaxation. Today, this beverage is made from freshly chopped roots (in Vanuatu) or dried roots (in Fiji, Samoa, or Tonga). Sometimes, coconut is used as an constituent, which improves the extraction of kavalactones. After consuming large amounts of this beverage, people were unable to remain upright and fell into a long slumber-like state. The difference between the effects of alcohol and kava is that with kava, the state of consciousness remains clear, and kava does not produce a hangover effect in its aftermath. On the contrary, people feel more refreshed. In this respect, similarities with tranquilizers are found.

From the time of colonial rule over many Pacific island states at the end of the 19th century, kava has been in frequent use in Germany and its effects have been studied pharmacologically and clinically. This research was intensified when kava's anxiolytic effect was noted and interest developed in its application with anxiety syndromes, also as a component of depressions.

Medicinal applications use the **kava roots and peeled root stock** (Piperis methystici rhizome).

▶ **Pharmacology.** Kava contains a variety of pharmacologically active substances, especially α-pyrones (kavapyrones, today usually referred to as kavalactones), chalcones, flavonoids, and small amounts of volatile oils.

Kava is a **sedative, sleep inducer,** and **muscle relaxant**, primarily due to its kavalactones: 100 g of kava contains between 3 and 12 g of kavalactones. These include kavain (K), dihydrokavain (DHK), methysticin (M), dihydromethysticin (DHM), yangonin (Y), and desmethoxyyangonin (DMY). Approved kava drug products, in Germany, contain a standardized kavalactone content of 60 to 120 mg. They act on the limbic system, likely through interaction with GABA receptors.

Patients who were given the drug showed significant increases in the number of high affinity GABA receptors, especially in the limbic system. This subdues emotional excitability without, for example, reducing the ability to concentrate or cognitive functions. This is a key difference compared to benzodiazepines.

Therapeutic use of kava in German-speaking countries suffered a serious setback at the beginning of the 21st century. After more than 100 years of successful use of kava drugs and extracts, a few isolated cases of hepatotoxic side effects were documented. This adverse effect was rare given the high level of usage but could not be ignored because some very serious cases were documented. In a phased process, the German Federal Agency for Drugs and Medical Products revoked the approval of kava preparations in 2002.

Without reflecting upon the potential cosequences, other regulatory institutions in a number of other countries followed the decision of the German authorities to revoke the approval of kava. This led to a severe economic crisis in several developing Pacific island nations whose entire economies depend largely on the export of this drug.

The decision by the German authorities also quickly invoked strong resistance from the medical and scientific communities. It was pointed out that the majority of case studies cited against kava were practically unviable. Several cases were listed twice, which artificially raised the number of cases. A number of cases listed co-medications that sufficiently explained the documented liver damage. Finally, several reports of liver damage referred to patients who appeared to be suffering from alcohol abuse. Deducting all of these questionable cases left only a handful of cases of reported liver damage where a cause other than kava was plausible.

Attempts by kava manufacturers to regain approval were not initially successful. The problem of hepatotoxicity could have been solved by requiring a prescription for kava. However, at that point, from the point of view of the German authorities, the problem had shifted from one of drug safety to one of drug efficacy. To regain approval, manufacturers were required to present current studies that reflected the state of science. However, all relevant studies of kava that had been used previously to gain approval of kava had been conducted before this regulatory standard had been issued and did not meet the current standards. Even though, as mentioned above, hepatotoxic side effects were reported for a very small number of cases relative to the number of prescribed dosages, the German authorities took the position that the efficacy of kava was not proven. This meant that even a slight possibility of hepatotoxic effects shifted the risk-benefit ratio into negative territory. At that point, manufacturers applied for permission to conduct new clinical studies. However, these studies were not approved because of the risk of hepatotoxic side effects for participants of the study. This circular logic prevented the rehabilitation of kava in the German market for years.

It took a protracted court case to fully rehabilitate kava in a legally binding judgment issued by the Higher Administrative Court in Münster in the spring of 2015 (Kuchta 2015). The court ruled that quality standards for clinical studies cannot be applied retroactively to studies used to gain prior drug approval. This means that the efficacy of kava preparations for clinical use is once again to be considered proven. On the issue of risk, the court viewed it as proven that the chemosynthetic drugs listed as alternatives for kava, such as benzodiazepines, carry a much higher risk of side effects and that revoking approval of kava drugs in 2002 not only did not benefit patients, but actually caused harm. Therefore, the revocation of approval was decided as unlawful and invalid. This decision became final in April of 2015 and restored the initial approval of kava in the German market. However, kava now requires a prescription and other requirements such as weekly liver tests, which make it practically impossible for practitioners to prescribe kava. Therefore, the manufacturers who hold the initial approval have gone back to court.

Meanwhile, there appears to be an explanation for the small number of hepatotoxic cases reported after taking kava preparations before the 1990s. A range of kava cultivars are grown on the South Pacific islands, which are used for different applications. For about 100 years, the kava drugs used to treat anxiety disorders were exclusively derived from kava cultivars belonging to the group of "noble kava" varieties. In the Pacific island states, these are used for daily kava consumption and are characterized by their particularly pleasant effect and their lack of a "hangover" effect (p. 268) following consumption. In the 1990s, the Melanesian country of Vanuatu—the main supplier of kava—began large-scale cultivation of kava for the European market. The kava cultivar chosen for export to Europe for the first time was a "two-day kava" variety because it provides higher yields. "Two-day kava" is characterized by pronounced aftereffects such as hangover, nausea, and headaches, and persons consuming this kind of kava cannot return to their normal responsibilities for 2 days. "Two-day kava" is rarely consumed in the South Pacific islands, which explains the lack of body of experience regarding potential liver toxicity. The use of "two-day kava" in phytotherapeutic preparations in Europe in the late 1990s historically represented the first application of this kava variety for treatment of anxiety disorders. This coincides with the appearance of all the cases of liver toxicity after taking kava preparations in the late 1990s that cannot be attributed to other causes.

There are precedents for dealing with cases where a certain medicinal plant cultivar does not meet the required therapeutic quality standards (for example, calamus). This problem should be solvable with relatively little regulatory effort. Systematic tests have shown that "noble kava" and "two-day kava" can be differentiated analytically.

▶ **Indications.** Of primary interest for kava's clinical application is its **anxiolytic effect**. Modern kava extract preparations, primarily due to their long-term tolerability, provide a rational alternative to the typical pharmaceuticals used in the treatment of anxiety disorders, such as benzodiazepines, antidepressants, opipramol, and buspirone. They also do not reduce concentration and cognitive functions. For this reason, kava has been called a phytotranquilizer, a not so well-chosen name.

The German Commission E monograph for kava lists the indications **nervous anxiety, stress, and restlessness**.

Anxiety disorders are becoming more frequent. The 10th revision of the International Statistical Classification of Diseases and Related Health Problems (ICD 10) includes social phobias, specific phobias, panic disorders, and generalized anxiety disorders. These disorders are further differentiated into types of anxiety, for example, panic disorders, persistent or object focused, or situational or diffuse phobias. Always, differential diagnosis needs to rule out underlying physical disorders (multiple sclerosis, epilepsy, hyperthyroidism, hypoglycemia, etc.).

The use of kava is documented by many trials and studies (Kuchta 2018).

▶ **Research.** Johnson et al. demonstrated in a single-blind study with healthy subjects that the quantitative EEG showed an increase in the α/β index typical for the pharmacological EEG profile of anxiolytics. The increase of β activity occurred primarily in the β2 area. This special extract did not have any sedative or hypnotic effects even at a maximum dose of 600 mg.

Emser and Bartylla examined kava's effect on **sleep quality** in healthy subjects (extract compared with placebo). They showed that kava increases sleep spindle density and the proportion of slow-wave (deep) sleep and caused no changes in REM sleep. Stage I sleep and sleep onset latency tended to be reduced and subjective sleep duration was increased.

Kinzler et al. examined the effectiveness of a special kava extract against a placebo in 58 patients with **anxiety, tension, and agitation** of non-psychotic genesis in a 4-week double-blind study. Treatment outcomes were measured on the Hamilton Anxiety Rating Scale (HAM-A), the German Adjective Word List (Eigenschaftswörterliste, EWL), and the Clinical Global Impression (CGI) scale. After only 1 week, the patients treated with kava showed a significant decrease in total HAM-A scores compared to the placebo group. This difference increased further after 4 weeks.

Warnecke showed good effects for kava in women with **psychoautonomic** and **psychosomatic symptoms during menopause**. In a randomized, placebo-controlled, double-blind study, 20 female patients received 3 × 100 mg kava extract or a placebo for 8 weeks. After only 1week, the kava group showed significant reductions in their total HAM-A scores compared to placebo. The differences between the kava group and the placebo group were significant. Other study parameters such as depressive mood, subjective feelings, severity of disorder, and menopause symptoms responded well to kava.

In an observational study, Siegers et al. studied the good to very good efficacy of a special kava extract in 4,086 patients with **nervous anxiety, tension, and restlessness**. All studies emphasize the good tolerability of the kava extract. Rare reported side effects included allergic skin reactions, accommodation disorders, enlarged pupils, and problems with oculomotor balance. Longer use of kava can also cause yellow skin pigmentation, which is known to the Indigenous population of the South Pacific islands as a harmless side effect

of frequent kava use. Interactions with substances that impact the central nervous system such as alcohol, barbiturates, and other psychopharmaceuticals need to be considered. Kava is contraindicated during pregnancy, lactation, and in patients with endogenous depression who are at risk for suicide.

In another very elaborate randomized, reference-controlled study, Mittmann et al. showed that the effects of a special kava-spissum extract as a **premedication for gynecological surgery** is comparable to that of benzodiazepines, without the significant increase in blood pressure during surgery frequently observed with benzodiazepines. The study also showed that the frequent assertion that kava takes 10 to 14 days to be effective is not true. When taken in sufficient dosages, kava can have acute (short-term) effects.

Bibliography

Bieniek D, Korte F. Neuere Ergebnisse zur Chemie und Pharmakologie des Haschisch. Dtsch Apoth Ztg. 1978; 118:1933–1935

Burchard JM. Opiumtherapie und moderne Psychopharmaka [Opium therapy and modern psychopharmacological agents]. Arzneimittelforschung. 1967; 17(5):557–561

Butterweck V, Jürgenliemk G, Nahrstedt A, Winterhoff H. Flavonoidfraktionen und Hyperosid aus Hypericum perforatum L. zeigen antidepressive Aktivität im Forced Swimming Test nach Porsolt. Zeitschr f Phytotherapie. 1999; 20:86–87

Dittmann J, Herrmann HD, Palleske H. Normalisierung des Glukose-Stoffwechsels von Hirntumor-Schnitten durch hyperosid [.Normalizing glucose metabolism in brain tumor slices by hyperoside]. Arzneimittelforschung. 1971; 21(12):1999–2003

Emser E, Bartylla K. Verbesserung der Schlafqualität. Neurol Psychiatr. 1991; 5:636–642

Friebel H. Zur Toxikologie der Muskatnuss. Med Klin. 1953; 42:1570

Friede M, Wüstenberg P. Johanniskraut zur Therapie von Angstsyndromen bei depressiven Verstimmungen. Zeitschr f Phytotherapie. 1998; 19:309–317

Gastpar M, Singer A, Zeller K. Efficacy and tolerability of hypericum extract STW3 in long-term treatment with a once-daily dosage in comparison with sertraline. Pharmacopsychiatry. 2005; 38 (2):78–86

Hall SD, Wang Z, Huang SM, et al. The interaction between St. John's wort and an oral contraceptive. Clin Pharmacol Ther. 2003; 74(6):525–535

Hänsgen KD, Vesper J, Ploch M. Multizentrische Doppelblindstudie zur antidepressiven Wirksamkeit des Hypericum-Extraktes LI 160. Nervenheilkunde. 1993; 12:285–289

Harrer G, Hübner WD, Podzuweit H. Wirksamkeit und Verträglichkeit des Hypericum-Präparates LI 160. Nervenheilkunde. 1993; 12:297–301

Harrer G, Sommer H. Therapie leichter/mittelschwerer Depressionen mit Hypericum. Munch Med Wochenschr. 1993; 22:305–309

Hölzl J. Johanniskraut, eine alte Arzneipflanze mit neuer Bedeutung. Therapeutikon. 1989; 10:540–547

Hübner WD, Arnoldt KH. Johanniskraut-Einjahresstudie. Z Phytother. 2000; 21:306–310

Johnson D, Frauendorf A, Stecker K, Stein U. Neurophysiologisches Wirkprofil und Verträglichkeit von Kava-Extrakt WS 1490. TW Neurol Psychiatr. 1991; 5:349–354

Kasper S, Anghelescu IG, Szegedi A, Dienel A, Kieser M. Superior efficacy of St. John's wort extract WS 5570 compared to placebo in patients with major depression: a randomized, double-blind, placebo-controlled, multi-center trial [ISRCTN77277298]. BMC Med. 2006; 4:14–27

Kinzler E, Krömer J, Lehmann E. Wirksamkeit eines Kava-Spezial-Extraktes bei Patienten mit Angst-, Spannungs- und Erregungs-zuständen nicht psychiatrischer Genese. Arzneimittelforschung. 1991; 41:584–588

Kretschmar R, Teschendorf HJ. Pharmakologische Untersuchungen zur sedativ-tranquillisierenden Wirkung des Rauschpfeffers (Piper methysticum Forst). Chemiker Zeitung. 1974; 98:24–28

Kuchta K, de Nicola P, Schmidt M. Randomized, dose-controlled double-blind trial: Efficacy of an ethanolic kava (Piper methysticum rhizome) extract for the treatment of anxiety in elderly patients. Tradit Kampo Med. 2018; 5(1):3–10

Kuchta K, Schmidt M, Nahrstedt A. German kava ban lifted by court: the alleged hepatotoxicity of kava (Piper methysticum) as a case of ill-defined herbal drug identity, lacking quality control, and misguided regulatory politics. Planta Med. 2015; 81(18):1647–1653

Meyer HJ. Untersuchungen über den antikonvulsiven Wirkungstyp der Kava-Pyrone Dihydromethysticin und Dihydrokavain mit Hilfe chemisch induzierter Krämpfe. Arch Int Pharmacodyn Ther. 1964; 150:118–131

Mittmann U, Schmidt M, Vrastyakova J. Akut-anxiolytische Wirksamkeit von Kava-Spissum-Spezialextrakt und Benzo-diazepinen als Prämedikation bei chirurgischen Eingriffen – Ergebnisse einer randomisierten, referenzkontrollierten Studie. Journal für Pharmakologie und Therapie. 2000; 9:99–108

Mück-Weymann M, Lukesch J, Kaltwasser A, Zeller K, Joraschky P. Verändert Johanniskrautextrakt bei depressiven Patienten autonome Funktionen? Zeitschr f Phytotherapie. 1999; 20:91–92

Pfrunder A, Schiesser M, Gerber S, Haschke M, Bitzer J, Drewe J. Interaction of St. John's wort with low-dose oral contraceptive therapy: a randomized controlled trial. Br J Clin Pharmacol. 2003; 56(6):683–690

Reuter H. Hypericum als pflanzliches Antidepressivum. Zeitschr f Phytotherapie. 1997; 18(1):45–52

Röder C, Schaefer M, Leucht S. Meta-Analyse zu Wirksamkeit und Verträglichkeit der Behandlung der leichten und mittelschweren Depression mit Johanniskraut [Meta-analysis of effectiveness and tolerability of treatment of mild to moderate depression with St. John's wort]. Fortschr Neurol Psychiatr. 2004; 72(6):330–343

Roth L. Untersuchung verschiedener Johanniskrautarten auf ihren Gehalt an Hypericin. Dtsch Apoth Ztg. 1953; 93:653–656

Scharfetter C. Anwendung der Psychopharmaka bei bestimmten In-dikationsgruppen [The use of psychopharmacologic agents in c-ertain indicated groups]. Med Klin. 1967; 62(22):861–863

Schmidt U, Harrer G, Kuhn U, Biller A. Äquivalenzvergleich: Johanniskrautextrakt LoHyp-57 vs. Fluoxetin-HCl. Z Phytother. 1999; 20:89–90

Schulz V, Johne A. Side effects and drug interactions. In: Müller WE, ed St. John's Wort and its Active Principles in Depression and Anxiety. Milestone in Drug Therapy. Basel: Birkhäuser; 2005: 145–160

Schulz V. Arzneimittelinteraktionen: Relevanz für Phytopharmaka? Z Phytother. 2004; 25:283–288

Schulz V. Johanniskraut ohne Photosensibilisierung. Weitere Studie mit 40 Probanden bestätigt Geringfügigkeit des Risikos nach Extrakteinnahme. Zeitschrift für Phytotherapie. 2006; 27(4): 178–179

Schulz V. Stellenwert von Hypericum-Extrakten in der Therapie leichter bis mittelschwerer Depressionen. In: Loew D, Blume H, Dingermann T, ed. Phytopharmaka. Vol V. Darmstadt: Steinkopff; 1999: 151–156

Siegers CP, Honold E, Krall B, Meng G, Habs M. Ergebnisse der Anwendungsbeobachtung L 1090 mit Laitan® Kapseln. Arztl Forsch. 1992; 39:7–11

Singer A, Wonnemann M, Müller WE. Hyperforin: Wichtigster Hemmstoff der Neurotransmitteraufnahme aus Hypericum perforatum. Z Phytother. 1999; 20:83–86

Szegedi A, Kohnen R, Dienel A, Kieser M. Acute treatment of moderate to severe depression with hypericum extract WS 5570 (St. John's wort): randomised controlled double-blind noninferiority-inferiority trial versus paroxetine. (Note: Dosage error in article text). BMJ. 2005; 330(7490):503–506

Trautmann-Sponsel RD. Johanniskraut in der Behandlung von Depressionen. Z Phytother. 1999; 20:87–88

Vorbach EU, Arnoldt KH, Mannel M. Johanniskraut als Phyto-Antidepressivum. Fundamenta Psychiatrica. 2000; 14:172–180

Vorbach EU, Hübner WD, Arnoldt KH. Wirksamkeit und Verträglichkeit des Hypericum-Extraktes LI 160 im Vergleich mit Imipramin. Nervenheilkunde. 1993; 12:290–296

Wagner H, Wiesenauer M. Phytotherapie: Phytopharmaka und pflanzliche Homöopathika. 2nd ed. Stuttgart: Wissenschaftliche Verlagsgesellschaft; 2003

Warnecke G. Psychosomatische Dysfunktionen im weiblichen Klimakterium. Klinische Wirksamkeit und Verträglichkeit von Kava-Extrakt WS 1490 [Psychosomatic dysfunctions in the female climacteric. Clinical effectiveness and tolerance of Kava Extract WS 1490]. Fortschr Med. 1991; 109(4):119–122

Wonnemann M, Schäfer C, Müller WE. Johanniskrautextrakt: Effekte auf GABA- und glutamaterge Rezeptorsysteme. Z Phytother. 1999; 20:77–82

Zeller K, Gastpar M. Hypericumextrakt STW3-VI im Vergleich zu Citalopram und Plazebo bei Patienten mit mittelschwerer Depression. Psychopharmakotherapie. 2007; 14:65–69

8.3 Psychophysical Exhaustion

> ### Medicinal Plants
>
> **Ginseng**, Panax ginseng
> Ginseng root, Ginseng radix
> **Eleuthero**, Eleutherococcus senticosus
> Eleuthero rootstock, Eleuterococci rhizoma
> **Yerba Mate**, Ilex paraguariensis
> Yerba Mate leaves, Mate folium
> **Kola Nut**, Cola nitida
> Kola nuts (seeds), Colae semen
> **Calamus**, Acorus calamus
> Calamus rootstock, Calami rhizoma
> **Rosemary**, Rosmarinus officinalis
> Rosemary leaves, Rosmarini folium

Many people suffer from exhaustion nowadays. Almost always, it is difficult to assess if this exhaustion has **physical-organic** or **mental–emotional causes**. The first step is to exclude serious, hidden, and chronic organ disorders, for example, adrenal insufficiency, hypothyroidism, chronic liver disease, which often leads to a characteristic dip in performance, or even undiagnosed cancer. On the other hand, it needs to be recognized that drive, initiative, and physical strength can only develop through mental and physical cooperation, which primarily originate in our psychic life. The term psychophysical exhaustion derives from a coming together of "psyche" and "somatic" and almost always provides a precise description of the situation. Psychophysical exhaustion has many diverse causes, sometimes mostly physical, and sometimes mostly mental–emotional.

How people experience states of exhaustion differs widely and is characterized by their living situation and the expectations, satisfaction, and disappointments associated with it. Many people invoke the abstract term "circulation disorder," and often people with constitutional hypotension carry this condition through life like a label that provides a ready-made excuse for their lack of performance. On the other hand, the relentless demand of our performance-oriented society for always present "power" and strength drives people to seek even more challenges and adventure.

What is often overlooked is that health results from the interplay of tension and relaxation, from waking and sleeping. Exhaustion is always an indication of disparity in this necessary balance or rhythm.

Psychophysical exhaustion needs to be differentiated from other types of exhaustion, for example, following a serious illness, prolonged excessive social obligations, and long-lasting isolation. These conditions are subject to different regularities. During **convalescence**, medicinal plant remedies can help patients to regain their strength.

8.3.1 Phytopharmaceuticals: Limits and Possibilities

Remedies used to treat exhaustion should never be stimulating. One example of a stimulating drug is pervitin (methamphetamine), which was frequently prescribed in the past. Instead, they should support and encourage the interaction of physical and mental activities. Phytopharmaceuticals with more **short-term acute action** need to be distinguished from those more suitable for **long-term treatment**.

Plants Used in Treatment

Ginseng (Panax ginseng)

Ginseng (▶ Fig. 8.6) is a member of the Araliaceae family. It is a perennial shrub with a thick, spindle-shaped, brownish-yellow root. Its flowers are small and inconspicuous, and its fruits are light-red berries. Chinese ginseng grows wild in the primeval forests of North Korea and Manchuria. **Ginseng root**, a drug that tastes slightly sweet and mildly aromatic, is cultivated as an undergrowth in shady forests or on plantations under a shade cover in North Korea, China, Japan, Ukraine, and the areas surrounding Moscow. Ginseng cultivation is an important part of North Korea's exports and creates tens of thousands of jobs.

Cultivated ginseng roots take at least 7 years to reach a harvest weight of 60–100 g. Ginseng roots growing in the wild take 150–200 years to reach the same size. The efficacy of young cultivated ginseng roots is reported to be one and a half to two times weaker than that of old roots growing in the wild. Ginseng roots fetch a high price, which makes its elaborate, time-consuming, and arduous cultivation worthwhile.

Ginseng roots are differentiated by color into red and white roots. When the perishable ginseng roots are sterilized and preserved using hot steam,

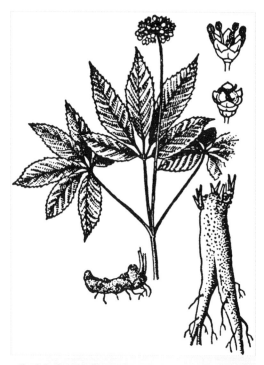

Fig. 8.6 Ginseng, Panax ginseng.

the color of the root turns from white to reddish while maintaining its chemical composition.

Eight types of ginseng are known to exist. In addition to Chinese ginseng, American ginseng (Panax quinquefolius) is also used medicinally. Its action is said to be weaker than that of Chinese ginseng. The remaining six types of ginseng are not used medicinally.

▶ **Note.** The Panax genus derives its name from Panacea, the Greek goddess of universal remedy. The Chinese name of this plant, *jin-sim*, which means "person plant root" because its roots, like those of the mandrake, resemble the shape of the human body.

Ginseng is one of the oldest remedies in East Asia, especially in China and North Korea. Ginseng root is held in high regard there and is used to treat a variety of disorders. It is said to preserve vitality into ripe old age, lengthen life expectancy, and is considered an aphrodisiac.

▶ **Pharmacology.** Ginseng root contains a minimum of 1.5% ginsenosides as well as volatile oil, phytosterols, and peptidoglycans.

▶ **Research.** Many studies have found a multitude of effects, primarily on the **central nervous system**, **endocrine** system, and **immune** system for ginseng extracts or the isolated ginsenosides.

According to Wagner and Wiesenauer, corticomimetic, central nervous system stimulating and suppressing, tranquilizing and stimulating effects have been documented for ginseng root. Cholinergic, serotonin-like effects, and histamine-like effects have also been documented. Different ginseng extracts or individual ginsenosides have different and sometimes opposing effects. It is not yet known which ginsenosides or other constituents are mainly responsible for ginseng's action and how they work.

▶ **Indications.** Medical experience with the support of clinical trial results has attributed primarily tonic and central nervous system stimulating effects to ginseng. This is why ginseng could also be called a **psychotonic**. It increases vitality and improves general health, age-related depression, and lack of concentration. For this reason, ginseng is primarily used as a tonic for **fatigue**, **overexertion**, **hypotension**, general and nervous **exhaustion**, especially in the elderly, and for **mild depression**.

Ginseng's primary application is as a general **phytogeriatric remedy**. Human trials have shown increased psychophysical performance and vitality as well as improved memory, intellect, ability of abstraction, verbal conceptualization, and coordination.

The Commission E monograph lists the following indications for ginseng: as a tonic for invigoration and fortification in times of fatigue and debility, for declining capacity for work and concentration, and during convalescence.

Eleuthero (Eleutherococcus senticosus)

Eleuthero is sometimes viewed as a "substitute" for ginseng and also originates from East Asia. It primarily grows wild and is plentiful in the eastern part of Siberia and is also called Siberian ginseng or devil's shrub.

Eleuthero extract is prepared from the **eleuthero rootstock** (Eleutheroccoci rhizoma).

▶ **Pharmacology.** Eleuthero is in the same Araliaceae family as ginseng, but its constituents are different. It contains very little ginsenoside. Instead, it contains oleanolic acid and sitosterol glucosides. Wagner and Wiesenauer list the main compounds as simple phenyl propanes, lignans, coumarins, and polysaccharides.

The mostly Russian experimental research results for eleuthero are similar to those for ginseng.

▶ **Indications.** The Commission E monograph lists the indications for eleuthero as a tonic in times of fatigue and debility, declining capacity for work or concentration, and during convalescence.

It remains to be seen whether eleuthero offers advantages and different therapeutic options compared to ginseng.

Preparation

- **Tea**
  Add 1 cup of boiling water to 1 teaspoon of the finely chopped drug. Steep for 15 minutes, then strain.
  Drink 2–3 cups warm every day.

Yerba Mate (Ilex paraguariensis)

This evergreen tree is also sometimes cultivated as a shrub. It grows and is also cultivated in Brazil between 30 and 20 degrees south latitude and is a member of the Aquifoliaceae family.

Medicinal applications use the **yerba mate leaves** (Mate folium).

▶ **Pharmacology.** The main constituents of yerba mate are caffeine as well as other purine and chlorogenic acid derivatives, triterpenes and triterpene saponins, and small amounts of volatile oil (Frohne). The action of the caffeine contained in the drug is primarily analeptic but also diuretic and positive inotrope and chronotrope as well glycogenolytic and lipolytic.

Preparation

- **Tea**
  Add 1 cup of hot water to 1 teaspoon of the chopped drug. Steep for 5 minutes, then strain.
  Drink 2 cups a day.

Kola Nut (Cola nitida, Cola aquinata)

The medium-size kola trees resemble chestnuts and grow to a height of about 20 m. Kola trees originate from coastal West Africa.

The kola tree trunk is smooth, and its alternate leaves have single, undivided, or sometimes trilobed leaves that are lancet shaped or oval, with curved edges, and a long, stretched tip. Its flowers form paniculate cymes. Its nut pods contain two to six flattened, cone-shaped seeds with parchment-like, brownish-red skin.

Medicinal applications use the **kola nuts** (seeds, Colae semen).

▶ **Pharmacology.** Kola nuts contain a minimum of 1.5% methylxanthines such as caffeine and theobromine. Their action is respiratory analeptic, stomach acid stimulating, lipolytic, motility increasing, mildly positive chronotrope, and mildly diuretic. These psychoanaleptic effects determine the therapeutic use of kola nuts.

Preparations

- **Dry Extract**
  For tablets or capsules.
  Take 0.25–0.75 g several times a day.
- **Fluid Extract**
  2.5 g 3 × a day.
- **Tincture**
  3 g several times a day.
  Maximum daily dosage: 30 g.

Calamus (Acorus calamus)

For more information about this plant, see Calamus (p. 59).

Preparation

- **Tincture**
  For a full bath, add 250 g of tincture to the bath water.
  Calamus baths are stimulating and should be taken in the morning, followed by 1 hour of rest.

Rosemary (Rosmarinus officinalis)

For more information about this plant, see Rosemary (p. 172).

Preparation
• **Infusion** For a full bath, add 1 L of hot water to 50 g of the drug. Steep covered for 30 minutes, then strain, and add to bath water. Rosemary baths are stimulating and should be taken in the morning, followed by a period of rest.

Bibliography

Frohne D. Mate-Ilex paraguariensis St.-Hil. Zeitschr f Phytotherapie. 1999; 20:53–58

Wagner H, Wiesenauer M. Phytotherapie: Phytopharmaka und pflanzliche Homöopathika. 2nd ed. Stuttgart: Wissenschaftliche Verlagsgesellschaft; 2003

8.4 Autonomic Dysregulation, Dysautonomia

Medicinal Plants

Kava, Piper methysticum
Kava rootstock, Piperis methystici rhizoma
Valerian, Valeriana officinalis
Valerian root, Valerianae radix
Lemon Balm, Melissa officinalis
Lemon Balm leaves, Melissae folium
Lavender, Lavandula angustifolia
Lavender flowers, Lavandulae flos
Bugleweed, Lycopus virginicus/europaeus
Bugleweed herb, Lycopi herba
Motherwort, Leonurus cardiaca
Motherwort herb, Leonuri cardiacae herba
Rosemary, Rosmarinus officinalis
Rosemary leaves, Rosmarini folium

8.4.1 Autonomic Dysregulation

Autonomic dysregulation was, for a long time, virtually discriminated against by labeling it vegetative dystonia. Unlike the states of nervous restlessness and sleep disorders described earlier, autonomic dysregulation is caused by imbalances in the **autonomic nervous system** (sympathetic and parasympathetic nervous system). Autonomic dysregulation is very typical with hyperthyroidism and chronic alcoholism. Its symptoms include attacks of sweating, tremors, diarrhea, and tachycardia as well as general irritability that erupts suddenly and aggressively. Imbalances of the central nervous system are more frequently caused by an overload of optical and acoustical sensory stimulation. Imbalances of the autonomic nervous system, on the other hand, are often caused by external stimuli that are not perceived consciously. Modern humans are subjected to many different stimuli that are almost impossible to escape. People who live in big cities "get used to" traffic noise that persists day and night, whereas people who live in the countryside and visit big cities find it unimaginable to live or sleep while surrounded by so much noise. However, this seeming adaptation to external stimuli can be highly damaging because the body no longer perceives them consciously and therefore does not "digest" them.

Autonomic dysregulation is now viewed as the main indication for **tranquilizers**. However, synthetic tranquilizers only cover up the symptoms of dysregulation and do not really protect against or resolve them.

Plants Used in Treatment

Kava (Piper methysticum),
Valerian (Valeriana officinalis),
Lemon Balm (Melissa officinalis),
Lavender (Lavandula angustifolia,
Lavandula officinalis),
Motherwort (Leonurus cardiaca),
Bugleweed (Lycopus europaeus)

People whose autonomic nervous system is overstimulated urgently need substances that used to be referred to as "nerve food." Newest research indicates that kava is effective in this regard. Other medicinal plants described in earlier parts of this book such as valerian (p. 253), lemon balm (Melissa officinalis) (p. 48), or lavender (p. 259) are also useful in this context.

The combination of bugleweed and motherwort provides an excellent remedy for states of autonomic restlessness.

Rosemary (Rosmarinus officinalis), Lavender (Lavandula angustifolia, Lavandula officinalis)

Preparation

- **Infusion**
  Prepare a tea infusion of each plant and add 1 L of the tea blend to a full bath that is the right temperature to allow the drug to be fully effective. Water temperature should be 37–39 °C (99–102 °F), depending on personal preference.

▶ **Therapy Recommendation.** Rosemary (p. 172) full or partial baths are very invigorating and should primarily be used in the morning. Lavender (p. 259) baths are primarily relaxing and are more suitable for the evening.

8.5 Degenerative Central Nervous System Disorders

Medicinal Plants 📄

Ginkgo, Ginkgo biloba
Ginkgo leaves, Ginkgo biloba folium
Saffron, Crocu sativus
Saffron, dried stigma, Croci stigma
Garlic, Allium sativum
Garlic bulb, Allii sativi bulbus
Hawthorn, Crataegus laevigata/monogyna
Hawthorn flowers, leaves, and fruit, Crataegi flos et folium et fructus
Strophanthus kombe
Strophanthus seeds, Strophanthi semen
Belladonna, Atropa belladonna
Belladonna root, Belladonnae radix
Henbane, Hyoscyamus niger
Henbane leaves, Hyoscyami folium
Jimsonweed, Datura stramonium
Jimsonweed leaves and jimsonweed seeds, Stramonii folium et semen

8.5.1 Cognitive Brain Dysfunctions

Degenerative disorders of the central nervous system, especially cognitive brain dysfunction, are among the most common disorders of our day. Cognitive brain dysfunction was formerly called brain sclerosis, but today these disorders are more commonly classified as **cerebral vascular insufficiency** or **cerebral atrophy** and present as various forms of **dementia**.

Symptoms of these disorders present as degenerative changes in the brain or **cognitive brain dysfunctions**. These include problems with concentration, memory, various types of vertigo, headaches, tinnitus, and finally psychoorganic syndrome (POS) and changes to personality (dementia). Alzheimer type dementia, which was formerly also referred to as presenile dementia, is a special variant of the group of disorders described here.

▶ **Note.** There are a large number of synthetic drugs (nootropics) available that claim to act on the central nervous system. However, these drugs have not yet shown any safe and reliable efficacy. The pharmacologist Kuschinsky (1975a, 1975b) refers to these drugs as "impure placebos" that undoubtedly produce some effects but seem unable to impact the underlying problem of the central nervous system's lack of regeneration. They seem only able to reduce certain symptomatic imbalances.

Plants Used in Treatment

Ginkgo (Ginkgo biloba)

For more information about this plant, see Ginkgo (p. 157). Ginkgo requires patient, long-term treatment to fully develop its impressive effects.

▶ **Indications.** Many evidence-based proofs of efficacy are now available for ginkgo leaf extracts. We present some older and some newer studies as evidence. This evidence is so conclusive that ginkgo must be termed a remedy of first choice for the treatment of dementia, also because of its extremely high long-term tolerability. The earlier ginkgo is started, the higher its efficacy is expected to be, and it is clearly a preventive. This is especially true for the commercial special extract (EGb 761), that has been used for most of the studies.

▶ **Research.** In a randomized, placebo-controlled double-blind study, Kanowski et al. tested the efficacy of 240 mg/d ginkgo special extract (EGb 761) in patients with Alzheimer type dementia and multi-infarct dementia for 24 weeks. The verum group registered higher scores for attention and memory than the placebo group. For severe cases, ginkgo reduced the level of nursing care required.

Wettstein showed in his studies that improvements in memory and orientation for patients with Alzheimer type dementia were achieved with EGb 761 and were comparable to the effects of acetylcholinesterase inhibitors.

Le Bars et al. showed in another randomized, placebo-controlled, double-blind study of 327 patients who were treated for 52 weeks with 120 mg/d EGb 761 or placebo that ginkgo produced significant improvements in memory, attention, temporal and location orientation, social behavior, and daily living skills.

Oken et al. conducted a meta-analysis of EGb 761 trials that met all requirements for assessing the efficacy of this substance for treating Alzheimer type dementia. They found significant effects resulting from 3 to 6 months of treatment with 120–240 mg/d EGb 761 on **cognitive performance** that were comparable to the effects of other antidementia drugs.

Newer studies also document the efficacy of EGb 761 with dementia (Napryeyenko and Borzenko). A randomized, double-blind, placebo-controlled, multicenter (16 centers) trial of 400 outpatients found statistically significant effects for ginkgo extract with all application criteria compared to placebo ($p < 0.001$). It also showed that tolerability of **long-term treatment** of dementia patients with ginkgo is markedly better and more than five times less expensive than treatment with standard synthetic acetylcholinesterase inhibitors. Ginkgo preparations that have been proven to be effective with dementia should be the remedy of first choice for treating dementia or cognitive brain dysfunction.

A randomized, placebo-controlled double-blind trial examined the ginkgo extract EGb 761 (240 mg a day) in 300 patients with very mild cognitive dysfunction (average age 55 years) for a period of 12 weeks. Testing included tests for memory and retention, for example, face recognition, and simple and complicated appointments as well as performance and attention. Validated questionnaires also recorded perceived physical health and self-assessment of quality of life. EGb 761 was significantly superior to placebo ($p > 0.0025$) in all areas and patients reported an improved sense of physical health (Grass-Kapanke et al.). A similar trial produced comparable results (Kaschel).

In another trial, 410 outpatients with Alzheimer type dementia, vascular dementia, or a mixture received 240 mg of EGb 761 or placebo for 24 weeks. This trial was also randomized, placebo-controlled, and double-blind. Patients suffered not only from cognitive dysfunctions but also from neuropsychiatric symptoms such as depressive moods, anxiety, and affective lability with increased irritability and aggressive behavior. Ginkgo was superior to placebo for all test parameters ($p > 0.001$). The tolerability of the extract was described as good (Herrschaft et al.).

Finally, we present an unusual long-term trial conducted by the University of Bordeaux for 20 years. This publicly funded trial tested brain aging and dementia development in 3,777 residents of communities in southern France who were older than 65. More than 800 study participants developed dementia. Those who decided to take EGb 761 experienced much slower decreases in mental performance than those who did not take any antidementia drugs. The authors of this study attributed these results to the specific effects of the ginkgo extract. These results provide another indication for the preventive effects of ginkgo (Amieva et al.).

A review of the antidementia effects of ginkgo extracts can be found in a supplement of International Psychogeriatrics (2012) (Lautenschlager et al.) and as a review in the Wiener Medizinischen Wochenschrift (Janßen et al.).

Saffron (Crocus sativus)

The dried stigmas and styles of saffron can be used to treat chronic nervousness and restlessness.

Saffron is a member of the Iridaceae family and is a perennial, tuberous plant. Saffron is the common name for the dried stigma of the plant (Croci stigma). Saffron is known as a spice and a dye but was also considered a medicinal in the past. Traditionally, it was used as an emmenagogue and to treat depression and digestive disorders. The Commission E listed it as a sedative and for spasms and asthma but issued a negative monography because it did not find any proof of efficacy and because of unresolved questions about toxicology.

More recently, several working groups have studied saffron and conducted foundational pharmacologic and clinical trials. These proved antioxidant, anti-inflammatory, antidiabetic and thrombocyte aggregation inhibiting effects. Evidence-based clinical trials show antidepressant effects. Berger et al. published a very good review of the current research about saffron. These authors conducted their own trials using a saffron extract they manufactured. They examined the topical and central issue of its neuroprotective effect, especially regarding cerebral infarction and neurodegenerative dementia. They showed that saffron, especially its constituent trans-crocetin, interacts in various ways with neurotransmitters and brain metabolism, for example, calcium metabolism. This provides antagonistic effects on NMDA and kainate receptors and influences the important glutamate metabolism. These multi-target effects were emphasized because degenerative changes also have a multitude of causes and are likely not influenced by a single effect. The views of Berger et al. views saffron as having great potential for the future treatment and prevention of neurodegenerative disorders, especially with a view to the proven bioavailability of its main constituents and their ability to pass through the blood-brain barrier. This outlines a path for this type of therapy, but several more steps are required to develop a generally available extract and to conduct clinical trials. However, the information about these possibilities needed to be included in this book and thus closes the circle of information provided by R.F. Weiss about this plant in the past.

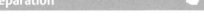

Preparation

- **Tea**
  Add boiling water to 2 teaspoons of the drug. Steep for 3 to 5 minutes, then strain. Drink 1 cup 3 × a day.

Hawthorn (Crataegus laevigata, Crataegus monogyna), Strophanthus (Strophanthus kombe)

For information about these plants, see Hawthorn (p. 137) and strophanthus.

▶ **Indications.** Many cognitive brain disorders involve latent congestive heart failure or circulatory dysregulation. Hawthorn and strophanthus are primary remedies for treating these disorders.

Parenteral use of the pure g-strophanthin and oily capsules have been shown to be useful.

▶ **Therapy Recommendation.** The use of finished pharmaceutical products is recommended. Hawthorne preparations should be dosed at, for example, 120–240 mg/d, which is lower than with congestive heart failure (p. 147).

Belladonna (Atropa belladonna)

For more information about this plant, see Belladonna (p. 69).

▶ **Indications.** Its **parasympaticolytic effects** make belladonna suitable for several indications, for example, as a spasmolytic in the gastrointestinal area. It also has strong effects on the central nervous system. In the past, belladonna was especially known for its impact on **chronic encephalitis**. It was noted that very large amounts that exceeded the maximum daily dose needed to be taken and that these doses were tolerated surprisingly well.

A key discovery involved the fact that belladonna's special therapeutic effects on the central nervous system were derived from the belladonna root. Normally, belladonna leaves are used medicinally.

Belladonna root extracts are therefore especially suitable for treating **parkinsonism**.

Parkinsonian syndrome therapy has benefited greatly from many specific synthetic drugs. Especially L-dopa and amantadine and a large number of synthetic anticholinergics effect rigor and tremor. This appears to make belladonna treatment outdated, particularly because postencephalitic Parkinsonism is rare nowadays and resulted primarily from serious flu epidemics. Today, parkinsonism occurs primarily as a result of degenerative (sclerotic) changes in the central nervous system. The belladonna therapy described above is also recommended for this condition, especially when synthetic drugs are not tolerated or are rejected or when they do not produce the desired results.

Henbane (Hyoscyamus niger)

Henbane grows to a height of about 0.5 m. It has sticky, villous leaves and dirty pale yellow flowers with violet dots at the bottom (▶ Fig. 8.7). It is found in inhospitable locations and along the edges of paths and is not native to Germany. The drug is derived through cultivation.

Medicinal applications use **henbane leaves** (Hyoscyami folium).

▶ **Pharmacology.** Henbane leaves contain hyoscyamine and other alkaloids.

▶ **Indications.** Henbane is an effective tremor remedy, especially for **Parkinson's disease** and **age-related (essential) tremor**. Its tolerability is surprisingly good. Experience has shown that—as with belladonna and synthetic neuroleptics—its tolerability in patients with organic brain changes is much higher than in healthy patients.

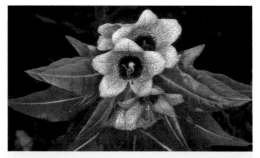

Fig. 8.7 Henbane, Hyoscyamus niger. Photo: Dr. Roland Spohn, Engen.

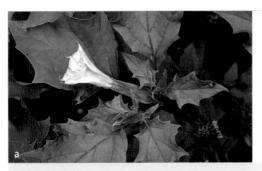
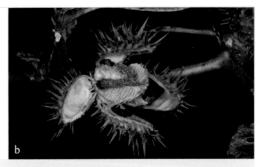

Fig. 8.8 a and b Jimsonweed, Datura stramonium. Photos: Dr. Roland Spohn, Engen.

Preparation ☞

- **Tincture**
  Relatively large doses must be given, up to 30 drops 3–4 × a day.

Jimsonweed (Datura stramonium)

Jimsonweed is a nightshade plant. Its stem can reach up to 1 m in height and is forked. Single large, white, cone-shaped flowers are located at the base of the forked branches of its stem. The spiny fruit that develops from these flowers has given this plant one of its names, thorn apple. The fruit is a rather large spherical capsule covered with soft spines and contains black seeds (▶ Fig. 8.8).

Jimsonweed likely originates from Asia. It is now found along garden fences and in inhospitable locations and has become a part of the German flora. As a typical ruderal plant, it prefers to grow near human settlements where the soil has been enriched by refuse, especially of a protein nature. The drug is mostly derived from cultivated plants.

Medicinal applications use the **jimsonweed leaves** and **jimsonweed seeds** (Stramonii folium, Stramonii semen).

▶ **Pharmacology.** Jimsonweed contains 0.03–0.5% alkaloids, primarily hyoscyamine.

▶ **Indications.** Jimsonweed provides good results for **Parkinson's disease** and other types of tremors, but these results are only symptomatic.

The Commission E has issued a **negative monograph** for jimsonweed because of the discrepancy between insufficiently documented efficacy and the unpredictable risk of toxicity from the alkaloids

L-hyoscyamine and L-scopolamine. Because jimsonweed has hallucinogenic properties, it presents the risk of dependency and abuse.

Preparation ☞

- **Tincture**
  Derived from the seeds.
  For age-related (essential) tremor, start with 15 drops/d and increase up to 40–60 drops/d, best taken in a single dose. If this dose is not sufficient, retain the jimsonweed dose as a base remedy and add one of the synthetic anti-Parkinson drugs.

Bibliography

Amieva H, Meillon C, Helmer C, Barberger-Gâteau P, Dartigues JF. Ginkgo biloba extract and long-term cognitive decline: a 20-year follow-up population-based study. PLoS One. 2013; 8(1): e52755

Berger F, Hensel A, Nieber K. Crocus sativus L. ist nicht nur ein Gewürz—Die neuroprotektive Wirkung eines Safranextraktes. Z Phytother. 2012; 33(6):263–271

Grass-Krapanke B, Busmane A, Lasmanis A, Hoerr R, Kaschel R. Effects of Ginkgo Biloba Special Extract EGb 761® in very mild Cognitive Impairment. Neurosci Med. 2011; 2(1):48–56

Herrschaft H, Nacu A, Likhachev S, Sholomov I, Hoerr F. Schlaefke S. Ginkgo biloba extract EGb®761 in dementia with neuropsychiatric features: a randomised, placebo-controlled trial to confirm the efficacy and safety dose of 240 mg. J Psychiatr Res. 2012; 46(6): 716–723

Heui S, Lavretsky H. The aging brain: current concepts, intervention strategies and the role of Ginkgo biloba extract EGb 761. Introduction. Int Psychogeriatr. 2012; 24 Suppl 1:S1–S2

Janssen IM, Sturtz S, Skipka G, Zentner A, Velasco Garrido M, Busse R. Ginkgo biloba in Alzheimer's disease: a systematic review. Wien Med Wochenschr. 2010; 160(21–22):539–546

Kanowski S, Herrmann WM, Stephan K, Wierich W, Hörr R. Proof of efficacy of the ginkgo biloba special extract EGb 761 in outpatients suffering from mild to moderate primary degenerative dementia of the Alzheimer type or multi-infarct dementia. Pharmacopsychiatry. 1996; 29(2):47–56

Kaschel R. Specific memory effects of Ginkgo biloba extract EGb 761 in middle-aged healthy volunteers. Phytomedicine. 2011; 18(14):1202–1207

Kuschinsky G. Homöopathie und ärztliche Praxis. Dtsch Ärztebl/Arztl Mitteilungen. 1975a; 8:496

Kuschinsky G. Homöopathie und ärztliche Praxis. Dtsch Ärztebl/Ärztl Mitteilungen. 1975b; 20:1425:1429

Lautenschlager NT, Ihl R, Müller WE. Ginkgo biloba extract EGb 761® in the context of current developments in the diagnosis and treatment of age-related cognitive decline and Alzheimer's disease: a research perspective. Int Psychogeriatr. 2012;24 Suppl 1:S46–S50.

Le Bars PL, Katz MM, Berman N, Itil TM, Freedman AM, Schatzberg AF. A placebo-controlled, double-blind, randomized trial of an extract of Ginkgo biloba for dementia. North American EGb Study Group. JAMA. 1997; 278(16):1327–1332

Napryeyenko O, Borzenko I. (GINDEM-NP Study Group). Ginkgo biloba special extract in dementia with neuropsychiatric features. A randomised, placebo-controlled, double-blind clinical trial. Arzneimittelforschung. 2007; 57(1):4–11

Oken BS, Storzbach DM, Kaye JA. The efficacy of Ginkgo biloba on cognitive function in Alzheimer disease. Arch Neurol. 1998; 55 (11):1409–1415

Schulz V. Risiken und Kosten bei der Therapie mit Antidementiva—Ginkgo-biloba-Extrakt im Vergleich mit Acetylcholinesterasehemmern. Zeitschr f Phytotherapie. 2007; 28(1):17–20

Wettstein A. Cholinesterasehemmer und Ginkgoextrakte in der Demenztherapie vergleichbar? Vergleich publizierter plazebokontrollierter Wirksamkeitsstudien von mindestens sechsmonatiger Dauer. Fortschr Med Orig. 1999; 117:11–18

8.6 Vascular Headache, Neuralgia

8.6.1 Migraines

Migraines and migraine-like vasomotor headaches and neuralgia are common disorders. **Trigeminal neuralgia** and classic **migraines** can severely impact well-being.

There are no typical plant-based analgesics that can provide the kind of reliable acute effects of synthetic drugs. However, aspirin, one of the first and very effective analgesics, is derived from willow bark and therefore has medicinal plant origins. The strongest analgesic effect is still provided by the opiate alkaloids of the poppy plant. However, today, this area is dominated by synthetic preparations and derivatives as isolated active constituents.

Some phytotherapeutics are suitable as a remedy of first choice for symptomatic treatment of primarily mild pain. Frequently, these remedies can preclude the need for synthetic analgesics. This includes **willow bark** extract preparations and **Indian snakeroot**, which is especially useful for headaches that occur in conjunction with latent hypertension.

Butterbur and **peppermint** are two newly researched plants whose efficacy has been documented.

▶ **Note.** In the past, monkshood (Aconitum napellus) was used to treat neuralgia, including trigeminal neuralgia. This prescription is now considered obsolete. The Commission E issued a negative monograph for monkshood due to insufficiently documented efficacy and its risk profile as an alkaloid drug. However, Tinctura Aconiti in its various potentiations is still used successfully in homeopathy.

Plants Used in Treatment

Butterbur (Petasites hybridus)

Butterbur (▶ Fig. 8.9) is a member of the Asteraceae family and is found all over Europe. In Germany, it grows abundantly along riverbanks and in moist, spring-saturated forest floors. Usually, large plant contingents are clustered together. Its reddish flower heads with narrow reddish involucral bracts and pale purple flower petals appear in the spring. In the summer, roundish leaves grow from the rootstock. Butterbur leaves are some of the largest leaves found in plants native to Germany. The name petasites comes from the Greek *petasos* means hat with a wide brim.

Medicinal applications use the **butterbur rootstock** (Petasitidis rhizoma).

▶ **Note.** Butterbur needs to be distinguished from coltsfoot (Tussilago farfara). Coltsfoot's golden yellow flowers look very different, but its leaves can also reach a very large size, although not as large as those of butterbur. Coltsfoot leaves feature white woolly hairs on the underside. The underside of butterbur leaves are more gray than white wholly hairs.

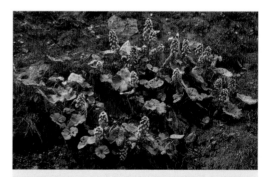

Fig. 8.9 Butterbur, Petasites hybridus. Photo: Dr. Roland Spohn, Engen.

Butterbur contains a significantly higher amount of pyrrolizidine alkaloids than coltsfoot, even though this can vary widely biologically.

▶ **Pharmacology.** The most important constituents of butterbur are **petasin** and **isopetasin**, which have spasmolytic as well as analgesic effects. However, butterbur (p. 352) also contains pyrrolizidine alkaloids with a 1,2-unsaturated necine structure. As discussed previously, from a toxicology perspective, these constituents present a **carcinogenic risk**.

▶ **Indications.** The Commission E listed only one indication it its monograph for butterbur root—supportive therapy for acute spastic pain in the urinary tract—and limited its use to 4 to 6 weeks a year.

Breeding and new extraction methods have made extracts possible that contain no or very little pyrrolizidine alkaloids (< 0.001%). This means that their use is no longer limited. The indication of **migraine** for butterbur is supported by a new study that has proven its efficacy.

▶ **Research.** In a randomized, placebo-controlled, double-blind trial, Grossmann and Schmidramsel studied 58 patients with migraines who received either 100 mg of a defined butterbur extract or a placebo for 12 weeks. They showed that the extract significantly reduced the frequency and duration of migraines. No adverse effects were documented. The authors state that its high efficacy and excellent tolerability makes butterbur especially suitable for prophylactic migraine treatment. Other authors reevaluated the results of this study and confirmed butterbur's superiority compared to placebo (Diener et al.) (see Bibliography (p. 284)).

Another randomized, placebo-controlled, double-blind trial involving 245 patients documented the preventive effects of a butterbur extract. Treatment of 4 months using 75 and 50 mg of the extract significantly reduced the frequency of migraines compared to placebo. There were few observed adverse effects and the extract was well tolerated (Lipton et al.).

Mentha piperita

For more information about this plant, see Peppermint (p. 46).

This section discusses only the use of **peppermint essential oil** (Menthae piperitae aetheroleum).

▶ **Indications.** Many studies document the efficacy of peppermint oil for vasomotor headaches.

▶ **Research.** In a very elaborate randomized, placebo-controlled, double-blind study, Göbel et al. researched the efficacy of 10% peppermint oil (LI 170) and paracetamol or aspirin compared to placebo in patients with episodic or chronic tension headaches. Statistical data was available for 105 patients.

Clinical improvements within 4 hours were seen in 30.5% of the placebo group, 54.3% of the paracetamol group and 56.2% of the peppermint oil group. When paracetamol was combined with peppermint oil applied to the temples and forehead, 66.7% of patients achieved improvements within that defined time frame. Tolerability was excellent.

In another trial, the same authors studied the peppermint oil solution LI 170 compared to 100 mg of paracetamol. They analyzed 408 migraine attacks in 102 patients. No differences were seen between peppermint oil, paracetamol, and placebo.

The authors also conducted a placebo-controlled trial of aspirin in patients with tension headaches and documented clinical improvements in 77.3% of the patients treated with peppermint oil compared to 86.4% for aspirin and 27.3% for the placebo.

Yellow Jessamine (Gelsemium sempervirens)

For a detailed description of this plant, see yellow jessamine (p. 165).

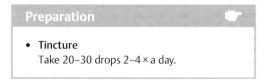

Preparation

- **Tincture**
  Take 20–30 drops 2–4 × a day.

Norway Spruce (Picea abies)

This preparation uses the needles and bark of these trees, primarily spruce. Younger, small branches from older trees (60–80 years) are preferred because they contain the highest level and best quality active constituents.

Natural spruce needle extract is created by distillation to obtain the spruce essential oil. The water-soluble constituents are extracted and then vacuum processed to the consistency of a syrup. Then the spruce needle essential oil is added back into the extract.

Fir or pine needle extracts are created in the same manner. Spruce needle is the most typical, which is why its preparations are described in this chapter.

Preparations

- **Spruce Needle Oil**
  For a full bath, add about a shot glass full to the bathwater.
- **Spruce Needle Whole Extract**
  The whole extract is derived from needles and small twigs. It contains volatile oil and 15–16% tannic acid. Add 50–100 mL of the whole extract for a full bath.
- **Tanbark Bath (Lohtannin)**
  This bath addition consists of the tree bark and contains 26–28% tannins, which provides increased stimulation. Add 20 mL of the preparation for a full bath.
- **Spruce Wood Bath**
  This bath addition consists of the wood of the tree and contains only small amounts of volatile oil.

  All spruce needle baths should be followed by at least a 1-hour rest period.

Special Treatments

All types of neuralgia benefit from applying **spirit inunctions** to the temples, which provide a mild **hyperemic** effect.

The following **types of spirit** are common:
- **Juniper spirit** (Spiritus Juniperi)
- **Stinging Nettle spirit** (Spiritus Urticae)
- **Rosemary spirit** (Spiritus Rosmarini)
- **Calamus spirit** (Spiritus Calami)

The following spirits are more **calming**:
- **Lemon Balm spirit** (Spiritus Melissae compositus)
- **Lavender spirit** (Spiritus Lavandulae)

Bibliography

Diener HC, Rahlfs VW, Danesch U. The first placebo-controlled trial of a special butterbur root extract for the prevention of migraine: reanalysis of efficacy criteria. Eur Neurol. 2004; 51 (2):89–97

Göbel H, Heinze A, Dworschak M, Heinze-Kuhn K, Stolze H. Placebokontrollierte, randomisierte und doppelblinde Studien zur Analyse der Wirksamkeit und Verträglichkeit von Oleum-menthae-piperitae-Lösung LI 170 bei Kopfschmerz vom Spannungstyp und Migräne. In: Rietbrock N, ed Phytopharmaka. Vol VI. Darmstadt: Steinkopff; 2002: 118–132

Grossmann M, Schmidramsl H. An extract of Petasites hybridus is effective in the prophylaxis of migraine. Int J Clin Pharmacol Ther. 2000; 38(9):430–435

Lipton RB, Göbel H, Einhäupl KM, Wilks K, Mauskop A. Petasites hybridus root (butterbur) is an effective preventive treatment for migraine. Neurology. 2004; 63(12):2240–2244

8.7 Addiction Recovery

8.7.1 Nicotine Addiction

Plants Used in Treatment

Oats (Avena sativa)

Oats is not only a well-known grain, but is also used as a medicinal plant. It is said to be sedative and sleep promoting based on the phenol glucoside vanilloside and the tryptamine derivative gramine it contains. However, this conclusion is based primarily on conclusion by analogy.

The frequently asserted and described effects of oats are likely very similar to passionflower and also very weak.

Medicinal applications use an alcoholic extraction of **oat fruit** (seeds/grains, Avenae fructus decorticatus).

Oat straw (Avenae stramentum) does not seem to contain the active substance or contains only minimal amounts. It contains mainly pectins and silicic acid.

▶ **Indications.** The Commission E monograph for oat straw lists a dermatological indication and took a very skeptical view of the sedative effects of oats.

However, an older report documents the efficacy of oats for the very special indication of nicotine withdrawal.

▶ **Research.** Anand reported in *Nature* magazine about a visit to India during which he was introduced to ancient Ayurvedic medicine, which uses decoctions of ordinary oats for opium withdrawal treatment. This made him realize that oats may be used for nicotine withdrawal. He prepared an alcoholic extract of fresh plants and gave it to a group of 26 heavy cigarette smokers.

A similar group of 26 received a placebo. Oats were significantly superior and this effect was unambiguously documented statistically. The number of cigarettes smoked in the oats group decreased significantly and this withdrawal effect persisted for 2 months after discontinuing the medication.

Bibliography

Anand CL. Effect of Avena sativa on cigarette smoking. Nature. 1971; 233(5320):496

Questions

1. Which medicinal plants are sleep promoting?
2. Which combination of two plants is especially well suited for this indication?
3. Which plant is well suited as a daytime sedative?
4. Formulate a sleep tea.
5. How seriously does one need to take the photosensitizing effects of therapeutic dosages of St.-John's-wort?
6. Which substance groups does St.-John's-wort interact with?
7. Are there plants that stimulate the central nervous system? If yes, what are they?
8. Which plant extract has unambiguous, evidence-based proof of efficacy for treatment of dementia, including Alzheimer type dementia?
9. Which external application of an essential oil has been proven in practice with vasomotor headaches?

Answers (p. 422) for Chapter 8.

9 Skin Disorders

The skin is referred to as the "mirror of the soul" for good reasons. It reflects the close correlation between body and psyche in many conspicuous ways. This makes skin disorders even harder to bear for many patients. Purely symptomatic therapy using synthetics often provides only temporary relief. This chapter provides an overview of the many reliable medicinal plant remedies that have been shown to be efficacious for treating skin disorders and that frequently provide holistic and even causal therapy.

The **skin** is one of the central organs of the human organism. Its surface spans about 2 m² and it weighs almost 4 kg. This makes the skin one of the largest and also one of the most varied organ systems—it not only fulfills sensory and metabolic functions but also functions as the interface that humans use to communicate with and to delineate themselves from the world. The skin is also an interesting organ from a psychosomatic point of view. The disfiguring effects of many eczematous skin disorders impact not only the skin as an organ but also cause mental distress. With chronic skin disorders, these two components are in a constant state of interdependence. Healthy, clear, beautiful skin is very important for our **well-being** and **sense of self**.

Modern dermatology has access to sophisticated and even morphological diagnostics. At the same time, it is impressive how experienced dermatologists can frequently arrive at a diagnosis based on clinical observation, without making use of any technical tools. Despite this comprehensive body of knowledge dermatology seems to have been bypassed by the whirlwind of synthetic therapeutic developments seen, for example, in cardiology or in gastroenterology. Dermatology offers only **symptomatic treatment systems** based on glucocorticoids, antibiotics, and antimycotics.

Phytotherapeutics offer a range of additional therapeutic possibilities for treating skin disorders. However, phytotherapeutic treatments require sufficient patience for long-term treatment and possible healing of the root causes. This patience is often lacking and patients/practitioners then again resort to the quick relief provided by corticosteroid ointments.

Willuhn (1992) has published a critical overview of plant-based dermatics that is worth reading.

Medicinal Plants

Acute Weeping Eczema
Common Oak (Quercus robur), Sessile Oak (Quercus petraea)
Mallow, Malva sylvestris
Heart's Ease, Viola tricolor
English Walnut, Juglans regia
Balloon Vine, Cardiospermum halicacabum
Common Mallow (Cheeseweed), Malva neglecta
German Chamomile, Matricaria recutita

Dry Eczema
Beech, Fagus sylvatica
Birch, Betula pendula, Betula pubescens, Betula verrucosa
Juniper, Juniperus communis
Pine, Pinus sylvestris
Woody Nightshade, Solanum dulcamara
Kidney Bean, Phaseolus vulgaris
Sand Sedge, Carex arenaria
Wheat, Triticum aestivum
Oats, Avena sativa

Atopic Dermatitis
Evening Primrose, Oenothera biennis
Wheat, Triticum aestivum
Oats, Avena sativa

Venous Ulcer (Ulcus cruris)
Comfrey, Symphytum officinale
St.-John's-wort, Hypericum perforatum
Horse Chestnut, Aesculus hippocastanum
Common Oak (Quercus robur), **Sessile Oak** (Quercus petraea)
German Chamomile, Matricaria recutita
Calendula, Calendula officinalis

Furunculosis
Flax, Linum usitatissimum
Hay Flower, Graminis flos
Common Oak (Quercus robur), Sessile Oak (Quercus petraea)
Arnica, Arnica montana

Chilblains
Common Oak (Quercus robur), Sessile Oak (Quercus petraea)

Tormentil, Potentilla tormentilla
Horsetail, Equisetum arvense

Lymphedema
Horse Chestnut, Aesculus hippocastanum

Wounds, Contusions, Distortions
Arnica, Arnica montana
Foxglove, Digitalis lanata/purpurea
Comfrey, Symphytum officinale
Purple Echinacea, Echinacea purpurea
Calendula, Calendula officinalis
Witch Hazel, Hamamelis virginiana
Horsetail, Equisetum arvense

9.1 Dermatitis and Eczema

9.1.1 Acute, Wet Eczema

Medicinal Plants

Common Oak (Quercus robur), **Sessile Oak**
(Quercus petraea)
Oak bark, Quercus cortex
Mallow, Malva sylvestris
Mallow leaves and flowers, Malvae folium
et flos
Heart's Ease, Viola tricolor
Heart's ease herb, Violae tricoloris herba
English Walnut, Juglans regia
Walnut leaves, Juglandis folium
Balloon Vine, Cardiospermum halicacabum
Balloon vine herb, Cardiospermi herba
Common Mallow, Malva neglecta
Mallow leaves and flowers, Malvae folium
et flos
German Chamomile, Matricaria recutita
German chamomile flowers, Matricariae flos

The treatment principle for wet eczema is "moist on moist." This disorder initially requires moist compresses, or better yet, moist **poultices**. Once the weeping and acute inflammation have resolved, treatment can progress first to pastes and then to ointments. This treatment principle applies to any type of wet eczema or dermatitis.

When applied correctly, this treatment causes acute symptoms to improve surprisingly quickly.

▶ **Application of Moist Poultices.** Linen cloths, gauze compresses, or absorbent washing mitts provide the most suitable material for **loose and breathable moist compresses**. Poultices are placed on the skin in the morning, midday, and evening for about 1–2 hours. They need to be replaced as soon as they become dry and warm, usually every 10 to a maximum of 20 minutes. Between treatments, the area is covered with a moist compress without active constituents and loosely wrapped.

Poultices should never be covered by non-breathable materials. Such materials, if they are used at all, should only be placed under the extremity being treated, for example, under the leg for wet eczema of the lower leg to protect pillows or sheets. Patients should be specifically instructed about this point and carefully instructed about the treatment method.

Oak bark and **mallow** are the main medicinal plants used for moist poultices.

Plants Used in Treatment

Common Oak (Quercus robur), Sessile Oak (Quercus patraea)

Oaks are well-known trees in the German landscape. In Germany, common oak (Quercus robur) (▶ Fig. 9.1) and sessile oak (Quercus petraea) are common.

Medicinal applications use the **oak bark** (Quercus cortex).

▶ **Pharmacology.** The drug contains large amounts of tannin. This provides the basis for its primarily **astringent effect**. Oak bark is also considered antiphlogistic and virostatic.

In addition to tannin, oak bark also contains quercetin (see Oak (p. 87)). Oak tannin is tolerated extremely well and there is no concern about skin irritation.

▶ **Indications. Contact eczema of the lower arms** in its fresh, weeping phase is a popular indication for oak bark. This treatment is also very suitable for weeping **eczema** surrounding ulcers **of the lower legs**. The ulcer itself will also be cleansed by this treatment and becomes more responsive to treatment with ointments.

The Commission E monograph for oak bark lists the indications inflammatory skin diseases (external use); nonspecific, acute diarrhea (internal use)

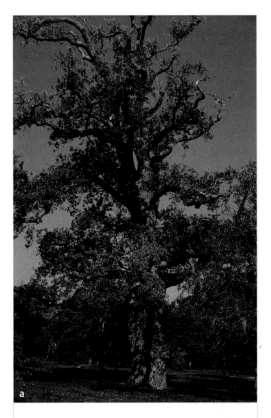

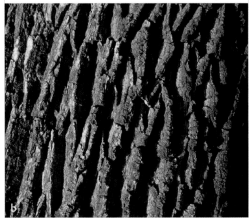

Fig. 9.1 a and b Common Oak, Quercus robur.
Photos: Dr. Roland Spohn, Engen.

- **Decoction**
  For poultices: boil 1–2 tablespoons of chopped oak bark in 500 mL of water for 15 minutes. Strain, cool, and then use this undiluted liquid for poultices. A stronger decoction can be prepared in the morning and then diluting it for use with poultices during the day. This decoction must be freshly prepared each day.
  To prepare a decoction for hand or foot baths, simmer a small handful of oak board in 1 L of water for 15 minutes. Strain and add to bath water. If a full bath is indicated, finished pharmaceutical products that are easy to dose should be used.

▶ **Therapy Recommendations.** This treatment should be limited to 2–3 weeks due to its tannic and drying effects.

Oak poultices should be immediately resumed in case of exacerbation of the eczema with renewed weeping. Partial or full baths may be indicated for eczema on large areas of the body.

Mallow (Malva sylvestris)

For more information about this plant, see Mallow (p. 185).

The effects of mallow are weaker than that of oak bark.

▶ **Indications.** Mallow leaves and flowers are indicated for patients with very sensitive skin. This treatment can precede a subsequent oak bark treatment.

- **Decoction**
  For poultice preparation and instructions, see oak bark above.
  This decoction is intended for short-term use. As a rule, treatment can progress fairly quickly to other, more substantial applications.

as well as local treatment of mild inflammation of the oral cavity and pharyngeal region, and genital and anal area.

Heart's Ease (Viola tricolor)

Two types of heart's ease are found in Germany: **Viola tricolor arvensis** has primarily yellowish-white flowers and is found mostly in agricultural fields. **Viola tricolor vulgaris** (▶ Fig. 9.2) is larger, has violet flowers, and is found more often in meadows. Both types are used medicinally in the same manner.

Medicinal applications use the **whole heart's ease herb** (above-ground parts, Violae tricoloris herba).

▶ **Pharmacology.** Heart's ease herb is a saponin drug that also contains flavonoids and methyl salicylate glycosides.

▶ **Indications.** Heart's ease has been proven effective for treating **mild seborrheic dermatitis** and **infantile eczema (cradle cap)**. However, **chronic adult eczema** also frequently responds well to the internal use of heart's ease tea. This therapy needs to be continued long term.

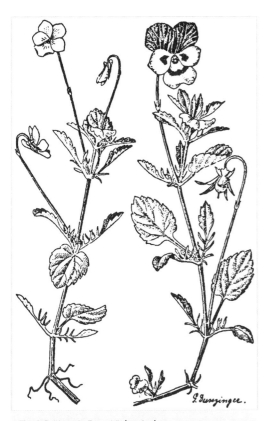

Fig. 9.2 Heart's Ease, Viola tricolor.

Preparation	

- **Tea**
  Add 1 cup of hot water to 1 teaspoon of the finely chopped drug. Steep for 5 minutes, then strain.
  Drink 1 cup several times a day.
  For moist warm poultices, soak gauze compresses in heart's ease tea. For this use, the tea can be less strong.

▶ **Therapy Recommendation.** Prescriptions for heart's ease should specify Violae tricoloris herba to prevent confusion with sweet violet (Viola odorata) (p. 190). Sweet violet root is used as an expectorant.

English Walnut (Juglans regia)

This large tree with its pinnate leaves (▶ Fig. 9.3) originates from the Middle East. In Germany, it is frequently planted in protected locations.

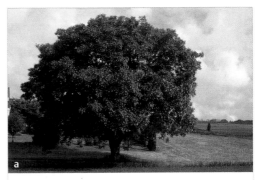

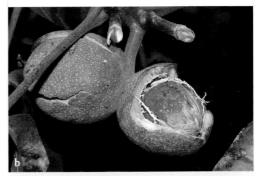

Fig. 9.3 a and b English Walnut, Juglans regia. Photos: Dr. Roland Spohn, Engen.

Medicinal applications use the **walnut leaves** (Juglandis folium).

▶ **Indications.** Walnut leaves are considered a remedy for **chronic eczema**, **scrofula**, and **marginal blepharitis**. However, its efficacy is much less reliable than that of heart's ease.

> **Preparations**
>
> - **Decoction**
>   For poultices, boil 2 teaspoons of the drug in 500 mL of water for 10–15 minutes, then strain.
>   Equal parts of heart's ease and walnut leaves provide a useful remedy.
> - **Tea**
>   Add 2 cups of cold water to 1 tablespoon of walnut leaves. Boil for 5 minutes, then strain. Drink 1–2 cups 2 × a day.

Balloon Vine (Cardiospermum halicacabum)

Medicinal applications use the above-ground, flowering parts of the **balloon vine plant** (Cardiospermi herba) and processed in accordance with the German standard homeopathic instructions for preparation into a mother tincture (as described in the *German Homoeopathic Pharmacopoeia (GHP)*).

▶ **Indications.** In a controlled study, Merklinger et al. documented very good treatment results for an ointment containing balloon vine (Cardiospermum halicacabum L.) in healing different types of **chronic dermatitis**.

Common Mallow (Cheeseweed, Malva neglecta)

This plant is common in meadows but is easily overlooked (or neglected, as its Latin name *neglecta* indicates). Its flowers are much smaller than those of the large, beautiful mallow (Malva sylvestris). Its corolla petals are less than the size of its calyx sepals and very inconspicuous, but they are also reddish, with more intense reddish-blue stripes.

Medicinal applications use the **common mallow leaves** (Malvae folium) and **flowers** (Malvae flos).

▶ **Indications.** Moist poultices can calm **exudative dermatitis** quickly in preparation for the use of stronger ointments.

> **Preparation**
>
> - **Decoction**
>   For poultices, add 2 teaspoons of the drug to 500 mL of water. Boil for 10 minutes, then strain.

German Chamomile (Matricaria recutita)

For more information about this plant, see German Chamomile (p. 42).

Chamomile is **anti-inflammatory**. An irritating effect during acute, weeping stages is explained by the stimulation of granulation.

▶ **Indications.** German chamomile is more suitable for use with **torpid ulcers** and less for extensive areas of skin inflammation.

> **Preparations**
>
> - **Infusion**
>   For poultices, add 1 cup of boiling water to 2 teaspoons of the drug. Steep for 5–10 minutes, then strain.
> - **Lotio Alba with German Chamomile Fluid Extract**
>   Subacute eczema that is no longer weeping when being treated with moist poultices then needs to be treated with lotio alba ("white lotion"). This white liquid suspension contains bentonite clay, zinc oxide, talc, propylene glycol, and water. The liquid is shaken and then brushed onto the skin areas to be treated. If a stronger lotion is desired, 2 g of German chamomile fluid extract can be added to 100 g of lotio alba.
> - **Zinc Paste with Chamomile Extract or St.-John's-wort Oil**
>   If the lotio alba treatment described above is well tolerated, treatment can proceed first to pastes and finally to ointments. Normally, 1% chamomile extract is added to the zinc paste. For very refractory torpid eczema, the addition of 2–5% of St.-John's-wort oil is recommended. Zinc paste works very well.

▶ **Therapy Recommendation.** Chamomile tea is less effective than oak bark, which is the remedy of first choice. If the area to be treated is very inflamed, treatment can alternate between oak bark decoction and chamomile tea.

9.1.2 Dry Eczema

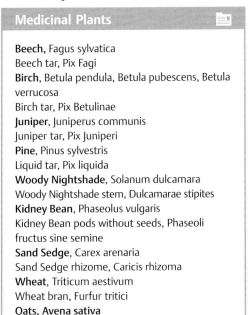

Medicinal Plants

Beech, Fagus sylvatica
Beech tar, Pix Fagi
Birch, Betula pendula, Betula pubescens, Betula verrucosa
Birch tar, Pix Betulinae
Juniper, Juniperus communis
Juniper tar, Pix Juniperi
Pine, Pinus sylvestris
Liquid tar, Pix liquida
Woody Nightshade, Solanum dulcamara
Woody Nightshade stem, Dulcamarae stipites
Kidney Bean, Phaseolus vulgaris
Kidney Bean pods without seeds, Phaseoli fructus sine semine
Sand Sedge, Carex arenaria
Sand Sedge rhizome, Caricis rhizoma
Wheat, Triticum aestivum
Wheat bran, Furfur tritici
Oats, Avena sativa
Oat straw, Avenae stramentum

Plants Used in Treatment

As soon as the eczema has transitioned to a dry, chronic stage, it can be treated externally with several types of wood tar derived from pine, beech, birch, or juniper. When applied correctly, tar therapy is one of the best treatment methods for chronic eczema.

▶ **Application of Tar Types.** All types of tar are applied by carefully increasing their concentration, from 0.25% to 0.5% and finally to 1% in dry preparations, which are then brushed on the eczema area, or in zinc paste. If these concentrations are well tolerated, they can be increased to 5–10% or even higher until finally, pure tar preparations are applied.

> **Caution** ⚠
>
> Tar treatments can cause kidney irritation. During long-term treatment or treatment of large areas of skin, the patient's urine should be repeatedly tested for proteins and sediments. Carboluria (presence of phenols in the urine) causes the urine to turn black when exposed to air for a longer period.

Beech, Fagus sylvatica

Beech tar (Pix Fagi, also called Oleum Fagi empyrheumaticum) is derived from beech trees. This blackish-brown, syrupy mass is lighter in color than pine tar (see below).

Beech tar is distilled into creosote.

Birch (Betula pendula, Betula pubescens, Betula verrucosa)

For more information about this plant, see Birch (p. 238).

Birch tar (Pix Betulinae or Oleum Rusci) is derived from this plant. It is lighter and greenish brown in color and exudes a peculiar odor. It contains a mixture of guaiacol, creosote, cresol, and a small amount of carbolic acid.

Birch tar is considered a mild plant-derived tar that is especially well suited for treating many types of chronic eczema.

Juniper (Juniperus communis)

For more information about this plant, see Juniper (p. 220).

Juniper tar (Pix Juniperi) is a brown, syrupy mass with a similar composition as birch tar. It also contains a small amount of phenol, and its disinfecting action is rather weak. Some dermatologists prefer juniper tar because it is well tolerated by the skin.

Pine (Pinus sylvestris)

Conifer or pine tar (Pix liquida) is derived from dry distillation of wood from various types of pine, usually from Scots pine (Pinus sylvestris).

Pine tar is a blackish-brown liquid that exudes an intense odor. It is largely insoluble in water but is soluble in alcohol. Its main constituents are phenols with keratoplastic and antiseptic actions.

Pine tar is a strong skin irritant. The other plant-derived tars discussed in this section are usually better tolerated and are therefore preferred.

Dermatotropic Antidyscratics

The close relationship between chronic eczema and metabolic disorders, in the most general sense, is known, but difficult to assess in individual cases. Gastrointestinal disorders, especially chronic constipation, are a good indicator. In the absence of such indicators, various therapeutic approaches need to be tried to see if they make a difference. Experience has shown that some chronic eczema conditions respond surprisingly well and quickly to **metabolic transposition**. Medical treatment of eczema is more successful when it is preceded by a diet or fasting. Other cases are refractory and there are many transitions between those two extremes.

Dermatotropic antidyscratics are a treatment option for this condition. This term refers to the plants described in Plants Used in Treatment: Internal Use for Treatment of Rheumatic Disorders (p. 237). They are described there as aquaretics in the most general sense: woody nightshade (Solanum dulcamara) (p. 238), kidney bean (Phaseolus vulgaris) (p. 239) and sand sedge (Carex arenaria) (p. 240).

Laxatives

Strong laxatives are also indicated for dry eczema, primarily senna leaves (see below for prescriptions). A strong "metabolic tea" with an added antidyscratic can be very efficacious for chronic eczema.

Proven Prescriptions

Prescriptions	

Rx
Sennae fol. 40.0 (senna leaves)
Carvi fruct. (caraway seeds)
Matricariae flos (German chamomile flowers)
Dulcamarae stipit. 20.0 (woody nightshade stems)
M. f. spec.
Add 1 cup of boiling water to 2 teaspoons of the blend. Steep for 20 minutes, then strain.
D.S.
Drink 1 cup in the morning and in the evening.

Prescriptions	

Rx
Dulcamarae stipit. (woody nightshade stems)
Caricis rhiz. (sand sedge rhizome)
Urticae herb. (stinging nettle herb)
Taraxaci rad. c. herb. (dandelion root and herb)
Sennae fol. (senna leaves)
Foeniculi fruct. āā ad 100.0 (fennel seeds)
M. f. spec.
Add 1 cup of boiling water to 1–2 teaspoons of the blend. Steep for 10 minutes, then strain.
D.S.
Drink 1 cup in the morning and in the evening for 4 weeks.

Additional Therapy Options

Wheat (Triticum aestivum)

This treatment uses wheat bran.

Preparation	

- **Full Bath**
  Use 150 g of wheat bran for a full bath.

Oats (Avena sativa)

This treatment uses oat straw (Avenae stramentum).

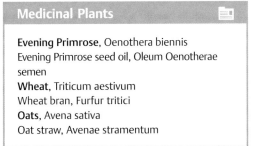

Preparation

- **Decoction**
  For a full bath, add 50 g of the drug to 2 L of water. Boil for 30 minutes, then strain, and add to the bath water.

9.2 Atopic Dermatitis

9.2.1 Neurodermatitis

Medicinal Plants

Evening Primrose, Oenothera biennis
Evening Primrose seed oil, Oleum Oenotherae semen
Wheat, Triticum aestivum
Wheat bran, Furfur tritici
Oats, Avena sativa
Oat straw, Avenae stramentum

The treatment of neurodermatitis or atopic dermatitis presents a profound therapeutic challenge, especially with young children. In our experience, cortisone ointments are used much too quickly. They provide transitory improvements, but used long term, tend to cause this type of eczema to become chronic.

This indication is especially conducive to being treated by making use of the full range of phytotherapy options. Of these, evening primrose seed oil is especially suitable.

Plants Used in Treatment

Evening Primrose (Oenothera biennis)

Evening primrose grows to a height of 1–2 m and has beautiful, bright yellow flowers. It was brought to Germany from North America about 400 years ago. It prefers sandy soils and, in Germany, is frequently found growing along railroad embankments. Its name is derived from the fact that its flowers first open in the evening and stay fully open the next day.

Newer research shows that evening primrose seeds contain high amounts of a fatty oil (**Oleum Oenothera semen**); its aromatic flavor is reminiscent of poppy seed oil.

▶ **Note.** In the past, the fleshy roots of evening primrose were harvested in the autumn and eaten as a vegetable. They were boiled in a type of broth containing vinegar and oil. Evening primrose seeds were recommended as a coffee substitute.

▶ **Pharmacology.** Evening primrose seed oil contains 70% linoleic acid and about 10% γ-linolenic acid (GLA).

There is a high likelihood that neurodermatitis is caused by metabolic disorders involving long-chain essential fatty acids. These fatty acids, in turn, are precursors of the highly active prostaglandins E_1 und E2. According to Willuhn (1992), there are numerous indicators that people suffering from neurodermatitis have lower δ-6-desaturase activity. This causes insufficient production of γ-linolenic acid, which can be supplemented by evening primrose seed oil.

Experience to date has shown that this **substitution therapy** can be helpful. However, it is not sufficient on its own for treating neurodermatitis.

▶ **Indications.** Essential omega-6 fatty acids are increasingly used orally and topically to treat **neurodermatitis**.

▶ **Therapy Recommendation.** To be successful, γ-linolenic acid needs to be substituted at a minimum rate of 240–320 mg/d. Skin improvements take 4 to 12 weeks to become apparent; 60–70% of patients treated in this manner should respond to this treatment.

Wheat (Triticum aestivum)

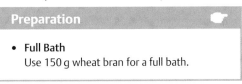

Preparation

- **Full Bath**
  Use 150 g wheat bran for a full bath.

Oats (Avena sativa)

Preparation

- **Decoction**
  For a full bath, add 50 g of the drug (oat straw, Avenae stramentum) to 2 L of water. Boil for 30 minutes, then strain, and add to the bath water. Oat straw contains primarily pectins and silicic acid.

9.3 Venous Ulcers (Ulcus cruris)

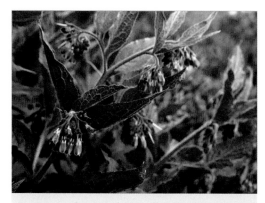

Fig. 9.4 Comfrey, Symphytum officinale. Photo: Thieme Verlagsgruppe, Stuttgart.

9.3.1 External Applications

The multitude of therapy recommendations for venous ulcers (also called leg ulcers, venous insufficiency ulceration, stasis ulcers, stasis dermatitis, varicose ulcers, or ulcus cruris) indicates that treatment of such chronic ulcers is difficult. Venous ulcers almost always occur in conjunction with arterial or venous vascular disorders. We present the following phytotherapy recommendations, but no single therapy can claim to be the sole valid therapy.

Plants Used in Treatment

Comfrey (Symphytum officinale)

Comfrey is an ancient medicinal plant. This tall plant with rough, hairy stems and leaves frequently grows wild in damp soil, for example, in damp meadows or along the edges of ditches. Its pendulous, bell-shaped flowers are reddish violet and sometimes white. Its narrow leaves are attached linearly along the stem (▶ Fig. 9.4).

Comfrey is a member of the Boraginaceae family. Its German name *Beinwell* (bein = leg) indicates its traditional use for treating leg disorders.

Medicinal applications use the **comfrey root, herb,** and **leaves** (Symphyti radix, herba, folium)

▶ **Note.** The traditional names for comfrey in English (boneset, knitbone) and the German *Beinwell*, which is derived from the Old High

German *Wallwurz* (wallen = knitting together of bones), all point to the fact that the callus-promoting and wound-healing power of this plant has been known for a long time. The Latin name *consolida* (*consolidare* = to tie together) used for this plant by the healer Hildegard von Bingen signifies a similar meaning. The English name comfrey refers to Symphytum officinale as well as to Symphytum peregrinum, also called Russian comfrey (*peregrinum* = from a foreign land). Russian comfrey is cultivated widely in the USA, Australia, and New Zealand as feedstock. In East Prussia (an area of east of present-day Pomerania), this plant was eaten as a vegetable by the so-called comfrey eaters. A comfrey tea prepared from the whole plant or the root and primarily from the leaves was used widely as a "blood cleansing remedy."

▶ **Pharmacology.** The comfrey drug contains allantoin and mucopolysaccharides (glycosaminoglycans or GAGs).

Comfrey's therapeutic effect is attributed primarily to allantoin, which promotes granulation and callus formation. Antimitotic effects have also been described.

Comfrey—like coltsfoot, butterbur, and plants in the Senecio genus—contain toxic pyrrolizidine alkaloids with a 1.2 unsaturated necine structure. Experiments have shown mutagenic and carcinogenic effects for these substances. However, no increases in cancer risk compared with the average population have been shown epidemiologically for the groups of comfrey eaters (mentioned above) compared to the average population or in animals fed comfrey, which were exposed to the alleged carcinogenic potential of comfrey. In addition, primary liver cancer that does not occur in conjunction with liver cirrhosis is rarely seen in Central European populations.

▶ **Note.** In the past, comfrey was also used to promote bone healing.

▶ **Indications.** Comfrey is used to treat refractory **varicose ulcers of the lower leg** and **chronic ulcerations**.

Comfrey is applied to venous ulcers as a paste. Experience has shown that this treatment reliably promotes granulation. However, care must be taken to avoid excessive granulation.

The Commission E decided—following long and frequently heated discussions—to approve only the external use of comfrey. The maximum daily dosage of toxic pyrrolizidine alkaloids is limited to 100 μg/d based on a pyrrolizidine alkaloid content of 5–7% in the drug or 1 ppm/g in finished pharmaceutical products. The products available today contain such reduced extracts of pyrrolizidine alkaloids that the recommended daily dose of less than 10 μg negates the posited health risks. This means that comfrey preparations can be used externally for as long as needed. Staiger published a very good review of the current state of comfrey research.

> ### Caution ⚠
>
> Internal use of comfrey is considered to be too risky by toxicologists.

Additional Therapy Options

St.-John's-wort (Hypericum perforatum)

For more information about this plant, see St.-John's-wort (p. 264).

▶ **Indications.** St.-John's-wort oil is recommended for the treatment of varicose vein disorders that tend toward venous ulcers.

> ### Preparation
>
> - **St.-John's-wort Oil**
>   Frequent external application of the oil to the legs is recommended.

Horse Chestnut (Aesculus hippocastanum)

For more information about this plant, see Horse Chestnut (p. 176).

Common Oak (Quercus robur), Sessile Oak (Quercus patraea)

For more information about this plant, see Oak (p. 287).

▶ **Indications.** Infected leg ulcers can be treated by applying moist poultices soaked in oak bark decoction. This can dry up weeping dermatitis. As mentioned earlier, oak bark is an astringent only and is never irritating or allergenic.

> ### Preparation
>
> - **Decoction**
>   For **poultices:** Add 1–2 tablespoons of the finely chopped drug to 500 mL of water. Boil for 15 minutes, then strain. Allow to cool and then use the undiluted liquid.
>   For **partial baths:** Add a small handful of oak bark to 1 L of water. Simmer for 15 minutes, then strain. Add to bath water.

German Chamomile (Matricaria recutita)

For more information about this plant, see German Chamomile (p. 42).

> ### Preparation
>
> - **Tea for Poultices:**
>   Add 1 cup of hot water to 2 teaspoons of the drug. Steep for 5–10 minutes, then strain.

Calendula (Calendula officinalis)

This member of the Asteraceae family is grown as a decorative plant in many gardens. Its beautiful large yellow-orange flowers have made this a very popular plant (▶ Fig. 9.5).

Medicinal applications use the **calendula flowers** (Calendulae flos), either whole flower heads including the green epicalyx, or the individual ray florets without the epicalyx (Isaac).

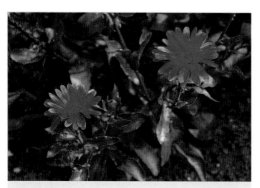

Fig. 9.5 Calendula, Calendula officinalis. Photo: Prof. Dr. Volker Fintelmann, Stuttgart.

▶ **Pharmacology.** Calendula contains triterpene glycosides, carotenoids, volatile oil, and bitters. Its effect is **antiphlogistic** and **granulation promoting**.

▶ **Indications.** Calendula is the treatment of first choice for initial treatment of **secondary infections** of leg ulcers.

The Commission E monograph for calendula lists the following uses: inflammation of the oral and pharyngeal mucosa, poorly healing wounds, and leg ulcers (ulcus cruris).

▶ **Research.** A randomized, single-blind, comparative study of 254 women receiving postoperative radiation for nonmetastasizing breast cancer showed that calendula ointment significantly reduced ($p < 0.001$) the intensity of substantial **radiation dermatitis** compared to a synthetic reference product commonly used in France. A total of 10 patients in the group treated with the synthetic, but no patients in the group treated with calendula ointment, had to stop radiation treatment due to the occurrence of severe radiation dermatitis. No cases of grade 4 radiation dermatitis with skin ulcerations were documented (Pommier et al.).

Preparations
• **Tea** For poultices: Add 1 tablespoon of the chopped drug to 500 mL of cold water. Bring to a brief boil, then strain. Apply poultices for 1–2 hours 2–3 × a day. • **Tincture** For rinsing: Add 2–4 mL of the tincture to 250–500 mL water that has been boiled and cooled.

9.4 Furunculosis

Medicinal Plants
Flax, Linum usitatissimum Flaxseeds, Lini semen **Grasses**, Gramineae (Poaceae) Hay flower, Graminis flos **Common Oak** (Quercus robur), **Sessile Oak** (Quercus patraea) Oak bark, Quercus cortex **Arnica**, Arnica montana Arnica flowers, Arnicae flos

9.4.1 Internal and External Applications

Refractory furunculosis (boils) is treated internally as well as externally using phytotherapeutic remedies. Treatment is primarily targeted at the digestive and metabolic systems. External poultices allow the boil to mature, which usually eliminates the need for the boil to be lanced. They also provide a significant reduction of symptoms for the patient.

Plants Used in Treatment: Laxative Drugs

Preparation
• **Tea** A mild laxative tea should be taken regularly and over a long period. An antidyscratic drug, for example, dandelion, can be added, similar to the treatment of chronic eczema. The tea can be made stronger by adding rosehips or other plants that contain vitamin C.

Prescriptions
Rx Urticae herb. (stinging nettle herb) Taraxaci rad. c. herb. (dandelion root and herb) Cynosbati fruct. (syn. Rosae pseudofructus, rosehips) Frangulae cort. (buckthorn bark) Sennae fol. (senna leaves) Anisi fruct. āā ad 100.0 (anise seeds) M. f. spec.

Add 1 cup of hot water to 2 teaspoons of the blend. Steep for 20 minutes, then strain.
D.S.
Drink 1 cup in the morning and in the evening.

▶ **Therapy Recommendation.** Laxative teas used to treat furunculosis should never be as strong as those used for chronic skin disorders. The amount of senna leaves used should be about half the amount used in a metabolic tea for treating chronic skin disorders.

Flax (Linum usitatissimum)

For more information about this plant, see Flax (p. 62).

▶ **Indications. Flaxseeds** (Lini semen) are a superior remedy for getting boils (furuncle) to mature.

Preparation

- **Poultice**
  Fill a small linen bag about one-third full of flaxseeds. Close the bag and briefly boil it in plenty of water. This will cause the flaxseeds to swell considerably and fill the entire bag. Remove the bag from the water and squeeze it carefully and briefly. Then quickly wrap the bag in a clean cloth and apply it as hot to the furuncle location as the patient can tolerate. Refill the linen bag with fresh flaxseeds and re-heat and re-apply the poultrice as frequently as possible.

Hay Flower (Graminis flos)

For more information about this plant, see Hay Flower (p. 245).

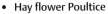
Preparation

- **Hay flower Poultice**
  See preparation of hay flower poultice (p. 246).
  Hay flower poultices are applied the same way as flaxseed (Lini semen) poultices (see above).

Common Oak (Quercus robur), Sessile Oak (Quercus patraea)

For more information about this plant, see Oak (p. 287).

Preparation

- **Decoction**
  For poultices: Add 1–2 tablespoons of the finely chopped drug to 500 mL of water. Boil for 15 minutes, then strain. Allow to cool to a tolerable temperature, soak the poultice in the undiluted liquid, and apply while warm.

Arnica (Arnica montana)

For more information about this plant, see Arnica (p. 144).

Preparation

- **Tincture**
  For poultices: Add 1 tablespoon of the drug to 1 L of cool water, soak the poultice in this liquid, and apply.

9.5 Chilblains

9.5.1 Astringents

Medicinal Plants

Common Oak (Quercus robur), **Sessile Oak** (Quercus patraea)
Quercus cortex
Tormentil, Potentilla tormentilla
Tormentil rhizome, Tormentillae rhizoma
Horsetail, Equisetum arvense
Equiseti herba

Plants Used in Treatment

Astringents are the treatment of first choice for chilblains.

Common Oak (Quercus robur), Sessile Oak (Quercus patraea)

For more information about this plant, see Oak (p. 287).

- **Decoction**
  For foot and hand baths: Add 200 g of the drug to 2 L of water. Boil for 15 minutes, strain, and use undiluted.

Tormentil (Potentilla tormentilla, Potentilla erecta)

For more information about this plant, see Tormentil (p. 84).

- **Tormentil Extract Blended with Glycerin**
  The following prescription can be brushed on the affected area.

Rx
Extr. Tormentill. sicc. 5.0 (tormentil extract)
Glycerin. 25.0 (glycerin)
D.S.
For external use; brush on the affected area.

- **Tormentil Tincture with Skin Stimulating Constituent**
  The following prescription is best applied to the skin immediately following baths.

Rx
Tinct. Tormentillae (tormentil tincture)
Spirit. Calami āā 25.0 (calamus spirit)
D.S.
For external application with chilblains.

Horsetail (Equisetum arvense)

For more information about this plant, see horsetail (p. 224).

- **Decoction**
  For partial baths: Add 2 tablespoons of the finely chopped drug to 500 mL of water. Boil for at least 30 minutes, then strain.
  This decoction activates the local connective tissue metabolism.

Additional Therapy Options

Taking a plant-derived bitter **tonic** starting several weeks before the period of frost can significantly increase peripheral circulation. Small amounts of a mild **cardiac remedy** can be added to support this effect.

Rx
Tinct. Nuc. Vomicae 10.0 (nux vomica tincture)
Tinct. Gentianae 20.0 (gentian tincture)
Tinct. Strophanthi 5.0 (strophanthin tincture)
D.S.
Take 30 drops 2 × a day in a little water shortly before meals.

9.6 Lymphedema

9.6.1 External Applications

Horse Chestnut, Aesculus hippocastanum
Horse chestnut seeds

Lymphedema and lymph stasis most frequently result from **trauma** and **inflammatory processes**. One well-known and difficult to treat example is lymphedema of the arm following breast amputation due to cancer. Lymphedema is frequently associated with **postthrombotic syndrome** (venous insufficiency) and can progress to severe swelling of the legs, also referred to as elephantiasis.

The main therapy options include exercise programs, compression dressing, and lymph drainage, according to Vodder. Local external application of lymph ointments that frequently contain horse chestnut can be used as supportive therapy.

Plants Used in Treatment

Horse Chestnut (Aesculus hippocastanum)

For more information about this plant, see Horse Chestnut (p. 176).

9.7 Wounds, Contusions, Distortions

9.7.1 External Applications

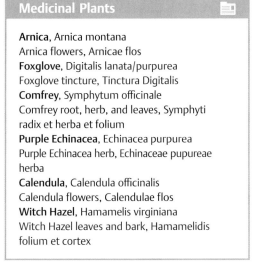

Medicinal Plants

Arnica, Arnica montana
Arnica flowers, Arnicae flos
Foxglove, Digitalis lanata/purpurea
Foxglove tincture, Tinctura Digitalis
Comfrey, Symphytum officinale
Comfrey root, herb, and leaves, Symphyti radix et herba et folium
Purple Echinacea, Echinacea purpurea
Purple Echinacea herb, Echinaceae pupureae herba
Calendula, Calendula officinalis
Calendula flowers, Calendulae flos
Witch Hazel, Hamamelis virginiana
Witch Hazel leaves and bark, Hamamelidis folium et cortex

The use of medicinal plants for treating wounds and skin suppuration is a very old tradition. Today, this type of treatment is dominated by chemotherapy using sulfonamides and antibiotics. However, phytotherapeutic remedies are still significant and will likely continue to play a role in the future. Ointments containing plant constituents strongly stimulate **granulation** and **epithelization**.

Wounds should first be **cleansed** using moist poultices. During the **healing phase**, ointments are then applied very thinly and primarily to the edges of wounds.

Plants Used in Treatment

Arnica (Arnica montana)

For more information about this plant, see Arnica (p. 144).

▶ **Indications.** Arnica is an excellent **wound healing remedy**. It is especially effective for torpid wounds that are coated in viscous fluids and exhibit poor tissue granulation.

Arnica together with consistent rest and elevation of the affected limbs is a very effective treatment for the early stages of lymphangitis and phlegmon and works better than conventional alcohol poultices.

Preparations

- **Tincture**
  For poultices: Add 1 tablespoon of tincture to 1 L of water at body temperature. Moisten gauze compresses in this liquid and place on the wound.

Woolly Foxglove (Digitalis lanata) Purple Foxglove (Digitalis purpurea)

Purple foxglove, also sometimes called lady's glove (▶ Fig. 9.6), is a member of the Plantaginaceae family. This plant is widespread in the temperate areas of Europe. It is one of the first plants to appear in forest clear-cuts. Its stem reaches a height of about 1 m, and in late summer, it develops bright purple flowers that bumble bees like to visit.

Woolly foxglove has smaller yellowish-white flowers. Its leaves are also smaller and more pointed, and the entire plant is covered in long, woolly hairs. Unlike purple foxglove, woolly foxglove can be cultivated in agricultural fields.

▶ **Indications.** Extensive observations by Weiss showed that moist compresses containing foxglove tincture very effectively promote **wound healing**. Older, torpid wounds of all types that are covered in viscous fluid as well as chronic skin ulcerations respond especially well to foxglove.

As with arnica, foxglove acts on the peripheral vessels. It promotes circulation in the area of the wound. Special saponins (digitonins) and glycosides contained in foxglove stimulate the skin in the wound area. Any digitalis preparation can be used to prepare the moist compresses.

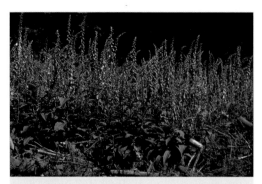

Fig. 9.6 Purple Foxglove, Digitalis purpurea. Photo: Dr. Roland Spohn, Engen.

Additional information about foxglove can be found in the chapter on chronic heart failure (p. 147).

Preparations

- **Tincture**
  For poultices: Add 1 teaspoon to 500 mL of water.
  Smaller torpid wounds can be treated by applying undiluted digitalis tincture directly to the wound and allowing it to dry before dry bandaging the wound. This process should be repeated once a day.
- **Ointment with foxglove tincture**

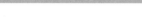

Prescriptions

Rx
Tinct. Digitalis 10.0 (foxglove tincture)
Eucerin. anhydric. 50.0
M. f. ungt.
D.S.
Ointment for external use

Comfrey (Symphytum officinale)

For more information about this plant, see Comfrey (p. 294).

▶ **Indications.** Studies show that the external application of comfrey extract is effective for treating ankle joint distortions.

▶ **Research.** In a randomized, placebo-controlled, double-blind study, Koll et al. showed that a comfrey extract ointment was superior to placebo for **ankle joint distortions**. Of the total, 142 patients experienced highly significant differences in the main study criteria of pain and swelling as well as in restoration of mobility. The tolerability of the preparation was good, both locally and in general.

Predel et al. confirmed these results in another study comparing the same comfrey extract ointment to a diclofenac gel, with equally positive results.

Purple Echinacea (Echinacea purpurea)

For more information about this plant, see Echinacea (p. 205).

▶ **Indications.** Purple Echinacea (coneflower) not only stimulates the immune system. It is also a preferred **wound healing remedy**.

Preparation

- **Tincture**
  For poultices: Add 15 drops of the drug to a glass of water.

Calendula (Calendula officinalis)

For more information about this plant, see Calendula (p. 295).

Caution ⚠

Due to calendula's strong granulation-promoting properties, care should be taken to prevent excessive granulation and subsequent keloid formation.

Preparation

- **Decoction**
  For poultices, especially for wound cleansing: Add 1 tablespoon of the drug to 500 mL of water. Bring to a brief boil, then strain.

Witch Hazel (Hamamelis virginiana)

For more information about this plant, see Witch Hazel (p. 100).

▶ **Indications.** The Commission E monograph for witch hazel lists the following indications: external use with **minor skin injuries**, local inflammation of the skin and mucous membranes, hemorrhoids, and varicose vein symptoms.

Studies have shown that tolerability of witch hazel by the skin is very good (Willms et al.).

Preparation

- **Infusion**
  For poultices: Add 1 tablespoon of the finely chopped drug to 1 cup of water. Bring to a boil, remove from heat, steep for 15 minutes, then strain.

Proven Wound Oils

Small localized torpid wounds often heal quickly when treated with wound oils.

St.-John's-wort Oil (Oleum Hyperici)

Saturate a gauze compress with the oil and apply as a wound dressing. This dressing needs to be changed frequently.

Wound Healing Oil Containing Arnica, St.-John's-wort, Calendula, and Crocus

Tampons saturated with a wound oil containing arnica, St.-John's-wort oil, calendula, and crocus (Colchicum autumnale) have been shown to be very effective, even for infected bone wounds. The oil-saturated dressings can be left in place for 5 days or longer and can be removed painlessly.

Advanced Therapy

Wound infections that are likely to spread require stronger remedies such as resin ointments. They can contain the infection by mobilizing a local immune response, similar to the action of ammonium bituminosulfonate ointment. Resin of the European larch (Larix decidua) is a proven remedy.

Prescriptions

Rx
Terebinthinae lariciae (larch turpentine)
Vaselini albi āā 50.0 (white Vaseline)
M. f. ungt.
Melt together to blend and stir well.

9.7.2 Herpes Labialis and Viral Warts
Thuja (Thuja occidentalis)

Preparation

- **Tincture**
  Brush on warts in the morning and evening for several weeks. This causes small warts to often disappear completely. However, this treatment is usually not sufficient to remove large tough warts.

Lemon Balm (Melissa officinalis)

Medicinal Plants

Lemon balm, Melissa officinalis

Lemon Balm Leaves

Should be prescribed as a finished pharmaceutical product.

Bibliography

Casetti F, Wölfle U, Seelinger G, Schempp CM. Beinwellsalbe. Klinischer Nutzen und Wirkmechanismus in der Haut. Z Phytother. 2014; 35(06):268–272

Isaac O. Die Ringelblume—eine alte Arzneipflanze, neu betrachtet. Z Phytother. 2000; 21(3):138–142

Koll R, Buhr M, Dieter R, et al. Wirksamkeit und Verträglichkeit von Beinwellwurzelextrakt (Extr. Rad. Symphyti) bei Sprunggelenksdistorsionen. Ergebnisse einer multizentrischen, randomisierten, plazebokontrollierten Doppelblindstudie. Z Phytother. 2000; 21(3):127–134

Mennet-von Eiff M, Meier B. Phytotherapie in der Dermatologie. Z Phytother. 1995; 16:201–210

Merklinger S, Messemer C. Niederle P. Ekzembehandlung mit Cardiospermum halicacabum. Z Phytother. 1995; 16:263–266

Pommier P, Gomez F, Sunyach MP, D'Hombres A, Carrie C, Montbarbon X. Phase III randomized trial of Calendula officinalis compared with trolamine for the prevention of acute dermatitis during irradiation for breast cancer. J Clin Oncol. 2004; 22(8):1447–1453

Predel HG, Giannetti B, Koll R, Bulitta M, Staiger C. Efficacy of a comfrey root extract ointment in comparison to a diclofenac gel in the treatment of ankle distortions: results of an observer-blind, randomized, multicenter study. Phytomedicine. 2005; 12 (10):707–714

Staiger C. Comfrey root: from tradition to modern clinical trials. Wien Med Wochenschr. 2013; 163(3–4):58–64

Welzel J, Walther C, Kieser M, Wolff HH. Hamamelis-Salbe in der Pflege der trockenen Altershaut. Z Phytother. 2005; 26 (1):6–13

Willms RU, Walther C, Funk P. Lokale Verträglichkeit von Hamamelis-Salbe. Z Phytother. 2006; 27(6):267–271

Willuhn G. Pflanzliche Dermatika. Dtsch Apoth Ztg. 1992; 132: 1873–1883

Willuhn G. Phytopharmaka in der Dermatologie. Z Phytother. 1995; 16:325–342

Questions

1. Which constituents make oak bark such a valuable remedy for skin disorders?
2. Which plant provides a good remedy for treating neurodermatitis?
3. Which plant is especially well suited for treating leg ulcers (ulcus cruris)?
4. Can foxglove also be used for wound healing? If yes, how is it applied?
5. Which plant is especially suited for quickly cleansing contaminated wounds?

Answers (p. 422) for Chapter 9.

10 Gynecological Disorders

In the past, gynecological disorders were not a focus area for phytotherapy except for certain palliative treatments of functional symptoms. This has changed completely since basic and clinical research has been conducted on two plants that have now gained importance as significant treatment alternatives for synthetic drugs, especially hormone replacement drugs: **chaste tree** (Vitex agnus castus) and **black cohosh** (Cimicifuga racemosa). These two plants demonstrate high tolerability, which makes them especially well suited for long-term treatment.

This chapter provides more information about these and other medicinal plants that hold promise for the successful treatment of gynecological disorders.

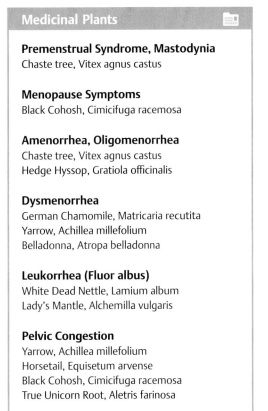

Medicinal Plants

Premenstrual Syndrome, Mastodynia
Chaste tree, Vitex agnus castus

Menopause Symptoms
Black Cohosh, Cimicifuga racemosa

Amenorrhea, Oligomenorrhea
Chaste tree, Vitex agnus castus
Hedge Hyssop, Gratiola officinalis

Dysmenorrhea
German Chamomile, Matricaria recutita
Yarrow, Achillea millefolium
Belladonna, Atropa belladonna

Leukorrhea (Fluor albus)
White Dead Nettle, Lamium album
Lady's Mantle, Alchemilla vulgaris

Pelvic Congestion
Yarrow, Achillea millefolium
Horsetail, Equisetum arvense
Black Cohosh, Cimicifuga racemosa
True Unicorn Root, Aletris farinosa

10.1 Hormonal Dysfunction

Numerous medicinal plants have traditionally been used to treat disorders of the primary and secondary sexual organs of women caused by hormone imbalance. These phytotherapeutics were of marginal importance in gynecology because hormone replacement therapy using synthetic hormones was considered a superior treatment approach. However, in the meantime, many women are rejecting synthetic hormones, especially in the wake of controversial public discussions about the side effects of synthetic hormone replacement therapy.

Phytotherapeutics can be successfully prescribed to treat **premenstrual syndrome (PMS)**, **menopause symptoms**, and **mastodynia**. Some of these plants feature constituents that are similar to human sex hormones in structure. This seems to be the theoretical foundation for their great practical success. As is typical for phytotherapeutics, the whole plant is more efficacious than the sum of its constituents.

Before prescribing the following medicinal plants, a gynecological examination should be conducted to exclude organic causes.

10.1.1 Premenstrual Syndrome, Mastodynia

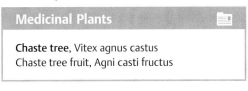

Medicinal Plants

Chaste tree, Vitex agnus castus
Chaste tree fruit, Agni casti fructus

Premenstrual syndrome (PMS) consists of a set of **serious symptoms** that usually start several days before the onset of menstruation: mood disorders, headaches, sleep disorders, nervous and often aggressive tenseness, and breast tension and tenderness. Abdominal symptoms can include meteorism, cramps, and premenstrual edema of the lower legs.

The cause is thought to be an imbalance between relatively increased levels of estrogen and decreased levels of progesterone. However, psychosomatic aspects also certainly play a role.

Chaste tree has been shown to be an excellent remedy for premenstrual syndrome. Clinical results also document its efficacy for mastodynia. Chaste tree is the remedy of first choice for these two indications.

Plants Used in Treatment

Chaste tree (Vitex agnus castus)

Chaste tree has recently been reclassified by botanists from the Verbenaceae family to the Lamiaceae family. This shrub can grow to a height of 3–5 m and is much larger and statelier than the common verbena (Verbena officinalis). Its leaves are finger-shaped and its flower paniculates are violet (▶ Fig. 10.1). It is found from the Mediterranean to central Asia.

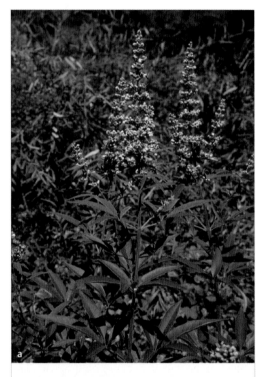

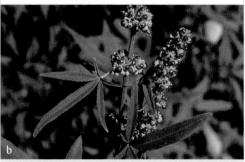

Fig. 10.1 a and b Chaste tree, Vitex agnus castus. Photos: Dr. Roland Spohn, Engen.

Medicinal applications use the **chaste tree fruit** (Agni casti fructus).

▶ **Note.** As the name chaste tree implies, this plant was considered an anaphrodisiac and has been in use for a long time (Mayer and Czygan).

▶ **Pharmacology.** Chaste tree fruit contains the iridoids aucubin and agnuside as well as flavonoids, volatile oil, the bitter constituent castin and fatty oil.

▶ **Research.** A working group including Gorkow and Wuttke is primarily responsible for documenting the pharmacological effects of chaste tree fruit (Gorkow et al. 1999a; 1999b).

Initially, chaste tree fruit was shown to have **prolactin inhibiting** effects (Jarry et al. 1991; 1994). Today, the efficacy of chaste tree fruit is attributed to its dopaminergic effect. Dopamine is a physiological inhibitor of prolactin. A connection is thought to exist between the **dopaminergic effect** of chaste tree fruit and bicyclic diterpenes. However, the whole extract has been shown to be more effective than a number of individual constituents that have been tested. These appear to include phytoestrogens, which have indeed been found in higher concentrations in the chaste tree leaves (Meier and Hoberg). Also of interest is the fact that the prolactin inhibiting effect only occurs with the increased secretion of prolactin. It does not occur when normal amounts of prolactin are secreted.

Brugisser et al. also showed that chaste tree binds to **opioid receptors**. This could provide another explanation for chaste tree's therapeutic efficacy because some of the symptoms of PMS are attributed to excessive decreases in central endorphin levels.

▶ **Indications.** The main indications for chaste tree fruit are **PMS**, mastodynia, and **menstrual disorders**. These are also the indications listed by the Commission E in its monograph for chaste tree fruit.

Many clinical studies have confirmed the efficacy of chaste tree fruit. This remedy and its preparations are very well tolerated. This is another factor in its favor compared to synthetic drugs.

▶ **Research.** Gorkow et al. (1999a; 1999b) and Beer (2015a; 2015b) provide good overviews of the most important clinical studies. Two randomized, placebo-controlled, double-blind studies showed the efficacy of a standardized chaste tree fruit extract for **mastodynia** and **mastalgia**. Although these symptoms are known to exhibit a high placebo effect, the differences in favor of chaste tree were still significant.

These earlier results have been confirmed in placebo-controlled studies more recently by Aydin et al. as well as Dinç and Coşkun.

A review by van Die et al. summarizes the research on PMS. It shows that chaste tree's efficacy for this indication is well documented by randomized and controlled studies. Beer (2015a) also characterizes the various research results using two different chaste tree extracts (BNO 1095, Ze 440) in his review. As is to be expected, the symptoms exhibit a high rate of placebo effects. Nevertheless, the differences between verum and placebo were significant, with improvement rates of 79.8% and 50%, respectively (He et al.; Schellenberg et al.).

Several evidence-based studies are also available now for the use of chaste tree to treat **menstrual disorders** (Milewicz et al.); Eltbogen et al.). They show high and reliable (reproducible) response rates of over 80% in one multicentric observational study of 211 female patients. At the beginning of the study, one-quarter of the study participants wishing to become pregnant was unfulfilled; during treatment, 23% of these participants became pregnant.

Interesting observations have also been made regarding the efficacy of chaste tree for **hyperprolactinemia** and potentially associated **subfertility** (Struck). The prolactin-lowering effects of chaste tree for stress induced hyperprolactinemia were demonstrated in animal experiments (Jarry et al. 1994) and clinically (Milewicz et al.). Struck reported several pregnancies following chaste tree treatment in patients who previously presented with subfertility associated with hyperprolactinemia. The study emphasizes the much higher tolerability and much lower daily treatment costs of chaste tree compared to synthetic dopamine antagonists.

It is important to highlight that studies have demonstrated that chaste tree extracts do not seem to affect patients suffering from estrogen-sensitive tumors negatively, as would be expected for an analogous estrogen substitution treatment. Various experimental studies have shown that chaste tree extracts do not bind with estrogen receptors that promote cell proliferation (ER∝). In fact, casticin, an important constituent of chaste tree extracts, inhibits the expression of ER∝ mRNA.

Cytotoxic effects of chaste tree extracts on human breast cancer cell lines have also been shown.

A clinical case study of more than 10,000 women in Germany found indications for reduced menopausal breast cancer risk in women who used chaste tree extracts (Obi et al.).

▶ **Therapy Recommendation.** When prescribing standardized finished pharmaceutical products, extract preparations that have been shown to produce the pharmacological and clinical effects should be given preference.

10.1.2 Menopause Symptoms

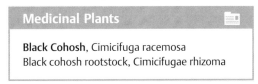

Medicinal Plants

Black Cohosh, Cimicifuga racemosa
Black cohosh rootstock, Cimicifugae rhizoma

Almost every woman experiences symptoms during menopause. Symptoms such as **hot flashes** and **mood imbalances** are especially characteristic. The level and duration of suffering associated with these symptoms varies widely from individual to individual.

Nowadays, these symptoms mostly prompt the prescription of synthetic female sex hormones. Many women resist taking these drugs because of the associated risks, such as thromboembolic complications, increased incidence of cancer, or liver function disorders.

Black cohosh provides an excellent herbal alternative. In the authors' experience over several decades, this medicinal plant is a remedy of first choice for the treatment of menopause symptoms. It also should be emphasized that it has additional striking effects on the psychological symptoms of menopause.

Plant Used in Treatment

Black Cohosh (Cimicifuga racemosa; syn. Actaea racemosa)

Black cohosh is a member of the Ranunculaceae family. This resilient plant originates from North America and can grow to a height of 2 m. Its upright stems carry large paripinnate leaves with pointed deeply lobed leaflets (▶ Fig. 10.2). Its small

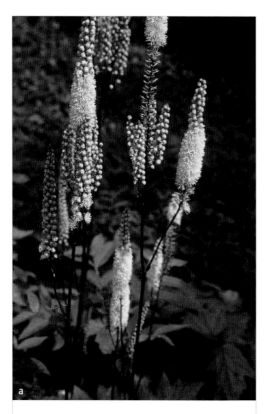

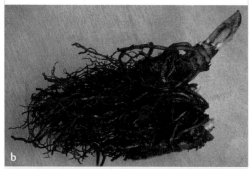

Fig. 10.2 a and b Black Cohosh, Cimicifuga racemosa. Photos: Dr. Roland Spohn, Engen.

whitish flowers are arranged into very long and narrow racemes and develop follicular fruit.

Like chaste tree, black cohosh was used traditionally without detailed knowledge of its mode of action.

Medicinal applications use the dried **black cohosh rootstock** (Cimicifugae rhizoma).

▶ **Pharmacology.** Black cohosh rootstock contains triterpene glycosides such as actein and cimifugoside along with isoflavones and resins of unknown chemical structure.

The effects and actions of individual constituents of black cohosh are not as well known as those for chaste tree. It is thought that black cohosh acts on the hypothalamic–pituitary–ovary axis. It possibly selectively inhibits luteinizing hormones (LH) in the pituitary gland but has no effect on follicle stimulating hormones (FSH) and prolactin.

▶ **Research.** A very extensive study that conformed to good clinical practice (GCP) showed no impact of low and high dosages of black cohosh on hormone levels of estradiol, prolactin, LH, FSH, and sex hormone binding globulin (SHGB). This indicates that black cohosh does not have estrogen-like effects (Liske et al. 2000). The current discussion favors selective estrogen receptor modulation (SERM), as has been shown in experiments on estrogen receptor-positive breast cancer cells (Freudenstein and Bodinet) and in the uterus.

Experiments on rats using two black cohosh types showed that experimentally induced bone mass reduction through lack of dietary calcium or ovariectomy was reduced by perorally administered black cohosh extracts or defined constituents, especially triterpene glycosides.

This casts an interesting light on adjuvant postmenopausal osteoporosis treatment using black cohosh rootstock.

A review discusses this question in reference to further pharmacological and clinical data (Seidlová-Wuttke). There are many indications for osteoprotective effects of black cohosh.

▶ **Indications.** In the authors' experience, **menopausal symptoms** are the most important indication for black cohosh. The Commission E lists the following indications in its monograph for black cohosh: premenstrual discomfort and dysmenorrhea or climacteric (menopausal) neurovegetative ailments.

Despite the uncertain pharmacological assessment of black cohosh, its therapeutic efficacy has been well established in practice and clinically for decades. More recently, controlled studies have also confirmed its efficacy (Boblitz et al.).

In their decades of experience, the authors have seen black cohosh continue to produce good results for adjuvant therapy of postmenopausal osteoporosis as measured primarily by subjective experience or radiological bone density scans. The animal experiment results described above confirm this clinical experience. There is a need for extensive long-term trials to systematically study these possibilities.

▶ **Research.** The study by Liske et al. (2000) cited above used several parameters—based on Kuppermann (1953; 1959)—to show highly significant improvements of **menopausal symptoms** following 24 weeks of therapy. These effects were seen after 2 weeks of treatment and reached a maximum after about 3 months. The high index at the beginning of treatments (31 and 31.5) was lowered to 7.0 and 8.0. Test participants received either the daily dose recommended by the Commission E (40 mg of drug equivalent) or a high daily dose of 127 mg. Tolerability was excellent in both groups.

A randomized, placebo-controlled, multicentric, double-blind trial studied the efficacy and safety of an isopropanolic extract of black cohosh for 12 weeks in 304 women whose most recent menstruation occurred at least 12 months before the beginning of the study. The trial showed significant superiority of black cohosh on the Menopause Rating Scale (MRS) compared to the placebo. The most significant effects were seen for **hot flashes** and associated **sleep disorders**. The subscores **psyche** and **vaginal atrophy** also showed significant improvements compared to the placebo, although not quite as pronounced. In summary, 50 patients reported adverse events for the verum compared to 47 for the placebo, but no serious adverse events were registered. Liver enzymes were not impacted at all.

The liver enzyme results are significant because toxic liver failure in a woman who had taken a black cohosh preparation along with other substances could have been attributed to black cohosh in 2002. Subsequent analysis showed this association to be unlikely (Osmers et al.). The authors have also never observed liver toxicity resulting from black cohosh prescriptions in their own hepatology practice.

Fixed combinations of **black cohosh** and **St.-John's-wort** are also of interest because menopause is often accompanied by depressive mood disorders.

In a randomized, placebo-controlled, double-blind, and multicentric trial of 301 women for 16 weeks, this combination was shown to have positive

effects in women with **menopausal symptoms with a pronounced psychological component**. During the second half of the trial, the initial dosage was cut in half. The resulting scores were highly significant ($p < 0.001$) on both the Menopause Rating Scale (MRS) and on the Hamilton Depression Scale (HAMD 17) with its 17 criteria (Uebelhack R, et al.).

Numerous other evidence-based trials showing the efficacy and tolerability of black cohosh root extracts have been published since the second edition of this book. The summation of these results prompted Beer to conclude that black cohosh rootstock extracts approved for medicinal use are efficacious, well tolerated, and safe. He compiled a review, including a table of data, of all the corresponding studies (Beer 2015b). The findings in his review and in another publication contradict the ambivalent statements made in a Cochran review that did not consider several important randomized, double-blind, and placebo-controlled trials showing significant proof of efficacy (Leach and Moore).

Earlier indications for bone protective effects of black cohosh have now also been clinically studied. García-Pérez et al. conducted a controlled clinical trial of 82 menopausal women to study the effects of black cohosh rootstock extract on various bone metabolism parameters. The trial results showed a significant improvement in inhibiting bone loss factors compared to an untreated control group of female patients. Unfortunately, the study does not include bone density measurements as originally planned in the study protocol. Stute and Pickartz compiled a very good overview about this specialized question of bone protective effects of black cohosh. They suggest black cohosh as an add-on therapy for standard hormone therapy and possibly to reduce the dosage of hormones and thereby reduce the risk of adverse effects of the synthetic drugs.

Another indication for black cohosh is the treatment of uterine fibroids. A randomized, double-blind, controlled trial of 244 menopausal Chinese women studied the effects of black cohosh versus tibolone on fibroid size. Twelve weeks of therapy using an isopropanolic black cohosh extract finished pharmaceutical product reduced fibroid volume by 30.3%. Fibroid size increased by 4.7% in the tibulone group. This represents a significant difference of $p = 0.016$ (Bai et al.). Liske et al. (2015) compiled a current overview of these results.

▶ **Therapy Recommendation.** The indications listed above should always be treated using approved finished pharmaceutical products. Untested extracts showed no effects in several studies.

10.2 Functional Menstrual Disorders

Phytotherapeutics can provide hormone substitution as well as purely regulating effects for functional menstrual disorders such as **amenorrhea**, **oligomenorrhea**, and **dysmenorrhea**. They can meet a multitude of requirements for successfully treating these frequent concomitant and secondary disorders.

10.2.1 Amenorrhea, Oligomenorrhea

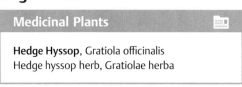

Medicinal Plants

Hedge Hyssop, Gratiola officinalis
Hedge hyssop herb, Gratiolae herba

Absent, infrequent, or light menstruation is not an actual disease, but is one symptom of a more comprehensive disorder. Treatment is dominated by prescription hormone replacement, especially for **primary amenorrhea**.

Secondary amenorrhea, on the other hand, can be very successfully treated by **emmenagogues**, i.e., menstruation promoting drugs.

Caution ⚠

All emmenagogues can have abortive effects and must always be used carefully based on a precise diagnosis, if possible, by a gynecological specialist.

Plants Used in Treatment

Hedge Hyssop (Gratiola officinalis)

This little-known plant grows sparsely in wet meadows and fens and is a member of the figwort family (Scrophulariaceae). It can reach a height of up to 30 cm. Its leaves are narrow and opposite and its white to reddish flowers are moderately large.

Medicinal applications use the **hedge hyssop herb** (Gratiolae herba). It is considered a very efficacious emmenagogue.

Preparation

- **Tea**
  Add 1 cup of boiling water to 1 teaspoon of the dried herb. Steep for 5–10 minutes, then strain.
  Drink 1 cup in the morning and in the evening.

10.2.2 Dysmenorrhea

Medicinal Plants

German Chamomile, Matricaria recutita
Chamomile flowers, Matricariae flos
Yarrow, Achillea millefolium
Yarrow herb and flowers, Millefolii herba et flos
Belladonna, Atropa belladonna
Belladonna leaves and root, Belladonnae folium et radix
Couch Grass, Elymus repens
Couch Grass rootstock, Graminis rhizoma

Dysmenorrhea symptoms can be treated successfully using a number of the pain-relieving and antispasmodic plants discussed in this book. In general, individualized prescriptions for teas or tinctures are preferred.

> ## Caution
>
> St. Germain tea has sometimes been recommended by herbalists in this indication. However, it is a purely laxative tea blend that also contains potassium tartrate and tartaric acid. Its use for the treatment of functional menstrual disorders is strongly discouraged.

> ## Preparation
>
> - **St. Germain tea**
>   Senna leaves (after 24 hours, pre-extraction with 90% Ethanol) 8 Loth
>   Elderflowers 5 Loth
>   Foeniculum vulgare var. dulce fruits 2,5 Loth
>   Anisi fructus (Aniseed) 2,5 Loth
>   Potassium bitartrate (cream of tartar) 1,5 Loth
>   Each day infuse and drink 4 Loth of the mixture with 5 cups of boiling water as tea.
>   According to: Michaelis: Über den Saint Germain-Thee. In: Journal der Chirurgie und Augenheilkunde. Band 14, 1830, Stück 2, S. 333–336.

Plants Used in Treatment

German Chamomile (Matricaria recutita)

For more information about this plant, see German Chamomile (p. 42).

It should be noted that the Latin name for the genus Matricaria is derived from *mater*, which is an ancient term for uterus.

German chamomile is soothing and provides rapid relief from spasms.

> ## Preparation
>
> - **Tea**
>   Add 1 cup of hot water to 2–3 teaspoons of the drug. Steep covered for 5–10 minutes, then strain.
>   Drink slowly while still comfortably warm.

Yarrow (Achillea millefolium)

For more information about this plant, see Yarrow (p. 108).

Yarrow's effect is similar to chamomile, but weaker. It is more suitable for chronic conditions and needs to be taken long term.

> ## Preparation
>
> - **Tea**
>   Add 1 cup of boiling water to 1 tablespoon of the drug. Steep for 5 minutes, then strain. Drink several cups throughout the day.

Belladonna (Atropa belladonna)

For more information about this plant, see Belladonna (p. 69).

Belladonna is **spasmolytic**.

▶ **Therapy Recommendation.** Treatment should always start with German chamomile. If its effects are not sufficient, treatment can transition to stronger remedies.

Proven Prescriptions: "Women's Tea" (Species gynaecologicae)

Dysmenorrhea requires treatment of mainly spastic conditions and usually concurrent constipation. Remedies to treat concomitant inflammation can also be added. The resulting "women's tea" (Species gynaecologica) contains antispasmodics, laxatives, and antidyscratics.
- **"Women's Tea Martin" (Species gynaecologica Martin, according to the German Prescription Formulas, DRF)**
  In this case, the saponin-containing couch grass (Elymus repens) rootstock, (Graminis rhizoma) provides the antidyscratic effect.

> ## Prescriptions
>
> Rx
> Frangulae cort. (buckthorn bark)
> Millefolii herb. (yarrow herb)
> Sennae fol. (senna leaves)
> Graminis rhiz. āā 25.0 (couch grass rootstock)
> M. f. spec.,
> D.S.
> Drink 2–3 cups a day.

Extract

- **Combination of Belladonna as Antispasmodic with a Mild Laxative**

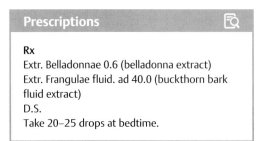

Prescriptions

Rx
Extr. Belladonnae 0.6 (belladonna extract)
Extr. Frangulae fluid. ad 40.0 (buckthorn bark fluid extract)
D.S.
Take 20–25 drops at bedtime.

Essential Oils

Local application of essential oils can relieve pain and spasms. A few drops can be applied to a sanitary napkin or rubbed into the lower abdominal area. A few drops of pure peppermint oil are usually sufficient.

- **Recommended Blend**

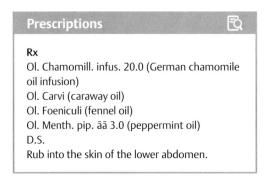

Prescriptions

Rx
Ol. Chamomill. infus. 20.0 (German chamomile oil infusion)
Ol. Carvi (caraway oil)
Ol. Foeniculi (fennel oil)
Ol. Menth. pip. āā 3.0 (peppermint oil)
D.S.
Rub into the skin of the lower abdomen.

10.3 Leukorrhea (Fluor albus)

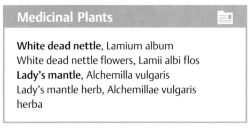

Medicinal Plants

White dead nettle, Lamium album
White dead nettle flowers, Lamii albi flos
Lady's mantle, Alchemilla vulgaris
Lady's mantle herb, Alchemillae vulgaris herba

10.3.1 Tea Preparations and Rinses

White vaginal discharge in women needs to be examined gynecologically to exclude **organic causes**. Phytotherapeutic treatment is only appropriate for leukorrhea with functional or constitutional causes.

Antidyscratics may be used (see Rheumatic Disorders (p. 235)). Internal use of yarrow (p. 108) or horsetail (p. 224) is useful, as is **white dead nettle** and **lady's mantle**.

Plants Used in Treatment

White Dead Nettle (Lamium album)

White dead nettle is a member of the mint family (Lamiaceae). This plant grows widely in Germany along paths, fences, shrubs, and the edges of forests. Its name is derived from the similarity between its leaves and that of the true stinging nettle. However, white dead nettle does not have stinging hairs. Its almost pure white flowers are located in the leaf axils and feature a small orange spot on the tiny, multilobed lower lip. Its upper lip is nicely curved (▶ Fig. 10.3).

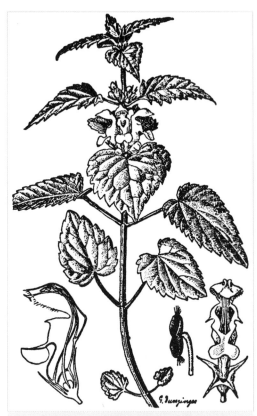

Fig. 10.3 White dead nettle, Lamium album.

Medicinal applications use the **white dead nettle flowers** (Lamii albi flos).

▶ **Pharmacology.** The flowers must be picked from the calyx one by one. They contain iridoid and secoiridoid glycosides, triterpene saponins, flavonoids, phenol carbonic acid, tannins, and mucilage.

▶ **Indications.** The Commission E has issued a positive monograph for white dead nettle for this indication.

Preparations

- **Tea**
  Add 1 cup of boiling water to 2 teaspoons of the finely chopped drug. Steep for 10 minutes, then strain.
  Drink 1 cup several times a day.
- **Infusion**
  For washing and rinsing, add 500 mL of hot water to 50 g of the finely chopped drug. Steep for 10 minutes, then strain.
  Use lukewarm or cold for washing and rinsing.

Lady's Mantle (Alchemilla vulgaris, Alchemilla xanthochlora)

Lady's mantle flowers are very inconspicuous and yellowish green. Its leaves are rather large and shaped almost like a half circle with several large lobes. This low-growing herb grows in Germany in meadows and is a member of the rose family.

In the morning, the leaves are folded like a funnel and bright drops of dew can be found inside. These drops are created by the flow of droplets expressed from the inside of the leaf. Another peculiar botanical aspect of this plant is that its seeds develop parthenogenically and its inconspicuous flowers are often not pollinated.

Medicinal applications use the entire **lady's mantle herb** (Alchemillae vulgaris herba).

▶ **Note.** Lady's mantle, like white dead nettle, is a popular folk remedy for gynecological disorders.

▶ **Pharmacology.** Lady's mantle herb contains tannins, bitters, and flavonoids.

Preparation

- **Infusion**
  For washing and rinsing, add 500 mL of boiling water to 50 g of the drug. Steep for 10 minutes, then strain.
  Use lukewarm for washing and rinsing.

Proven Prescriptions for Vaginal Rinses

Prescriptions

Mucilaginous Decoction
Rx
Malvae fol. 50.0 (mallow leaves)
M. f.
Add 2–3 tablespoons of the drug to 1 L of water. Bring to a brief boil.

Prescriptions

Anti-Inflammatory Infusion
Rx
Matricariae flos (German chamomile flowers)
Salviae fol. āā 50.0 (sage leaves)
M. f.
Add 1 L of hot water to 2–3 tablespoons of the blend. Steep for 15 minutes, then strain.

Prescriptions

Astringent Infusion
Rx
Quercus cort. (oak bark)
Matricariae flos āā 50.0 (German chamomile flowers)
M. f.
Add 1 L of hot water to 2–3 tablespoons of the blend. Steep for 15 minutes, then strain.

Prescriptions

Aromatic Infusion

Rx

Lavandulae flos (lavender flowers)

Serpylli herb. āā 50.0 (Serpylli herba,wild thyme herb)

M. f.

Add 1 L of hot water to 1 tablespoon of the blend. Steep for 15 minutes, then strain.

10.4 Pelvic Congestion

Medicinal Plants

Yarrow, Achillea millefolium
Yarrow herb and flowers, Millefolii herba et flos
Horsetail, Equisetum arvense
Horsetail herb, Equiseti herba
Black Cohosh, Cimicifuga racemosa
Black cCohosh rootstock, Cimicifugae rhizoma
True Unicorn Root, Aletris farinosa
True Unicorn root, Aletris radix

Pelvic congestion, also called pelipathia vegetativa or parametritis posterior, is an important medical condition. It has also been called vegetative dystonia of the small pelvis. The condition is characterized primarily by spasms and muscle tension caused by **neurovegetative** (i.e., functional) **disorders**. From all women who consult a gynecologist, 10–20% suffer from this disorder. It presents as a multitude of symptoms, primarily spastic pelvic pain that is hard to localize, back pain, leukorrhea, pruritus vulvae, mastodynia, and dysmenorrhea. The gynecological findings for this disorder do not reflect the severity of symptoms and the intensity with which they are presented.

This psychosomatic condition can be treated with a therapy of focused counseling supported by phytotherapeutics. The treatment goal is to balance the autonomic nervous system, relieve spasms, and provide general toning.

10.4.1 Plants Used in Treatment

Yarrow (Achillea millefolium)

For more information about this plant, see Yarrow (p. 108).

This condition is a primary indication for yarrow. Like chamomile, yarrow contains antispasmodic and anti-inflammatory constituents and its bitter principle acts as a tonic.

Preparations

- **Tea**
  Add 1 cup of hot water to 1 teaspoon of the finely chopped drug. Steep covered for 5 minutes, then strain through a tea strainer.
  Drink 1 cup several times a day.
- **Infusion**
  For a sitz bath: Add 1 L of hot water to 50 g of yarrow flowers. Steep for 5 minutes, then strain, and add to 20 L of bath water. Bathe 1–2 × a day.
- **Fresh Pressed Plant Juice**
  Take 1 tablespoon 3 × a day with meals.

▶ **Therapy Recommendation.** Yarrow is most effective when used as a long-term regimen.

Horsetail (Equisetum arvense)

For more information about this plant, see Horsetail (p. 224).

This plant is used to strengthen connective tissues.

Preparations

- **Tea**
  Add 1 cup of boiling water to 2 teaspoons of the chopped drug. Steep for 15 minutes, then strain.
  Drink 1 cup several times a day. This remedy should be used as a series of repeated long-term regimens.
- **Decoction for Sitz Baths**
  Add 50 g of the finely chopped drug to 500 mL of water. Boil for 30 minutes. Strain and add to 20 L of bath water. Bathe 1–2 × a day.
  These baths are frequently very effective due to horsetail's silicic acid content.

Black Cohosh (Cimicifuga racemosa)

Preparation

- **Tea**
  Add 1 cup of hot water to 1 teaspoon of the chopped drug. Steep for 10 minutes, then strain.
  Drink 1 cup 2–3 × a day.

▶ **Therapy Recommendation.** Black cohosh should be used consistently as a series of repeated long-term regimens.

True Unicorn Root (Aletris farinose)

True unicorn root is a member of the lily family and originates from North America. Its fresh tubers (**Aletris radix**) contain bitters that provide tonic effects. These seem to be especially suited to treating lower abdominal organs.

▶ **Indications.** True unicorn root is reported to have positive effects on **pelvic floor weakness** and **genital prolapse**, especially in older women. It is also used to treat **back pain** associated with symptoms of prolapse.

Bibliography

Amann W. Amenorrhoe: Günstige Wirkung von Agnus castus (Agnolyt) auf Amenorrhoe. Z Allgemeinmed. 1978; 58:228–231

Amann W. Extr. Fruct. Agni casti sicc., ein pflanzliches Mittel mit vielfältiger Anwendungsmöglichkeit. Therapeutikon. 1988; 11: 627–632

Aydin I, Baltaci D, Türkyilmaz S, Öncu M. Comparison of Vitex agnus castus with meloxicam and placebo in treatment of patients with cyclical mastalgia. Düzce Tip Dergisi. 2012; 14:1–5

Bai W, Henneicke-von Zepelin HH, Wang S, et al. Efficacy and tolerability of a medicinal product containing an isopropanolic black cohosh extract in Chinese women with menopausal symptoms: a randomized, double-blind, parallel-controlled study versus tibolone. Maturitas. 2007; 58(1):31–41

Becela-Deller C. Ruta graveolens L.—Weinraute. Z Phytother. 1995; 16(5):275–281

Beer AM, Osmers R, Schnitker J, Bai W, Mueck AO, Meden H. Efficacy of black cohosh (Cimicifuga racemosa) medicines for treatment of menopausal symptoms—comments on major statements of the Cochrane Collaboration report 2012 "black cohosh (Cimicifuga spp.) for menopausal symptoms (review)." Gynecol Endocrinol. 2013; 29(12):1022–1025

Beer AM. Cimicifuga racemosa bei klimakterischen Beschwerden. Zeitschr f Phytotherapie. 2015b; 36(01):10–17

Beer AM. Vitex agnus castus: Evidenz-basierte Therapie bei zyklusabhängigen Beschwerden. Zeitschr f Phytotherapie. 2015a; 36(1):4–9

Beuscher N. Cimicifuga racemosa L.—Die Traubensilberkerze. Z Phytother. 1995; 16(5):301–310

Boblitz N, Liske E, Wüstenberg P. Traubensilberkerze. Dtsch Apoth Ztg. 2000; 140:107–114

Brugisser R, Burkard W, Simmen U, Schaffner W. Untersuchungen an Opioid-Rezeptoren mit Vitex agnus castus L. Z Phytother. 1999; 20:140–158

Dinç T, Coşkun F. Comparison of fructus agni casti and flurbiprofen in the treatment of cyclic mastalgia in premenopausal women. Ulus Cerrahi Derg. 2014; 30(1):34–38

Eltbogen R, Litschgi M, Gasser UE, et al. Vitex agnus castus extract (Ze 440) improves symptoms in women with menstrual cycle irregularities. Planta Med. 2014; 80:19)

Freudenstein J, Bodinet C. Influence of an isopropanolic acqueous extract of Cimicifugae racemosae rhizoma on the proliferation of MCF-7 cells. Poster. 23. Internationales LOF-Symposium "Phyto-Oestrogens" in Gent, Belgien im Januar 1999

García-Pérez MA, Pineda B, Hermenegildo C, Tarín JJ, Cano A. Isopropanolic Cimicifuga racemosa is favorable on bone markers but neutral on an osteoblastic cell line. Fertil Steril. 2009; 91(4) Suppl:1347–1350

Gorkow C, Wuttke W, März RW. Evidence of efficacy of Vitex agnus castus preparations. In: Loew D, Blume H, Dingermann T, ed Phytopharmaka. Vol V. Darmstadt: Steinkopff 1999b; 189–208

Gorkow C. Klinischer Kenntnisstand von Agni-casti fructus. Z Phytother. 1999a; 20:159–168

He Z, Chen R, Zhou Y, et al. Treatment for premenstrual syndrome with Vitex agnus castus: A prospective, randomized, multi-center placebo-controlled study in China. Maturitas. 2009; 63 (1):99–103

Jarry H, Leonhardt S, Gorkow C, Wuttke W. In vitro prolactin but not LH and FSH release is inhibited by compounds in extracts of Agnus castus: direct evidence for a dopaminergic principle by the dopamine receptor assay. Exp Clin Endocrinol. 1994; 102(6):448–454

Jarry H, Leonhardt S, Wuttke W, Behr B, Garkow C. Agnus castus als dopaminerges Wirkprinzip in Mastodynon® N. Z Phytother. 1991; 12:77–82

Kubista E, Müller G, Spona J. Behandlung der Mastopathie mit zyklischer Mastodynie: Klinische Ergebnisse und Hormonprofile [Treatment of mastopathy with cyclic mastodynia: clinical results and hormone profile]. Gynakol Rundsch. 1986; 26(2):65–79

Kupperman HS, Blatt MH, Wiesbader H, Filler W. Comparative clinical evaluation of estrogenic preparations by the menopausal and amenorrheal indices. J Clin Endocrinol Metab. 1953; 13(6):688–703

Kupperman HS, Wetchler BB, Blatt MHG. Contemporary therapy of the menopausal syndrome. J Am Med Assoc. 1959; 171:1627–1637

Leach MJ, Moore V. Black cohosh (Cimicifuga spp.) for menopausal symptoms. Cochrane Database Syst Rev. 2012; 9(9):CD007244

Li JX, Kadota S, Li HY, et al. Effects of Cimicifugae rhizoma on serum calcium and phosphate levels in low calcium dietary rats and on bone mineral density in ovariectomized rats. Phytomedicine. 1997; 3(4):379–385

Liske E, Boblitz N, Henneicke-von Zepelin HH. Therapie klimakterischer Beschwerden mit Cimicifuga racemosa – Daten zur Wirkung und Wirksamkeit aus einer randomisierten kontrollierten Doppelblindstudie. In: Rietbrock N, ed Phytopharmaka. Vol VI. Darmstadt: Steinkopff; 2000: 246–257

Liske E, Henneicke-von Zepelin HH, Pickartz St., Meden H. Wirkung des isopropanolischen Cimicifuga-racemosa-Extrakts iCR auf Uterusmyome bei Frauen mit klimakterischen Beschwerden. Zeitschr f Phytotherapie. 2015; 36(01):23–26

Mayer JG, Czygan FC. Vitex agnus castus L., der oder das Keuschlamm. Ein kulturhistorischer Essay. Z Phytother. 1999; 20:177–182

Meier B, Hoberg E. Agni-casti fructus. Neue Erkenntnisse zur Qualität und Wirksamkeit. Z Phytother. 1999; 20:140–158

Milewicz A, Gejdel E, Sworen H, et al. Vitex agnus castus-Extrakt zur Behandlung von Regeltempoanomalien infolge latenter Hyperprolaktinämie. Ergebnisse einer randomisierten Plazebo-kontrollierten Doppelblindstudie [Vitex agnus castus extract in the treatment of luteal phase defects due to latent hyperprolactinemia. Results of a randomized placebo-controlled double-blind study]. Arzneimittelforschung. 1993; 43(7):752–756

Obi N, Chang-Claude J, Berger J, et al. The use of herbal preparations to alleviate climacteric disorders and risk of postmenopausal breast cancer in a German case control study. Cancer Epidemiol Biomarkers Prev. 2009; 18(8):2207–2213

Osmers R, Friede M, Liske E, Schnitker J, Freudenstein J, Henneicke-von Zepelin HH. Efficacy and safety of isopropanolic black cohosh extract for climacteric symptoms. Obstet Gynecol. 2005; 105(5 Pt 1):1074–1083

Schellenberg R, Zimmermann C, Drewe J, Hoexter G, Zahner C. Dose-dependent efficacy of the Vitex agnus castus extract Ze 440 in patients suffering from premenstrual syndrome. Phytomedicine. 2012; 19(14):1325–1331

Seidlová-Wuttke D. Schützt Cimicifuga-Spezialextrakt vor Osteoporose? NaturaMed. 2009; 1:12–16

Sourgens H, Winterhoff H, Gumbinger HG, Kemper FH. Antihormonal effects of plant extracts. TSH- and prolactin-suppressing properties of Lithospermum officinale and other plants. Planta Med. 1982; 45(2):78–86

Stoll W. Phytotherapeutikum beeinflußt atrophisches Vaginalepithel. Therapeutikon. 1987; 1:23–31

Struck D. Hyperprolaktinämie und Subfertilität. Z Phytother. 2005; 26(3):130–131

Stute P, Pickartz St. Zusatznutzen eines isopropanolischen Cimicifuga-racemosa-Extrakts (iCR). Z Phytother. 2015; 36(01): 18–22

Trunzler G, de Rossi M.. Phytotherapeutika in der Gynäkologie. Ärztez Naturheilverfahren. 1990; 31:460

Uebelhack R, Blohmer JU, Graubaum HJ, Busch R, Gruenwald J, Wernecke KD. Black cohosh and St. John's wort for climacteric complaints: a randomized trial. Obstet Gynecol. 2006; 107(2 Pt 1):247–255

van Die MD, Burger HG, Teede HJ, Bone KM. Vitex agnus castus extracts for female reproductive disorders: a systematic review of clinical trials. Planta Med. 2013; 79(7):562–575

Wagner H, Hörhammer L, Frank U. Lithospermsäure, das antihormonale Wirkprinzip von Lycopus europaeus L. (Wolfsfuss) und Symphytum officinale L. (Beinwell) [.Vitex agnus castus extract in the treatment of luteal phase defects due to latent hyperprolactinemia. Results of a randomized placebo-controlled double-blind study]. Arzneimittelforschung. 1970; 20(5):705–713

Weiss RF. Phytotherapie bei Frauenkrankheiten. Ärztez Naturheilverfahren. 1986; 27:579–584

Winterhoff H, Gorkow C, Behr B. Die Hemmung der Laktation bei Ratten als indirekter Beweis für die Senkung von Prolaktin durch Agnus castus. Z Phytother. 1991; 12(6):175–179

Winterhoff H, Gumbinger HG, Sourgens H. On the antigonadotropic activity of Lithospermum and Lycopus species and some of their phenolic constituents. Planta Med. 1988; 54(2):101–106

Winterhoff H. Endokrinologisch wirksame Phytopharmaka. Z Phytother. 1987; 8:169–171

Questions

1. Which two phytotherapeutic plants are predominantly used for gynecological indications?
2. Which plant can be used to prepare a tea for treating leukorrhea?
3. What is the effect of yarrow on pelvic congestion?
4. Are there evidence-based studies about the efficacy of phytopharmaceuticals for hormone disorders?

Answers (p. 422) for Chapter 10.

11 Geriatric Disorders

Experience has shown that phytotherapeutics are especially suitable for treating geriatric disorders. The factors that make phytotherapeutics so well suited for this area of medicine is on the one hand their comprehensive therapeutic range and good tolerability, and on the other hand the issue of prevention. Some of the areas of applicability include sclerosis and deposition disorders, many types of benign tumors, degenerative heart and vascular disorders, and benign prostatic hyperplasia (BPH). Phytotherapeutics such as hawthorn, ginkgo, garlic, and the urologic remedies are able to fill therapeutic gaps and provide true alternatives to synthetics. The therapy options described in this book for specific disorders also apply to geriatric disorders.

This chapter provides an overview of how phytotherapy is used to treat geriatric disorders. This includes aspects such as dosage, long-term therapy, which can often become continuous therapy, and special sensitivities of the older organism to medications. Some medicinal plants could even be characterized as typical geriatric drugs.

Geriatrics is clearly developing into a **medical specialty**. We have learned that the organism develops special needs as it ages and that these needs must be addressed. The organism becomes more sensitive to medications in old age than in middle age—similar to the sensitivity to medications in childhood. In general, there are many commonalities between old age and childhood, even though disease patterns differ.

One might assume that practitioners dedicated to geriatric medicine would be open to and even excited about natural medicine and phytotherapeutics. Surprisingly, this is not the case. While physical therapy, ergotherapy, and art therapy play an important role in geriatrics, when it comes to medications, geriatrics mainly rely on **synthetic drugs**.

At the 12th Continuing Education Conference for Practical Geriatrics, in 1992, in the German town of Lübeck, Nehen introduced the topic of "Natural Medicine in Geriatrics" as follows: "For the past few years the term 'multiple morbidities' has come into general use in geriatrics. Many geriatric patients discover for themselves that they suffer from several very different disorders. At the same time, they discover that their treating physician is somewhat helpless in the face of this problem. These patients feel subjected to 'polypharmacy.' They are often prescribed four, five, or more medications. On the other hand, patients are informed in the media about the potential dangers and adverse effects of medications. This leaves patients feeling unsettled by the experience of their own frailty, the helplessness of their helpers, and their ambivalence about the treatments they receive. In the search for healing and well-being, natural medicine seems to be a possible alternative (Nehen)."

Warning differentiates between harmonious aging in concordance with senile changes and disharmonious aging resulting from the divergent involution processes of individual organ groups and mental behavior patterns. Physically, aging always involves involution or degeneration as well as a decline of life force and of sensory capabilities such as vision and hearing. These physical changes are associated with mental and emotional responses, including age-related mental confusion. We need to differentiate between **age-related physiological changes** and true **geriatric disorders**. This requires a holistic approach that meets the special needs of the aging with regards to diagnosis and therapy.

Understanding the process of aging requires that we view aging as an integral part of the human biography. Suppressing this process or attaching a social stigma to it means denying an integral part of being human. "Advanced age" is the phase of life during which human beings most fully develop their individual spirit. This phase starts much earlier than is commonly recognized. The phase of life known as aging and studied by the special field of geriatrics means the age or period, which is predominantly characterized by **degenerative processes** (Fintelmann 2005a). At the same time, individuality can produce increasing mental and emotional youthfulness during this period of life.

The following overview is intended to provide orientation for the **possibilities of phytotherapy**. Detailed information about the individual plants can be found in the respective chapters of this book.

Prescriptions for adults should generally focus on finished pharmaceutical products with specific dosage instructions. However, for seniors, prescriptions for medicinal teas or tinctures are frequently easier to introduce and tolerability is better. The intent is not to achieve quick acute results but to create long-term effects, also frequently in a preventive sense. This is an area where the practitioner can rediscover the joy of formulating individualized prescriptions. This book contains many examples for prescriptions, but there are no limits to a practitioner's imagination when it comes to meeting the needs of individual patients.

Medicinal Plants

Sclerotic Heart and Vascular Disorders
Hawthorn, Crataegus laevigata, Crataegus monogyna
Ginkgo, Ginkgo biloba
Garlic, Allium sativum
Artichoke, Cynara cardunculus
Lily-of-the-Valley, Convallaria majalis
Squill, Drimia maritima (syn. Scilla maritima, syn. Urginea maritima)
Arnica, Arnica montana
Bishop's weed, Ammi visnaga

Digestive Disorders
Gentian, Gentiana lutea
Centaury, Centaurium minus
Bogbean, Menyanthes trifoliata
Calamus, Acorus calamus
Angelica Root, Angelica archangelica
Blessed Thistle, Cnicus benedictus, syn. *Carduus benedictus*; syn. *Centaurea benedicta*
Ginger, Zingiber officinale
Galangal, Alpinia officinalis
Turmeric, Curcuma longa
Fumitory, Fumaria officinalis
Dandelion, Taraxacum officinale
Papaya, Carica papaya
Pineapple, Ananas comosus

Respiratory Tract Disorders
See Respiratory Disorders (p. 181)

Kidney, Efferent Urinary Tract and Prostate Disorders
Juniper, Juniperus communis
Lovage, Levisticum officinale
Spiny restharrow, Ononis spinosa
Parsley, Petroselinum crispum
Horsetail, Equisetum arvense

Java tea, Orthosiphon aristatus
Goldenrod, Solidago virgaurea
Pumpkin, Cucurbita pepo
Saw palmetto, Serenoa repens
Stinging nettle, Urtica dioica, Urtica urens

Metabolic Disorders
Dandelion, Taraxacum officinale
Stinging Nettle, Urtica dioica, Urtica urens
Birch, Betula pendula, Betula pubescens, Betula verrucosa

Anxiety, Insomnia, Depression
Passionflower, Passiflora incarnata
Valerian, Valeriana officinalis
Hops, Humulus lupulus
St.-John's-wort, Hypericum perforatum

Avolition, Exhaustion
Ginseng, Panax ginseng

11.1 Sclerotic Heart and Vascular Disorders

Medicinal Plants

Hawthorn, Crataegus laevigata, Crataegus monogyna
Hawthorn leaves, flowers and fruit, Crataegi folium et flos et fructus
Ginkgo, Ginkgo biloba
Ginkgo leaves, Ginkgo biloba folium
Garlic, Allium sativum
Garlic bulbs, Allii sativi bulbus
Artichoke, Cynara cardunculus
Artichoke leaves, Cynarae folium
Lily-of-the-Valley, Convallaria majalis
Lily-of-the-Valley herb, Convallariae herba
Motherwort, Leonurus cardiaca
Squill, Drimia maritima syn. Scilla maritima, syn. Urginea maritima
Squill bulb, Scillae bulbus
Arnica, Arnica montana
Arnica flowers, Arnicae flos
Bishop's weed, Ammi visnaga
Bishop's weed fruit, Ammeos visnagae fructus

11.1.1 Aging Heart and Arteriosclerosis

Prevention (see Degenerative Heart and Vascular Disorders (p. 137)) is a key consideration in the treatment of degenerative changes of the heart and vascular system, especially the arteries. The decision to initiate therapy should not wait until the end stages of these disorders are reached. This is especially important for early-stage arteriosclerosis and also for treating the **aging heart**.

The following five medicinal plants play a key role in this context: **Hawthorn** (Crataegus laevigata, Crataegus monogyna), **motherwort** (Leonurus cardiaca), **ginkgo** (Ginkgo biloba), **garlic** (Allium sativum), and **artichoke** (Cynara cardunculus). "Digitaloids" (heart glycosides), arnica (Arnica montana), Bishop's weed (Ammi visnaga), and periwinkle (Vinca minor) are mentioned here as examples for the many other options.

Plants Used in Treatment

Hawthorn (Crataegus laevigata, Crataegus monogyna)

For more information about this plant, see Hawthorn (p. 137).

▶ **Indications.** Hawthorn is the ideal remedy for treating the **aging heart**. Symptoms of the aging heart include decreasing muscle strength, tendency toward hypertension, mild arrhythmia, and, frequently, also bradycardia and mild angina pectoris resulting from insufficient coronary circulation. Each of these symptoms on its own is not serious enough to manifest a grave diagnosis, but together they significantly impact organ function and well-being. Hawthorn's pharmacology has demonstrated effects on all the above areas.

The Commission E views the main indication for hawthorn to be chronic heart failure as per NYHA II. However, antianginal (coronary circulation increasing), mild antihypertensive, and antiarrhythmic effects need also to be demonstrated. Hawthorn should be prescribed when one or more of these symptoms develop, even if no manifest diagnosis can be established. It is best taken as **interval therapy**, but never for less than 3 months. Its compelling efficacy, however, frequently causes patients to not want to stop taking this remedy.

It is important to note that experience has shown that the increased sensitivity or intolerance of the aging heart to digitalis drugs can be improved by simultaneous administration of hawthorn.

Hawthorn is also especially useful in combination with motherwort (Leonurus cardiaca) for treating the aging heart.

▶ **Therapy Recommendation.** Due to the complexity of constituents, only standardized extract preparations should be prescribed.

Ginkgo (Ginkgo biloba)

For more information about this plant, see Ginkgo (p. 157).

▶ **Indications.** There is very good evidence for the therapeutic efficacy of ginkgo leaf extract for brain dysfunction based on **cerebral vascular insufficiency** and for early stages of peripheral arterial occlusive disease.

The tolerability of ginkgo preparations is excellent. Adverse effects are rarely to be expected with the exception of local phlebitides with parenteral administration. The ginkgo dosage must be **sufficiently high** and started during the **early stages** of symptoms. Once the stage of complete vascular occlusion is reached, vascular surgery is unavoidable.

In the early stages, therapy should be long term, but not continuous. Practical experience has shown repeatedly that **interval therapy** can be more effective than continuous therapy. However, in the late stages of dementia, continuous therapy is indicated.

▶ **Note.** Other well-documented indications for ginkgo are **tinnitus** and **sudden hearing loss**. These conditions are primarily treated with ginkgo infusion therapy.

Garlic (Allium sativum)

For more information about this plant and its pharmacological effects, see Garlic (p. 154).

▶ **Indications.** For a long time, garlic was considered the best preventive medicinal plant remedy for **arteriosclerosis**. This seems plausible given its well-documented pharmacological efficacy, even if the results of epidemiological long-term trials are not yet available. Meanwhile, study results with an artichoke leaf extract finished pharmaceutical product have become available that exceed the efficacy of garlic for this indication (Gebhardt).

Garlic should not be considered a lipid-lowering or fibrinolytic remedy. Instead, it acts on several important points involved in the pathogenesis of arteriosclerosis. Each individual therapeutic factor has significantly weaker effects than the corresponding selective synthetic drugs, but garlic is unsurpassed in its complexity of action.

Regarding the unavoidable odor associated with garlic therapy, which many people consider unpleasant, it should be noted that **odorless** or **low odor preparations** are not sufficiently effective. There are galenic preparations available that reduce the direct odor in the mouth. However, the sulfuric odor will always be noticeable with effective preparations because garlic's therapeutic efficacy is derived from its sulfur-containing constituents.

Garlic is only prescribed for oral use.

▶ **Therapy Recommendations.** Garlic is suitable for long-term and continuous therapy. The authors' experience confirms that interval therapy is more effective than continuous therapy to prevent rapid habituation.

Artichoke (Cynara cardunculus, Cynara scolymus)

For more information about this plant, see Artichoke (p. 106).

▶ **Indications.** Artichoke is a very effective preventive remedy for **arteriosclerosis**.

Studies with an aqueous special artichoke leaf (p. 106) extract have demonstrated that the resulting finished pharmaceutical product is effective for treating hypercholesteremia, which is a key factor in the development of arteriosclerosis (Gebhardt). Artichoke leaf extract acts on different, but very complementary locations to effectively lower cholesterol. It promotes choleresis to increase the elimination of cholesterol and it inhibits the biosynthesis of cholesterol in the liver.

The most important result of these studies is that the high **antioxidant potential** of artichoke leaf extract can prevent oxidation of LDL cholesterol. This is viewed as the most important factor in the development of intima changes in the arteries that lead to arteriosclerosis.

▶ **Therapy Recommendations.** The idea of early prevention of age-related vascular changes by regularly taking a sufficiently dosed artichoke leaf extract preparation is outweighed by the aspiration of rational medical treatment to act only when necessary. Practitioners should conduct the necessary diagnostics to assess the individual risk factors of each patient before prescribing such remedies. This includes a constitutional and family anamnesis, palpatory and auscultatory examination of vascular status and assessment of the ocular fundus vessels. If these diagnostic measures provide clear indications of early stage vascular changes, the **preventive prescription** of the standardized artichoke leaf extract described above is indicated.

Preventive therapy should also be administered as **interval therapy** based on serum cholesterol and especially LDL cholesterol values. Since artichoke leaf extract and standardized garlic extract preparations have different effects, they can be alternated for long-term interval therapy.

Motherwort (Leonurus cardiaca)

▶ **Pharmacology.** Although several antiarrhythmic drugs of chemical origin have been in clinical use for decades, their application is often limited by their adverse effects and especially by their inherent proarrhythmic risk, which can lead to a significantly increased mortality in patients receiving these compounds.

On the other hand, aqueous extracts from the aerial parts of the European medicinal plant motherwort, Leonurus cardiaca L. (Lamiaceae), have traditionally been used as a remedy against tachyarrhythmias, heart failure, and other cardiac disorders for centuries (Barnes et al.). These were extensively described in European herbals dating from the 15th and 16th centuries such as *Gart der Gesundheit* (1485) or in the writings (as of 1544) of Pietro Andra Matthioli (Aber). Few attempts to understand the action of L. cardiaca, such as bradycardic effects observed in the therapy of children (Orlandi) or negative chronotropic and weak hypotensive effects of the single constituent lavandulifolioside (Milkowska et al.), have not yet been able to explain the complex cardiac effects of the Leonuri cardiacae herba (LCH) extract.

In order to enrich the active constituents from the primary extract that test as the most cardioactive, namely the aqueous Soxhlet extraction, and to eliminate undesired substances such as the dichloromethanic fraction or potassium, a bioassay-guided fractionation procedure was applied. The resulting development was a Leonurus cardiaca refined extract (LCRE), which was characterized together with Leonurus crude extracts by a newly developed gradient elution high performance liquid chromatography (HPLC) fingerprint analysis for separation and quantification of six major phenolics as well as by qNMR for determining the stachydrine content. This refined extract was applied intracoronarily in isolated rabbit hearts perfused according to the Langendorff technique.

Mapping experiments with electrodes on the heart surface showed a reduction of left ventricular pressure and an increase of relative coronary flow. Furthermore, the PQ-interval was prolonged, and both the basic cycle length and the activation recovery interval increased. In addition, voltage clamp measurements were performed on the following cell models in order to characterize the electrophysiological profile of LCRE: neonatal rat ventricular cardiomyocytes to investigate the effect on I(Na) and I(Ca.L), sinoatrial node cells and ventricular myocytes isolated from adult guinea pigs to test the effects on I(f) and action potential (AP) duration as well as HERG-transfected HEK 293 cells to analyze the influence on the I (K.r). In these voltage clamp experiments, LCRE exerted a calcium antagonistic activity by I(Ca.L) blockade, reduced the repolarizing current I(K.r), and prolonged the AP duration, while I(Na) was not affected. Although LCRE displayed only weak effects on the I(f) amplitude and voltage dependence, it significantly prolonged the activation time constant of I(f). Thus, LCRE acts on multiple electrophysiological targets–specifically I(Ca.L), I(K.r), and I(f)–observed both at whole organ and single cell level, lending support to the traditional antiarrhythmic indication of the LCH drug (Ritter).

The positive effects of Leonuri cardiacae herba (LCH) extract in cases of heart disease are, however, not limited to its direct effect on the heart. A main traditional use of Leonurus cardiaca L. in Western herbalism (Keller) and of the closely related L. japonicus Houtt. (Lamiaceae) in traditional East Asian Medicine (Li) is the treatment of neurological disorders such as anxiety, nervousness, depression, and as a sedative for insomnia. Within the context of Central European phytotherapy, these indications were especially signalized by A. Nahrstedt (Nahrstedt). In the eclectic school of traditional medicine in the United States, L. cardiaca aerial parts have been described as "having considerable control over the nervous system, advised

in nervous debility with irritation and unrest (Felter)." Especially in Russian folk medicine, the above-ground parts of L. cardiaca are regarded as an equal replacement for the roots of Valeriana officinalis L. (Caprifoliaceae) in the treatment of anxiety disorders (Kozo-Poljanskij). The similarity to valerian, especially under long-term therapy, was also noted by R.F. Weiss as within the context of the German herbal tradition, and described by him in an earlier edition of this book (Weiss 1960).

Anxiety and depressive disorders are increasingly being recognized as connected to dysfunctions of the gamma-aminobutyric acid system. Therefore, the in vivo effects of standardized L. cardiaca and L. japonicus extracts as well as five of their isolated constituents–the labdane-type isoleosibirin, the iridoid 7R-chloro-6-desoxy-harpagide, the phenylethanoid lavandulifolioside, and the N-containing compounds stachydrine and leonurine–on this type of neuronal receptor were investigated. Extracts of L. cardiaca and L. japonicus, characterized by reversed-phase high-performance liquid chromatography determination, as well as their above-named isolated possible active constituents of different chemical nature, were tested in several receptor binding assays on rat $GABA_A$ receptors using [3H]-SR95 531 and [3H]-Ro-15–1788 (flumazenil/diazepam control). The L. cardiaca and L. japonicus extracts as well as leonurine inhibited the concentration dependent binding of [3H]-SR95 531 to the gamma-aminobutyric acid site of the gamma-aminobutyric acid type A receptor with a high binding affinity: IC_{50} values of 21 µg/mL, 46 µg/mL, and 15 µg/mL, respectively. In contrast, binding to the benzodiazepine site of the rat gamma-aminobutyric acid type A receptor had a 15 to 30 times lower binding affinity than to the gamma-aminobutyric acid site.

The presented experiments provide hints that the neurological mechanism of action of L. cardiaca and L. japonicus may essentially be based on their interaction to the gamma-aminobutyric acid site of the gamma-aminobutyric acid type A receptor, while the benzodiazepine site most probably does not contribute to this effect. In the case of L. japonicus, these effects can be at least partially be explained by its leonurine constituent, whereas the active principle of L. cardiaca, which does not contain leonurine, is subject to further research as none of the other investigated individual constituents displayed significant activity in the applied test system (Rauwald).

Other Phytotherapeutics

Lily-of-the-Valley (Convallaria majalis)

For more information about this plant, see Lily-of-the-Valley (p. 149).

Lily-of-the-valley is indicated for declining heart muscle performance.

Squill (Drimia maritima, syn. Scilla maritima, syn. Urginea maritima)

For more information about this plant, see Squill (p. 147).

Squill is used to treat **declining heart muscle performance** and **tendency toward edema**.

Arnica (Arnica montana)
Bishop's Weed (Ammi visnaga)

For more information about these plants, see Arnica (p. 144) and Bishop's weed (p. 202).

Arnica and bishop's weed are used to treat **anginous symptoms**.

Bibliography

Arber A. Herbals: their origin and evolution. A chapter in the history of botany 1470–1670. Cambridge: Cambridge University Press; 1938

Barnes J, Anderson LA, Phillipson JD. Monograph motherwort. Herbal medicines. London: Pharmaceutical Press; 2002: 354–356

Felter HW. The eclectic materia medica, pharmacology and therapeutics. Cincinnati: John K Scudder; 1922: 251–252

Fintelmann V. Alterssprechstunde. Ein Ratgeber zum Umgang mit dem Alter. 3. ed. Stuttgart: Verlag Urachhaus; 2005

Gebhardt R. Artischockenextrakt: In-vitro-Nachweis einer Hemmwirkung auf die Cholesterin-Biosynthese. Med Welt. 1995; 46:348–350

Keller K. Assessment report on Leonurus cardiaca L. Herba. EMA/HMPC/127430/2010/Community herbal monograph on Leonurus cardiaca L. Herba. EMA/HMPC/127428/2010

Kozo-Poljanskij BM. Motherwort—the new pharmaceutical and technical crop from the Voronezh region. Voronezh 1945:1–10

Li S. Bencao Gangmu (1593). Luo X, translator. Compendium of Materia Medica, Book III, Vol. 15, category of herbs (IV). Beijing: Foreign Languages Press; 2003: 1637–1644

Miłkowska-Leyck K, Filipek B, Strzelecka H. Pharmacological effects of lavandulifolioside from Leonurus cardiaca. J Ethnopharmacol. 2002; 80(1):85–90

Nahrstedt A. Drogen und Phytopharmaka mit sedierender Wirkung. Zeitschr f Phytotherapie. 1985; 6:101–109

Nehen HG. Naturheilkunde im Alter. Einleitung. In: Schütz RM, ed. Praktische Geriatrie 12. Lübeck; 1992

Orlandi E. [Application of Leonurus cardiaca in therapy of children]. Lattante. 1950; 21(9):582–586

Rauwald HW, Savtschenko A, Merten A, Rusch C, Appel K, Kuchta K. GABAA Receptor Binding Assays of Standardized Leonurus cardiaca and Leonurus japonicus Extracts as Well as Their Isolated Constituents. Planta Med. 2015; 81(12–13):1103–1110

Ritter M, Melichar K, Strahler S, et al. Cardiac and electrophysiological effects of primary and refined extracts from Leonurus cardiaca L. (Ph.Eur.). Planta Med. 2010; 76(6):572–582

Weiss RF. Lehrbuch der Phytotherapie. 2nd ed. Stuttgart: Hippokrates; 1960: 213

Warning A. Naturheilkunde im Alter. Naturheilkunde bei multimorbiden älteren Patienten. In: Schütz RM, ed Praktische Geriatrie 12. Lübeck; 1992

11.2 Digestive Disorders

Medicinal Plants

Tonic Bitters
Gentian, Gentiana lutea
Gentian root, Gentianae radix
Centaury, Centaurium minus
Centaury herb, Centaurii herba
Bogbean, Menyanthes trifoliata
Bogbean leaves, Menyanthis folium

Aromatic Bitters
Calamus, Acorus calamus
Calamus rootstock, Calami rhizoma
Angelica, Angelica archangelica
Angelica root, Angelicae radix
Blessed thistle, Cnicus benedictus, syn.
Carduus benedictus; syn. Centaurea benedicta
Blessed thistle herb, Cnici benedicti herba
Ginger, Zingiber officinale
Ginger rootstock, Zingiberis rhizoma
Galangal, Alpinia officinarium
Galangal rootstock, Galangae rhizoma

Cholagogues
Turmeric, Curcuma longa
Turmeric rootstock, Curcuma rhizoma
Fumitory, Fumaria officinalis
Fumitory herb, Fumariae herba
Dandelion, Taraxacum officinale
Dandelion herb and root, Taraxaci herba cum radix

Pancreatic Remedies
Papaya, Carica papaya
Papaya leaves, Caricae papayae folium
Pineapple, Ananas comosus
Pineapple juice, Ananas succus

11.2.1 Decline in Digestive Capacity

A **decline in capacity of the digestive organs** is a typical physiological characteristic of aging. It presents as increased food intolerance. Symptoms can include a **feeling of fullness** after meals, increased **meteorism**, including Roemheld syndrome, and mild **constipation**. True maldigestion is not the focus here.

The process of physical digestion requires a complex collaboration of different organs, including the stomach, gallbladder, and pancreas. Poor digestion, therefore, is an indication for plant remedies that stimulate appetite, choleresis, and enzyme production. The most important plant remedies are grouped into the categories of bitters, cholagogues, and carminatives. Carminatives can also have spasmolytic effects. Plants that substitute exocrine pancreas functions are also presented.

Plants Used in Treatment: Tonic Bitters

This section first introduces several bitters used to treat poor digestion. Bitters are drugs that contain bitter principles. Bitters are grouped into tonic bitters, aromatic bitters, and acrid bitters (p. 52). Bitter principles promote secretion of digestive juices, especially in the stomach, but also in other areas.

The primary symptom focus for bitters in treating poor digestion is to **stimulate appetite**, but their more important effect is to **promote digestion**. A large number of plants are suitable for this purpose.

Of the **stomachics** or **aperitifs** presented here, gentian has the highest bittering value (20,000); centaury is weaker (3,500), and bogbean is the weakest (1,500).

Practitioners should consider the patient's age and symptoms when determining prescription strength. This is yet another example that the highest strength is not always the best choice. **Mild prescriptions** can often be more effective longer term.

Gentian (Gentiana lutea)

For more information about this plant, see Gentian (p. 54).

Gentian is the most well-known plant with bittering effects. Its bittering power is exceeded by artemisia, but the slightly milder gentian is more suitable for geriatric prescriptions.

Preparation

- Tincture
  Add 20–40 drops to 1 glass of water.
  Drink before each meal.

Centaury (Centaurium minus, Centaurium erythraea)

For more information about this plant, see Centaury (p. 53).

> **Preparation**
>
> - **Tea**
>   Add 1 cup of boiling water to 1–2 teaspoons of the drug. Steep for 15 minutes, then strain.
>   Drink 1 cup at room temperature before each meal.

Bogbean (Menyanthes trifoliate)

For more information about this plant, see Bogbean (p. 56).

> **Preparations**
>
> - **Tea**
>   Add 1 cup of boiling water to 1 teaspoon of the finely chopped drug or add the drug to cold water and bring to a brief boil. Steep for 10 minutes, then strain.
>   Drink unsweetened 15–30 minutes before meals.
> - **Tincture**
>   Add 20–40 drops to half a glass of water and drink slowly.

Aromatic Bitters

Aromatic bitters contain volatile oils in addition to bittering principles. This provides additional **spasmolytic**, **carminative**, or **cholagogue** effects.

Calamus (Acorus calamus)

For more information about this plant, see Calamus (p. 59).

> **Preparation**
>
> - **Tincture**
>   Add 20–30 drops to 1 glass of water.
>   Drink 3 × a day before meals.

Angelica Root (Angelica archangelica)

For more information about this plant, see angelica root (p. 57).

> **Preparation**
>
> - **Tea**
>   Add 1 teaspoon of the drug to 1 cup of cold water and bring to a brief boil, then strain. Alternatively, add 1 cup of boiling water to 1 teaspoon of the drug, then strain.
>   Drink 1 cup before meals.

Blessed Thistle (Cnicus benedictus, Carduus benedictus, syn. Centaurea benedicta)

For more information about this plant, see Blessed Thistle (p. 58).

> **Preparation**
>
> - **Tea**
>   Add 1 cup of boiling water to 2 teaspoons of the drug. Steep for 30 minutes, then strain.
>   Drink 2–3 cups 20–30 minutes before meals.

Acrid Bitters (Amara acria)

Acrid bitters contain acrid constituents in addition to bitter principles. They are rarely used in geriatrics.

Ginger (Zingiber officinalis)

For more information about this plant, see Ginger (p. 60).

> **Preparation**
>
> - **Tincture**
>   Add 10–20 drops to 1 glass of water and drink before meals.

Galangal (Alpinia officinarium)

For more information about this plant, see Galangal (p. 61).

Galangal rootstock has pronounced spasmolytic effects and can also relieve **mild biliary colics**.

Proven Prescriptions: Stomachic Teas (Species stomachicae)

> **Prescriptions**
>
> **Rx**
> Centaurii herb. (centaury herb)
> Trifolii fibrini fol. (bogbean leaf)
> Calami rhiz. āā 20.0 (calamus rootstock)
> M. f. spec.
> Add 1 tablespoon of the blend to 1 L of water.
> Boil for 15 minutes, then strain.
> D.S.
> Drink 1 cup warm 1 hour before each main meal.

> **Prescriptions**
>
> **Rx**
> Foeniculi fruct. (fennel seeds)
> Menth. pip. Fol (peppermint leaves)
> Melissae fol. (lemon balm leaves)
> Calami rhiz. āā 20.0 (calamus rootstock)
> M. f. spec.
> Add 1 cup of boiling water to 1 teaspoon of the blend. Steep for 10 minutes, then strain.
> D.S.
> Drink while warm in small sips 2–3 × a day.

Stomachic Tinctures (Tincturae stomachicae)

> **Prescriptions**
>
> **Rx**
> Tinct. Gentianae (gentian tincture)
> Tinct. Absinthiii āā 20.0 (wormwood tincture)
> Tinct. Menth. pip. 10.0 (peppermint tincture)
> D.S.
> Add 15–30 drops to 1 glass of water and drink 3 × a day shortly before meals.

> **Prescriptions**
>
> **Rx**
> Tinct. Belladonnae 5.0 (belladonna tincture)
> Tinct. Gentianae (gentian tincture)
> Tinct. Absinthii āā 20.0 (wormwood tincture)
> D.S.
> Add 15–30 drops to 1 glass of water and drink 3 × a day shortly before meals.

Additional Therapy Options: Cholagogues

For a detailed description of cholagogues and choleretics from the perspective of phytotherapy, see Plant Cholagogues (p. 111).

Stimulating biliary function, especially biliary secretion, is an essential prerequisite for effective digestion. Many gastroenterologists are critical in their assessment of phytotherapeutics in this area because these remedies are viewed rather one-sidedly from an experimental perspective. However, these remedies have a long history of successful use in practice.

Turmeric (Curcuma longa, Curcuma domestica)

For more information about this plant, see Turmeric (p. 122).

Turmeric rootstock is highly significant for the indications discussed in this section. This has been confirmed by typical observational studies (Thamlikitkul et al.). Furthermore, the fact that curcumin promotes apoptosis of activated hepatic stellate cells by inhibiting protein expression of the MyD88 pathway might hint to the usefulness of this drug in preventing liver fibrosis (He et al.).

Fumitory (Fumaria officinalis)

For more information about this plant, see Fumitory (p. 114).

Fumitory has a somewhat milder effect than turmeric.

▶ **Therapy Recommendation.** We like to use fumitory in prescriptions that represent the characteristic trio of cholagogues, spasmolytics, and carminatives.

Dandelion (Taraxacum officinale)

For more information about this plant, see Dandelion (p. 124).

Dandelion is a typical antidyscratic that is of special interest for geriatric patients because it acts as a **cholagogue** and is also a plant-based **diuretic** (aquaretic). Dandelion stimulates elimination via the kidneys. From the perspective of traditional medicine, this promotes the excretion of substances that would otherwise tend to be deposited in the organism. As discussed elsewhere in this book, this also makes dandelion a suitable remedy for patients with a tendency toward gallstone formation.

Preparation

- **Tea**
  Add 1–2 teaspoons of the finely chopped drug to 1 cup of cold water. Bring to a brief boil and steep for 15 minutes.
  Drink 1 cup each morning and evening for 4–6 weeks.

Proven Prescriptions: Cholagogue Teas (Species cholagogae)

Prescriptions

Rx
Cnici benedicti herb. (blessed thistle herb)
Absinthii herb. (wormwood herb)
Menth. pip. fol. (peppermint leaves)
Cardui Mariae fruct. (milk thistle seeds)
Taraxaci rad. c. herb. āā ad 100.0 (dandelion root and herb)
M. f. spec.
Add 1–2 cups of boiling water to 1 teaspoon of the blend. Steep for 20 minutes, then strain.
D.S.
Drink 3 cups a day for 3–4 weeks.

Prescriptions

Rx
Carvi fruct. 10.0 (caraway seeds)
Menth. pip. fol. (peppermint leaves)
Absinthii herb. āā 30.0 (wormwood herb)
Frangul. cort. (buckthorn bark)
Sennae fol. conc. āā 15.0 (senna leaves)
M. f. spec.
Add 1 cup of hot water to 1–2 teaspoons of the blend. Steep for 10 minutes, then strain.
D.S.
Drink 1 cup in the morning and in the evening.

Cholagogue Tinctures (Tinctura cholagoga)

Prescriptions

Rx
Ol. Carvi 5.0 (caraway oil)
Tinct. Absinthii (wormwood tincture)
Tinct. carminativ. (see Carminative tinctures (p. 79))
Tinct. Belladonnae āā 10.0 (belladonna tincture)
Tinct. Valerian. aeth. 15.0 (ethereal valerian tincture)
D.S.
Take 15–30 drops 3 × a day after meals.

Additional Therapy Options: Pancreatic Remedies

Papaya and pineapple are included here as remedies that support the digestive function of the pancreas.

Proof of efficacy is strongest for the enzyme-like action of papain, the milky juice of unripe papaya fruits. However, the efficacy of bromelain derived from pineapple is also well documented. In any case, these well-tolerated plant enzymes can play a supportive role in geriatrics. As of the date of this writing, it remains to be seen if these remedies offer significant advantages compared with defined pancreatic preparations.

Papaya (Carica papaya)

For more information about this plant, see Papaya (p. 126).

Pineapple (Ananas comosus)

For more information about this plant, see Pineapple (p. 127).

Bibliography

Ali T, Shakir F, Morton J. Curcumin and inflammatory bowel disease: biological mechanisms and clinical implication. Digestion. 2012; 85(4):249–255

He YJ, Kuchta K, Deng YM, et al. Curcumin Promotes Apoptosis of Activated Hepatic Stellate Cells by Inhibiting Protein Expression of the MyD88 Pathway. Planta Med. 2017; 83(18):1392–1396

He YJ, Kuchta K, Lv X, et al. Curcumin, the main active constituent of turmeric (Curcuma longa L.), induces apoptosis in hepatic stellate cells by modulating the abundance of apoptosis-related growth factors. Z Natforsch C J Biosci. 2015; 70(11–12):281–285

Thamlikitkul V, et al. Randomized Double-Blind Study of Curcuma domestica Val. for Dyspepsia. J Med Assoc Thai. 1989; 72(11):613–620

11.3 Respiratory Disorders

The special application areas of phytotherapeutics for acute and chronic respiratory disorders are described in Chapter 5. The classifications and descriptions in that chapter also apply to prescribing these remedies for geriatric patients.

Medicinal plant demulcents, expectorants, and antitussives are especially valuable for older people because of their therapeutic range, good tolerability, and milder effects. In addition, synthetic alternatives cannot be considered sufficiently proven and superior to be given preference in every case.

▶ **Note.** Sufficient and plentiful fluid intake is an important prerequisite for effective expectoration, especially for older people with respiratory disorders. Sometimes, not following this basic rule is the only reason that phytotherapeutic expectorants are not sufficiently efficacious.

For references corresponding to the preceding section, see Chapter 11.7 Bibliography.

11.4 Kidney, Efferent Urinary Tract, and Prostate Disorders

Medicinal Plants
Juniper, Juniperus communis
Juniper berries, Juniperi fructus
Lovage, Levisticum officinale
Lovage root, Levistici radix
Spiny restharrow, Ononis spinosa
Spiny Restharrow root, Ononidis radix
Parsley, Petroselinum crispum
Parsley herb and root, Petroselini herba et radix
Horsetail, Equisetum arvense
Horsetail herb, Equiseti herba
Java tea, Orthosiphon aristatus
Java tea leaves, Orthosiphonis folium
Goldenrod, Solidago virgaurea
Goldenrod herb, Solidaginis herba
Pumpkin, Cucurbita pepo
Pumpkin seeds, Cucurbitae semen
Saw palmetto, Serenoa repens
Saw palmetto fruit, Sabalis serrulati fructus
Stinging nettle, Urtica dioica, Urtica urens
Stinging nettle root, Urticae radix

11.4.1 Benign Prostatic Hyperplasia (BPH)

A wide variety of options are available for the treatment of **benign prostatic hyperplasia** (BPH), a seemingly obligate disorder for men. Relieving the symptoms associated with this benign prostate growth—for example, nocturia—provides significant improvements in quality of life.

Phytotherapeutics that stimulate kidney excretion are especially suitable for older people. Schilcher refers to them as **aquaretics.**

▶ **Note.** The efficacy of phytotherapeutics with this condition also depends on sufficient fluid intake.

Plants Used in Treatment

For descriptions, indications, and dosage information for the phytotherapeutics discussed in this section, see Chapter 6, Kidney, Urinary Tract, and Prostate Disorders.

Juniper (Juniperus communis), Lovage (Levisticum officinale), Spiny Restharrow (Ononis spinose), Parsley (Petroselinum crispum), Horsetail (Equisetum arvense)

These medicinal plants specifically **promote excretion.**

Java Tea (Orthosiphon spicatus/stamineus/aristatus), Goldenrod (Solidago virgaurea)

Both plants also enhance **kidney function**. Phytotherapeutics play an important role for this physical function because it declines with age.

Pumpkin (Cucurbita pepo), Saw Palmetto (Serenoa repens, Sabal serrulata), Stinging Nettle (Urtica dioica), Dwarf Nettle (Urtica urens)

These plants predominate in the treatment of **benign prostatic hyperplasia (BPH)**. They are also a good preventive.

For references corresponding to the preceding section, see Chapter 11.7 Bibliography.

11.5 Metabolic Disorders

Dandelion, Taraxacum officinale
Dandelion herb and root, Taraxaci herba cum radix
Stinging nettle, Urtica dioica, Urtica urens
Stinging Nettle herb and leaves, Urtica herbae et folium
Birch, Betula pendula, Betula pubescens, Betula verrucosa
Birch leaves, Betulae folium

11.5.1 Deposition Disorders

The antidyscratics described here are phytotherapeutics used to treat chronic metabolic disorders, especially those exhibiting a tendency toward deposition (see Section 7.1.1 Arthritis and Arthrosis (p. 235)). These remedies have a natural affinity with aging because aging is associated with a slowing metabolism and a tendency toward deposition. The aging organism can therefore benefit from support of excretion.

Plants Used in Treatment

Dandelion (Taraxacum officinale), Stinging Nettle (Urtica dioica, Urtica urens), Dwarf Nettle (Urtica urens), Birch (Betula pendula, Betula pubescens, Betula verrucosa)

For more information about these plants and information about their use, see Dandelion (p. 124) and Stinging Nettle (p. 237).

Proven Prescriptions

Rx
Urticae herb. (nettle herb)
Dulcamar. stipit. (woody nightshade stems)
Caricis rhiz. (sand sedge rhizome)
Sennae fol. (senna leaves)
Foenicul. fruct. āā 20.0 (fennel seeds)
M. f. spec.
Add 500 mL of boiling water to 1–2 tablespoons of the blend. Steep for 10–15 minutes, then strain.
D.S.
Drink 1 cup in the morning and in the evening.

Rx
Taraxaci rad. c. herb. (dandelion root and herb)
Juniperi fruct. (juniper berries)
Sennae fol. (senna leaves)
Frangul. cort. (buckthorn bark)
Carvi fruct. āā 20.0 (caraway seeds)
M. f. spec.
Add 500 mL of boiling water to 1–2 tablespoons of the blend. Steep for 10–15 minutes, then strain.
D.S.
Drink 1 cup in the morning and in the evening.

▶ **Therapy Recommendation.** This therapy should be prescribed as a recurring **course of treatment**, especially in the spring and autumn. Each course usually lasts no longer than 1–2 months, which indicates that this treatment is more preventive in nature.

This type of treatment has also been referred to as detoxification and patients experience it as helpful, reviving, and refreshing.

For references corresponding to the preceding section, see Chapter 11.7 Bibliography (p. 329).

11.6 Anxiety, Insomnia, Depression

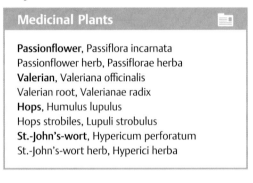

Medicinal Plants

Passionflower, Passiflora incarnata
Passionflower herb, Passiflorae herba
Valerian, Valeriana officinalis
Valerian root, Valerianae radix
Hops, Humulus lupulus
Hops strobiles, Lupuli strobulus
St.-John's-wort, Hypericum perforatum
St.-John's-wort herb, Hyperici herba

11.6.1 First-Line Therapy Phytopharmaceuticals

A subtle approach is required for prescribing synthetic psychopharmaceuticals in geriatrics. Treatment using phytotherapeutics or a suitable combination should always precede the use of synthetic drugs. Of course, this does not apply to acute psychotic confusional states.

Plants Used in Treatment

Passionflower (Passiflora incarnate)

For more information about this plant, see Passionflower (p. 258).

Passionflower serves as a daytime sedative (possibly also combined with a low dose of valerian).

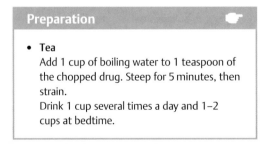

Preparation

- **Tea**
  Add 1 cup of boiling water to 1 teaspoon of the chopped drug. Steep for 5 minutes, then strain.
  Drink 1 cup several times a day and 1–2 cups at bedtime.

Valerian (Valeriana officinalis), Hop (Humulus lupulus)

For more information about these plants, see Valerian (p. 253) and Hop (p. 255).

These two phytotherapeutics are **sleep promoting**. A sufficiently dosed combination of both plants is especially effective.

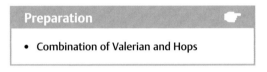

Preparation

- **Combination of Valerian and Hops**

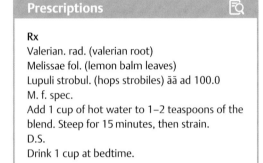

Prescriptions

Rx
Valerian. rad. (valerian root)
Melissae fol. (lemon balm leaves)
Lupuli strobul. (hops strobiles) āā ad 100.0
M. f. spec.
Add 1 cup of hot water to 1–2 teaspoons of the blend. Steep for 15 minutes, then strain.
D.S.
Drink 1 cup at bedtime.

St.-John's-wort (Hypericum perforatum)

For more information about this plant, see St.-John's-wort (p. 264).

Our experience has shown St.-John's-wort to be the **antidepressant** of first choice in geriatrics. Synthetic antidepressants often have severe side effects, especially excessive sedation or cardiotoxicity.

However, St.-John's-wort extract preparations are not immediately effective. They require a ramp up period of 8 to 14 days and develop their full efficacy after 4 to 8 weeks.

This medicinal plant antidepressant does not create dependency or produce personality changes, which makes it especially valuable.

For references corresponding to the preceding section, see Chapter 11.7 Bibliography (p. 329).

11.7 Exhaustion, Avolition

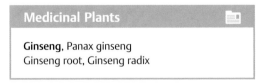

Medicinal Plants

Ginseng, Panax ginseng
Ginseng root, Ginseng radix

11.7.1 Phytogeriatric Remedies

It has been said repeatedly: There is no cure for aging. At the same time, as has been shown in this chapter, a number of useful phytotherapeutics can be used preventively to deal with certain processes of aging and the symptoms—primarily a decline in well-being—associated with them.

Phytogeriatrics are plants that have special strengthening and tonic effects. **Ginseng** is the most well studied of these plants.

Plants Used in Treatment

Ginseng (Panax ginseng)

For more information about Chinese ginseng, see Ginseng (p. 272).

Based on what we know today, ginseng is the only phytogeriatric remedy with proven efficacy.

Bibliography

Fintelmann V. Altersprechstunde. Ein Ratgeber zum Umgang mit dem Alter. 3. ed. Stuttgart: Verlag Urachhaus; 2005a

Fintelmann V. Praktische Teetherapie. Stuttgart: Wissenschaftliche Verlagsgesellschaft; 2005b

Fintelmann V. Therapie mit Phytopharmaka. In: Platt D, Mutschler E, ed Pharmakologie im Alter. Ein Lehrbuch für Praxis und Klinik. Stuttgart: Wissenschaftliche Verlagsgesell-schaft; 1999: 456–476

Gebhardt R. Artischockenextrakt: In-vitro-Nachweis einer Hemm-wirkung auf die Cholesterin-Biosynthese. Med Welt. 1995; 46: 348–350

Nehen HG. Naturheilkunde im Alter. Einleitung. In: Schütz RM, ed. Praktische Geriatrie 12. Lübeck; 1992

Pfister-Holz G. Phytotherapie in der Geriatrie. Z Phytother. 1997; 18(3):163–169

Schilcher H. Pflanzliche Urologika. Dtsch Apoth Ztg. 1984; 124: 2429–2436

Trunzler G.. Phytopharmaka in der Geriatrie. Ärztez Naturheilver-fahren. 1987; 28:85–99

Warning A. Naturheilkunde im Alter. Naturheilkunde bei multimorbiden älteren Patienten. In: Schütz RM, ed Praktische Geriatrie 12. Lübeck; 1992

Zoch E. Über die Inhaltsstoffe des Handelspapains [Contents of commercial papain]. Arzneimittelforschung. 1969; 19(9):1593–1597

Questions

1. What makes phytotherapeutics so valuable for the treatment and prevention of geriatric disorders?
2. Which plant is especially indicated for treatment of the "aging heart"?
3. Formulate a tea (Species stomachicae) that stimulates appetite and is a mild laxative.
4. Which combination of medicinal plant drugs has good sleep-promoting effects without adverse effects the next day?
5. Which plant is considered a special phytogeriatric remedy?

Answers (p. 423) for Chapter 11.

12 Pediatric Disorders

Especially during the early and late stages of life—childhood and old age—the human organism is particularly sensitive to external stimuli, including medications. This sensitivity is also a factor in immunology, since the mechanisms to defend against exogenous effects and substances need to be learned during childhood and generally decline in old age.

This chapter presents more information about medicinal plants that are especially well suited for treating pediatric disorders based on their wide therapeutic range and good tolerability.

The ability to use medicines that are more familiar to the organism's metabolic pathways than modern synthetics invented during the 20th and 21st centuries is of great advantage. The therapeutic range and tolerability of many phytotherapeutics makes them excellent remedies during childhood and advanced age. However, there is one important difference between these two phases of life: A child's organism possesses a high potential for self-healing, which is usually lacking in advanced age. Consider the healing process for bone fracture in childhood! The regenerative element of organ development is also much more pronounced in childhood than in advanced age.

When treating pediatric disorders, the primary objective for practitioners needs to be to promote and support the organism's **self-healing powers**. When these powers are too intense, they may even need to be dampened, but they should never be counteracted. This objective is certainly more easily accomplished by using phytotherapeutics than by using most specialized synthetic drugs that carry a high potential for adverse effects.

As with the phytotherapeutics recommended in the chapter on geriatric disorders, the effects and characteristics of each of the medicinal plants described in the respective chapters still pertain. In this chapter, however, we present medicinal plants that are especially suitable for pediatrics. Where applicable, we indicate special dosage considerations for children and indications that may differ from those for adults.

Medicinal Plants

Dyspeptic Symptoms
German chamomile, Matricaria recutita
Lemon balm, Melissa officinalis
Peppermint, Mentha piperita
Fennel, Foeniculum vulgare

Lack of Appetite
Calamus, Acorus calamus
Bitter orange, Citrus aurantium ssp. amara
Angelica, Angelica archangelica
Centaury, Centaurium minus

Flatulence
Caraway, Carum carvi

Diarrhea
Bilberry, Vaccinium myrtillus
Uzara, Xysmalobium undulatum

Constipation
Flax, Linum usitatissimum
Psyllium seed, Plantago psyllium
Alder buckthorn, Rhamnus frangula
Castor bean, Ricinus communis
Rhubarb, Rheum palmatum/officinale

Respiratory Disorders
Marshmallow, Althaea officinalis
Narrowleaf plantain, Plantago lanceolata
Iceland moss, Cetraria islandica
Cowslip primrose, Primula veris

Convulsive Cough and Whooping Cough
Thyme, Thymus vulgaris
Roundleaf sundew, Drosera rotundifolia
Ivy, Hedera helix
Meadowsweet, Filipendula ulmaria

Colds
Linden, Tilia cordata/platyphyllos
European elderberry, Sambucus nigra
Purple Echinacea, Echinacea purpurea
Thuja (white cedar), Thuja occidentalis
Boneset, Eupatorium perfoliatum

Kidney and Urinary Tract Disorders
See Chapter 6

Anxiety, Restlessness, Sleep Disorders
Passionflower, Passiflora incarnata
Lemon balm, Melissa officinalis
California poppy, Eschscholtzia californica
Lavender, Lavandula angustifolia

Depression
St.-John's-wort, Hypericum perforatum

Dermatitis
German chamomile, Matricaria recutita
Calendula, Calendula officinalis
Heart's ease, Viola tricolor
English walnut, Juglans regia

Contusions, Hematomas, Sprains
Arnica, Arnica montana
Yarrow, Achillea millefolium
Peruvian balsam, Myroxylon balsamum
Rosemary, Rosmarinus officinalis

Burns, Scalding
St.-John's-wort, Hypericum perforatum

Herpes Simplex
Lemon balm, Melissa officinalis

▶ **Dosage.** Dosage represents a special consideration in pediatrics. The type of research that determines the usually precise dosage and effect relationship in adults is frequently not available for children. One of the reasons for this lack of research is that much stricter rules apply for clinical and experimental research with children. This also fully applies to phytopharmaceuticals. The Commission E monographs also do not list specific differences in dosages for adults and children.

In view of this fact, the German Cooperative on Phytopharmaceuticals (Kooperation Phytopharmaka) deserves special credit for its report on pediatric dosages for phytopharmaceuticals [Dorsch et al.]. The authors of this report computed plausible pediatric dosages for phytopharmaceuticals they considered especially useful in pediatrics. Based on the criteria of body surface, age, and body weight, they computed dosages for four **age groups**. These calculations form the basis for the dosages given in the chapter at hand. All dosages in Dorsch et al. are computed for the whole drug, which allows for easy comparison with the dosage information provided in the Commission E monographs. However, dosages for extracts require further conversions.

Most pharmaceutical manufacturers list pediatric dosages on their product labels or patient leaflets. For infusions or teas, which are the key dosage form for children up to the age of 4, the indicated dosages are directly applicable.

At the end of January 2007, the European Union enacted its **regulation on medicinal products for pediatric use** (EG 1901/2006, modified by EG 1902/2006). At the same time, the European Medicines Agency (EMEA) established a pediatric committee (PDCO). Its goal is to increase the safety of medications that are especially suitable for children and to investigate their usefulness without initiating unnecessary studies in children. However, pharmaceutical manufacturers are still expected to provide comprehensive data for all pediatric remedies. This applies to synthetic drugs as well as to special therapeutic remedies, which includes phytotherapeutics. The German Federal Ministry of Health also constituted a commission on medicinal products for children and youths. All medicinal products that are **approved for use in children** are required to display a special symbol on their label.

▶ **Research.** The computation of pediatric dosing is supported by the results of a survey of 1,000 pediatricians about age-dependent differences in dosage for the finished pharmaceutical product Esberitox (a finished pharmaceutical extract product of Thuja occidentalis leaf, Echinacea purpurea root, Echinacea pallida root, and Baptisia tinctoria root), which is commonly prescribed for children. In approximately 250,000 treatments of 141,400 children, almost identical dosages were matched to those computed by the German Cooperative on Phytopharmaceuticals (Kooperation Phytopharmaka) (Köhler et al.). It is also important that indications for use in infants were only found for 36 of the 101 drugs for which dosage was computed.

▶ **Preparation.** One advantage of phytotherapeutics is that its medications frequently require preparation. Preparing a tea or administering an ointment, poultice, or bath requires physical contact. This therapeutic application promotes human communication and strengthens the relationship between the adult and the child.

Tea preparations are more suitable for young children than for any other age group. For this reason, they should always be given preference. Other suitable preparations include infusions, decoctions, and macerations. The choice of preparation depends on the type of drug used and its main constituents. For example, constituents can be hydrophilic or lipophilic. Other relevant preparations include **fresh plant juices**, provided the child tolerates their flavor. Juices that taste less pleasant can be mixed with juices that taste more pleasant, such as grape juice. We would like to warn against the use of instant teas due to their high sugar content and associated risk of tooth decay.

However, some phytotherapeutics are less advisable for use with children. This is especially true for **alcoholic extractions**. These should be prescribed for children under the age of 4 only for very strict indications because the elimination of alcohol from the organism takes significantly longer in children than in adults. With older children and youths, the alcohol content in prescription drops is not a concern. Even the consumption of larger amounts of fruit juice concentrate involves the intake of many times over the amount of alcohol in medications (Kauert, Gorgus 2016).

Likewise, care should be exercised with drugs that have aggressive effects such as wormwood, ginger, galangal, and drastic, senna-type laxatives.

Phytotherapeutics **used externally** play a special role for children. A child's skin is still very open to all environmental impacts. This characteristic allows for a very different use of remedies than is the case of older people.

Special care must be exercised with the external and internal application of **essential oils,** for example, menthol. Inappropriate use of medications that contain menthol can cause respiratory depression and even respiratory paralysis (Kratschmer's reflex).

12.1 Digestive Disorders

12.1.1 Dyspeptic Symptoms

> **Medicinal Plants**
>
> **German Chamomile**, Matricaria recutita
> German hamomile flowers, Matricariae flos
> **Lemon Balm**, Melissa officinalis
> Lemon Balm leaves, Melissae folium
> **Peppermint**, Mentha piperita
> Peppermint leaves, Menthae piperitae folium
> **Fennel**, Foeniculum vulgare
> Fennel seeds, Foeniculi fructus

Plants Used in Treatment

German Chamomile (Matricaria recutita)

For more information about this plant, see German chamomile (p. 42).

▶ **Indications.** German chamomile appears to have been created especially for treating children. The protective, nourishing, and healing effect of **chamomile flowers** (Matricariae flos) on the boundary layers of skin and mucous membranes is unparalleled. This is especially true for internal use in treating the upper digestive tract. German chamomile is a very effective remedy for all **inflammatory mucous membrane changes** in this area. Its combination of antiphlogistic and spasmolytic effects can be described as ideal.

> **Preparation**
>
> • **Tea**
>   Add 1 cup of hot water to an appropriate dose of the drug. Steep covered for 5–10 minutes, then strain.
>   Drink 1 cup of freshly prepared tea in small sips several times a day.

▶ **Therapy Recommendation.** Medicinal applications should use the fresh German chamomile flowers from the living plant. If this is not possible, one should obtain the pure drug. Packaged teas and teabags often contain a poor-quality drug. Sometimes, they even contain chamomile herb instead of flowers (Schilcher 2006).

Lemon Balm (Melissa officinalis)

For more information about this plant, see Lemon Balm (p. 48).

▶ **Indications. Lemon balm leaves** (Melissae folium) are calming for **gastrointestinal symptoms** of a mostly **nervous** and **spasmodic** nature. They also promote falling sleep and are therefore especially suited for symptoms that occur primarily at night.

Preparation

- **Tea**
  Add 1 cup of hot water to the appropriate amount of the drug. Steep covered for 10–15 minutes, then strain. May be sweetened with honey.
  Drink 1–2 cups of the freshly prepared tea in small sips.

Peppermint (Mentha piperita)

For more information about this plant, see Peppermint (p. 46).

▶ **Indications. Peppermint leaves** (Menthae piperita folium) have spasmolytic, choleretic, and carminative effects, but can also frequently irritate mucous membranes. This can lead to heartburn. Peppermint leaves are more suitable for older children and youths for treating primarily **spastic upper abdominal pain that is functional in origin**.

Preparation

- **Tea**
  Add 1 cup of hot water to the appropriate amount of the drug. Steep covered for 10–15 minutes, then strain.
  Drink while warm in small sips.

- **Digestive Tea Containing Peppermint Leaves and Other Mild Medicinal Plants**

Prescriptions

Rx
Foeniculi fruct. cont. (crushed fennel seeds)
Menth. pip. fol. conc. (chopped peppermint leaves)
Melissae fol. conc. āā 20.0 (chopped lemon balm leaves)
M. f. spec.
Add 1 cup of hot water to 1 teaspoon of the drug. Steep covered for 10 minutes, then strain.
D.S.
Drink 1 cup in small sips while warm 2–3 × a day.

Fennel (Foeniculum vulgare)

For more information about this plant, see Fennel (p. 76).

▶ **Indications. Fennel seeds** (Foeniculi fructus) are primarily a carminative, but also a mild expectorant. Antispasmodic and even mild narcotic effects have also been attributed to fennel seeds. The carminative effect of fennel seeds is not as strong as that of caraway, but the distinctive fennel flavor is an advantage.

Fennel tea is frequently used to treat **dyspepsia** and **diarrhea in infants** during the initial fasting period. It decreases meteorism and intestinal spasms.

Preparation

- **Tea**
  Add 1 cup of hot water to the appropriate amount of freshly crushed fennel seeds. Steep covered for 5 minutes, then strain. May be sweetened with honey.

12.1.2 Lack of Appetite

Medicinal Plants

Calamus, Acorus calamus
Calamus rootstock, Calami rhizoma
Bitter orange, Citrus aurantium ssp. amara
Bitter orange peel, Aurantii pericarpium
Angelica, Angelica archangelica
Angelica root, Angelicae radix
Centaury, Centaurium minus
Centaury herb, Centaurii herba

Plants Used in Treatment

Calamus (Acorus calamus)

For more information about this plant, see Calamus (p. 59).

▶ **Indications. Calamus rootstock** (Calami rhizoma) is an aromatic bitter (Amarum aromaticum) and works especially well for **lack of appetite associated with asthenia and neuropathy in young girls**, and for **anorexia nervosa**.

A few drops of calamus root tincture taken before meals are also frequently extremely effective for **umbilical colics** and associated lack of appetite in young children. The small amount of alcohol contained in the tincture has to be accepted for this treatment.

<table><tr><td>**Caution** ⚠</td></tr><tr><td>Only beta-asaron free calamus rootstock obtained from the North American diploid acorus calamus race must be used. Tetraploid calamus races of Indian or Chinese origin contain up to 80% beta-asaron in their volatile oil. This has been shown in animal experiments to cause malignant tumors of the upper small intestine.</td></tr></table>

Preparation

- **Tincture**
  Add 3–10 drops to a small amount of water or fennel tea and drink several times a day.

Bitter Orange (Citrus aurantium ssp. amara)

This orange subspecies is very common in the Mediterranean. In the past, preparations using bitter orange flowers, leaves, and unripe fruit played an important role in therapy. Medicinal applications use the **bitter orange peel** (Aurantii pericarpium).

Bitter orange is very popular with young children. It has a pleasant taste and is a mild sedative.

Preparation

- **Tea**
  Add 1 cup of boiling water to about 2 g of bitter orange peel, then strain.
  Drink 1 cup 3 × a day.

Angelica (Angelica archangelica)

For more information about this plant, see Angelica (p. 57).

Preparation

- **Tea**
  Add 1 teaspoon of the drug to 1 cup of cold water. Bring to a brief boil. Or add 1 cup of boiling water to 1 teaspoon of the drug, then strain.
  Drink 1 cup before meals.

Centaury (Centaurium minus, Centaurium erythraea)

Of the **tonic bitters**, Centaury (p. 53) is the most suitable for use in pediatrics.

Preparation

- **Tea with yarrow and peppermint**

Prescriptions

Rx
Centaurii herb. (centaury herb)
Millefolii herb. (yarrow herb)
Menth. pip. fol. āā 20.0 (peppermint leaves)
M. f. spec.
Add 1 cup of boiling water to 1 teaspoon of the blend. Steep for 5 minutes, then strain.
D.S.
Drink lukewarm or cold before meals.

12.1.3 Flatulence

Medicinal Plants

Caraway, Carum carvi
Caraway seeds, Carvi fructus

Plants Used in Treatment

Caraway (Carum carvi)

For more information about this plant, see Caraway (p. 75).

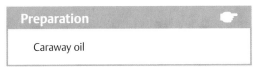

Preparation ☞

Caraway oil

Prescriptions 🔍

Rx
Ol. Carvi 5.0 (caraway oil)
Ol. Olivarum ad 10.0 (olive oil)
D.S.
Massage 10–20 drops into the skin of the abdomen using a circular motion.

- **Anise, Fennel, and Caraway Tea**

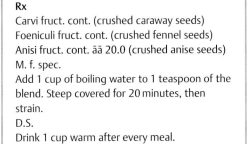

Prescriptions 🔍

Rx
Carvi fruct. cont. (crushed caraway seeds)
Foeniculi fruct. cont. (crushed fennel seeds)
Anisi fruct. cont. āā 20.0 (crushed anise seeds)
M. f. spec.
Add 1 cup of boiling water to 1 teaspoon of the blend. Steep covered for 20 minutes, then strain.
D.S.
Drink 1 cup warm after every meal.

12.1.4 Diarrhea

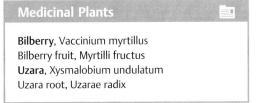

Medicinal Plants 📄

Bilberry, Vaccinium myrtillus
Bilberry fruit, Myrtilli fructus
Uzara, Xysmalobium undulatum
Uzara root, Uzarae radix

Plants Used in Treatment

All plants listed for treatment of diarrhea in Chapter 3.3.4, Diarrhea (p. 84), can be used. **Bilberry** and

Uzara root are the most significant plants for pediatric use.

In Germany, a finished pharmaceutical product combining apple pectin and chamomile flower extract has also been established as a very effective remedy, especially for use with children.

▶ **Research.** In 1997, a double-blind study showed the reliable and high tolerability of this remedy. A newer, randomized, double-blind, placebo-controlled study of 241 preschool children (average age: 33 months) with acute, nonspecific diarrhea showed a statistically significant superiority of this remedy compared to placebo, although a high placebo effect was observed for this indication and rehydration therapy on the first day (Becker et al.). Independent of evidence-based studies, this remedy has been shown to be reliable in practice for many years.

Bilberry (Vaccinium myrtillus)

For more information about this plant, see Bilberry (p. 86).

▶ **Bilberry Diet.** In infants, the bilberry diet is **initiated** following a brief tea fast by administering a 5% suspension every day (150–200 g/kg body weight). This solution is gradually replaced by one of the standard therapeutic foods. To **stabilize bowel movements** in intestinally sensitive children, especially during intercurrent infections, a 10–20% suspension is given in which 15% rice flower can be added to provide texture and volume to bowel movements. Without the addition of rice flower, bowel movements will be low in substance and relatively wet as a result of the bilberry diet.

Infants prefer a cooked suspension of bilberries because the raw product is somewhat grittier. The bilberry suspension is deep violet blue in color and tastes like raw bilberries: sweet-sour, tart, and not at all unpleasant. Its dark color rarely irritates infants. Its taste can be improved by adding a saccharin tablet to 100 g of bilberry suspension. The calorie content of this preparation is negligible.

- **Decoction**
  Add 2–3 teaspoons of dried bilberries to 500 mL of water. Boil for 30 minutes, then strain. Take 1 teaspoon a day. This decoction can be added to cream of wheat or cottage cheese.
- **Dried Bilberry Powder**
  Bilberry powder derived from dried, finely ground and sieved bilberries. A suspension is prepared by adding this powder to water or tea.
- For the **bilberry diet** with infants and young children, 1–2 teaspoons of the raw or cooked suspension is given per day (see above).
- **Tea**
  Add the indicated amount of dried bilberries to 500 mL of water. Boil for 10 minutes, then strain.
  Drink 1 glass warm several times a day.

▶ **Therapy Recommendations.** Young children with diarrhea can quickly come into a critical situation because of dehydration and the associated loss of sodium. **Sufficient amounts of fluid replacement** are important.

Small amounts of **salt** should also always be provided, either by adding it to tea if the child tolerates it, or, for example, by giving the child pretzel sticks.

Uzara (Xysmalobium undulatum)

For more information about this plant, see Uzara (p. 87).

12.1.5 Constipation

Flax, Linum usitatissimum
Flax seeds, Lini semen
Psyllium, Plantago psyllium
Psyllium seeds, Psyllii semen
Alder buckthorn, Rhamnus frangula
Alder buckthorn bark, Frangulae cortex
Castor bean, Ricinus communis
Castor oil, Oleum ricini
Rhubarb, Rheum palmatum/officinale
Rhubarb root, Rhei radix

Habitual constipation always requires diagnostics to identify its causes. These can include poor eating habits, a low-fiber diet, or psychosomatic factors.

Plants Used in Treatment

Flaxseeds (Linum usitatissimum)

For more information about this plant, see Flax (p. 62).

▶ **Therapy Recommendation.** Flaxseeds used to treat constipation should be of good medicinal quality, i.e., increasing to 5 times in volume following soaking. Flaxseed cultivars that are specially bred to increase 6–10 times in volume following soaking are especially recommended.

Psyllium Seeds (Plantago psyllium)

For more information about this plant, see Psyllium (p. 97).

Psyllium seeds are a stronger bulking agent than flaxseeds and should be prescribed for **older children** and **youths**.

- **Psyllium Seeds**
  Take 1 teaspoon of the drug mixed in 1 cup of cold water before meals.

Alder Buckthorn (Rhamnus frangula)

For more information about this plant, see Alder Buckthorn (p. 93).

With more **acute constipation**, saline laxatives and alder **buckthorn bark** (Frangulae cortex)—one of the anthranoid laxatives—provide quick relief.

- **Tea**
  Add 1 cup of boiling water to 2 teaspoons of the chopped drug. Steep for 10 minutes, then strain.
  Drink 1–2 cups in the evening, and if needed, also in the morning.

Additional Therapy Options

Castor Bean (Ricinus communis)

For more information about this plant, see Castor Bean (p. 97).

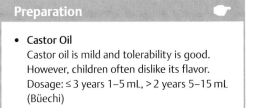

Preparation

- **Castor Oil**
  Castor oil is mild and tolerability is good. However, children often dislike its flavor. Dosage: ≤ 3 years 1–5 mL, > 2 years 5–15 mL (Büechi)

Rhubarb (Rheum palmatum, Rheum officinale)

For more information about this plant, see Rhubarb (p. 92).

Preparation

- **Syrup**
  Take 1–2 teaspoons a day.

12.2 Respiratory Disorders

12.2.1 Colds

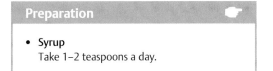

Medicinal Plants

Marshmallow, Althaea officinalis
Marshmallow root, Althaeae radix
Narrowleaf plantain, Plantago lanceolata
Plantain herb, Plantaginis lanceolatae herba
Cowslip primrose, Primula veris
Cowslip primrose root, Primulae radix
Iceland moss, Cetraria islandica
Iceland moss, Lichen islandicus

Respiratory infections occur frequently in children. In the past, antibiotics were prescribed much too readily because children quickly develop fever in response to infections. Fever is an expression of the immune system's increased **self-healing activity**. Serious bacterial infections must be treated with antibiotics, even in children. However, simple colds respond well to phytotherapeutic treatments.

Schapowal provides a detailed overview of special dosages for children.

Caution ⚠

Coltsfoot should not be prescribed to children because of its toxic pyrrolizidine alkaloid content.

Plants Used in Treatment

Marshmallow (Althaea officinalis)

For more information about this plant, see Marshmallow (p. 183).

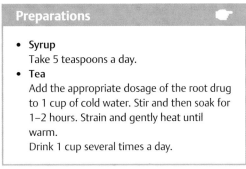

Preparations

- **Syrup**
  Take 5 teaspoons a day.
- **Tea**
  Add the appropriate dosage of the root drug to 1 cup of cold water. Stir and then soak for 1–2 hours. Strain and gently heat until warm.
  Drink 1 cup several times a day.

Narrowleaf Plantain (Plantago lanceolate)

For more information about this plant, see Plantain (p. 186).

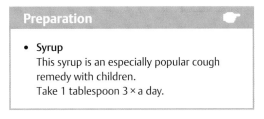

Preparation

- **Syrup**
  This syrup is an especially popular cough remedy with children.
  Take 1 tablespoon 3 × a day.

Cowslip Primrose (Primula veris)

For more information about this plant, see Primrose (p. 187).

Cowslip primrose root is the remedy of first choice for promoting **expectoration**. In addition to saponins, the roots of this plant also contain glycosides and volatile oil.

- **Cowslip Primrose Root Tea with Anise and Fennel**

Rx
Primulae rad. 20.0 (cowslip primrose root)
Anisi fruct. (anise seeds)
Foeniculi fruct. ad 50.0 (fennel seeds)
M. f. spec.
Add 1 cup of boiling water to 2 teaspoons of the blend.
D.S.
Drink 1 cup several times a day.

- **Tincture**
  For older children, 10–20 drops 4 × a day.
  For more formulation suggestions, see (p. 188).

Iceland Moss (Cetraria islandica)

For more information about this plant, see Iceland Moss (p. 61).

12.2.2 Spasmodic Coughs and Whooping Cough

Thyme, Thymus vulgaris
Thyme herb, Thymi herba
Roundleaf sundew, Drosera rotundifolia
Roundleaf sundew herb, Droserae herba
Ivy, Hedera helix
Ivy leaves, Hederae helicis folium

With whooping cough, the symptom "spasmodic cough" develops into a nosological unit.

Plants Used in Treatment

Thyme (Thymus vulgaris)

For more detailed information about thyme and its effects and constituents, see Thyme (p. 194).

▶ **Indications.** In an application study of 200 infants aged 6–12 months in pediatric practices, a finished pharmaceutical product containing a fixed combination of **thyme herb** and **cowslip primrose** extracts was shown to be a reliable cough remedy. The study demonstrated good tolerability, with a high rate of acceptance by both parents and infants (Schmidt).

A newer, open, prospective, randomized cohort study of 54 children showed significant improvements of symptoms of acute respiratory tract infections for a finished pharmaceutical product containing a combination of thyme and ivy leaves extracts when used in addition to standard therapy compared to only standard therapy alone (Safina). The study for this phytopharmaceutical product demonstrated good tolerability.

- **Tea**
  Add 1 cup of hot water to the appropriate dose of the finely chopped drug. Steep covered for 5 minutes, then strain.
  Drink 1 cup several times a day.
- **Syrup**
  Take 1 teaspoon 3 × a day.

Roundleaf Sundew (Drosera rotundifolia)

For more information about this plant, see Roundleaf Sundew (p. 195).

- **Tincture**
  Add 5 drops to a small amount of water.
  Drink 3 × a day.

Ivy (Hedera helix)

For more information about this plant, see Ivy (p. 197).

Medicinal applications use the **ivy leaves** (Hederae helicis folium). They contain saponins and glycosides. Ivy leaves are spasmolytic and secretolytic, and act as a mild sedative.

▶ **Indications.** Several studies have shown very good therapeutic efficacy of a finished pharmaceutical product containing a **refined extract** of ivy leaves for indications in children.

▶ **Research.** Application observations (Lässig et al.) as well as controlled studies (Gulyas et al.; Mansfeld et al.) showed the efficacy of this extract for obstructive respiratory disorders, including plethysmography.

These studies also once again documented the excellent tolerability and associated patient compliance for this extract.

12.3 Uncomplicated Infections

12.3.1 Colds

> **Medicinal Plants**
>
> **Linden**, Tilia cordata/platyphyllos
> Linden flower, Tiliae flos
> **European elderberry**, Sambucus nigra
> European elderberry flower, Sambuci flos
> **Meadowsweet**, Filipendula ulmaria
> Meadowsweet flowers and herb, Spireae flos et herba (syn. Filipendulae ulmariae flos et herba)
> **Purple Echinacea**, Echinacea purpurea
> Purple Echinacea herb, Echinaceae purpureae herba
> **Thuja**, Thuja occidentalis
> Thuja branch tips, Thujae summitates
> **Boneset**, Eupatorium perfoliatum
> Boneset herb, Eupatorium perfoliati herba

Plants Used in Treatment

Littleleaf Linden (Tilia cordata), Bigleaf Linden (Tilia platyphyllos)

For more information about this plant, see Linden (p. 207).

> **Preparation**
>
> • **Tea**
>   Add 1 cup of hot water to 1 teaspoon of the drug. Steep for 10 minutes, then strain. Drink slowly and as hot as possible.

European Elderberry (Sambucus nigra)

For more information about this plant, see European Elderberry (p. 206).

> **Preparation**
>
> • **Tea**
>   Add 1 cup of boiling water to 2 teaspoons of the drug. Steep for 15 minutes, then strain. Drink 1 cup several times a day.

Meadowsweet (Filipendula ulmaria)

This plant with its white blossoms is native to Germany and grows in damp meadows. It has been introduced and naturalized in North America. It is said to have mild **fever-reducing effects** due to its salicyl content. The drug is referred to as **Spireae ulmariae flos et herba** (syn. Filipendulae ulmariae flos et herba).

> **Preparations**
>
> • **Tea**
>   Add 150 mL of boiling water to 1 tablespoon of the drug. Steep for 10 minutes, then strain.
>   Drink as hot as possible. This tea has diaphoretic effects and should therefore be taken in ample quantities.
> • **Tea blend according to Schilcher**

> **Prescriptions**
>
> **Rx**
> Tiliae flos conc. 70.0 (linden flowers, cut)
> Spireae flos (syn. Filipendulae ulmariae flos) conc. 10.0 (meadowsweet flowers, cut)
> Menth. pip. fol. conc. 15.0 (peppermint leaves, cut)
> Aurantii pericarp. conc. 5.0 (bitter orange peel, cut)
> M. f. spec.
> Add 1 cup of hot water to 1–2 teaspoons of the blend. Steep for 10 minutes, then strain.
> D.S.
> Drink 1 cup several times a day.

Purple Echinacea (Echinacea purpurea)

For information about Echinacea's immunogenic effects, see Pharmacology p. 205-206.

> ### Preparation ☞
>
> • Pressed juice (extract)

▶ **Therapy Recommendation.** Echinacea can also be used preventively with children who frequently suffer from infections. Depending on the age of the child, 20–50 drops of a finished pharmaceutical product is taken in a small amount of water in the morning for several weeks or months.

Thuja (Thuja occidentalis), Boneset (Eupatorium perfoliatum)

These plants are used as supportive treatments for colds. They are found in several proven combination remedies.

12.4 Kidney and Urinary Tract Disorders

Please also see Chapter 11.4 Kidney, Efferent Urinary Tract, and Prostate Disorders (p. 326). No special instructions for children are needed. This also applies to dosage instructions for which only the tolerated amounts of fluids vary. The information in this book about bed-wetting (see Section 6.4.1 Bed-Wetting (p. 227)) and treatment of irritable bladder (p. 227) (Section 6.4.2 Irritable Bladder and Prostatopathy) is also relevant in this context.

▶ **Therapy Recommendation.** Unlike many other therapeutic teas, "kidney teas" frequently need to be consumed in large quantities and should **not** be sweetened with sugar. If a child rejects the unsweetened tea, the tea can be sweetened with a small amount of honey.

12.5 Anxiety, Restlessness, Sleep Disorders, Depression

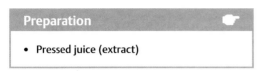

> ### Medicinal Plants 📄
>
> **Lemon balm**, Melissa officinalis
> Lemon balm leaves, Melissae folium
> **Passionflower**, Passiflora incarnata
> Passionflower herb, Passiflorae herba
> **California poppy**, Eschscholtzia californica
> California poppy herb, Eschscholtziae herba
> **Lavender**, Lavandula angustifolia
> Lavender flowers, Lavandulae flos
> **St.-John's-wort**, Hypericum perforatum
> St.-John's-wort herb, Hyperici herba

12.5.1 Herbal Sedatives

Herbal sedatives are extremely effective for treatment of anxiety and restlessness in children. This cannot be emphasized enough. The experience of using these sedatives will show that there is very little need for synthetic psychopharmaceutical drugs and their serious disadvantages.

The remedies of first choice for children are **passionflower** and **lemon balm**, whereas for adults, valerian is the remedy of first choice.

Plants Used in Treatment

Lemon Balm (Melissa officinalis)

For more information about this plant, see Lemon Balm (p. 48).

▶ **Indications.** The primary indications for lemon balm are nervous heart and gastric symptoms and problems related to falling asleep. This plant is especially helpful when children experience problems falling asleep due to unpleasant **heart sensations** or **gastric distress**.

▶ **Research.** An application observation of 918 children under the age of 12 demonstrated very good efficacy of a finished pharmaceutical product containing a fixed combination of **lemon balm leaves** and **valerian root** extracts against hyperkinesis and sleep disorders (Müller and Klement).

The application observation of this preparation demonstrated good tolerability, with a high rate of acceptance.

Preparations

- **Tea**
  Add 1 cup of hot water to the appropriate amount of the drug. Steep covered for 10–15 minutes, then strain.
  Drink while still warm and sweetened with a little honey in small sips after dinner and right before bedtime.
  If gastric symptoms are predominant, a small amount of peppermint leaves can be added.
- **Lemon Balm Oil**
  For a full bath, add 1–2 tablespoons to the bath water.

Passionflower (Passiflora incarnate)

For more information about this plant, see Passionflower (p. 258).

▶ **Indications.** Passionflower is an effective **daytime sedative** for restless, anxious children.

▶ **Research.** An application observation of 324 children age 3 to 12 showed a finished pharmaceutical product containing a fixed combination of **passionflower herb**, **valerian root**, and **hops strobiles** extracts to have good therapeutic efficacy and tolerability for states of restlessness and sleep disorders (Staiger et al. 2006).

Preparation

- **Tea**
  Add 1 cup of boiling water to the appropriate dosage. Steep for 5 minutes, then strain.
  Drink 1 cup in the morning and at noon and, if needed, 1 cup in the evening.

California Poppy (Eschscholtzia californica)

For more information about this plant, see California poppy (p. 260).

California poppy is used for **pediatric neuropathy** and **nocturnal enuresis** (bed-wetting).

Lavender (Lavandula angustifolia, Lavandula officinalis)

For more information about this plant, see Lavender (p. 259).

Lavender is helpful with sleep disorders.

▶ **Note.** Careful practical experience is needed to determine whether young children presenting with especially pronounced autonomic nervous system symptoms can be prescribed kava (Piper methysticum). Nevertheless, kava is certainly as useful for young adults as it is for adults. In all cases, standardized extract preparations as finished pharmaceutical products should be used.

Preparation

- **Lavender Oil**
  Add 20–30 mL to an evening bath. Bathe for 10–20 minutes.

St.-John's-wort (Hypericum perforatum)

For more information about this plant, see St.-John's-wort (p. 264).

Treating depression in juveniles is difficult. Psychotherapy is the first-line treatment, but with increasing severity, medication therapy becomes increasingly unavoidable.

In the USA, selective serotonin reuptake inhibitors (SSRIs) are the drug of choice, despite the fact that warnings have been issued about an increased risk of suicide and self-harm with the use of these drugs. In contrast, in Germany, **St.-John's-wort preparations** are the remedy of first choice (they made up 56% of all prescriptions for antidepressants in 2000). Several open studies document the efficacy and safety of prescribing this remedy to children and youths. However, evidence-based, controlled studies are still somewhat lacking (Seelinger and Mannel).

▶ **Indications.** In youths, the use of St.-John's-wort should be limited to **mild to moderate depression** without discernible suicide risk. The fact that tolerability of this remedy is good should make it highly acceptable for juveniles and their parents.

▶ **Therapy Recommendation.** Only finished pharmaceutical products (daily dosage: 450–600 mg) should be used.

12.6 Skin Disorders

12.6.1 Dermatitis

Medicinal Plants

German chamomile, Matricaria recutita
German chamomile flowers, Matricariae flos
Calendula, Calendula officinalis
Calendula flowers, Calendulae flos
Heart's ease, Viola tricolor
Heart's ease herb, Violae tricoloris herba
English walnut, Juglans regia
English walnut leaves, Juglandis folium

Plants Used in Treatment

German chamomile (Matricaria recutita)

For more information about this plant, see German Chamomile (p. 42).

German chamomile is the treatment of first choice for all types of **dermatitis**.

Preparation

- **Decoction**
  For poultices: Add 1 cup of boiling water to 1 tablespoon of the drug. Steep covered for 5–10 minutes, then strain.
  German chamomile is indicated for severe eczema.

Calendula (Calendula officinalis)

For more information about this plant, see Calendula (p. 295).

Calendula is more effective than chamomile for the treatment of **purulent dermatitis**, for example, diaper rash. It works surprisingly quickly. Once healing has begun, treatment can be switched to chamomile.

Preparations

- **Essence**
  For poultices: Add 1 teaspoon to 500 mL of lukewarm water.
  Apply for 30–60 minutes several times a day.
- **Calendula Baby Oil**
  Apply several times a day.

Heart's Ease (Viola tricolor)

For more information about this plant, see Heart's Ease (p. 289).

Heart's ease herb reduces irritation of **mild seborrheic skin disorders** and can also be used for **cradle cap**.

Preparation

- **Infusion**
  For compresses: Add 150 mL of boiling water to 1.5 g of the drug. Steep for 5 minutes, then strain.

English Walnut (Juglans regia)

For more information about this plant, see English Walnut (p. 289).

Preparation

- **Decoction**
  For poultices: Add 2 teaspoons to 500 mL of water. Boil for 10–15 minutes, then strain.

12.6.2 Contusions, Hematomas, Sprains

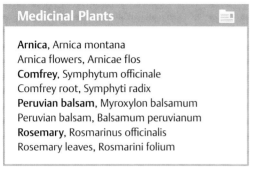

Medicinal Plants

Arnica, Arnica montana
Arnica flowers, Arnicae flos
Comfrey, Symphytum officinale
Comfrey root, Symphyti radix
Peruvian balsam, Myroxylon balsamum
Peruvian balsam, Balsamum peruvianum
Rosemary, Rosmarinus officinalis
Rosemary leaves, Rosmarini folium

Plants Used in Treatment

Arnica (Arnica montana)

For more information about this plant, see Arnica (p. 144).

Arnica flowers are the remedy of choice for these disorders. They also provide extremely fast pain relief.

Preparation

- **Tincture**
  For compresses: Dilute tincture with 3 to 10 times the amount of water.

Comfrey (Symphytum officinale)

For more information about this plant, see Comfrey (p. 294).

▶ **Indications.** Comfrey preparations are very reliable remedies for these indications.

▶ **Research.** An application observation of 306 children (average age: 7.7 years) showed very good therapeutic efficacy and tolerability for comfrey with contusions, strains, and sprains (Staiger and Wegener 2008).

▶ **Therapy Recommendation.** Only standardized, finished pharmaceutical products should be used.

Peruvian Balsam (Myroxylon balsamum)

"Balsam of Peru" is a natural balsam harvested in El Salvador from the tree Myroxylon balsamum or "Santos mahogany" in English. In the colonial period, Spanish traders exported it to Peru, from where it was in turn exported to Europe – hence the geographically misleading name. "Balsam of Peru" is well documented in German traditional herbal medicine books as a treatment for skin diseases since the early 17th century. It should best be used in the form of a finished pharmaceutical skin care product such as Peru-Lenicet®.

Rosemary (Rosmarinus officinalis)

For more information about this plant, see Rosemary (p. 172).

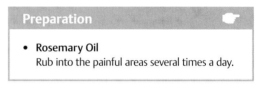

Preparation

- **Rosemary Oil**
  Rub into the painful areas several times a day.

12.6.3 Burns, Scalding

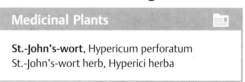

Medicinal Plants

St.-John's-wort, Hypericum perforatum
St.-John's-wort herb, Hyperici herba

Plants Used in Treatment

St.-John's-wort (Hypericum perforatum)

For more information about this plant, see St.-John's-wort (p. 264).

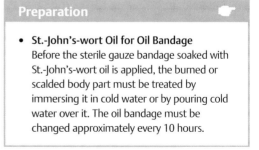

Preparation

- **St.-John's-wort Oil for Oil Bandage**
  Before the sterile gauze bandage soaked with St.-John's-wort oil is applied, the burned or scalded body part must be treated by immersing it in cold water or by pouring cold water over it. The oil bandage must be changed approximately every 10 hours.

12.6.4 Herpes Simplex (Cold Sores)

Medicinal Plants

Lemon balm, Melissa officinalis
Lemon balm leaves, Melissae folium

Plants Used for Treatment

Lemon Balm (Melissa officinalis)

For more information about this plant, see Lemon Balm (p. 48).

Bibliography

Becker B, Kuhn U, Hardewig-Budny B. Double-blind, randomized evaluation of clinical efficacy and tolerability of an apple pectin-chamomile extract in children with unspecific diarrhea. Arzneimittelforschung. 2006; 56(6):387–393

Biller A. Pflanzliche Therapie kindlicher Durchfallerkrankungen. Wien Med Wochenschr. 2007; 157(13–14):308–311

Büechi P. Rizinusöl. Z Phytother. 2000; 21:312–318

De la Motte S, Böse-O'Reilly S, Heinisch M, Harrison F. Doppelblind-Vergleich zwischen einem Apfelpektin/Kamillenextrakt-Präparat und Plazebo bei Kindern mit Diarrhoe [Double-blind comparison of a preparation of pectin/chamomile extract and placebo in children with diarrhea]. Arzneimittelforschung. 1997; 47(11): 1247–1249

Dorsch W, Loew D, Meyer-Buchtela E, Schilcher H. Kinderdosierungen von Phytopharmaka. Hrsg.: Kooperation Phytopharmaka GbR, 3. überarb. und erw. ed, Bonn 2002

Gorgus E, Hittinger M, Schrenk D. Estimates of Ethanol Exposure in Children from Food not Labeled as Alcohol-Containing. J Anal Toxicol. 2016; 40(7):537–542

Gulyas A, Repges R, Dethlefsen U. Konsequente Therapie chronisch obstruktiver Atemwegserkrankungen bei Kindern. Atemwegs-Lungenkr. 1997; 23:291–294

Kauert G. Sind ethanolhaltige Phytopharmakazubereitungen in der Pädiatrie toxikologisch bedenklich? In: Loew D, Rietbrock N, ed Phytopharmaka. Vol IV. Darmstadt: Steinkopff; 1998: 95–100

Köhler G, Elosge M, Hasenfuß J, Wüstenberg P. Kinderdosierungen von Phytopharmaka. Z Phytother. 1998; 19:318–322

Lässig W, Generlich H, Heydolph F, Patitz E. Wirksamkeit und Verträglichkeit efeuhaltiger Hustenmittel. TW Pädiatrie. 1996; 9: 489–491

Mansfeld HJ, Höhre H, Repges R, Dethlefsen U. Sekretolyse und Bronchospasmolyse. Klinische Studie: Behandlung von Kindern mit chronisch obstruktiven Atemwegserkrankungen. TW Pädiatrie. 1997; 10:155–157

Müller SF, Klement S. A combination of valerian and lemon balm is effective in the treatment of restlessness and dyssomnia in children. Phytomedicine. 2006; 13(6):383–387

Phytopharmaka K, Ed. Kinderdosierungen von Phytopharmaka. 3. ed Bonn; 2002

Safina AI. Treatment of young children with recurrent acute respiratory tract infections with a herbal combination of thyme herb and ivy leaf. Zeitschr f Phytotherapie. 2014; 35(06):262–267

Schapowal A. Phytopharmaka bei Atemwegsinfekten in der Pädiatrie. Z Phytother. 2007; 28(4):174–180

Schilcher H. Phytotherapie in der Kinderheilkunde. 4th ed. Stuttgart: Wissenschaftliche Verlagsgesellschaft; 2006

Schilcher H. Sinnvolle Darreichungsformen von Phytopharmaka in der kinderärztlichen Praxis sowie in der Selbstmedikation bei Kindern unter besonderer Berücksichtigung der Frischpflanzenpresssäfte. In: Loew D, Rietbrock N, ed Phytopharmaka. Vol IV. Darmstadt: Steinkopff; 1998: 73–80

Schmidt M. Fixe Kombination aus Thymiankraut- und Primelwurzel-Flüssigextrakt bei Husten. Zeitschr f Phytotherapie. 2008; 29(1): 7–14

Seelinger G, Mannel M. Antidepressiva bei Kindern und Jugendlichen—welchen Stellenwert hat Johanniskraut? Zeitschrift für Phytotherapie. 2007; 28(4):162–168

Staiger C, Wegener T, Tschaikin M. Pflanzliche Dreierkombination zur Behandlung von Unruhezuständen und Schlafstörungen bei Kindern. Zeitschr f Phytotherapie. 2006; 27:P32

Staiger C, Wegener T. Beinwell in der Therapie stumpfer Traumen: Anwendung bei Kindern. Zeitschr f Phytotherapie. 2008; 29(2): 58–64

Questions

1. In phytotherapeutics, are there special dosages recommended for children that differ from those recommended for adults?

2. What characterizes the special tolerability of phytotherapeutics in pediatrics?

3. What is the medicinal plant remedy of first choice for mucous membrane disorders in children?

4. Which plant is useful for stimulating appetite in children with "nervous" eating disorders?

5. Which plant should **not** be prescribed to children with respiratory tract infections because of safety concerns?

6. Which are the most suitable medicinal plants for treating nervous restlessness in children?

Answers (p. 423) for Chapter 12.

13 Oncologic Disorders

There are no phytotherapeutics for treating onco-logic disorders that ensure verifiable tumor regression or complete healing. This chapter provides an overview of the medicinal plant remedies that can play a supportive role in cancer therapy and provide valuable assistance to patients in dealing with their serious health challenges. These treatments are therefore referred to as "adjuvant tumor therapy."

Medicinal plants that have the potential to heal cancer have been searched for time and again. One of the most well-known examples of this is mistletoe, which became known as a cancer remedy in anthroposophical medicine rather than in phytotherapy. Rudolf Steiner, the founder of anthroposophy, first mentioned the possibility of treating cancer with special mistletoe preparations. Medical science considers this treatment method as controversial.

Certain plants or isolated plant constituents have been adopted for **cytostatic therapy**. Examples include the vinca alkaloids vinblastine (VBL) and vincristine (VCR). They are still considered important components of polychemotherapy, unlike substances such as podophyllin or colchicine. More recently, Pacific yew (Taxus brevifolia) was recognized as a plant with cancer treatment potential. The cancer drug Taxol (also referred to by its chemical name, paclitaxel) is derived from this plant.

Plant constituents in the first category are not discussed in this book. They are frequently synthetic derivatives.

Plants in the second category are receiving increased interest in the context of immunologic considerations. However, in order for these plants to become a fixed component of modern oncology, cancer needs to be recognized as a **holistic problem** rather than a morphologic problem. Focusing only on tumors as the expression of cancer activity and labeling the destruction of tumors as healing will increasingly be recognized as a one-sided approach that prevents true recovery or healing. The scientific approach to oncology needs to include the patient's personality, their biographical situation, how they deal with disease, and comprehensive questions about quality of life as factors that are equal to that of tumor biology.

There are many holistic scientific approaches: One especially significant approach to be mentioned here is **psycho-oncology**. Without a doubt, phytopharmaceuticals play a role in this holistic ("psychosomatic") view of oncologic disorders.

13.1 Adjuvant Therapy

 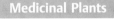
13.1.1 Plants Used in Treatment

Mistletoe (Viscum album)

Mistletoe has been in use as a medicinal remedy for a long time. This hemiparasite grows on several deciduous trees and conifers. Its indication for tumor therapy was not known until Rudolf Steiner, the founder of anthroposophy, referred to mistletoe as a specific remedy for this indication. **Anthroposophical** and pharmaceutical mistletoe preparations have been available since 1917. They were developed using a special manufacturing process and are used in cancer therapy.

Definition

Plants and plant constituents used in oncology can be classified into **two categories**:
1. Plant constituents for which **cytostatic efficacy** have been documented: vinca alkaloids, paclitaxel, and cytostatic drugs derived from lower-level plants, including antibiotics such as daunorubicin, mitomycin C, bleomycin, and mithramycin.
2. Medicinal plants that are recognized as havinh **adjuvant efficacy** for treatment of cancer: mistletoe (Viscum album) and pau d'arco (Tabebuia impetiginosa) as well as purple Echinacea (Echinacea purpurea) and thuja (Thuja occidentalis), the latter two because of their immunogenic properties.

Phytotherapeutic mistletoe preparations are represented by the **extract preparation** Lektinol (Meda). This drug was derived from the original preparation Plenosol (Madaus). **Plenosol** was primarily derived from mistletoe growing on poplars (Viscum populi), which is still the case today for the extract preparation, Lektinol.

▶ **Note.** Initially, Iscador (Iscador AG, formerly Weleda), about which a comprehensive body of literature exists, was the most well-known anthroposophical medical mistletoe preparation. Other mistletoe preparations manufactured according to anthroposophical medical methods include Helixor (Helixor), Abnobaviscum (Abnoba), and Iscucin (Wala).

All the above preparations are **injectables**. They are administered subcutaneously, intramuscular, or as intravenous infusions. They are also instilled into body cavities (for example, pleura and peritoneum), or injected directly into tumors. None of these preparations can be considered a phytotherapeutic in the narrower sense.

▶ **Pharmacology.** Important mistletoe constituents include mistletoe lectins (ML-1, ML-2, ML-3), viscotoxins, polysaccharides, amino acids, flavonoids, and certain membrane lipids (vesicles).

It is now known that mistletoe lectins play a significant role, but they are not the only constituents that determine the efficacy of mistletoe. Studies showed that low-lectin or lectin-free mistletoe preparations produce strong immunogenic effects. This appears to be another example of the effect of individual constituents in a total extract being stronger than when applied in isolation.

▶ **Note.** Plenosol was used very successfully as an adjuvant for advanced tumor stages until the 1950s, whereby primarily improvements in quality of life were achieved. This indication was successively lost as alternative methods were pushed out by the dominance of chemotherapy and radiation.

The interest in mistletoe was revived as **oncoimmunology** developed as a field of medicine. This initiated intensive research into mistletoe constituents, with a focus on mistletoe lectins, especially ML-1. This also led to the development and use of genetically engineered synthetic ML-1. Phytotherapeutically labeled mistletoe extract preparations are mostly standardized according to their ML-1 content.

▶ **Effects.** A comprehensive description of the available data and the research that produced it would fill a separate book (see for example, Fintelmann 2006; Kienle and Kiene; Fintelmann and Treichler). The following list summarizes the main effects of mistletoe herb:

- Immune modulation
- Antitumor effects (experimental)
- DNA stabilization

Immune modulation is the most well-documented effect. Mistletoe herb activates the innate ("nonspecific") immune response by stimulating macrophages, neutrophilic and eosinophilic granulocytes, and natural killer cells/large granular lymphocytes (NK/LGL cells). C-reactive protein and other acute-phase proteins increase temporarily (Berg and Stein; Stein et al.). Mistletoe also impacts the "humoral" immune system. It causes the creation of antibodies, for example, against mistletoe lectin, and the expression of various cytokines, including interferon-alpha and interleukin 2, 6, and 10.

We do not yet understand the role that these phenomena play clinically, that is, for patients and their cancer situation. Studying *in vivo* immunology in humans is extremely difficult because each of the many parts of the immune system reacts differently. For example, it can respond with activity in plasma, but with suppression in the area of the tumor, or vice versa. For every action, there is also a reaction. The immune system regulates individual immunologic processes to enable antagonistic parts to respond to activated parts. This immune response is also highly individualized and directly dependent on, for example, the psychological state of the organism (psychoneuroimmunology). Individual "positive" immune responses in humans provide very little or no information about the correlation with individual disease progression.

All research results to date are based on parenteral administration of mistletoe extracts. Peroral administration seems to have no effect. The standard treatment is subcutaneous injection.

Mistletoe's antitumor effect has been studied in numerous experimental animal and cell line models, with very contradictory results (Beuth et al.; Rostock). Results may be dosage dependent and antitumor effects were only observed with higher dosages. Clinical experiments showed individual cases of antitumor effects resulting from intratumoral administration and from instillations, for example, into the pleura cavity.

A third and possibly very important effect of mistletoe relates to DNA repair. It was shown that in certain circumstances, spontaneous or cyclophosphamide induced **DNA damage** in peripheral monocyte cells was significantly **reduced** following incubation in extracts from mistletoe grown on fir trees (Büssing). Practitioners have observed for a long time that adjuvant or interval injections of mistletoe extracts make radiation or certain cyclical courses of polychemotherapy more tolerable for patients. More long-term studies are needed to show a direct correlation, which would represent a meaningful expansion of the indication for mistletoe herb.

The last aspect of mistletoe herb to be discussed here is its **apoptosis-inducing effect** (Büssing). One essential prerequisite for the "uncontrolled," nondifferentiated cell proliferation in tumor development appears to be that the cancerous growth "switches off" or evades apoptosis. Can mistletoe extracts counter this effect, and would this process be of clinical relevance?

An abundance of questions constitute mistletoe as a current area of research, but many decisive answers are needed before the significance of mistletoe therapy can be considered proven on a phytotherapeutic basis in contrast to its current and mostly anthroposophical basis. This area of study is one of the more obvious demonstrations of the challenges of applying pharmacological and experimental data directly to the (individual) course of disease.

▶ **Indications.** Phytotherapy considers mistletoe as palliative or at most adjuvant therapy for cancer treatment. This sets it apart from anthroposophical medicine, which views mistletoe as a specific cancer therapy drug (Fintelmann 1994). Practical and clinical research to establish mistletoe extract preparations as a component of evidence-based medicine and as a therapeutic alternative or complementary therapy for recognized conventional cancer treatment did not begin until the end of the 20th century (Beuth).

Several randomized controlled trials with this objective have been initiated and some of them have been concluded (see overview compiled by Rostock). Even in the case of conventional oncology, it was a challenging task—despite incredible mental and material efforts—to arrive at a verified treatment standard for oncologic disorders. It is therefore no surprise that phytotherapy-based mistletoe treatments may, unfortunately, also require decades to create a comparable "verified" state of knowledge. However, the role of mistletoe therapy in oncology may be found much more quickly if the focus of research shifts away from tumor regression and full remission to "how" patients can live with their disease, including how to live with a tumor. Studies are also needed to examine the effects of mistletoe therapy on **secondary prevention** and cancer recurrence. Based on what we know today, this may be a possible key area of mistletoe's therapeutic efficacy.

Finally, we need to mention that effective mistletoe therapy requires knowledge and experience. This is especially true more for anthroposophy-based mistletoe preparations than for phytotherapeutic preparations. For the former, selection of the host tree that grows the mistletoe and dosage—including grams of drug equivalence in high-dosage infusions and high potency preparations (D30–60)—is of utmost importance.

The Commission E lists the following indications for mistletoe: **palliative therapy** for malignant tumors through nonspecific stimulation and degenerative inflammation of the joints. This indication illustrates, once again, that mistletoe is not considered to have direct antitumor effects and that phytotherapeutic mistletoe preparations are viewed only as adjuvants for improving quality of life and not as competition for conventional oncotherapy (see overview by Büssing). Unfortunately, neither the Commission E nor Büssing take the plethora of pharmacology and immunology research results that have been compiled on this topic for the past two decades into account.

Lapacho (syn. Pau d'arco; syn. Taheebo) (Tabebuia impetiginosa; syn. Handroanthus impetiginosus)

This tree is native to Central and South America and is also known as pau d'arco or taheebo. It reaches a height of 20–30 m and is a member of the trumpet flower (Bignoniaceae) family. The trumpet flower tree and the jacaranda, one of the landmarks of Buenos Aires, are other well-known members of this family.

Medicinal applications use the **tree bark** (Tabebuiae cortex).

▶ **Pharmacology.** Pau d'arco bark contains numerous naphthoquinones, the primary compounds lapachole and lapachone, anthraquinone, and dimeric tabebuin (Wagner and Seitz).

Pharmacological actions that have been documented include antimicrobial, antiviral, antitumor, cytotoxic, cancer-preventive, immune-stimulating, and anti-inflammatory effects. Folk medicine in Central and South America considers pau d'arco bark to be a cancer remedy and is used widely there. More recently, this drug arrived in Europe and is ingested as a tea.

▶ **Indications.** The available data about immune-modulating effects at a low dosage (Wagner and Seitz) make the above-described effects plausible. However, there is no clinical proof for its efficacy with oncologic disorders. We nevertheless decided to include pau d'arco in this chapter because of its potential as an immunagogue. Its most likely effect is **preventive**.

> ## Preparation
>
> - Tea
>   Add 1 L of boiling water to 2 teaspoons of the chopped drug. Simmer for 5 minutes, then steep covered for 15 minutes, then strain.
>   Drink in several portions in the course of a day.

Purple Echinacea (Echinacea purpurea)

For more information about this plant, see Purple Echinacea (p. 205).

▶ **Indications.** Purple Echinacea has immunogenic effects, especially stimulation of the innate immune response, and it has the proven ability to increase interferon production. This supports the working hypothesis that Echinacea is a suitable **adjuvant treatment** for tumors. At the very least, studies are needed to determine whether this remedy, which demonstrates good tolerability in practice, can contribute to improving general quality of life by stabilizing the immune system, improving a patient's general condition, and strengthening the ability to fight infections. Direct antitumor effects should not be expected.

▶ **Therapy Recommendation.** Medicinal applications should use only finished pharmaceutical products.

Thuja (Thuja occidentalis)

Medicinal applications of thuja use the tips of new shoots (Thujae summitates). They contain volatile oil (thujone), tannins, and resins.

Thuja can be found as an constituent in various finished pharmaceutical products. There is scant newer research about its specific effects or efficacy.

The Commission E has not issued a monograph for thuja.

> ## Preparation
>
> - Tincture
>   Take 20 drops several times a day in a small amount of water.

Chaga Mushroom (Inonotus obliquus)

"Chaga" is the Russian folk name given to the mushroom Inonotus obliquus. It is a member of the Hymenochaetaceae family and grows parasitically primarily on birch trees. The mushroom mycelium appears as a massive growth on the trunk of the tree. Its color and consistency are reminiscent of charcoal, which is due to the presence of large amounts of melanin. This growth on live trees is not the fruiting body of the mushroom. The fruiting body does not begin to form until the host tree has died.

The medicinal use of chaga has been well documented in Russia since the 16th century. Regrettably, clinical research of chaga's oncological indication—which is the main indication for this drug—is rather scarce. For this reason, it is not possible to draw any definite scientific conclusions about chaga's effects and efficacy (Nomura et al.). However, *in vivo* experiments showed a number of very promising effects for cancer therapy (Rzymowska; Mizuno et al.; Kim et al. 2006) as well as immune modulation (Kim et al. 2005) and anti-inflammatory effects (Park et al.; Mishra et al.) for chaga extracts and chaga constituents. Another very promising study of 50 patients (Dosychev and Bystrova) document the use of chaga for autoimmune disorders such as psoriasis.

This indication also represents a traditional use of chaga in Russian folk medicine.

Independent of the current state of clinical research, the use of this medicinal mushroom for cancer therapy in Russia is so well known that it made its way into world literature. In his semi-autobiographical novel *Cancer Ward* (1967), literature Nobel laureate Alexander Solschenizyn (1918–2008) devotes two pages to a description of cancer therapy using chaga mushrooms that is based on his own experience as a cancer patient in a hospital in Tashkent.

Bibliography

Berg PA, Stein G. Misteltherapie. Mistelextrakte—wirksame Modulatoren des natürlichen und des spezifischen Immunsystems? Inf Arzt. 1994; 15:769–776

Beuth J, ed. Grundlagen der Komplementäronkologie. Stuttgart: Hippokrates; 2002: 195–202

Beuth J, Lenartz D, Uhlenbruck G. Lektinoptimierter Mistelextrakt. Experimentelle Austestung und klinische Anwendung. Z Phytother. 1997; 18(2):85–91

Büssing A, Jurin M, Zarkovic N, Azhari T, Schweizer K. DNA-stabilisierende Wirkungen von Viscum album L. Sind Mistelextrakte als Adjuvans während der konventionellen Chemotherapie indiziert? Forsch Komplementaermed. 1996; 3 Suppl I:244–248

Büssing A. Apoptose-Induktion and DNA-Stabilisierung durch Viscum album L. Forsch Komplementarmed. 1998; 5(4):164–171

Dosychev EA, Bystrova VN. Lechenie psoriaza preparatami griba "Chaga" [Treatment o psoriasis using "Chaga" fungus preparations]. Vestn Dermatol Venerol. 1973; 47(5):79–83

Fintelmann V, ed. Loseblattwerk Onkologie auf anthroposophischer Grundlage. Stuttgart: Mayer; 2006

Fintelmann V, Treichler M. Die Mistel als Krebsheilmittel. Frankfurt/Main. Info3 2014 Band 2

Fintelmann V. Intuitive Medizin. Einführung in eine anthroposophisch ergänzte Medizin. 6th ed. Stuttgart: Hippokrates; 20-16:232–257

Fintelmann V. 1994

Franz G. Phytotherapie in der Tumorbehandlung. Dtsch Apoth Ztg. 1990; 130:1443–1450

Frohne D. Die Eibe—Taxus baccata L. Portrait einer Arzneipflanze. Z Phytother. 1998; 19(3):168–174

Holleb AI, Ed. Das Krebsbuch. Reinbek: Rowohlt; 1990

Kiene H. Klinische Studien zur Misteltherapie karzinomatöser Erkrankungen. Therapeutikon. 1989; 3:347–353

Kienle GS, Kiene H. Die Mistel in der Onkologie. Stuttgart: Schattauer; 2003

Kim YO, Han SB, Lee HW, et al. Immuno-stimulating effect of the endo-polysaccharide produced by submerged culture of Inonotus obliquus. Life Sci. 2005; 77(19):2438–2456

Kim YO, Park HW, Kim JH, Lee JY, Moon SH, Shin CS. Anticancer effect and structural characterization of endo-polysaccharide from cultivated mycelia of Inonotus obliquus. Life Sci. 2006; 79 (1):72–80

Luther P, Becker H. Die Mistel: Botanik, Lektine, medizinische Anwendung. Berlin: Springer; 1987

Mishra SK, Kang JH, Kim DK, Oh SH, Kim MK. Orally administered aqueous extract of Inonotus obliquus ameliorates acute inflammation in dextran sulfate sodium (DSS)-induced colitis in mice. J Ethnopharmacol. 2012; 143(2):524–532

Mizuno T, Cun Z, Kuniaki A, et al. Antitumor and Hypoglycemic Activities of Polysaccharides from the Sclerotia and Mycelia of Inonotus obliquus (Pers.: Fr.) Pil. (Aphyllophoromycetideae). Int J Med Mushrooms. 1999; 1(4):301

Nagel GA. Schulmedizin—Alternative Verfahren. Klinikarzt. 1994; 10:435–438

Nomura M, Takahashi T, Uesugi A, Tanaka R, Kobayashi S. Inotodiol, a lanostane triterpenoid, from Inonotus obliquus inhibits cell proliferation through caspase-3-dependent apoptosis. Anticancer Res. 2008; 28 5A:2691–2696

Park YM, Won JH, Kim YH, Choi JW, Park HJ, Lee KT. In vivo and in vitro anti-inflammatory and anti-nociceptive effects of the methanol extract of Inonotus obliquus. J Ethnopharmacol. 2005; 101(1–3):120–128

Rostock M. Misteltherapie: ihr aktueller Stellenwert bei der Behandlung von Tumorerkrankungen. In: Rietbrock N, ed Phytopharmaka. Vol VI. Darmstadt: Steinkopff; 2000: 167–180

Rzymowska J. The effect of aqueous extracts from Inonotus obliquus on the mitotic index and enzyme activities. Boll Chim Farm. 1998; 137(1):13–15

Scheer R, Bauer R, Becker H, Berg PA, Fintelmann V, Eds. Die Mistel in der Tumortherapie. Grundlagenforschung und Klinik. Essen: KVC; 2001

Scheer R, Becker H, Berg PA. Grundlagen der Misteltherapie. Stuttgart: Hippokrates; 1996

Solschenizyn A. Cancer Ward. London: Bodley Head, 1968

Stein G, Henn W, von Laue H, Berg P. Modulation of the cellular and humoral immune responses of tumor patients by mistletoe therapy. Eur J Med Res. 1998; 3(4):194–202

Steinhoff B. Fortschritte in der Misteltherapie. Z Phytother. 2000; 21:211–212

Wagner H, Seitz R. Lapacho (Tabebuia impetiginosa). Porträt einer südamerikanischen Urwalddroge. Z Phytother. 1998; 19:226–238

Wrba H, Ed. Kombinierte Tumortherapie. 2. ed Stuttgart: Hippokrates; 1995

Questions

1. Is there a scientifically verified phytotherapeutic treatment strategy for oncologic disorders?
2. Which known cytostatic (chemotherapeutic) drugs were originally derived from plants?
3. Which plant has been demonstrated experimentally and clinically to have immunogenic and tumor growth-inhibiting effects for oncologic disorders?

Answers (p. 423) for Chapter 13.

14 Critical Assessment of R.F. Weiss Treatment Concepts

In this chapter, the reader will find a virtual treasure trove of possible answers regarding historical aspects and special therapeutic options without needing to refer to previous editions of this book. The recommendations in this chapter are to be viewed from a historical perspective as they no longer meet today's requirements.

If one follows the development of this textbook about phytotherapy from its first iteration in 1944 until today, one recognizes the profound changes phytotherapy and its position in medicine have undergone during that time. Weiss continuously revised his representations as new scientific findings became available. However, he also rejected them if his practical experience as a physician did not correlate with these mostly experimental findings.

In the 21st century, modern phytotherapy is subject to requirements that no longer allow for some of Weiss's recommendations. Nevertheless, a summary is presented in this chapter in order to preserve his work and to make some of his experience and suggestions available for future research. One of Weiss's most characteristic presentations, a chapter on eye disorders, is presented here in its entirety, although none of the remedies described meet today's treatment standards.

14.1 Digestive and Metabolic Disorders

14.1.1 Hemorrhoids

Plants Used in Treatment

Water Pepper (Polygonum hydropiper; syn. Persicaria hydropiper)

This inconspicuous plant with narrow tender leaves and small, green to reddish flowers located in the leaf axils is native to Germany. It thrives in wet habitats, along ditches, and in meadows. The herb has a pepper-like biting flavor, which gave it its name.

Medicinal applications use the **water pepper herb** (Polygoni hydropiperis herba).

▶ **Pharmacology.** Water pepper contains volatile oils and tannins.

▶ **Indications.** Water pepper is especially indicated for the treatment of bleeding hemorrhoids. The mechanism of its action is not yet known. It cannot stanch severe hemorrhoid bleeding. Its primary indication is for treating **mild** and more **refractory chronic bleeding**.

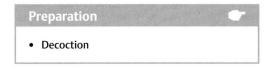

Preparation

- **Tea**
  Add 1 cup of boiling water to 2 teaspoons of the drug. Steep for 5 minutes, then strain. Drink 1–2 cups in the morning and in the evening, alternating with "Hemorrhoid tea" (p. 102), which is taken in the evening.

14.1.2 Diabetes Mellitus

Plants Used in Treatment

Sarcopoterium (Sarcopoterium spinosum, syn. Poterium spinosum)

This small, thorny shrub grows wild in the Mediterranean and in the Middle East. A decoction of **sarcopoterium roots** (Poterii radix) is said to be a well-known diabetes remedy among Bedouin.

▶ **Pharmacology.** Sarcopoterium's constituents are not known. It is speculated that they stimulate endogenous insulin production, similar to oral antidiabetes drugs (sulfonylurea).

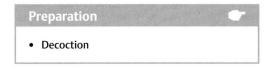

Preparation

- **Decoction**

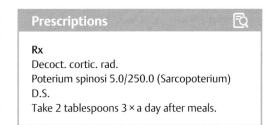

Prescriptions

Rx
Decoct. cortic. rad.
Poterium spinosi 5.0/250.0 (Sarcopoterium)
D.S.
Take 2 tablespoons 3 × a day after meals.

Copalchi (Hintonia latiflora, syn. Coutarea latiflora)

Copalchi is a member of the Rubiaceae family. It originates from Mexico and Brazil and is said to have antidiabetic effects. Medicinal applications use the **copalchi bark** (Copalchi cortex).

▶ **Pharmacology.** The main constituents of copalchi are neoflavonoid glycosides, including coutareoside, bitters, and mannitol.

14.2 Heart and Circulatory System Disorders

14.2.1 Degenerative Heart and Vascular Disorders

Plants Used in Treatment

Onion (Allium cepa)

Ordinary culinary onions have been shown to impact blood lipids and can be considered **mildly lipid lowering**, similar to garlic. However, this has only been documented for freshly pressed onion juice.

> **Preparation**
>
> - **Pressed Juice**
>   Take 50 g of raw pressed onion juice daily.

14.2.2 Vascular System Disorders

Plants Used in Treatment

Rue (Ruta graveolens)

Rue is a shrub-like plant that is planted in gardens and has also been naturalized in Germany (▶ Fig. 14.1). It originates from the Mediterranean. Its oddly grayish-green bipinnate leaves exude a very strong fragrance of volatile oil.

Rue is in the Rutaceae family, which also counts lemons, oranges, and mandarin oranges among its members.

▶ **Pharmacology.** Rue contains rutin, bitters, tannins, and volatile oil.

Older botanical nomenclature referred to rue as Ruta hortensis, which provided the name for its constituent **rutin**. The chemical name for rutin is

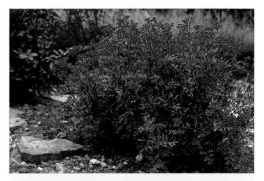

Fig. 14.1 Rue, Ruta graveolens. Photo: Dr. Roland Spohn, Engen.

quercetin-3-O-rutinoside, one of a group of bioflavonoids that has been shown to have antihemorrhagic effects.

This group of substances is found in many plants. It is characterized by its free radical scavenging properties. Of interest in the context of this chapter are its **edema-protecting** and **antihemorrhagic** effects. These substances are not very water-soluble. To make use of their properties medicinally, their water solubility needs to be increased through partial synthesis. The most well known of these substances is hydroxyl ethyl rutin. Most pharmacological studies have been conducted using this substance.

For practical use, flavonoid preparations, for example, those derived from buckwheat (Fagopyrum esculentum) are significantly less effective than horse chestnut seeds or sweet clover (Melitotus officinalis). Frequently, they are **synthetic derivatives** of plant substances and no longer meet the definition of phytotherapeutics.

▶ **Indications.** The Commission E has issued a negative monograph for the rue drug, which consists of **rue leaves** (Rutae folium) and **rue herb** (Rutae herba). The reasons given are that rue's efficacy for the application areas indicated is not sufficiently documented. More importantly, rue's risk potential makes its use not advisable.

Rue oil can cause **contact dermatitis** in humans. **Phototoxic reactions** (polymorphous light eruptions [PMLE]) have also been reported. Therapeutic dosages of rue have been observed to cause melancholic moods, sleep disorders, fatigue, vertigo, and spasms. For these reasons, rue is no longer recommended for use as a phytotherapeutic.

14.3 Respiratory Disorders

14.3.1 Cough

Plants Used in Treatment

Butterbur (Petasites hybridus)

For more information about this plant, see Butterbur (p. 282).

▶ **Indications.** In Germany, butterbur as a **cough remedy** has largely been replaced by coltsfoot. The demulcents contained in coltsfoot form a protective layer on the pharyngeal mucous membranes and reduce the urge to cough. Butterbur's effects, on the other hand, are **spasmolytic**. Its constituents petasin and isopetasin impact the smooth bronchial muscles. This explains why butterbur has been considered a good remedy for whooping cough and bronchial asthma since antiquity and during the Middle Ages.

The Commission E has issued a negative monograph for butterbur leaves.

▶ **Note.** Butterbur is also very suitable for treating neurovegetative conditions of the stomach and biliary tract.

14.3.2 Whooping Cough

Plants Used in Treatment

Common Butterwort (Pinguicula vulgaris)

This delicate carnivorous plant grows in bogs and swamps. It bears a single blue flower with a small spike on a thin stem. Its longish ovate leaves form a basal rosette. The edges of the leaves are curled up and excrete a proteolytic ferment.

Medicinal applications use the **butterwort herb** (Pinguiculae herba).

▶ **Indications.** Christen and Gordoneff discovered a highly aromatic cinnamic acid ester (trans-cinnamic acid) that exhibits spasmolytic properties. They viewed this as an explanation for butterwort's use in treating whooping cough by stipulating that "butterwort's effects mirrored the active principle isolated from roundleaf sundew (Drosera rotundifolia), which is also characterized by spasmolytic properties."

Preparation

- **Tea**
  Add 1 cup of boiling water to 1 teaspoon of the drug. Steep for 5 minutes, then strain. Drink 2–3 cups a day.

Blue Eryngo (Eryngium planum)

Blue eryngo, also known as flat sea holly, is a close relative of the beautiful sea holly (Eryngium maritinum). In spite of its thorny appearance, this plant is a member of the Apiaceae family.

Blue eryngo is much more inconspicuous than sea holly and grows far inland, especially in southeastern Europe. It is also found on the shores of the Oder and Vistula rivers.

Medicinal applications use the entire **blue eryngo herb** (Eryngii plani herba).

▶ **Indications.** Pater was the first person to draw attention to blue eryngo. He discovered that this plant was considered to be an old folk remedy against whooping cough in Transylvania. His inquiries showed that this plant does indeed have calming cough reducing and spasmolytic effects in **children with whooping cough**. This plant is easily cultivated and does not require collecting in the wild.

Today, thyme and roundleaf sundew are more widely used than blue eryngo as effective and reliable cough remedies. It is rarely prescribed today.

Preparation

- **Tea**
  Add 1 cup of hot water to 1 teaspoon of the drug. Steep for 15 minutes, then strain. Drink 2–3 cups a day.

Bibliography

Christen K, Gordonoff T. [The active principle of Pinguicula vulgaris L]. Arzneimittelforschung. 1960; 10:560–561

Pater B. Erungium planum L. als Heilpflanze. Heil- u. Gewürzpfl. 1932; 14:112–114

14.3.3 Bronchial Asthma

Plants Used in Treatment

Jimsonweed (Datura stramonium)

For more information about this plant, see Jimsonweed (p. 280).

▶ **Indications.** Alkaloids in jimsonweed can relieve bronchial spasms. This effect can be enhanced by adding saltpeter.

However, this effect is not sufficiently reliable compared to modern reliable β-sympathomimetic drugs. The Commission E therefore issued a negative monograph.

Jimsonweed is no longer prescribed for bronchial asthma today.

> **Preparations**
>
> - **Folia Stramonii nitrata (Jimsonweed leaves and nitrate)**
>   This smoking powder also contains saltpeter.
> - **Tincture** This tincture was usually prescribed in combination with other cough remedies such as ephedra as well as belladonna and lobelia.

14.3.4 Lung Tuberculosis

Before synthetic tuberculosis drugs became available to provide causal (antibacterial) treatment for tuberculosis, phytotherapeutics, along with light therapy, played some role in the treatment of this disease. In those days, tuberculosis therapy primarily involved **silicic acid preparations**. They were thought to increase resistance to the disease, primarily in the lungs.

Three plants that contain silicic acid were used as a rule: horsetail (Equisetum arvense), knotweed (Polygonum aviculare) and hempnettle (Galeopsis ochroleuca). These plants were also constituents in a well-known remedy of the time, Kobert's Lung Tea (p. 354).

Today, these plants are no longer important for tuberculosis treatment, although with the ever-increasing problem of multidrug resistance, they may very well become relevant again in the future. The question whether and to what extent they are a preventive remains open. It is also up to the practitioner whether to use the Kobert's Lung Tea

described below (p. 354) as a follow-up treatment for tuberculosis.

Plants Used in Treatment

Horsetail (Equisetum arvense)

Horsetail is the most potent silicic acid drug. Its contain 6% silicic acid, 06% of which is soluble in decoction. Medicinal applications use the **horsetail herb** (Equiseti herba).

▶ **Indications.** It has been shown that silicic acid administration induces leukocytosis. Practical experience confirms that this remedy has general **performance-enhancing effects**.

Hempnettle (Galeopsis ochroleuca)

Hempnettle grows abundantly in light-filled forests and often covers entire mountain slopes. It can reach a height of up to 0.5 m. Its leaves are opposite, and its yellowish-white flowers are grouped in the leaf axils.

Medicinal applications use the entire **hempnettle herb** (Galeopsidis herba).

▶ **Pharmacology.** Hempnettle contains 0.8% silicic acid, 0.03% of which is soluble in decoction. In addition to silicic acid, hempnettle contains saponins and tannins.

Knotweed (Polygonum aviculare)

Knotweed, also called knotgrass, is one of the most common plants in Germany. However, it is inconspicuous and often overlooked. This low-growing plant snakes along the ground and only rises up in areas where it has access to light. Its small leaves are opposite and feature a membranous sheath at their base.

Medicinal applications use the entire **knotweed herb** (Polygoni avicularis herba).

▶ **Pharmacology.** Knotweed herb contains 1% silicic acid, 0.08% of which is soluble in decoction. It is said to have diuretic effects, but this has not been proven.

▶ **Indications.** Knotweed is still being prescribed for respiratory tract colds, but it is of minor importance.

Historical Prescription

Kobert's Lung Tea

Rx

Equiseti herb. 75.0 (horsetail herb)

Polygoni aviculare herb. 150.0 (knotweed herb)

Galeopsidis herb. 50.0 (hempnettle herb)

M. f. spec.

Add 4 teaspoons of the blend to 6 cups of cold water. Simmer until reduced by half (3 cups).

D.S.

Drink 3 cups a day for several months.

14.4 Nervous and Psychological Disorders

14.4.1 Anxiety, Restlessness

This section introduces plants and plant preparations that are considered sedatives but are no longer considered important in modern phytotherapy: **avens** (Geum urbanum) and **asafetida** (Ferula assa-foetida). They are included for practitioners interested in developing their own individualized prescriptions.

Bitter orange (Citrus aurantium ssp. amara) also has significant sedative effects and is discussed in some detail in this section.

In the past, **opium poppy** was the most important medicine for this indication. Synthetic alternatives and prescription restrictions imposed by narcotics regulations make its use in phytotherapy obsolete.

Plants Used in Treatment

Avens (Geum urbanum)

Avens is a largely inconspicuous plant that is frequently found in damp forests. Its flowers are small and yellow, and its leaves are lyrate and pinnate. Avens is a member of the Rosaceae family.

Medicinal applications use the **avens root** (traditional name: **Radix Caryophyllatae**). Avens is used in a similar manner as valerian root (Valerianae radix), but it is significantly weaker than valerian.

Asafetida (Ferula assa-foetida)

This remedy is derived from a shrub that grows wild in the Middle East, especially in Iran.

Asafetida was used to impart a suggestive effect, for example, with **bed-wetting** in children, or to treat **hysteria**.

- **Tea**
  Add boiling water to 2 teaspoons of the drug. Steep for 3–5 minutes, then strain. Drink 1 cup 3 × a day.
- **Tincture**
  Dosage varies according to the age of the individual (see avens).
- **Combination with Valerian Tincture**
  In the past, asafetida tincture was sometimes combined with valerian tincture because of asafetida's strong unpleasant odor.

Bitter Orange (Citrus aurantium ssp. amara)

For more information about this plant, see Bitter Orange (p. 334).

▶ **Indications.** Bitter orange is a pleasant tasting aromatic bitter. It is said to be a mild **sedative** and a useful **remedy to promote falling asleep** in people suffering from anxiety and restlessness.

- **Tea**
  Add 1 cup of boiling water to 1–2 teaspoons of bitter orange peel. Steep for 10 minutes, then strain.
  Drink 1–2 cups slowly as a soporific at bedtime.
- **Combination with Valerian Tea**
  Prepare valerian tea as a decoction (using cold water, see Valerian Tea (p. 254)) in the morning. Steep until evening. In the evening, mix 1 cup of valerian tea with freshly prepared warm bitter orange tea and drink before bedtime.
- **Combination with Valerian Tincture**
  Add 1 teaspoon of valerian tincture to 1 cup of freshly prepared, warm bitter orange tea.
- **Tincture**
  Take 30 drops 3 × a day.
- **Orange Syrup (Sirupus Aurantii)**
- **Orange Flower Syrup (Sirupus Aurantii Florum)**
  In the past, both types of syrup were used, primarily as a flavor corrigent for sedative mixtures.

Opium Poppy (Papaver somniferum)

For more information about this plant, see Opium Poppy (p. 87).

Opium is derived from the dried milky sap of unripened opium poppy seed capsules. The main opium alkaloid is morphine. It is unsurpassed as a pain-relieving remedy.

Opium is a type of forte-phytotherapeutic (powerful phytotherapy) in the area of nervous disorders. It is subject to narcotics regulations (e.g., Controlled Substances Act in the USA). Consequently, prescribing is limited.

The following provides a summary of the traditional phytotherapeutic use of opium. It remains to be seen if opium will ever regain practical significance.

▶ **Indications.** Opium therapy was at one time one of the best remedies for depression, especially for severe and chronic cases of true melancholia with hypochondria and obsessive guilt. As it was known that this group of patients was not prone to addiction, the greatest spontaneous reservation about the use of opium was negated. Scharfetter wrote in 1967: "For patients with purely psychotic anxiety, the efficacy of opium pills, such as those that are rarely used today for opium therapy, is to date unsurpassed by any other pharmaceutical. Opium therapy is primarily indicated for patients with endogenous depression. Experience has shown that these patients are not prone to addiction." Burchard also pointed out that opium was used as a psychopharmaceutical for a very long time. Its success rate of 66% with reference to treating depression, especially endogenous depression, was excellent and not significantly different from the success rates usually achieved with modern synthetic psychopharmaceuticals.

Opium likely acts on the brain stem. However, unlike neuroleptic drugs, opium does not induce parkinsonism. When opium treatment is stopped, psychosomatic symptoms worsen in the same way as when psychopharmaceutical drugs are stopped. The most frequent side effects seen with opium are nausea, lack of appetite, and constipation. Interestingly, the well-known constipating effect of opium is more pronounced at the beginning of treatment but decreases progressively during the course of treatment. If necessary, it can be counteracted by adding small amounts of rhubarb to the prescription.

If for very individual reasons, treatment of depression using small amounts of opium is desired, practitioners should formulate their own prescriptions and combine opium with other phytotherapeutic remedies corresponding to the predominant organic symptoms.

Instead of referring to this remedy as opium tincture, the nomenclature used by physicians of the past—**Thebaica Tincture**—should be used to avoid the stigma associated with the word "opium."

Preparation

- **Tincture**
  For opium treatment ("opium cure"), start with 3 × 5 drops on day 1; increase to 2 × 5 drops and 1 × 10 drops on day 2; on day 3, increase to 3 × 10 drops, then carefully increase to 3 × 20 drops a day. Maintain this dosage for a while, then decrease in the same manner.

- **Combination for Heart Phobias**

Prescriptions

Rx
Tinct. Thebaic. 1.0/2.0 (opium tincture)
Tinct. Strophant. 5.0 (strophanthin tincture)
Tinct. Convallar. 10.0 (lily-of-the-valley tincture)
Tinct. Valerian. 20.0 (valerian tincture)
D.S.
Take 10 drops 3–4 × a day.

- **Combination for Gastric Pain, also Nausea and Urge to Vomit (said to help ease symptoms and relieve pain even with inoperable stomach cancer)**

Prescriptions

Rx
Tinct. Thebaic. 1.0 (opium tincture)
Tinct. Menth. pip. 2.0 (peppermint tincture)
Tinct. Gentianae 3.0 (gentian tincture)
Tinct. Valerianae 4.0 (valerian tincture)
D.S.
Take 10 drops 3 × a day before meals.

For references corresponding to the preceding section, see Bibliography following 14.4.2 (p. 357)

14.4.2 Avolition (Lack of Motivation)

Plants Used in Treatment

Nux Vomica (Strychnos nux vomica)

Nux vomica is derived from the seeds of a tall tree that is native to Java, the Malaysian Islands, and northern Australia; it is also cultivated in some of those areas. Its seeds (Strychni semen) contain a number of alkaloids, with strychnine being the most well known. Nux vomica is a tonic bitter, similar to bitters native to Germany, but stronger in its effect. It is also more toxic.

▶ **Pharmacology.** Pharmacologists advise against using the pure strychnine alkaloid in strychnine pills and instead recommend use of the whole drug (Strychni semen). This confirms what we also know about other medicinal plants. In many cases, use of the whole drug is preferable to using pure substances. In the case of nausea, the effect of the whole drug develops more slowly, but more evenly than that of strychnine.

Some patients are suspicious about being prescribed strychnine because the name is representative of a strong poison. This perception can be avoided by prescribing **nux vomica seeds** (nux vomicae semen) and **nux vomica tincture** (**Tinctura Nucis vomicae**) instead of using the term Strychni semen.

▶ **Indications.** In the past, nux vomica was considered the most efficacious stimulant for the nervous system. It was especially useful as a tonic for **old people** because it also reduces pain sensitivity in patients suffering from nervous gastric disorders.

The Commission E issued a negative monograph for nux vomica because it considered its efficacy to be insufficiently documented and because of concerns about a serious risk of inducing central nervous system spasms with the uncontrolled use of nux vomica alkaloids.

In serious cases, nux vomica was combined with native bitter drugs that also provided useful tonic and roborant effects.

Preparation

- Tonic Tincture for Pale Children with Lack of Appetite

Prescriptions

Rx
Tinct. Nuc. vomic. 5.0 (nux vomica tincture)
Tinct. Chinae 10.0 (cinchona composite tincture, see Cinchona (p. 55))
Tinct. Ferri pomat. 15.0 (ferri pomatum tincture, ferrated apple tincture)
D.S.
Take 3 drops 3 × a day, carefully increase if needed.

- **Combination with Bitter Drugs**

Prescriptions

Rx
Tinct. Calami (calamus tincture)
Tinct. Gentianae (gentian tincture)
Tinct. Nuc. vomic. āā 10.0 (nux vomica tincture)
D.S.
Take 20 drops 3 × a day.

Khat (Catha edulis)

Khat grows in Ethiopia and Somalia and from there was introduced into Yemen and southern Saudi Arabia. The fresh leaves of this small shrub are chewed similarly to the way the Indigenous peoples of the Americas chewed tobacco leaves prior to European colonization. Its active substance is **cathine (formerly referred to in German-language literature as** nor-Iso-ephedrine, which is very similar to the well-known active substance in ephedra and closely related to central nervous system stimulants such as amphetamines and pervitin).

Only fresh leaves contain the fully active substance. This substance is less effective or mostly lost when the leaves are dried.

▶ **Indications.** In the regions listed above, khat is used as a geriatric remedy.

Caution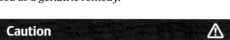

The chewing of khat can result in habituation and addiction, which needs to be considered before prescribing this substance.

Preparation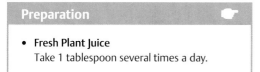

- **Fresh Plant Juice**
  Take 1 tablespoon several times a day.

Black Hellebore (Helleborus niger)

For a long time, **black hellebore rootstock** (Hellebori rhizoma) was known to contain cardioactive glycosides that are very similar to digitalis glycosides. In German, this root is also referred to as "sneezing root," which indicates that the powder derived from the black hellebore rootstock is a substantial local irritant. In the past, it was also used as a sneezing powder.

Phytochemical research by Martinek brought to light some interesting results. He found a previously unknown glycoside in the dried **leaves** of fresh plants that was easily crystalized. This sheds new light on information imparted by Paracelsus, who recommended a dried black hellebore leaf preparation as a geriatric remedy and "elixir for a long life." At the time, this geriatric remedy was well known and widely used and likely involved the administration of small amounts of a heart glycoside. It appears that Paracelsus had rightly discovered that the tolerability of dried hellebore leaves is better than that of rootstock preparations.

▶ **Indications.** Hellebore rootstock (Hellebori rhizoma) is sometimes still used as a **stimulating geriatric remedy**.

Its frequent use as a heart remedy in the past is now obsolete because the tolerability of this remedy is not relatively poor.

Preparation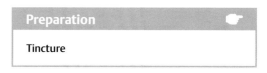

Tincture

Other Plants

Borage (Borago officinalis)

This well-known garden spice is said to have undefined mood stimulating effects, for example, with reference to depression during menopause. These effects have not been confirmed. No significant constituents have been found, only demulcents and tannins. Borage cannot be considered a psychotropic medicinal plant.

Lotus (Nelumbo nucifera), White Egyptian Lotus (Nymphaea lotus), European White Water Lily (Nymphaea alba)

The nutritious seeds of these plants are considered tranquilizers. The roots of these plants are also used and are said to possess an antiemetic principle.

These rather exotic plants have not found any practical use in phytotherapy.

Bibliography

Burchard JM. Opiumtherapie und moderne Psychopharmaka [Opium therapy and modern psychopharmacological agents]. Arzneimittelforschung. 1967; 17(5):557–561

Martinek A. Ranuncosid als Inhaltsstoff der getrockneten Blätter, Stengel und Blüten von Helleborus niger [Ranuncoside in dried stems, leaves and flowers of Helleborus niger]. Planta Med. 1974; 26(3):218–224

Scharfetter C. Anwendung der Psychopharmaka bei bestimmten Indikationsgruppen [The use of psychopharmacologic agents in certain indicated groups]. Med Klin. 1967; 62(22):861–863

14.4.3 Neuralgia

Plants Used in Treatment

Monkshood (Aconitum napellus)

In Germany, this beautiful, large plant with its striking blue flowers grows wild in damp meadows, in bogs, and in mountain forests. Medicinal applications use the **monkshood root tubers (Aconiti tubera)**. They contain various alkaloids, primarily aconitine.

▶ **Indications.** In the past, monkshood was used as the initial remedy in the attempt to treat trigeminal neuralgia. Today, phytotherapeutic preparations of monkshood are no longer available. If needed, homeopathic preparations are available.

The Commission E issued a negative monograph for monkshood.

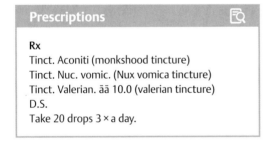

Preparation 👉

- **Tincture**
  Take 5–10 drops several times a day in increasing and decreasing dosages.

- **Combination with Nux Vomica and Valerian (for example, for nausea or restlessness)**

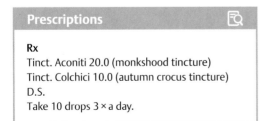

Prescriptions 📝

Rx
Tinct. Aconiti (monkshood tincture)
Tinct. Nuc. vomic. (Nux vomica tincture)
Tinct. Valerian. āā 10.0 (valerian tincture)
D.S.
Take 20 drops 3 × a day.

- **Combination of Monkshood and Autumn Crocus (Colchicum autumnale) Tincture (for a combination of arthritis or gout and neuralgia pain)**

Prescriptions 📝

Rx
Tinct. Aconiti 20.0 (monkshood tincture)
Tinct. Colchici 10.0 (autumn crocus tincture)
D.S.
Take 10 drops 3 × a day.

14.5 Skin Disorders

14.5.1 Chronic Eczema

In the past, chronic eczema was frequently treated with **irritating substances** to make it acute and then to treat it as acute eczema with moist compresses and similar methods. This approach is based on the experience that acute eczema conditions are more susceptible to treatment than chronic or very torpid conditions.

Various irritants can be used for this purpose. Weiss recommended parsley and cypress spurge.

Plants Used in Treatment

Parsley (Petroselinum crispum)

Weiss primarily used fresh juice or a strong decoction of **parsley herb** (Petroselini herba) or, better yet, parsley herb and **parsley root** (Petroselini radix).

Cypress Spurge Sap (Euphorbia cyparissias, Wolf's Milk)

Weiss recommended brushing fresh cypress spurge sap onto skin, in a way similar to the treatment for warts.

14.5.2 Psoriasis

No specific phytotherapeutics are available to treat refractory chronic bouts of psoriasis. However, reliable observations indicate that saponin drugs can have positive effects for refractory psoriasis.

Plants Used in Treatment

Sarsaparilla (Smilax aristolochiifolia, syn. Smilax medica)

In folk medicine, sarsaparilla root, the strongest of the saponin drugs, is still considered a psoriasis remedy. However, no pharmacologic or clinical justifications are available.

Medicinal applications use the **sarsaparilla root** (Sarsaparillae radix).

▶ **Pharmacology.** The main active constituents of the drug are considered to be the steroid saponins sarsaparilloside, smilacin and parillin. Corticomimedic and/or immunosuppressive actions are possible.

▶ **Indications.** The Commission E has issued a negative monograph for sarsaparilla root because it can induce gastric and kidney irritation and can increase or inhibit the effects of other important drug constituents.

Preparation

- **Tea**
  Add 1 L of cold water to 1 tablespoon of the drug in the evening. The next morning, boil for 20 minutes.
  Drink half of the tea immediately and the other half cold in the evening.
  Continue the regimen for several weeks.

Rupturewort (Herniaria glabra, Herniaria hirsuta)

Rupturewort (p. 219) is a saponin drug that is native to Germany.

Preparation

- **Cold Decoction**
  For preparation, see sarsaparilla root (p. 393).

14.5.3 Warts (Verruca vulgares)

Plants Used in Treatment

Celandine (Chelidonium majus)

For more information about this plant, see Celandine (p. 113).

Common warts (Verrucae vulgares) can be removed by applying the **fresh milky sap of the celandine plant** (Chelidonii succus). Celandine grows wild as a weed in the garden and along the edges of forests and is easy to find. Its yellow milky sap contains alkaloids that are considered Chelidonine.

▶ **Note.** The white milky sap of cypress spurge (Euphorbia cyparissias, "wolf's milk") is used in the same manner. It is high in skin irritants such as lactone, euphorbone, and resins. Its efficacy is considered less reliable, likely because it lacks virus-inhibiting effects.

Preparation

- **Milky Sap**
  Apply the milky sap to the wart. Allow to dry and leave in place as long as possible. Repeat daily for a long period.

Garlic (Allium sativum)

For more information about this plant, see Garlic (p. 154).

Preparation

- **Fresh Garlic**
  Applying slices of fresh garlic to warts is a known remedy, especially for warts on the hands. Garlic is often a reliable remedy when other remedies have failed.

Milk Thistle (Silybum marianum, Carduus marianus)

For more information about this plant, see Milk Thistle (p. 103).

Preparation

- **Tincture**
  Take 5 drops 3 × a day.

Genital Warts (Condylomata acuminate)

Mayapple (Podophyllum peltatum), Indian Podophyllum (Podophyllum emodi)

Mayapple, also called American mandrake, is a member of the Berberidaceae family. Mayapple (Podophyllum peltatum) originates from the southern United States (Texas, Mississippi) and Indian podophyllum originates from India. In the past, podophyllum was primarily known as a strong laxative. Its laxative effects are due to the resin derived from its **rootstock** (Podophylli rhizoma).

▶ **Indications.** Podophyllum resin can be used **externally** to treat **genital warts** (Condylomata acuminate). The treated skin area should not be larger than 25 cm² because of possible toxic effects. The podophyllotoxins contained in the drug have antimitotic effects. Use during pregnancy is contraindicated.

Preparation

- **Alcoholic Resin Solution (5–25%)**
  For external application.

14.5.4 Hair Loss (Alopecia)

Plants Used in Treatment

Stinging Nettle (Urtica dioica, Urtica urens), Dwarf Nettle (Urtica urens), Birch (Betula pubescens, Betula pubescens, Betula verrucosa), Burdock (Arctium lappa, Lappa major)

Hair loss should be treated with remedies that stimulate the scalp and thereby promote hair growth. This provides strong support for regeneration of hair growth, for example, following serious bouts of the flu, other infections, and surgery.

▶ **Indications.** The best results are achieved with **symptomatic alopecia following exhausting illnesses**.

Preparations

- **Hair Tonic**
  Hair tonics that stimulate the scalp can be prepared, for example, from stinging nettle herb, birch leaves, and burdock root. These tonic spirits are vigorously massaged into the scalp.
- **Burdock Root Oil**
- With **dry seborrhea of the scalp**, massaging burdock root oil into the scalp has been shown to be a reliable remedy. It is referred to by its old-fashioned name Oleum Bardanae.
  The following prescription has been proven in practice.

Prescriptions

Rx
Ol. Lavandulae (lavender oil)
Ol. Calami āā 1.0 (calamus oil)
Tinct. Gentianae 10.0 (gentian tincture)
Spirit. Rosmarini ad 100.0 (rosemary spirit)
M. f.
Use as a hair tonic. Shake before use.

14.6 Eye Disorders

14.6.1 Acute and Subacute Eye Inflammation

Plants Used in Treatment

Eyebright (Euphrasia officinalis)

The name of this plant already points to its traditional use for treating eye disorders.

Eyebright flowers in late summer and early autumn in large clusters in dry meadows, mountain slopes, and forests, from plains to alpine regions. Its small, pretty, pale violet flowers feature dark violet veins and a yellow spot on the lower lip. This plant grows up to a height of 25–30 cm. In poor soils, diminutive rudimentary forms of this plant can frequently be found that feature only a single flower.

Medicinal applications use the **entire eyebright herb** (Euphrasiae herba).

▶ **Pharmacology.** The drug contains iridoid glycosides, lignans, and phenylpropanoid glycoside. It is not known which of these constituents are responsible for the plant's effects.

▶ **Indications.** Eyebright is used primarily to treat **conjunctivitis** and **blepharitis** as well as **recent eye injuries** at risk of serpiginous ulcers of the cornea (ulcus serpens corneae) and **scrofulous eye disorders in children**.

Preparation

- **Tea for Eye Poultices**

Rx
Euphrasia herb. 200.0 (eyebright herb)
M. f. spec.
Add 1 tablespoon of the drug to 500 mL of
water. Boil for 10 minutes, then strain.
D.S.
Allow to cool and use full strength to soak poultices.
This tea can simultaneously be used internally.
Drink 1 cup several times a day.

- **Combination with Walnut Tea, Chamomile Tea or Fennel Tea for Scrofulous Eye Disorders in Children**
- **Tea for Eye Poultices to Treat Stye (hordeolum)**

Prescriptions

Rx
Euphrasia herb. (eyebright herb)
Matricariae flos āā 150.0 (German chamomile
flowers)
M. f. spec.
Add 2–3 teaspoons of the blend to 250 mL
of boiling water. Steep for 5 minutes, then
strain.
D.S.
Allow to cool and use full strength to soak poultices.
This tea can simultaneously be used internally.
Drink 1 cup several times a day.

Common Oak (Quercus robur), Sessile Oak (Quercus patraea)

For more information about this plant, see Oak
(p. 287).

▶ **Indications.** Oak bark is effective for treating
acute inflammatory eye disorders, especially **acute
blepharitis** and **conjunctivitis.**

Preparation

- **Decoction**
  Add 500 mL of water to 1–2 tablespoons of
  the drug. Boil for 15 minutes, then strain.
  Use undiluted for moist poultices.

14.6.2 Inner Eye Disorders

Plants Used in Treatment

Pasque Flower (Pulsatilla vulgaris, Pulsatilla pratensis)

Pasque flower, also known as pulsatilla, is one of
the most beautiful spring flowers in the Central
Uplands of Germany. Pulsatilla vulgaris has large
upright, blue-violet flowers and Pulsatilla pratensis has smaller drooping black-violet flowers. Medicinally, both plants are used in the same way.

Medicinal applications use the **pasque flower
herb** (Pulsatillae herba).

▶ **Indications.** Pasque flower is used internally for
treating **iritis, scleritis,** and **retinal disorders,** and
especially for **cataracts** and **glaucoma.**

Preparations

- **Extract**
- **Pilulae antamauroticae**
  The famous ophthalmologist von Graefe
  (1828–1870) developed the following
  recommendation for treating glaucoma:

Prescriptions

Rx
Pulsatillae pulv. herb. (pasque flower herb powder)
Extr. Pulsatillae āā 5.0 (pasque flower extract)
f. pil. Nr. 75
D.S.
Take 1–3 pills 3 × a day.

• Infusion

Preparation

Rx
Infus. Pulsatillae herb. 6.0/150.0 (pasque flower herb infusion)
Sir. Aurant. 30.0 (syrup of orange peel)
D.S.
Take 1 tablespoon 3 × a day

Silver Ragwort (Jacobaea maritima, syn. Cineraria maritima, syn. Senecio cineraria)

This subshrub grows wild in the Mediterranean. In Germany, it is also frequently cultivated as a potted plant. This plant is a member of the Asteraceae family and is characterized by densely tomentose, silver-gray leaves.

Medicinal applications use the **juice** of the whole plant, which is a mild irritant.

▶ **Indications.** This remedy is used to treat **chronic conjunctivitis**, early stages of **cataracts,** and **general asthenopia** caused by constitutional factors or following acute consuming illnesses.

Applying the juice to the eye causes mild burning that disappears quickly. This juice is used to induce mild hyperemia, which promotes healing for many different eye disorders.

Preparation

• Juice

Bibliography

von Graefe CF. Repertorium augenärztlicher Heilformeln. Berlin: Realschulbuchhandlung; 1817. 69

14.6.3 Outer Eye Disorders

Plants Used in Treatment

Barberry (Berberis vulgaris)

Barberry is a thorny shrub with tufted clusters of yellow flowers and red berries. It grows along the edges of forests and shrubberies from the Northern Lowland to the Alps in Germany, and it is also cultivated in gardens.

Medicinal applications primarily use the **barberry root bark** (Berberis cortex) and the **barberry berries** (Berberis fructus).

▶ **Pharmacology.** Barberry contains the alkaloid berberine, which is considered an eye tonic.

▶ **Indications.** Barberry can help to resolve **disorders of the outer eye** which are harmless but protracted and those which are perceived by patients as very bothersome.

Proven Prescriptions

Eye tonics (Aquae ophthalmicae) are still very popular. They are said to "strengthen" the eyes and eyesight. This wealth of experience and knowledge should not be ignored.

Eye tonics are very simple to formulate and very economical since they only require the mixing of aromatic waters that are inexpensive and readily available in pharmacies (preferably chamomile or fennel).

Eye compresses soaked with these aromatic waters are very soothing for **eyestrain** as well as for **inflammation along the edges of the eyelid**. Some types of **conjunctivitis** also respond well to this treatment.

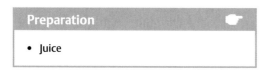

Prescriptions

Eye Tonic: Combination of Fennel and Chamomile
Rx
Aqu. Chamomillae (chamomile water)
Aqu. Foeniculi āā 150.0 (fennel water)
M. f.
Eye tonic for eye rinses and eye poultices.

• **Eye Poultices with Fennel Water**
Indicated for **general weak eyesight** to "strengthen" the eyes.
The volatile oil contained in fennel makes these poultices very soothing and gentle.

14.7 Gynecological Disorders

14.7.1 Uterine Bleeding

Plants Used in Treatment

Ergot (Claviceps purpurea)

Ergot is the sclerotium (Secale cornutum), the dormant stage of the filamentous fungus Claviceps purpurea, which grows on rye. It consists of thin square rods of 2–4 cm in length that grow out of the rye ovaries. They are usually incurved, somewhat horn shaped, and almost black.

In the past, ergot was the main remedy for gynecological bleeding and postpartum bleeding; witch hazel and goldenseal were also used. However, goldenseal is rarely used as a drug anymore since synthetic hydrastinine became available.

▶ **Pharmacology.** The active constituents of ergot are various alkaloids with different structures and effects, all derived from lysergic acid. The primary hemostatic action develops during uterine contraction induced by ergometrine and methylergometrine.

▶ **Indications.** The main action of ergometrine and methylergometrine develops only during the **postpartum period**. They are not very effective for the nongravid uterus.

Even isolated ergot alkaloids are not truly reliable as hemostatics. The Commission E considered the use of whole ergot extracts as too risky and no longer justified; a negative monograph for ergot was issued.

The use of ergot for uterine bleeding is obsolete.

Senecio Herb (Senecio fuchsia)

Senecio herb is a tall plant with bright yellow and fragrant flowers. It typically grows in clear-cuts, similar to digitalis, and is a member of the Asteraceae family. Senecio means "old man." In Germany, this ancient medicinal plant grows in mountain forests at higher elevations, primarily in the Black Forest and in the Alps. Of the many native Senecio species found in the German flora, Senecio fuchsii seems to be the best and most useful.

▶ **Pharmacology.** Senecio herb primarily contains the alkaloid senecionine and substantial amounts of flavonol (rutin).

Senecio plants contain varying amounts and compositions of toxic pyrrolizidine alkaloids. Whereas pyrrolizidine alkaloid limits were established for coltsfoot and comfrey, the Commission E issued a **negative monograph** for Senecio species. It considered its efficacy as not sufficiently documented and its risk of possible mutagenic or even carcinogenic effects as not acceptable.

Future research will show if this assessment is justified or if the results of animal experiments (using dosages that exceed those that would have been used with humans) also demonstrate a toxicological risk to humans. Applying results shown in animals to humans remains problematic even if it is widely accepted in toxicology.

Based on the current state of knowledge, use of Senecio herb is not recommended.

Scotch Broom (Cytisus scoparius, syn. Sarothamnus scoparius)

Scotch broom's (p. 163) effect is similar to that of quinine and quinidine. This led to the logical conclusion to prescribe Scotch broom for gynecological bleeding. This treatment primarily made use of Scotch broom's main alkaloid, sparteine.

Phytotherapeutic prescriptions can make use of an extract of **Scotch broom herb** (Sarothamni scoparii herba), which is available commercially, but is only recommended for heart arrhythmia.

Shepherd's Purse (Capsella bursa pastoris)

Shepherd's purse is one of the most common weeds in Germany. It derives its name from the shape of its diminutive fruit and is a member of the Brassicaceae family. Its hemostatic effect has often been questioned and is likely not very strong.

Medicinal applications use the **shepherd's purse herb** (Bursae pastoris herba).

▶ **Pharmacology.** The drug contains flavonoids and large amounts of potassium salts.

▶ **Indications.** The Commission E approved shepherd's purse for the indication areas **menorrhagia** and **metrorrhagia**.

Preparations

- **Tea**
  Add 1 cup of simmering water to 1 tablespoon of the drug. Steep for 15 minutes, then strain.
  Drink warm, freshly prepared tea up to 4 × a day between meals.
- **Fluid Extract**
  Add 25 drops in 1 glass of water and drink 3 × a day.
- **Tinctura Bursae pastoris Rademacher**
  Take 20–30 drops several times a day

Common Storksbill (Erodium cicutarium)

Common storksbill, also known as red-stem filaree, is a small plant that is common in Germany in fields, particularly dry and sandy fields, and along the edges of paths. It derives its name from the shape of its fruit. Its flowers are small and reddish, and its leaves are deeply lobed and pinnately cleft.

Medicinal applications use the **storksbill herb** (Erodii cicutarii herba).

▶ **Pharmacology.** The constituents of this plant are not yet well known. Its hemostatic effect is attributed to its substantial content of potassium salts.

Preparation

- **Infusion**
  Add 1 cup of water to 1 teaspoon of the drug. Bring to a brief boil and strain.
  Drink 1 cup several times a day.

Water Pepper (Polygonum hydropiper, Persicaria hydropiper)

For more information about this plant, see Water Pepper (p. 350).

▶ **Indications.** Reports document the hemostatic effects of water pepper. It has been recommended

for **atonic postpartum bleeding, postabortion bleeding** and **menopausal bleeding**. Its tolerability is said to be excellent, with no known adverse effects.

Preparation

- **Tea**
  Add 1 cup of hot water to 1–2 teaspoons of the drug, then strain.
  Drink 1 cup several times a day.

Proven Prescriptions for Hemostatic Teas

When prescribing formulations containing water pepper, **Polygoni hydropiperis herba** has to be specified to avoid confusion with Polygoni avicularis herba.

Prescriptions

Rx
Polygoni hydropip. herb. (water pepper herb)
Equiseti herb. (horsetail herb)
Millefolii herb. āā ad 100.0 (yarrow herb)
M. f. spec.
Add 1 cup of water to 2 teaspoons of the blend. Bring to a brief boil, steep for 20 minutes, then strain.
D.S.
Drink 1 cup 3 × a day.

Prescriptions

Rx
Sarothamni scop. Flos (Scotch broom flowers)
Bursae pastor. herb. (shepherd's purse herb)
Millefolii herb. āā ad 100.0 (yarrow herb)
M. f. spec.
Add 1 cup of hot water to 1 teaspoon of the blend. Steep for 20 minutes, then strain.
D.S.
Drink 1 cup 3 × a day.

14.7.2 Hormone Imbalances

Plants Used in Treatment

Bugleweed (Lycopus europaeus)

For more information about this plant, see Bugleweed (p. 134).

In addition to its antithyroid action, **bugleweed herb** (Lycopi herba) is also an antigonadotropin. These effects are most likely attributable to oligomers of caffeic or rosemarinic acid of the type lithospermic acid. This plant appears to have prolactin inhibiting effects. Today, there are reliable and effective drugs available for this indication, for example, derived from chaste tree (Vitex agnus castus), and bugleweed is mentioned only for historical reasons.

Siberian Rhubarb (Rheum rhaponticum)

Siberian rhubarb is related to the official rhubarb (Rheum officinalis), which is used as a laxative and described in that section (p. 92). Siberian rhubarb also contains anthraquinone glycosides and an additional constituent, rhaponticin, which is a stilbenoid glycoside that is chemically similar to diethylstilbestrol (DES).

The use of Siberian rhubarb is obsolete because of possible adverse effects, for example, endometrial hyperplasia.

European Stoneseed (Lithospermum officinale)

This plant derives its name from its seeds, which are as hard as stones. Stoneseed can grow to a height of 1 m in alluvial forests and on sunny slopes. Its flowers are small and greenish. The entire plant is characterized by appressed stiff hairs. Stoneseed is a member of the Boraginaceae family. All the members of this family are similarly covered in rough hairs.

Medicinal applications use the **stoneseed seeds** (Lithospermi semen, also referred to as Semen Millii solis) as well as the **stoneseed leaves** (Lithospermi folium), or the **entire plant.**

▶ **Pharmacology.** The active principle of stoneseed is hormonal in nature. Sourgens et al. showed experimentally that this plant has antigonadotropic effects. Wagner et al. examined aqueous extracts of stoneseed leaves that were gently processed. They were able to isolate lithospermic acid in those extracts and this constituent was shown to be efficacious. The effects of leaf extracts and root extracts were the same.

Rue (Ruta graveolens)

For more information about this plant, see Rue (p. 351).

This plant is said to have a mildly calming and sedative effect, but it is not very pronounced. When administered in larger dosages, its emmenagogue effect is considerable.

▶ **Indications.** The Commission E issued a negative monograph for rue because its therapeutic efficacy was considered insufficiently documented for the claimed indications and because its furanocoumarin content presents a defined toxicological risk.

Preparation

- **Tea**
  Add 1 cup of boiling water to 1–2 teaspoons of the dried drug. Steep for 5 minutes, then strain.
  Drink 1 cup in the morning and in the evening.

Bibliography

Sourgens H, Winterhoff H, Gumbinger HG, Kemper FH. Antihormonal effects of plant extracts. TSH- and prolactin-suppressing properties of Lithospermum officinale and other plants. Planta Med. 1982; 45(2):78–86

Wagner H, Hörhammer L, Frank U. Lithospermsäure, das antihormonale Wirkprinzip von Lycopus europaeus L. (Wolfsfuss) und Symphytum officinale L. (Beinwell) [Lithospermic acid, the antihormonally active principle of Lycopus europaeus L. and Symphytum officinale. 3. Ingredients of medicinal plants with hormonal and antihormonal-like effect]. Arzneimittelforschung. 1970; 20(5):705–713

14.8 Oncologic Disorders

14.8.1 Adjuvant Therapy

Plants Used in Treatment

Mayapple (Podophyllum peltatum, Podophyllum emodi)

For more information about this plant, see Mayapple (p. 359).

▶ **Indications.** Mayapple and Indian podophyllum (which originate from India) were considered useful cytostatic drugs for a period of time, especially for ovarian cancer. Frequently described adverse effects included leucopenia, hair loss, and erythema as well as gastrointestinal and orthostatic dysfunctions.

Mayapple is no longer used in practice.

Part 3

Appendices

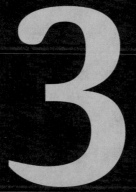

15 An A to Z of Indications

This book is intended to serve as a long-term companion for practitioners, therapists, and pharmacists in order to enable them to consistently expand their knowledge about medicinal plants and phytotherapy—both their possibilities and their limitations—as a component of comprehensive pharmacotherapy. These objectives can be reached by continually studying the comprehensive information in the individual chapters and, in specific cases, referring to the suggested references at the end of the chapters. We invite our readers to "live" with this book, to open it again and again in order to familiarize themselves with a particular plant or to simply refresh their knowledge.

Nevertheless, in daily practice, and in light of a patient's complaints or a diagnosis, the optimal prescription, for example, a phytopharmaceutical or an individualized prescription, is required without delay. This appendix addresses the need for a quick reference and complements the detailed information contained in the practice section of this book. Readers can search alphabetically by indication to quickly find appropriate therapies for each indication. This includes typical plants and drugs corresponding to the indication as well as recommendations for preparations, single prescriptions, and finished pharmaceutical products.

15.1 A

15.1.1 Aging Heart

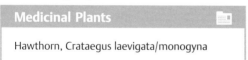

Medicinal Plants

Hawthorn, Crataegus laevigata/monogyna

Hawthorn Flowers, Leaves and Fruit

Prescribe a finished pharmaceutical product.

15.1.2 Amenorrhea, Oligomenorrhea

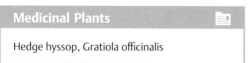

Medicinal Plants

Hedge hyssop, Gratiola officinalis

Hedge Hyssop

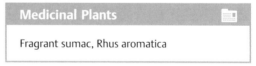

Preparation

- **Tea**
  This tea is best combined with a strong laxative and possibly with rue (ruta graveolens) and fennel.

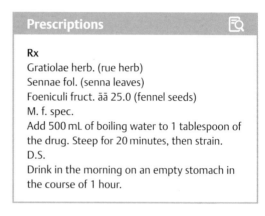

Prescriptions

Rx
Gratiolae herb. (rue herb)
Sennae fol. (senna leaves)
Foeniculi fruct. āā 25.0 (fennel seeds)
M. f. spec.
Add 500 mL of boiling water to 1 tablespoon of the drug. Steep for 20 minutes, then strain.
D.S.
Drink in the morning on an empty stomach in the course of 1 hour.

15.2 B

15.2.1 Bed-wetting

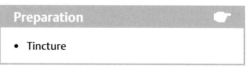

Medicinal Plants

Fragrant sumac, Rhus aromatica

Fragrant Sumac Bark

Preparation

- Tincture

- Proven prescription:

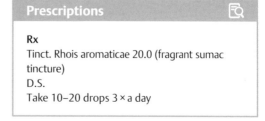

Prescriptions

Rx
Tinct. Rhois aromaticae 20.0 (fragrant sumac tincture)
D.S.
Take 10–20 drops 3 × a day

15.2.2 Brain Disorders

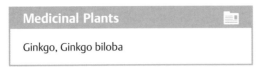

Medicinal Plants

Ginkgo, Ginkgo biloba

Ginkgo Leaves

Prescribe a finished pharmaceutical product.

15.3 C

15.3.1 Chilblains

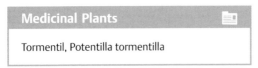

Medicinal Plants

Tormentil, Potentilla tormentilla

Tormentil Rootstock

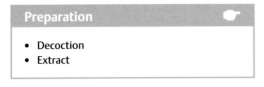

Preparation

- Decoction
- Extract

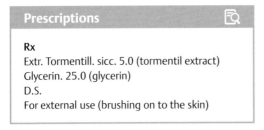

Proven Prescriptions

- Decoction
  Add 2 L of water to 200 g of the drug. Boil
  for 15 minutes and use undilated for partial
  baths.

- **Tormentil Extract** (Extractum Tormentillae)
  A mixture of tormentil extract and glycerin is
  suitable for brushing on to the skin.

Prescriptions

Rx
Extr. Tormentill. sicc. 5.0 (tormentil extract)
Glycerin. 25.0 (glycerin)
D.S.
For external use (brushing on to the skin)

Tormentil Tincture (Tinctura Tormentillae)
(1:10)
For external rubs, which are best done immediately following a bath, tormentil tincture is prescribed with skin stimulating additions.

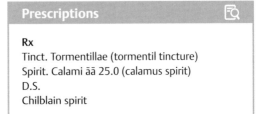

Prescriptions

Rx
Tinct. Tormentillae (tormentil tincture)
Spirit. Calami āā 25.0 (calamus spirit)
D.S.
Chilblain spirit

15.3.2 Constipation, Chronic Slow Transit

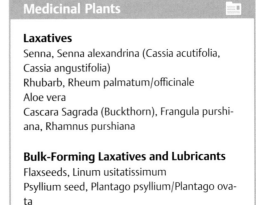

Medicinal Plants

Laxatives
Senna, Senna alexandrina (Cassia acutifolia,
Cassia angustifolia)
Rhubarb, Rheum palmatum/officinale
Aloe vera
Cascara Sagrada (Buckthorn), Frangula purshi-
ana, Rhamnus purshiana

Bulk-Forming Laxatives and Lubricants
Flaxseeds, Linum usitatissimum
Psyllium seed, Plantago psyllium/Plantago ova-
ta

Senna Fruit and Leaves

Only suitable for short-term use.
A finished pharmaceutical product should be
given preference.

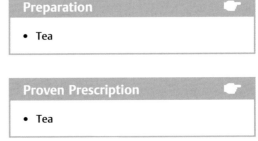

Preparation

- Tea

Proven Prescription

- Tea

Rhubarb Root

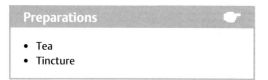

Preparations

- Tea
- Tincture

Proven Prescriptions

- Tea
  Add 1 cup of hot water to 1 teaspoon of the
  coarsely powdered drug. Steep for
  10 minutes, then strain.
  Drink 2 cups in the evening.
- **Aqueous Tincture of Rhubarb (Tinctura
  Rhei aquosa** [DAB 6])
  Take 1 tablespoon 2–3 × a day

Aloe Vera

Finished pharmaceutical products should be given
preference.

Cascara Sagrada Bark (Buckthorn)

Finished pharmaceutical products should be given
preference.

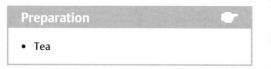

Preparation

- Tea

Proven Prescription

- Tea
  Add 1 cup of boiling water to 1 heaping
  teaspoon of the finely chopped drug. Steep
  for 10 minutes, then strain.
  Drink 1–2 cups in the evening at bedtime.

Flaxseeds

Suitable for long-term use.
- Proven prescription:

Prescriptions

Rx
Lini sem. cont. 200.0 (crushed flaxseeds)
D.S.
Stir 2–4 tablespoons into stewed fruit or similar
foods 1–2 × a day.

Psyllium Seeds, Psyllium Seed Husks

Prescribe a finished pharmaceutical product.

15.3.3 Contusions

Medicinal Plants

Arnica, Arnica montana
Comfrey, Symphytum officinale
St.-John's-wort, Hypericum perforatum

Arnica Flowers

Finished pharmaceutical products should be given
preference.

Comfrey Root, Herb, and Leaves

Prescribe finished pharmaceutical products.

St.-John's-wort

Prescribe finished pharmaceutical products.

15.3.4 Dermatitis

Medicinal Plants

Common Oak (Quercus robur), Sessile Oak (Quercus petraea)
Heart's ease, Viola tricolor
English walnut, Juglans regia

Oak Bark

Preparation

- **Decoctions**
  For the preparation of poultices and full or partial baths.

Proven Prescription

- **Decoction**
  Boil 1–2 tablespoons of chopped oak bark in 500 mL water for 15 minutes, then pour off or strain. Allow to cool. This liquid is used undiluted for poultices or added to baths.
  Use twice the amount of the chopped oak bark for a full bath.

Heart's Ease Herb

Preparation

- **Tea**
- **Decoction**
  For the preparation of compresses.

Proven Prescription

- **Tea**
  Add 1 cup of hot water to 1 teaspoon of the finely chopped drug. Steep for 5 minutes, then strain.
  Several times a day, drink 1 cup and/or apply moist and warm compresses.

Walnut Leaves

Preparations

- **Tea**
- **Decoction**
  For the preparation of compresses.

Proven Prescriptions

- **Tea**
  Add 1 tablespoon of the finely chopped drug to cold water. Heat to a simmer, steep for 3–5 minutes, then strain.
  Drink 2–3 cups a day.
- **Compresses**
  Add about 5 teaspoons of the finely chopped drug to cold water and prepare as above.

15.3.5 Depressive Mood Disorders

Medicinal Plants

St. John's wort, Hypericum perforatum
Kava, Piper methysticum

St.-John's-wort

Prescribe a finished pharmaceutical product.

Kava Rootstock

Prescribe finished pharmaceutical products.

15.3.6 Diabetes Mellitus

Medicinal Plants

Bilberry, Vaccinum myrtillus
White kidney bean, Phaseolus vulgaris
Goat's rue, Galega officinalis

Bilberry Leaves

Preparation

- **Tea**

- "Diabetes Tea" According to R.F. Weiss

Rx
Myrtilli folia (bilberry leaves)
Phaseoli concis. legumin. (chopped kidney bean pods)
Galegae herb. (goat's rue herb)
Galegae sem. (goat's rue seeds)
Menth. pip. fol. āā ad 200.0 (peppermint leaves)
M. f. spec.
Add 1 L of hot water to 2 tablespoons of the blend. Steep for 20 minutes, then strain.
D.S.
Drink 1 cup 3–4 × a day.

White Kidney Bean Pods

- Tea

- Tea
  Add 1 cup of boiling water to 1 tablespoon of the drug. Steep covered for 10 minutes, then strain.
  Drink 1 cup of freshly prepared tea between meals.

Goat's Rue Herb and Seeds

- Tea

- See **Diabetes Tea** above.

15.3.7 Diarrhea

Tormentil, Potentilla tormentilla
Bilberry (European Blueberry), Vaccinium myrtillus
Uzara, Xysmalobium undulatum
Poppy, Papaver somniferum
Myrrh, Myrrha

Tormentil Rootstock

- Tea
- Tincture

- **Tea**
  Add 1 teaspoon of the chopped drug to 1 cup of cold water. Bring to a brief simmer, then strain immediately.
  Drink 1 cup 3 × a day.
- **Tormentil Tincture** (Tinctura Tormentillae) (1:10)
  Take 10–30 drops in 1 shot glass of water several times a day (or with acute conditions, every hour).
- **Combination**
  With Carminative Tincture (see Carminative Tinctures (p. 79)).

Rx
Tinct. Tormentillae (tormentil tincture)
Tinct. carminativ. āā 25.0 (see Carminative Tinctures (p. 79))
D.S.
Take 30–40 drops in warm chamomile tea 3–5 × a day.

- For Diarrhea with **Spasms** and **Cholic**

Prescriptions

Rx
Tinct. Tormentillae 30.0 (tormentil tincture)
Tinct. Belladonnae 5.0 (belladonna tincture)
Tinct. carminativ. ad 50.0 (see Carminative Tinctures (p. 79))
D.S.
Take 30 drops in a small amount of water 3 × a day.

Bilberry Fruit

These remedies are also very well suited for children.

Preparations

- Tea
- Dried fruit

Proven Prescription

- Tea
  Add 3 tablespoons of the drug to 500 mL of water. Boil for 10 minutes, then strain. Drink 1 cup warm several times a day.
- Dried bilberry fruit
  Chew 1 tablespoon several times a day.

Uzara Root

Prescribe finished pharmaceutical products.

Poppy Tincture

Preparation

- Tincture

Proven Prescriptions

- **Opium Tincture** (Tinctura Opii)
  In accordance with the German Pharmacopoeia DAB 10: 5–10 drops every 1–2 hours until the diarrhea stops.
  Attention: According to the Betäubungsmittelgesetz, BtMG (the German Controlled Substances Act): The highest possible amount of opium that can be legally given out to a single patient on a single day is 5.0 g. This is equivalent to 300 drops of Tinctura Opii.

- **Tincture Blend**

Prescriptions

Rx
Tinct. Opii 5.0 (opium tincture)
Tinct. Belladonnae 10.0 (belladonna tincture)
Tinct. Tormentillae 20.0 (tormentil tincture)
D.S.
Take 10 drops in water 2–3 × a day.

Combination of Myrrh, Coffee Charcoal, and Chamomile Flowers

Prescribe finished pharmaceutical products.

15.3.8 Dysmenorrhea

Medicinal Plants

German chamomile, Matricaria recutita
Yarrow, Achillea millefolium

Chamomile Flowers

Preparation

- Tea

> **Proven Prescription**
>
> - Tea
>   Add 1 cup of hot water to 2 teaspoons of the drug. Steep for 5–10 minutes, then strain. Drink 1 cup several times a day while still warm, slowly in small sips.

Yarrow Herb and Flowers

These remedies are suitable for long-term use.

> **Preparation**
>
> - Tea

> **Proven Prescription**
>
> - Tea
>   Add 1 cup of hot water to 2 teaspoons of the finely chopped drug. Steep covered for 5 minutes, then strain. Drink 2–3 cups a day.

15.3.9 Dyspepsia, Functional

> **Medicinal Plants**
>
> Turmeric, Curcuma longa
> Artichoke, Cynara cardunculus
> Wormwood, Artemisia absinthium
> Peppermint, Mentha piperita
> Bitter Candytuft, Iberis amara

Turmeric Rootstock

> **Preparation**
>
> - Tea
> - Tincture

Artichoke Leaves

Finished pharmaceutical products should be given preference.

Wormwood Herb

> **Preparation**
>
> - Tea

> **Proven Prescription**
>
> - Tea
>   Add 1 cup of boiling water to 2 teaspoons of the finely chopped drug. Steep 1 to a maximum of 2 minutes, then strain. Drink 1 cup warm several times a day.

Peppermint Leaves

> **Preparation**
>
> - Tea

> **Proven Prescription**
>
> - Tea
>   Add 1 cup of hot water to 1–2 teaspoons of the drug. Steep for 5 minutes, then strain. Drink 1 cup warm several times a day.

Bitter Candytuft Flower

Prescribe only finished pharmaceutical products.

15.3.10 Dysuria Symptoms

> **Medicinal Plants**
>
> Juniper, Juniperus communis
> Lovage, Levisticum officinale
> Parsley, Petroselinum crispum
> Spiny Restharrow, Ononis spinosa
> Horsetail, Equisetum arvense

Juniper Berries

> **Preparation**
>
> - Tea

Proven Prescription

- Tea
  Add 1 cup of hot water to 1 teaspoon of the crushed drug. Steep covered for 5 minutes, then strain.
  Drink 1 cup 3 × a day.

Proven Prescription

- Tea
  Add 1 cup of boiling water to 1 teaspoon of the chopped drug. Steep for 30 minutes, then strain.
  Drink 1 cup several times a day.

Lovage Root

Preparation

- Tea

Horsetail Herb

Preparation

- Tea

Proven Prescription

- Tea
  Add 1 cup of boiling water to 1–2 teaspoon of the finely chopped drug. Steep covered for 10–15 minutes, then strain.
  Drink 1 cup warm several times a day before meals.

Proven Prescription

- Tea
  Add 1 cup of boiling water to 2 teaspoons of the chopped drug. Steep for 15 minutes, then strain.
  Drink 1 cup several times a day.

Parsley Herb, Parsley Root

Preparation

- Tea

Other Proven Prescriptions

Prescriptions

Rx
Juniperi fruct. (juniper berries)
Ononidis rad. (spiny restharrow root)
Liquiritiae rad. āā ad 200.0 (licorice root)
M. f. spec.
Add 1 cup of hot water to 1–2 teaspoons of the blend. Steep for 20 minutes, then strain.
D.S.
Drink 3 cups a day.

Proven Prescription

- Tea
  Add 1 cup of boiling water to 1–2 teaspoons of the finely chopped drug. Steep covered for 10–15 minutes, then strain.
  Drink several cups in the course of a day.

Spiny Restharrow Root

Preparation

- Tea

Prescriptions

Rx
Juniperi fruct. (juniper berries)
Petroselini fruct. (parsley seeds)
Equiseti fruct. (horsetail herb)
Ononidis rad. (spiny restharrow root)
Foeniculi fruct. (fennel seeds)
Menth. fol. pip. āā ad 200.0 (peppermint leaves)
M. f. spec.

Add 1 cup of hot water to 1–2 teaspoons of the blend. Steep for 20 minutes, then strain.
D.S.
Drink 3 cups a day.

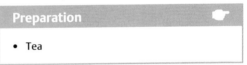

Proven Prescription

- Tea
  Add 1 cup of hot water to 1 teaspoon of the chopped drug. Steep for 5 minutes, then strain.
  Drink 2 cups a day.

15.4 E

15.4.1 Eczema, Atopic

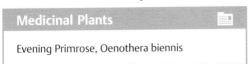

Medicinal Plants

Evening Primrose, Oenothera biennis

15.5 F

15.5.1 Flu, Colds

Medicinal Plants

Elderberry, Sambucus niger
Littleleaf linden, Tilia cordata
Purple Echinacea, Echinacea purpurea

Evening Primrose Oil

Prescribe finished pharmaceutical products.

Elderberry Flower

Preparation

- Tea

15.4.2 Exhaustion, in Geriatric Patients

Medicinal Plants

Ginseng, Panax ginseng

Proven Prescription

- Tea
  Add 1 cup of boiling water to 2 teaspoons of the drug. Steep for 15 minutes, then strain. To increase immunity, drink 1 cup several times a day. For a sweating regimen, drink 500 mL. The effects of the sweating regimen can be enhanced by simultaneously taking a hot bath.

Ginseng Root

Use finished pharmaceutical products.

15.4.3 Exhaustion, Psychophysical

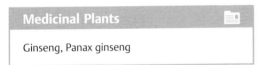

Medicinal Plants

Ginseng, Panax ginseng
Yerba mate, Ilex paraguariensis

Linden Flowers

Preparation

- Tea

Ginseng Root

See Chapter 11.7, Exhaustion (p. 328), Geriatrics for recommendations regarding use.

Yerba Mate Leaves

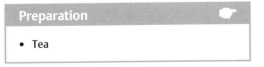

Preparation

- Tea

Proven Prescriptions

- Tea
  Add 1 cup of boiling water to 1–2 teaspoons of the drug. Steep for 10 minutes, then strain. Drink slowly in small sips, as hot as possible.

- **Tea Blend**

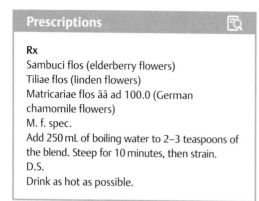

Prescriptions

Rx
Sambuci flos (elderberry flowers)
Tiliae flos (linden flowers)
Matricariae flos āā ad 100.0 (German chamomile flowers)
M. f. spec.
Add 250 mL of boiling water to 2–3 teaspoons of the blend. Steep for 10 minutes, then strain.
D.S.
Drink as hot as possible.

- This tea blend with Jaborandi leaves has a stronger **diaphoretic** effect.

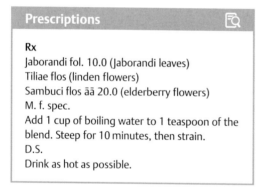

Prescriptions

Rx
Jaborandi fol. 10.0 (Jaborandi leaves)
Tiliae flos (linden flowers)
Sambuci flos āā 20.0 (elderberry flowers)
M. f. spec.
Add 1 cup of boiling water to 1 teaspoon of the blend. Steep for 10 minutes, then strain.
D.S.
Drink as hot as possible.

- The following is a proven prescription for **children.**

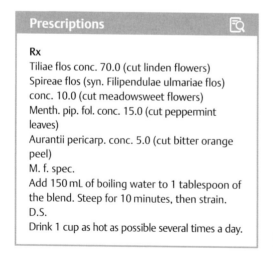

Prescriptions

Rx
Tiliae flos conc. 70.0 (cut linden flowers)
Spireae flos (syn. Filipendulae ulmariae flos) conc. 10.0 (cut meadowsweet flowers)
Menth. pip. fol. conc. 15.0 (cut peppermint leaves)
Aurantii pericarp. conc. 5.0 (cut bitter orange peel)
M. f. spec.
Add 150 mL of boiling water to 1 tablespoon of the blend. Steep for 10 minutes, then strain.
D.S.
Drink 1 cup as hot as possible several times a day.

Echinacea Herb and Root

Very well suited for **children.**
Prescribe finished pharmaceutical products.

15.6 G

15.6.1 Gallbladder Symptoms

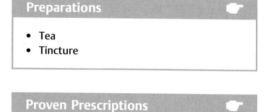

Medicinal Plants

Celandine, Chelidonium majus
Turmeric, Curcuma longa/domestica
Fumitory, Fumaria officinalis
Dandelion, Taraxacum officinale
Wormwood, Artemisia absinthium

Celandine Herb

Preparations

- **Tea**
- **Tincture**

Proven Prescriptions

- **Tea**
  Add 1 cup of hot water to 2 teaspoons of the finely chopped drug. Steep for 5–10 minutes, then strain.
  Drink warm between meals 3 × a day for 3 weeks as a regimen.

- **Celandine Tincture** (Tinctura chelidonii) (**1:10**)
  Add 20 drops to a small amount of water and drink 3 × a day.
- **With a Spasmolytic Component**

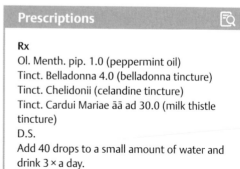

Prescriptions

Rx
Ol. Menth. pip. 1.0 (peppermint oil)
Tinct. Belladonna 4.0 (belladonna tincture)
Tinct. Chelidonii (celandine tincture)
Tinct. Cardui Mariae āā ad 30.0 (milk thistle tincture)
D.S.
Add 40 drops to a small amount of water and drink 3 × a day.

Turmeric Rootstock

Preparations

- Tea
- Tincture

Proven Prescriptions

- Tea
  Add 1 cup of hot water to 1–2 teaspoons of the finely chopped drug. Steep for 5 minutes, then strain.
  Drink 1 cup before each meal.
- **Turmeric Tincture** (Tinctura Curcumae) **(1:10)**
  Add 10–15 drops to a small amount of water and drink 3 × a day.

Fumitory Herb

Preparation

- Tea

Proven Prescription

- Tea
  Add 1 cup of hot water to 2 teaspoons of the chopped fumitory herb. Steep for 10 minutes, then strain.
  Drink 1 cup several times a day with meals.

Dandelion Root and Herb

Preparation

- Tea

Proven Prescription

- Tea
  Add 1–2 teaspoons of the finely chopped drug to 1 cup of cold water. Bring to a brief boil and steep for 15 minutes, then strain.
  Drink 1 cup in the morning and in the evening for 4–6 weeks.

Wormwood Herb

Preparations

- Tea
- Tincture

Proven Prescriptions

- Tea
  Add 1 cup of boiling water to 1 teaspoon of the finely chopped drug. Steep up to a maximum of 5 minutes, then strain. Drink 3 × a day.
- **Wormwood Tincture** (Tinctura Absinthii) **(1:10)**
  Add 10–30 drops to a sufficient amount of water and drink 3 × a day (the bitter taste improves with increased dilution).

15.6.2 Gastric and Duodenal (Peptic) Ulcers

Medicinal Plants

Licorice, Glycyrrhiza glabra
German chamomile, Matricaria recutita

Licorice Root

Prescribe finished pharmaceutical products.

German Chamomile Flowers
15.6.3 Gastric Disorders, Acute

Medicinal Plants

German chamomile, Matricaria recutita
Peppermint, Mentha piperita
Lemon balm, Melissa officinalis

German Chamomile Flowers

Preparation

- Tea

• Proven Prescription:

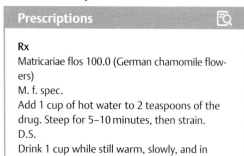

Prescriptions

Rx
Matricariae flos 100.0 (German chamomile flowers)
M. f. spec.
Add 1 cup of hot water to 2 teaspoons of the drug. Steep for 5–10 minutes, then strain.
D.S.
Drink 1 cup while still warm, slowly, and in small sips several times a day.

Peppermint Leaves

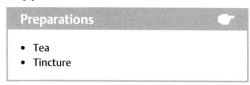

Preparations

• Tea
• Tincture

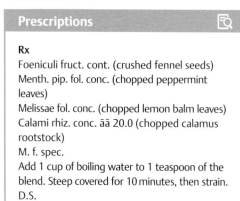

Proven Prescriptions

• Tea
Add 1 cup of hot water to 1–2 teaspoons of the drug. Steep covered for 10–15 minutes, then strain.
Drink 1 cup warm several times a day in small sips; best after or between meals.

• **Tea Blend**, also proven very effective with children:

Prescriptions

Rx
Foeniculi fruct. cont. (crushed fennel seeds)
Menth. pip. fol. conc. (chopped peppermint leaves)
Melissae fol. conc. (chopped lemon balm leaves)
Calami rhiz. conc. āā 20.0 (chopped calamus rootstock)
M. f. spec.
Add 1 cup of boiling water to 1 teaspoon of the blend. Steep covered for 10 minutes, then strain.
D.S.
Drink warm and in small sips 2–3 × a day.

• **Peppermint Tincture** (Tinctura menthae piperitae) (**1:10**)
Take 10–20 drops in a small amount of water.

Lemon Balm Leaves

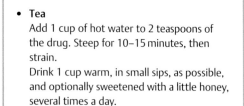

Preparation

• Tea

Proven Prescription

• Tea
Add 1 cup of hot water to 2 teaspoons of the drug. Steep for 10–15 minutes, then strain.
Drink 1 cup warm, in small sips, as possible, and optionally sweetened with a little honey, several times a day.

15.6.4 Gastric Disorders, Chronic

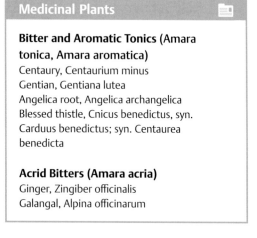

Medicinal Plants

Bitter and Aromatic Tonics (Amara tonica, Amara aromatica)
Centaury, Centaurium minus
Gentian, Gentiana lutea
Angelica root, Angelica archangelica
Blessed thistle, Cnicus benedictus, syn. Carduus benedictus; syn. Centaurea benedicta

Acrid Bitters (Amara acria)
Ginger, Zingiber officinalis
Galangal, Alpina officinarum

Centaury Herb

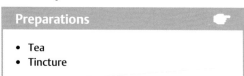

Preparations

• Tea
• Tincture

- **Tea**
  Add 1 cup of boiling water to 1–2 teaspoons of the drug. Steep for 15 minutes, then strain. Drink 1 cup at room temperature before each meal.

- **Tea Blend**
  This remedy is also proven to be very effective for children.

Rx
Centaurii herb. (centaury herb)
Millefolii herb. (yarrow herb)
Menth. pip. fol. āā 20.0 (peppermint leaves)
M. f. spec.
Add 1 cup of boiling water to 1 teaspoon of the blend. Steep for 10 minutes, then strain.
D.S.
Drink cold or lukewarm before meals.

- **Centaury Tincture** (Tinctura centaurii) **(1:10)**
  Add 10–20 drops to a small amount of warm water and drink 3 × a day before meals.

Gentian Root

- **Tea**
- **Tincture**

- **Tea**
  Add 1 teaspoon of the drug to 1 cup of cold water. Bring to a boil, steep for about 5 h, then strain.
  Or add 1 cup of boiling water to 1 teaspoon of the finely chopped drug. Steep for 5 minutes, then strain.
  Drink 1 cup before each meal.
- **Gentian Tincture** (Tinctura gentianae) **(1:10)**
  Add 20–40 drops to 1 glass of water and drink before each meal.

Angelica Root

- **Tea**
- **Tincture**

- **Tea**
  Add 1 teaspoon of the drug to 1 cup of cold water, bring to a boil, then strain.
  Or add 1 cup of boiling water to 1 teaspoon, then strain.
  Drink 1 cup before each meal.
- **Angelica Tincture** (Tinctura angelicae) **(1:5)**
  Add 10–30 drops to ½–1 glass of water and drink several times a day.

Blessed Thistle Herb

- **Tea**
- **Tincture**

- **Tea**
  Add 1 cup of boiling water to 2 teaspoons of the drug. Steep for 30 minutes, then strain.
  Drink 2–3 cups 15–30 minutes before meals.

- **Combination with Wormwood and Lemon Balm**

Rx
Cnici benedicti herb. (blessed thistle herb)
Absinthii herb. (wormwood herb)
Melissae fol. āā 20.0 (lemon balm leaves)
M. f. spec.
Add 1 cup of hot water to 1 teaspoon of the blend. Steep for 20 minutes, then strain.
D.S.
Drink 1 cup 3 × a day.

- Blessed Thistle Tincture (Tinctura cnici benedicti) **(1:5)**
Add 10–30 drops to a small amount of water and drink several times a day.

Ginger Rootstock

Preparations
• Tea • Tincture

Proven Prescriptions
• Tea Add 1 cup of hot water to 1 teaspoon of the coarsely powdered drug. Steep covered 5–10 minutes, then strain. Drink 1 cup several times a day, 15–30 minutes before meals. • **Ginger Tincture** (Tinctura zingiberis) **(1:5)** Add 10–20 drops to ½–1 glass of water and drink before meals.

Galangal Rootstock

Preparations
• Tea • Tincture

Proven Prescriptions
• Tea Add 1 cup of boiling water to 1 teaspoon of the finely cut or coarsely powdered drug. Steep covered for 5–10 minutes, then strain. Drink 1 cup before meals. • **Galangal Tincture** (Tinctura galangae) **(1:10)** Add 10 drops to a small amount of lukewarm water and drink 3 × a day, 15 minutes before meals.

15.6.5 Gout

Medicinal Plants
Autumn crocus, Colchicum autumnale

Autumn Crocus Seeds and Bulbs

Prescribe finished pharmaceutical products.

15.7 H

15.7.1 Hair Loss

- Proven Prescription:

Prescriptions
Rx Ol. Lavandulae (lavender oil) Ol. Calami āā 1.0 (calamus oil) Tinct. Gentianae 10.0 (gentian tincture) Spirit. Rosmarini ad 100.0 (rosemary spirit) D.S. Shake before use. Use as a hair tonic.

15.7.2 Headache, Vasomotor

Medicinal Plants
Butterbur, Petasites hybridus Peppermint, Mentha piperita

Butterbur Rootstock

Prescribe finished pharmaceutical products.

Peppermint Leaves

Prescribe finished pharmaceutical products.

15.7.3 Heart and Vascular Disorders, Degenerative

Medicinal Plants
Hawthorn, Crataegus laevigata/monogyna Bishop's weed, Ammi visnaga Arnica, Arnica montana

Hawthorn Leaves and Flowers

Preparations
• Tea • Tincture

Proven Prescriptions

- **Tea**
  Add 1 cup of hot water to 2 teaspoons of the drug. Steep for 20 minutes, then strain. Sweeten with 1–2 teaspoons of honey. Drink 1 cup in the morning and evening. In the beginning, also drink 1 cup at midday.

- **Combination with Lemon Balm**

Prescriptions

Rx
Crataegi flos (hawthorn flowers)
Crataegi fol. (hawthorn leaves)
Melissae fol. āā ad 100.0 (lemon balm leaves)
M. f. spec.
Add 1 cup of hot water to 1–2 teaspoons of the blend. Steep for 10 minutes, then strain.
D.S.
Drink 1 cup in the morning and in the evening.

- **Combination with Mistletoe**

Prescriptions

Rx
Crataegi flos (hawthorn flowers)
Crataegi fol. (hawthorn leaves)
Visci albi āā ad 100.0 (mistletoe herb)
M. f. spec.
Add 1 cup of hot water to 1–2 teaspoons of the blend. Steep for 10 minutes, then strain.
D.S.
Drink 1 cup in the morning and in the evening.

- **Hawthorn Tincture** (Tinctura crataegi) **(1:10)**
  Take 10–20 drops 3 × a day.

Arnica Flowers

Preparations

- Tea
- Tincture
- Essence

Proven Prescriptions

- **Tea**
  Add 1 cup of boiling water to 2 teaspoons of the drug. Steep for 10 minutes, then strain. Drink 1 cup, slowly, and in small sips 2 × a day.
- **Arnica Tincture** (Tinctura arnicae) **(1:10)**
  With acute angina pectoris symptoms, take 50 drops in 1 glass of lukewarm water. Drink slowly and in small sips over the course of 15 minutes.
- **Essence** (for external application)
  With oppressive heart symptoms, place a moist, warm arnica compress over the area of the heart.

Bishop's weed Fruit

Prescribe finished pharmaceutical products.

15.7.4 Heart Arrhythmia

Medicinal Plants

Scotch broom, Cytisus scoparius (Sarothamnus scoparius)
Yellow jessamine, Gelsemium sempervirens

Scotch Broom Herb

Finished pharmaceutical products should be given preference.

Primarily indicated for functional tachycardia arrhythmia.

Preparation

- Tea

Proven Prescription

- **Tea**
  Add 1 cup of boiling water to 1 teaspoon of the drug. Steep for 10 minutes, then strain. Drink 1 cup of freshly prepared tea 3–4 × a day.

Yellow Jessamine Rootstock

Indicated for functional heart symptoms with extrasystoles.

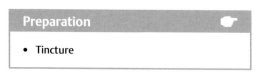

Preparation 👉

• Tincture

• Proven prescriptions:

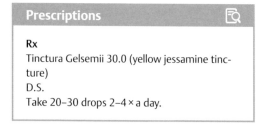

Prescriptions 🔍

Rx
Tinctura Gelsemii 30.0 (yellow jessamine tincture)
D.S.
Take 20–30 drops 2–4 × a day.

Prescriptions 🔍

Rx
Tinct. Gelsemii 10.0 (yellow jessamine tincture)
Tinct. Valerian. aeth. ad 30.0 (ethereal valerian tincture)
D.S.
Take 20–30 drops 3 × a day.

Prescriptions 🔍

Rx
Tinct. Gelsemii 10.0 (yellow jessamine tincture)
Extr. Adonidis fluid. 10.0 (pheasant's eye fluid extract)
Tinct. Valerianae ad 30.0 (valerian tincture)
D.S.
Take 20–40 drops 3 × a day.

Prescriptions 🔍

Rx
Tinct. Gelsemii 12.0 (yellow jessamine tincture)
Extr. Crataegi fluid. ad 30.0 (hawthorn fluid extract)
D.S.
Take 20 drops 3 × a day.

15.7.5 Heart Failure, Congestive (CHF) (NYHA II–III)

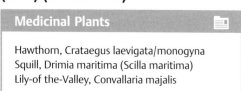

Medicinal Plants 📄

Hawthorn, Crataegus laevigata/monogyna
Squill, Drimia maritima (Scilla maritima)
Lily-of the-Valley, Convallaria majalis

Hawthorn Leaves and Flowers

Prescribe finished pharmaceutical products.

Lily-of-the-Valley Herb

Prescribe finished pharmaceutical products.

15.7.6 Hemorrhoids

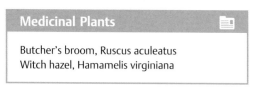

Medicinal Plants 📄

Butcher's broom, Ruscus aculeatus
Witch hazel, Hamamelis virginiana

Butcher's Broom Rootstock

Prescribe finished pharmaceutical products.

Witch Hazel Leaves

Prescribe finished pharmaceutical products.

15.7.7 Hepatitis, Chronic

Milk Thistle Seeds

Prescribe only finished pharmaceutical products.

15.7.8 Hypertension, Arterial

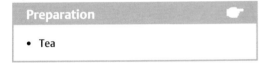

Medicinal Plants

Mistletoe, Viscum album

Mistletoe Herb

Preference should be given to finished pharmaceutical products.

Preparation

- Tea

Proven Prescriptions

- Tea

Prescriptions

Rx
Viscum alb. herb. conc. 100.0 (cut mistletoe herb)
M.f. spec.
Add 1 L of cold water to 2–4 teaspoons to the drug. Soak overnight. In the morning, prepare 1 cup in the same manner to drink in the evening.
D.S.
Drink in the morning (on an empty stomach) and in the evening.

- "Blood Pressure Tea" according to R.F. Weiss

Prescriptions

Rx
Visci albi herb. (mistletoe herb)
Crataegi fol. et flos (hawthorn leaves and flowers)
Melissae fol. āā ad 100.0 (lemon balm leaves)
M. f. spec.
Add 1 cup of hot water to 2 teaspoons of the blend. Steep for 5–10 minutes, then strain.
D.S.
Drink warm in small sips.

15.7.9 Hyperthyroidism

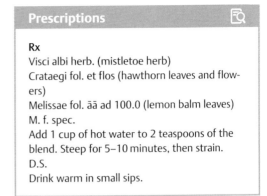

Medicinal Plants

Bugleweed, Lycopus virginicus/europaeus
Motherwort, Leonurus cardiaca

Bugleweed Herb

Prescribe finished pharmaceutical products.

Motherwort Herb

Finished pharmaceutical products should be given preference.

Preparation

- Tea

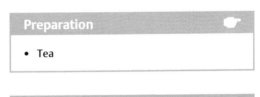

Proven Prescription

- Tea
  Add 1 cup of hot water to 1 teaspoon of the finely cut drug. Steep for 5 minutes, then strain.
  Drink 2–3 cups a day.

15.7.10 Hypotension

Medicinal Plants

Rosemary, Rosmarinus officinalis
Motherwort, Leonurus cardiaca
Camphor, Cinnamomum camphora

Rosemary Leaves

Preparations ☞

- Tea
- Tincture
- Bath Additive

Proven Prescriptions ☞

- Tea
  Add 1 cup of hot water to 1 teaspoon of the finely chopped drug. Steep covered for 5 minutes, then strain.
  Drink 1 cup warm in the morning and midday before meals.
- **Rosemary Tincture** (Tinctura Rosmarini) (1:5)
  Take 5 drops in a small amount of warm water 3 × a day, 15 minutes before meals.
- **Bath Additive**
  Add 1 L of hot water to 50 g of the drug. Steep covered for 30 minutes, then strain, and add to a full bath or sitz bath.

Motherwort Herb

Preparation ☞

- Tea

Proven Prescription ☞

- **Tea with Lily-of-the-Valley and the Sedative Effects of Lemon Balm**

Prescriptions

Rx
Leonur. card. herb. (motherwort herb)
Convallar herb. (lily-of-the-valley herb)
Melissae fol. āā 100.0 (lemon balm leaves)
M. f. spec.
Add 1 cup of hot water to 2 teaspoons of the blend. Steep covered for 5 minutes, then strain.
D.S.
Drink 1 cup in the morning and midday for several weeks.

Camphor

Prescribe finished pharmaceutical products.

15.8 I

15.8.1 Irritable Bladder

Medicinal Plants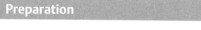

Saw palmetto, Serenoa repens
Pumpkin, Cucurbita pepo

Saw Palmetto Fruit

Prescribe finished pharmaceutical products.

Pumpkin Seeds

Prescribe finished pharmaceutical products.

15.8.2 Irritable Colon

Medicinal Plants

Peppermint, Mentha piperita

Peppermint Leaves

Prescribe finished pharmaceutical products.

15.9 L

15.9.1 Leukorrhea (Fluor Albus)

Medicinal Plants

White dead nettle, Lamium album

White Dead Nettle Flowers

Preparation

- Tea

Proven Prescriptions

- **Tea**
  Add 1 cup boiling water to 2 teaspoons of the finely chopped drug. Steep for 10 minutes, then strain.
  Drink 1 cup several times a day.
- **For vaginal rinses**
  Add 500 mL of hot water to 50 g of the finely chopped drug. Steep for 10 minutes, then strain. Rinse should be lukewarm to cold before using.

Proven Prescriptions for Vaginal Rinses

Prescriptions

Demulcent
Rx
Malvae fol. 50.0 (mallow leaves)
D.S.
Brief decoction of 2–3 tablespoons in 1 L of water.

Prescriptions

Anti-inflammatory
Rx
Matricariae flos (German chamomile flowers)
Salviae fol. āā 50.0 (sage leaves)
D.S.
Infusion of 2–3 tablespoons in 1 L of water

Prescriptions

Astringent
Rx
Anserinae herb. (potentilla herb)
Matricariae flos āā 50.0 (German chamomile flowers)
D.S.
Infusion of 2–3 tablespoons in 1 L of water.

Prescriptions

Aromatic
Rx
Lavandulae flos (lavender flowers)
Serpilli herb. āā 50.0 (Serpylli herba, wild thyme herb)
D.S.
Add 1 L of hot water to 1 tablespoon of the blend. Steep for 15 minutes, then strain.
Drink it.

15.9.2 Lipometabolic Disorders (Hyperlipoproteinemia, Dyslipoproteinemia)

See Section Metabolic Disorders (p. 388).

15.9.3 Liver Disorders, Toxic

Medicinal Plants

Milk thistle, Silybum marianum
Artichoke, Cynara cardunculus

Milk Thistle Seeds

Prescribe finished pharmaceutical products.

Artichoke Leaves

Prescribe finished pharmaceutical products.

15.10 M

15.10.1 Maldigestion, Dyspepsia

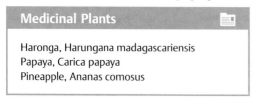

Medicinal Plants

Haronga, Harungana madagascariensis
Papaya, Carica papaya
Pineapple, Ananas comosus

Haronga Leaves

Prescribe finished pharmaceutical products.

Papaya Fruit

Prescribe finished pharmaceutical products.

Pineapple

Prescribe finished pharmaceutical products.

15.10.2 Mastodynia

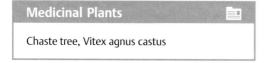

Medicinal Plants

Chaste tree, Vitex agnus castus

Chaste Tree Fruit

Prescribe finished pharmaceutical products.

15.10.3 Menopause Symptoms

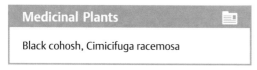

Medicinal Plants

Black cohosh, Cimicifuga racemosa

Black Cohosh Rootstock

Finished pharmaceutical products should be given preference.

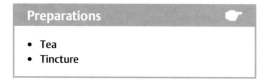

Preparations

- **Tea**
- **Tincture**

Proven Prescriptions

- **Tea**
  For mild symptoms, add 1 cup of hot water to 1 teaspoon of the chopped drug. Steep 10 minutes, then strain.
  Drink 1 cup 2–3 × a day.
- **Black Cohosh Tincture** (Tinctura cimicifugae racemosae) **(1:10)**
  Place 10 drops on 1 sugar cube. Dissolve slowly in the mouth 3 × a day.

15.10.4 Metabolic Disorders

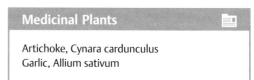

Medicinal Plants

Artichoke, Cynara cardunculus
Garlic, Allium sativum

Artichoke Leaves

Prescribe finished pharmaceutical products.

Garlic Bulb

Prescribe finished pharmaceutical products.

15.10.5 Meteorism

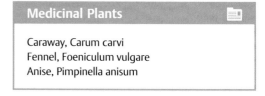

Medicinal Plants

Caraway, Carum carvi
Fennel, Foeniculum vulgare
Anise, Pimpinella anisum

Caraway Seeds

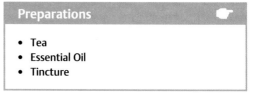

Preparations

- **Tea**
- **Essential Oil**
- **Tincture**

Proven Prescriptions

- **Tea**
  Add 1 cup of hot water to 1 teaspoon of freshly crushed caraway seeds. Steep covered for 5 minutes, then strain.
  Drink warm with meals 3 × a day.
- **Essential Oil**
  This remedy is also very suitable for children.

Prescriptions

Rx
Ol. carvi 5.0 (caraway essential oil)
Ol. Olivarum ad 50.0 (olive oil)
D.S.
Massage 10–20 drops into the skin of the abdomen using a circular motion.

- **Carminative Tincture (Tinctura carminative) (1:10)**

Prescriptions

Rx
Ol. Carvi 5.0 (caraway essential oil)
Tinct. carminativ. Erg. B (see Carminative Tinctures (p. 79))
Tinct. Valerian. aeth. āā 20.0 (ethereal valerian tincture)
D.S.
Add 20 drops to a small amount of water and drink 3 × a day after meals.

Caution ⚠

Do not rub into the navel; it can cause a burning sensation!

Fennel Seeds

Preparations

- **Tea**
- **Essential Oil**

Proven Prescriptions

- **Tea**
  Add 1 cup of hot water to 1 teaspoon of freshly crushed fennel seeds. Steep covered 5 minutes, then strain.
  Drink 1–2 cups several times a day.
- **Fennel Oil** (Oleum Foeniculi)
  Add 2–4 drops to a small amount of water and drink several times a day.

Anise Seeds

Preparation

- **Tea**

Proven Prescriptions

- **Tea**
  Add 1 cup of boiling water to 1 heaping teaspoon of the crushed or coarsely powdered drug. Steep covered for 10–15 minutes, then strain.
  Drink 1 cup several times a day.
- **Anise-Fennel-Caraway (AFC) Tea**
  This remedy is also very suitable for children.

Prescriptions

Rx
Carvi fruct. cont. (crushed caraway seeds)
Foeniculi fruct. cont. (crushed fennel seeds)
Anisi fruct. cont. āā 20.0 (crushed anise seeds)
M. f. spec.
Add 1 cup of boiling water to 1 teaspoon of the blend. Steep covered for 20 minutes, then strain.
D.S.
Drink 1 cup warm after every meal.

- For additional **dyspeptic** symptoms, a bitter or cholagogue type of plant can be added.

Prescriptions

Rx
Carvi fruct. (caraway seeds)
Foeniculi fruct. (fennel seeds)
Absinthii herb. (wormwood herb)
Millefolii herb. āā 25.0 (yarrow herb)
M. f. spec.
Add 1 cup of boiling water to 1 teaspoon of the
blend. Steep covered for 15 minutes, then strain.
D.S.
Drink 1 cup warm after every meal.

- **Combination with a Laxative for Insufficient
  Evacuation of the Bowels as an Adjuvant
  Symptom**

Prescriptions

Rx
Carvi fruct. (caraway seeds)
Foeniculi fruct. āā 20.0 (fennel seeds)
Menth. pip. fol. (peppermint leaves)
Sennae fol. āā 30.0 (senna leaves)
M. f. spec.
Add 1 cup of boiling water to 1–2 teaspoons of
the blend. Steep covered for 20 minutes, then
strain.
D.S.
Drink 1 cup in the morning and evening.

15.10.6 Mucous Membrane Disorders of the Mouth and Pharynx

Medicinal Plants

Sage, Salvia officinalis
German Chamomile, Matricaria recutita
Tormentil, Potentilla tormentilla

Sage Leaves

Preparations

- Tea
- Tincture

Proven Prescriptions

- **Tea**
  Add 1 cup of boiling water to 1 tablespoon
  of the cut drug. Steep for 5–10 minutes,
  then strain.
  Rinse or gargle several times a day.
- **Sage Tincture** (Tinctura salviae) **(1:10)**
  Use undiluted several times a day for
  brushing on to the area of treatment.

German Chamomile Flowers

Preparations

- Tea
- Extract

Proven Prescriptions

- **Tea**
  Add 1 cup of boiling water to 1 tablespoon
  of the cut drug. Steep for 5–10 minutes,
  then strain.
  Rinse or gargle several times a day.
- **Extract with Topical Antiphlogistic Effect**

Prescriptions

Rx
Extr. Salviae fluid. (sage fluid extract)
Extr. Chamomill. fluid. āā 20.0 (German
chamomile fluid extract)
D.S.
Add 20–30 drops to 1 glass of water and
gargle several times a day.

Tormentil Rootstock

Preparations

- Tea
- Tincture

- **Tea**
  Add 2–3 tablespoons of the drug to 1 L of cold water. Bring to a boil, then strain. Rinse or gargle several times a day.

- **Tormentil Tincture (Tinctura Tormentillae)**

Rx
Tinct. Tormentillae 20.0 (tormentil tincture)
D.S.
Add 1 teaspoon to 1 glass of water. Rinse several times a day.

- The following formulations have **astringent** effects:

Rx
Tinct. Tormentillae (tormentil tincture)
Tinct. Salviae āā 10.0 (sage tincture)
D.S.
Add 1 teaspoon to 1 glass of water. Rinse several times a day.

Rx
Tinct. Tormentillae (tormentil tincture)
Tinct. Myrrhae āā 20.0 (myrrh tincture)
D.S.
Use undiluted for brushing on to gums several times a day.

15.11 N

15.11.1 Nervous Restlessness

Valerian, Valeriana officinalis
Hops, Humulus lupulus
Lemon balm, Melissa officinalis
Passionflower, Passiflora incarnata

Valerian Root

- **Tea**
- **Tincture**
- **Infusion**

- **Tea**
  Add 1 cup water to 2 teaspoons of the drug. Bring to a brief boil, steep for 10 minutes, then strain. Drink 1 cup warm 2–3 × a day. Valerian tea can be fortified by adding 1 teaspoon of valerian tincture per cup.
- **Valerian Tincture** (Tinctura valerianae) **(1:10)**
  Take 1–2 teaspoons several times a day.
- **Infusion**

Rx
Infus. Valerian. rad. 15.0/150.0 (valerian root infusion)
Aqu. Menth. pip. ad 200.0 (peppermint water)
D.S.
Take 1 tablespoon 3 × a day.

Hops Strobiles

- **Tea**
- **Tincture**

- **Tea**
  Add 1 cup of boiling water to 1 heaping teaspoon of chopped hops strobiles. Steep covered for 10–15 minutes, then strain. Drink 1 cup warm several times a day.
- **Tincture**

Rx
Extr. Lupuli (hops extract)
Tinct. Valerian. āā 20.0 (valerian tincture)
D.S.
Take 30 drops in the evening at bedtime.

- Tea
  Add 1 cup of boiling water to 1 teaspoon
  of the finely chopped drug. Steep for
  5–10 minutes, then strain.
  Drink warm, 2–3 cups a day.

- For **Nervous Gastric Disorders**

Rx
Extr. Lupuli (hops extract)
Tinct. Carminativ. āā 10.0 (see Carminative
Tinctures (p. 79))
D.S.
Place 30 drops on to a teaspoon of sugar or a
sugar cube and allow to dissolve in mouth
before meals.

Lemon Balm Leaves

- Tea
- Bath Additive

Additional Proven Prescriptions

- **Nerve Tea (Species nervinae)**

Rx
Valerian. rad. (valerian root)
Melissae fol. (lemon balm leaves)
Lupul. strobul. āā ad 100.0 (hops strobiles)
M. f. spec.
Add 1 cup of hot water to 1–2 teaspoons of the
blend. Steep for at least 15 minutes, then
strain.
D.S.
Drink 1 cup in the evening at bedtime.

- Tea
  Add 1 cup of hot (but not boiling!) water to
  2–3 teaspoons of the drug. Steep for
  15 minutes, then strain. Drink 1 cup in the
  morning and evening, may be optionally
  sweetened with a little honey.
- Full Bath
  Add 2 L of hot water to 10 g of the drug.
  Steep covered for 5 minutes, then strain, and
  add to the bath water.

Passionflower Herb

- Tea

- **Tincturae nervinae**

Rx
Tinct. Gelsemii (yellow jessamine tincture)
Tinct. Valerianae āā 10.0 (valerian tincture)
D.S.
Add 30 drops to a small amount of water and
drink 3–4 × a day.

Rx
Tinct. Valerianae (valerian tincture)
Tinct. Convallariae āā 10.0 (lily-of-the-valley
tincture)
D.S.
Take 20 drops 3–4 × a day.

15.12 P

15.12.1 Pelvic Congestion

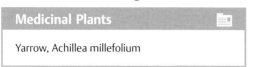

Medicinal Plants

Yarrow, Achillea millefolium

Yarrow Herb and Flowers

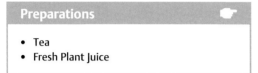

Preparations

- Tea
- Fresh Plant Juice

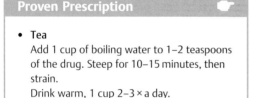

Proven Prescription

- Tea
  Add 1 cup of boiling water to 1–2 teaspoons of the drug. Steep for 10–15 minutes, then strain.
  Drink warm, 1 cup 2–3 × a day.

15.12.2 Premenstrual Syndrome

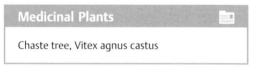

Medicinal Plants

Chaste tree, Vitex agnus castus

Chaste Tree Fruit

Prescribe finished pharmaceutical products.

15.12.3 Prostatic Hyperplasia, Benign (BPH)

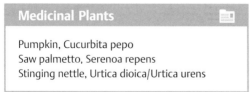

Medicinal Plants

Pumpkin, Cucurbita pepo
Saw palmetto, Serenoa repens
Stinging nettle, Urtica dioica/Urtica urens

Pumpkin Seeds

Prescribe finished pharmaceutical products.

Saw Palmetto Fruit

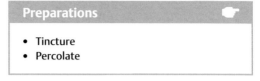

Preparations

- Tincture
- Percolate

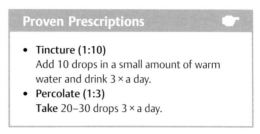

Proven Prescriptions

- Tincture (1:10)
  Add 10 drops in a small amount of warm water and drink 3 × a day.
- Percolate (1:3)
  Take 20–30 drops 3 × a day.

Stinging Nettle Root

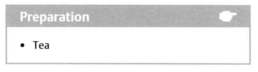

Preparation

- Tea

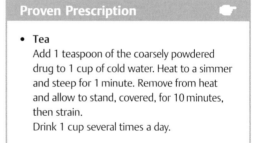

Proven Prescription

- Tea
  Add 1 teaspoon of the coarsely powdered drug to 1 cup of cold water. Heat to a simmer and steep for 1 minute. Remove from heat and allow to stand, covered, for 10 minutes, then strain.
  Drink 1 cup several times a day.

15.12.4 Prostatitis, Nonbacterial

See Irritable Bladder (pp. 227-229).

15.12.5 Psoriasis

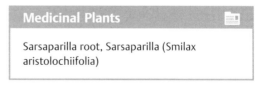

Medicinal Plants

Sarsaparilla root, Sarsaparilla (Smilax aristolochiifolia)

Sarsaparilla Root

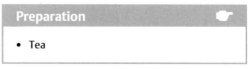

Preparation

- Tea

Proven Prescription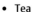

- **Tea**
  Add 1 tablespoon of the drug to 1 L of cold water in the evening and soak overnight. The next morning, boil for 20 minutes, then strain.
  Drink one-half in the morning and the other half in the evening.

Proven Prescriptions

- **Tea**
  Add 1 cup of cold water to the root drug. Soak for 1–2 hours, stirring frequently, then strain, and warm gently.
  Drink 1 cup several times a day. This tea is especially suitable for children.
- **Syrup**

15.13 R

15.13.1 Respiratory Tract Infections, Acute and Chronic

Medicinal Plants

Demulcents
Marshmallow, Althaea officinalis
Coltsfoot, Tussilago farfara
Narrowleaf plantain, Plantago lanceolata
Iceland moss, Lichen islandicus

Expectorants
Cowslip primrose, Primula veris
Pimpinella, Pimpinella saxifraga
Anise, Pimpinella anisum

Spasmolytic Cough Remedies
Thyme, Thymus vulgaris
Roundleaf sundew, Drosera rotundifolia
Ivy, Hedera helix

Prescriptions

Rx
Sir. Althaeae 30.0 (marshmallow syrup)
Liqu. Ammon. anisat. 5.0 (anisated solution of ammonia)
Aqu. dest. ad 200.0 (distilled water)
D.S.
Shake before use. Take 1 tablespoon every 2 hours.

Prescriptions

Rx
Sir. Althaeae (marshmallow syrup)
Sir. Plantaginis lanc. (plantain syrup)
Mel. Foeniculi āā ad 100.0 (fennel honey)
D.S.
Take 1 tablespoon every 2 hours.

Coltsfoot Leaves

Preparation

- **Tea**

Marshmallow Root and Leaves

This remedy is also very well suited for cough and bronchitis in children.

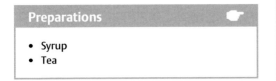

Preparations

- **Syrup**
- **Tea**

Proven Prescription

- **Tea**
  Add 1 cup of water to 1–2 teaspoons of the drug. Bring to a brief boil, steep for 10 minutes, then strain.
  Drink 1 cup 3 × a day.

Plantain Herb

This remedy is also very well suited for cough and bronchitis in children.

Prescribe a finished pharmaceutical products.

Preparation

- Syrup

Iceland Moss

Preparation

- Tea

Proven Prescription

- Tea
  Add 1 cup of boiling water to 1–2 teaspoons of the finely chopped drug. Steep for 10 minutes, then strain.
  Drink 2–3 cups a day for several months.

Cowslip Primrose Root

This remedy is also very well suited for cough and bronchitis in children.

Preparations

- Tea
- Tincture
- Fluid Extract

Proven Prescriptions

- Tea
  Add ¼ teaspoon of the finely chopped drug to 1 cup of cold water. Bring to a simmer, remove from heat, steep for 5 minutes, then strain.
  Drink 1 cup every 2–3 hours sweetened with a small amount of honey.
- Tea blend
  This tea blend is also highly recommended for children.

Prescriptions

Rx
Primulae rad. 20.0 (cowslip primrose root)
Anisi fruct. (anise seeds)
Foeniculi fruct. (fennel seeds)
Farfarae fol. āā ad 50.0 (coltsfoot leaves)
D.S.
Add 2 teaspoons of the blend to 1 cup of water.
Drink X

- **Cowslip Primrose Tincture (Tinctura Primulae) (1:10)**
  Take 20 drops 4 × a day.
- **Cowslip Primrose Fluid Extract (Extractum Primulae fluidum)** (even stronger and highly recommend)
  Take 20 drops several times a day.

This fluid extract is also well suited for combining with other cough remedies.

Prescriptions

Rx
Extr. Primul. fluid. (cowslip primrose fluid extract)
Extr. Thymi fluid. āā 20.0 (thyme fluid extract)
D.S.
Take 20 drops 3 × a day.

Pimpinella Root

Preparations

- Tea
- Tincture

Proven Prescriptions

- Tea
  Add 2 tablespoonsof the finely chopped drug to 1 cup of cold water. Bring to a brief boil, then strain.
  Drink 1 cup several times a day sweetened with a small amount of honey.
- **Pimpinella Tincture (Tinctura Pimpinellae) (1:10)**
  This remedy is well suited for combining with other cough remedies.

Anise Fruit

Preparations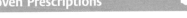

- Tea
- Essential Oil

Proven Prescriptions

- Tea
  Add 1 cup of boiling water to 1 heaping teaspoon of the crushed or coarsely powdered drug. Steep covered for 10–15 minutes, then strain.
  Drink 1 cup several times a day.
- Essential Oil
  Place 3 drops on a sugar cube and allow to dissolve in mouth several times a day.
- With Pimpinalla Tincture (Tinctura Pimpinellae)

Prescriptions

Rx
Ol. Anisi 0.2(–0.4) (anise essential oil)
Tinct. Pimpinellae 30.0 (pimpinella tincture)
D.S.
Take 10–30 drops 4 × a day.

Thyme Herb

This remedy is also very well suited for spasmodic cough and whooping cough in **children**.
For children, prescribing a finished pharmaceutical product is preferable.

Preparations

- Tea
- Tincture

Proven Prescriptions

- Tea
  Add 1 cup of hot water to 2 teaspoons of the finely chopped drug. Steep covered for 5 minutes, then strain.
  Drink 1 cup several times a day.
- **Thyme Tincture (Tinctura Thymi) (1:10)**
  Take 5–10 drops in a small amount of water or place on a sugar cube and allow to dissolve in month several times a day.

Roundleaf Sundew Herb

This remedy is also very well suited for **spasmodic cough** and **whooping cough** in **children**.
For children, prescribing a finished pharmaceutical product is preferable.

Preparations

- Fluid Extract
- Tincture

Proven Prescriptions

- Fluid Extract

Prescriptions

Rx
Extr. Droserae fluid. 5.0 (roundleaf sundew fluid extract)
Tinct. Pimpinellae 15.0 (pimpinella tincture)
D.S.
Take 5–20 drops 3 × a day.

- **Tinctura Droserae (1:10)**
  Adults: take 10 drops in a small amount of water several times a day. The dosage for children is lower: 5 drops 2 × a day.

Ivy Leaves

This remedy is also very well suited for **spasmodic cough** and **whooping cough** in **children.**

For children, prescribing a finished pharmaceutical product is preferable.

Preparation

- Tea

Proven Prescription

- Tea
  Add 1 cup of hot water to ½ teaspoon of the finely chopped drug. Steep for 10–15 minutes, then strain.
  Drink 1 cup up to 3 × a day, sweetened with honey.

African Geranium (Pelargonium sidoides DC)

Prescribe finished pharmaceutical products.

Combination of Nasturtium Herb and Horseradish Root

Prescribe finished pharmaceutical products.

Proven Cough Teas

Prescriptions

For Acute Throat Irritation (Urge to Cough, Acute Tracheobronchitis)
Rx
Verbasci flor. (mullein flowers)
Farfarae fol. (coltsfoot leaves)
Althaeae rad. (marshmallow root)
Anisi fruct. āā ad 100.0 (anise seeds)
M. f. spec.
Add 1 cup of boiling water to 2 teaspoons of the blend. Steep for 20 minutes, then strain.
D.S.
Drink 1 cup hot several times a day, optionally sweetened with honey.

Prescriptions

Stimulation of Expectoration With Subacute or Chronic Bronchitis
Rx
Primulae rad. (cowslip primrose root)
Thymi herb. (thyme herb)
Plantagin. herb. lanc. āā ad 100.0 (narrowleaf plantain herb)
M. f. spec.
Add 1 cup of boiling water to 1 heaping teaspoon of the blend. Steep for 20 minutes, then strain.
D.S.
Drink 3 cups a day.

Prescriptions

For Chronic, Recurring Bronchitis With Poor General Health
Rx
Helenii rad. (elecampane root)
Island. Lichen (Iceland Moss)
Farfarae fol. (coltsfoot leaves)
Pulmonariae herb. āā ad 100.0 (lungwort herb)
M. f. spec.
Add 1 cup of hot water to 1 teaspoon of the blend. Boil for 15 minutes, then strain.
D.S.
Drink 3 cups a day.

Prescriptions

For Spasmodic Cough, Whooping Cough, and Chronic Obstructive Pulmonary Disease (COPD)
Rx
Thymi herb. (thyme herb)
Droserae herb. (roundleaf sundew herb)
Eryngii herb. plan. (blue eryngo herb)
Anisi fruct. āā ad 100.0 (anise seeds)
M. f. spec.
Add 1 cup of boiling water to 1 teaspoon of the blend. Steep for 20 minutes, then strain.
D.S.
Drink 1 cup several times a day.

Proven Balms and Ointments

Prescriptions

Balm for Adults and Children 7 Years and Older
Rx
Ol. Thymi (thyme oil)
Ol. Rosmarin. (rosemary oil)
Ol. Eucalypt. āā 2.0 (eucalyptus oil)
Ol. Camphorat. ad 50.0 (camphor oil)
D.S.
Rub into chest and neck.

15.13.2 Rheumatic Disorders

Medicinal Plants

Dandelion, Taraxacum officinale
Stinging Nettle, Urtica dioica/urens
Birch, Betula pendula, Betula pubescens, Betula verrucosa
White kidney bean, Phaseolus vulgaris
Woody nightshade, Solanum dulcamara
Devil's claw, Harpagophytum procumbens
Comfrey, Symphytum officinale
Hay flower, Graminis flos
Calamus, Acorus calamus
St.-John's-wort, Hypericum perforatum

Dandelion Root and Leaves

Preparations

- Tea
- Extract

Proven Prescriptions

- Tea
  Add 1–2 teaspoons of the drug to 1 cup of cold water. Bring to a brief boil, steep for about 10 minutes, then strain.
  Drink 1–2 cups in the morning and evening for several weeks.
- Extract

Prescriptions

Rx
Extr. Taraxaci 30.0 (dandelion extract)
Aqu. Melissae ad 300.0 (lemon balm water)
D.S.
Take 1 tablespoon 3 × a day after meals.

Stinging Nettle Herb and Leaves

Preparations

- Tea
- Pressed Juice

Proven Prescription

- Tea
  Add 1 cup of hot water to 2 teaspoons of cut stinging nettle leaves and/or herb. Steep for 10 minutes, then strain.
  Drink 1 cup several times a day up to a total of 1 L a day.

Birch Leaves

Preparation

- Tea

Proven Prescription

- Tea
  Add 1 cup of hot water to 2 tablespoons of the drug, chopped medium fine. Steep for 10 minutes, then strain.
  Drink 1 cup warm several times a day, up to a total of 1 L a day.

Kidney Bean Pods

Preparation

- Tea

Proven Prescription

- **Tea**
  Add 1 cup of boiling water to 1 tablespoon of the drug. Steep covered for about 10 minutes, then strain.
  Drink 1 cup of freshly prepared tea several times a day between meals.

Woody Nightshade Stems

Preparations

- Tea
- Extract

Proven Prescriptions

- **Tea**
  Add 1–2 teaspoons of the drug to 1 cup of water. Bring to a brief boil, steep for 5 minutes, then strain.
  Drink 1 cup in the morning and evening for a longer period of time.
- Extract

Prescriptions

Rx
Extr. Dulcamarae 5.0 (woody nightshade extract)
Syrup. Juniperi ad 150.0 (juniper berry syrup)
D.S.
Take 1 teaspoon 3 × a day

Devil's Claw Root

Finished pharmaceutical products should be given preference.

Preparation

- Tea

Proven Prescription

- **Tea**
  Add 2 cups of boiling water to 1 tablespoon of the finely cut or coarse powdered drug. Soak at room temperature for 8 hours, then strain.
  Drink warm in 3 portions shortly before meals.

Hay Flower

Preparations

- Poultice
- Bath

Proven Prescriptions

- **Compress:** To prepare a "hay sack," fill a flat linen bag with dry hay flowers, place it in a pot, and pour enough boiling water over the hay sack to moisten it. Steep covered for 10 minutes, squeeze out the excess liquid, and place the sack on the body region to be treated. The hay sack should be applied as hot and as snugly as possible. Cover with a wool or flannel cloth and keep in place for 40–50 minutes.
  Apply 1–2 × a day. The hay sack can be reused multiple times.
- **Bath:** Add boiling water to 500 g hay flower. Steep for 10 minutes, then strain, and add the liquid to the bath.

Comfrey Root

Prescribe finished pharmaceutical products.

Calamus Rootstock

Preparation

- Essential Oil

Proven Prescription

- **Combination** with Angelica Root

Prescriptions

Rx
Ol. Calami 2.0 (calamus oil)
Spirit. Angelicae comp. ad 100.0 (angelica spirit composite)
D.S.
Inunction

St.-John's-wort

Preparation

- Essential Oil

Proven Prescription

- Essential Oil

Additional Proven Prescriptions

- Tea Blends

Prescriptions

Rx
Urticae herb. (stinging nettle herb)
Dulcamar. stipit. (woody nightshade stems)
Caricis rhiz. (sand sedge rhizome)
Sennae fol. (senna leaves)
Foenicul. fruct. āā 20.0 (fennel seeds)
M. f. spec.
Add 2 teaspoons of the blend to 1 cup of water and bring to a boil. Steep for 10 minutes, then strain.
D.S.
Drink 1 cup warm 2–3 × a day.

Prescriptions

Rx
Taraxaci rad. c. herb. (dandelion root and herb)
Juniperi fruct. (juniper berries)
Sennae fol. (senna leaves)
Frangul. cort. (buckthorn bark)
Carvi fruct. āā 20.0 (caraway seeds)
M. f. spec.
Add 2 teaspoons of the blend to 1 cup of water and bring to a boil. Steep for 10 minutes, then strain.
D.S.
Drink 1 cup warm 2–3 × a day.

- **Strong Laxative Tea for Antidyscratic Impact Therapy ("Stoss Therapy")**

Prescriptions

Rx
Sennae fol. (senna leaves)
Taraxaci rad. c. herb. āā 40.0 (dandelion root and herb)
Menth. pip. fol. (peppermint leaves)
Foenicul. fruct. āā 20.0 (fennel seeds)
M. f. spec.
Add 500 mL of boiling water to 1–2 tablespoons of the blend. Steep for 15 minutes, then strain.
D.S.
Drink 250 mL in the morning and in the evening (500 mL a day).

Prescriptions

Rx
Extr. Gramin. (hay flower extract)
Extr. Taraxaci (dandelion extract)
Extr. Frangulae fluid. āā 10.0 (buckthorn bark fluid extract)
Aqu. Foeniculi (fennel water)
Aqu. Petroselini āā ad 150.0 (parsley water)
D.S.
Take 1 tablespoon 2–3 × a day.

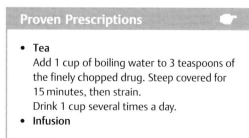

Proven Analgesic Combination Remedy ☞

- **Phytodolor Tincture** (with quaking aspen bark and leaves, goldenrod herb, and ash tree bark)
  D.S.
  Take 20–30 drops (40 drops for strong pain) 3–4 × a day.

15.14 S

15.14.1 Sleep Disorders

See Section 15.11.1 Nervous Restlessness (p. 391).

15.15 U

15.15.1 Ulcer, Venous

Medicinal Plants 📰

Comfrey, Symphytum officinale
Calendula, Calendula officinalis

Comfrey Root, Herb and Leaves

Prescribe finished pharmaceutical products.

Calendula Flowers

Indicated in the early stages of treating secondary infections.
  Prescribe finished pharmaceutical products.

15.15.2 Urinary Tract Infections

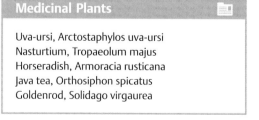

Medicinal Plants 📰

Uva-ursi, Arctostaphylos uva-ursi
Nasturtium, Tropaeolum majus
Horseradish, Armoracia rusticana
Java tea, Orthosiphon spicatus
Goldenrod, Solidago virgaurea

Uva-ursi Leaves

Preparation ☞

- Tea

Proven Prescriptions ☞

- **Maceration**
  Add 2 teaspoons of the drug to 1 cup of cold water. Steep for several hours, heat briefly, then strain.
- **Infusion**
  Add 1 cup of hot water to 2 teaspoons of the drug. Steep for 5 minutes, then strain. Drink 1 cup of either preparation several times a day.

Nasturtium Herb

Prescribe finished pharmaceutical products.

Horseradish Root

Prescribe finished pharmaceutical products.

Java Tea Leaves

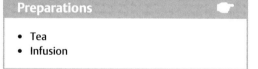

Preparations ☞

- Tea
- Infusion

Proven Prescriptions ☞

- **Tea**
  Add 1 cup of boiling water to 3 teaspoons of the finely chopped drug. Steep covered for 15 minutes, then strain. Drink 1 cup several times a day.
- **Infusion**

15.16 V

15.16.1 Vascular Disorders, Peripheral and Cerebral

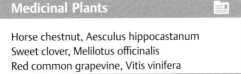

Medicinal Plants 📄

Garlic, Allium sativum
Ginkgo, Ginkgo biloba

Goldenrod Herb

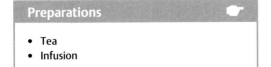

Preparations 👉

- Tea
- Infusion

Garlic Bulb

Prescribe finished pharmaceutical products.

Ginkgo Leaves

Prescribe finished pharmaceutical products.

15.16.2 Venous Disorders

Medicinal Plants 📄

Horse chestnut, Aesculus hippocastanum
Sweet clover, Melilotus officinalis
Red common grapevine, Vitis vinifera

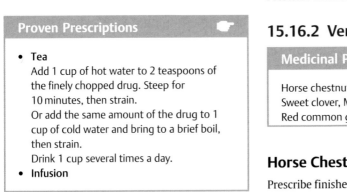

Proven Prescriptions 👉

- Tea
  Add 1 cup of hot water to 2 teaspoons of
  the finely chopped drug. Steep for
  10 minutes, then strain.
  Or add the same amount of the drug to 1
  cup of cold water and bring to a brief boil,
  then strain.
  Drink 1 cup several times a day.
- Infusion

Horse Chestnut Seeds

Prescribe finished pharmaceutical products.

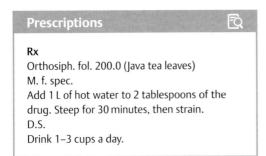

Sweet Clover Herb

- Tea
- Cataplasm

- Tea
  Add 1 cup of simmering water to
  1–2 teaspoons of the finely chopped drug.
  Steep for 10 minutes, then strain.
  Drink 1 cup 2–3 × a day.
- Cataplasm
  Moisten the drug well with an equal amount
  of simmering water. Allow to cool and use
  externally.

Red Common Grapevine Leaves

Prescribe finished pharmaceutical products.

15.17 W

15.17.1 Wounds

Medicinal Plants

Arnica, Arnica montana
German chamomile, Matricaria recutita
Purple Echinacea, Echinacea purpurea
Calendula, Calendula officinalis
Witch hazel, Hamamelis virginiana

Arnica Flowers

Finished pharmaceutical products should be given
preference.

German Chamomile Flowers

Finished pharmaceutical products should be given
preference.

Echinacea

Finished pharmaceutical products should be given
preference.

Calendula Flowers

Finished pharmaceutical products should be given
preference.

Witch Hazel Leaves

Finished pharmaceutical products should be given
preference.

16 An A to Z of Medicinal Plants

The designation of "positive" or "negative" in the column "Monograph" always refers to the Commission E monographs.

ESCOP = European Scientific Cooperative on Phytotherapy

HMPC = Herbal Medicine Products Commission of the European Union

WHO = World Health Organization

Table 16.1

Botanical Name	English Name	Drug	Indication(s)	Monograph
Abies alba	Fir	Fir Essential Oil (Abieti aetherolum)	Vasomotor headaches, neuralgia (balneology)	None
Achillea millefolium	Yarrow	Yarrow herb, flowers	Lack of appetite, dyspeptic symptoms, mild spastic gastrointestinal symptoms, pelvic congestion	Positive; HMPC
Aconitum napellus	Monkshood	Monkshood root tubers (Aconiti tubera)	Neuralgia, for example, trigeminal neuralgia	Negative
Acorus calamus	Calamus	Calamus rootstock	Lack of appetite	Positive
Adonis vernalis	Pheasant's Eye	Pheasant's Eye herb	Nervous restlessness, heart conditions, hypotonic dysregulation	Positive
Aesculus hippocastanum	Horse Chestnut	Horse Chestnut seeds	Chronic venous insufficiency with pain and feeling of heaviness in the legs, nocturnal cramping of the calves (charley horse), itching or swelling of the legs	Positive; ESCOP, HMPC
Alchemilla vulgaris/ xanthochlora	Lady's Mantle	Lady's Mantle herb	Diuretic, spasmolytic, for nonspecific diarrhea	Positive
Aletris farinosa	True Unicorn Root	True unicorn root tubers	Pelvic floor weakness, genital prolapse (especially in older women), back pain due to symptoms of ptosis	None
Allium cepa	Onion	Onion	Lack of appetite, prevention of age-related vascular changes	Positive; HMPC, WHO
Allium sativum	Garlic	Garlic bulb	Lowering of blood lipids, prevention of age-related vascular changes	Positive; HMPC monograph draft
Aloe vera	Aloe Vera	Aloe Vera leaf juice	Constipation, facilitating defecation with anal fissures, hemorrhoids, and after anorectal procedures	Positive; ESCOP, HMPC, WHO

(Continued)

Table 16.1 (*Continued*)

Botanical Name	English Name	Drug	Indication(s)	Monograph
Alpinia officinarum	Galangal	Galangal rootstock	Dyspeptic symptoms, lack of appetite, spastic abdominal pain, Roemheld complex	Positive
Althaea officinalis	Marshmallow	Marshmallow root, leaves	Mucous membrane irritation in the mouth and pharynx, dry irritating cough	Positive; HMPC
Althaea rosea	Hollyhock	Hollyhock flowers	Dry cough	Positive
Ammi visnaga	Bishop's Weed	Bishop's weed seeds	Mild stenocardia symptoms, support for mild types of obstructive respiratory tract disorders (spastic, asthmatic bronchial disorders)	Negative
Ananas comosus	Pineapple	Raw bromelain	Digestive disorders due to pancreas diseases, traumatic edema	Positive
Angelica archangelica	Angelica	Angelica root	Lack of appetite, dyspeptic symptoms, mild gastrointestinal cramps, bloating, flatulence	Positive
Anthemis nobilis (Chamaemelum nobile)	Roman Chamomile	Roman chamomile flowers (Anthemis flos, Chamomillae romanae flos)	Acute gastritis	None
Anthoxanthum odoratum	Sweet Vernal Grass	Hay flower (Graminis flos)	Rheumatic disorders, lumbago, stimulates circulation (balneology, external use)	Positive
Arctium lappa (Lappa major)	Greater Burdock	Burdock rootstock	Diuretic, diaphoretic	Negative; HMPC
Arctium tomentosum	Woolly Burdock			
Arctostaphylos uva-ursi	Uva-ursi	Uva-ursi leaves	Inflammation of efferent urinary tract	Positive; ESCOP, HMPC assessment report
Armoracia rusticana	Horseradish	Horseradish root	Upper respiratory catarrh, support for efferent urinary tract infections	Positive
Arnica montana	Arnica	Arnica flowers	For external application with injuries, hematomas, distortions, bruises, contusions, fracture edemas, rheumatic muscle and joint symptoms, inflammation of	Positive; ESCOP, HMPC

(Continued)

Table 16.1 (*Continued*)

Botanical Name	English Name	Drug	Indication(s)	Monograph
			the mouth and pharyngeal mucous membranes, furunculosis, superficial phlebitis	
Artemisia absinthium	Wormwood	Wormwood herb	Lack of appetite, dyspeptic symptoms, biliary tract dyskinesia	Positive; ESCOP; HMPC
Atropa belladonna	Belladonna	Belladonna leaves, root	Spasms and colic-type pain in the gastrointestinal tract, biliary tract, and urinary tract	Positive
Avena sativa	Oat	Oat straw	External application: inflammatory and seborrheic skin disorders, especially with itching	Negative; HMPC
Berberis vulgaris	Barberry	Barberry root bark, berries	External eye symptoms	Negative; WHO
Beta vulgaris	Beet	Betaine	Hepatopathy	None
Betula pendula/ verrucosa	Birch	Birch leaves	Flushing therapy with bacterial and inflammatory disorders of the efferent urinary tract and kidney gravel, rheumatic symptoms	Positive; ESCOP, HMPC
Betula pubescens	Downy Birch (Moor Birch)			
Boswellia serrata	Frankincense	Frankincense resin	Adjuvant for chronic polyarthritis, remission treatment of inflammatory flare-ups of ulcerative colitis and Crohn's disease	None
Calendula officinalis	Calendula	Calendula flowers	Inflammatory changes of the mouth and pharyngeal mucous membranes, wound healing, venous leg ulcers (Ulcus cruris)	Positive; ESCOP, HMPC
Capsella bursa pastoris	Shepherd's Purse	Shepherd's purse herb	Mild menorrhagia and metrorrhagia, nose bleeds, superficial bleeding skin injuries	Positive; HMPC
Capsicum anuum	Paprika	Paprika fruit	Rheumatic spectrum disorders	Positive; HMPC
Capsicum frutescens	Cayenne Pepper	Cayenne pepper fruit		
Cardiospermum halicacabum	Balloon Vine	Balloon vine herb	Chronic dermatitis	None
Carduus marianus (see Silybum marianum)				
Carex arenaria	Sand Sedge	Sand sedge rootstock	Dry eczema, rheumatic disorders	None

(Continued)

Table 16.1 (Continued)

Botanical Name	English Name	Drug	Indication(s)	Monograph
Carica papaya	Papaya	Papaya fruit	Digestive disorders due to pancreas insufficiency	Positive
Carum carvi	Caraway	Caraway seeds (fruit)	Dyspeptic symptoms such as mild gastrointestinal spasms, flatulence, bloating (feeling of fullness)	Positive; ESCOP
Cassia acutifolia/ angustifolia (see Senna alexandrina)				
Catha edulis	Khat	Khat leaves (Cathae edulis folium)	Avolition (lack of motivation)	None
Centaurium minus/ erythraea	Centaury	Centaury herb	Lack of appetite, dyspeptic symptoms	Positive; ESCOP, HMPC
Cephaelis ipecacuanha	Ipecac	Ipecac root	Expectorant	Negative
Cetraria islandica	Iceland Moss	Iceland moss	Mucous membrane irritations of the mouth and pharynx, dry irritating cough, lack of appetite	Positive; ESCOP, HMPC
Chelidonium majus	Celandine	Celandine herb	Biliary and gastrointestinal spasms	Positive; HMPC assessment report
Chondrus crispus	Irish Moss	Carrageen (Fucus irlandicus)	Acute and chronic respiratory tract inflammation, cough-calming remedy	None
Cimicifuga racemosa (Actaea racemosa)	Black Cohosh	Black cohosh rootstock	Premenstrual, neurovegetative premenstrual, dysmenorrhea, and menopause symptoms	Positive; HMPC
Cinchona pubescens/ succirubra	Cinchona	Cinchona bark	Lack of appetite, dyspeptic symptoms such as flatulence, bloating (feeling of fullness)	Positive
Cinnamomum camphora	Camphor	Camphor	Hypotonic circulatory system dysregulation, respiratory catarrh External use for muscular arthritis (myositis)	Positive
Citrus aurantium	Bitter Orange	Bitter orange peel	Lack of appetite, dyspeptic symptoms	Positive
Citrus limon	Lemon	Lemon juice	Supportive treatment for colds	None
Claviceps purpurea	Ergot	Ergot (Secale cornutum)	Gynecological and obstetric uterine bleeding	Negative

(Continued)

Table 16.1 (*Continued*)

Botanical Name	English Name	Drug	Indication(s)	Monograph
Cnicus benedictus, syn. Carduus benedictus, syn. Centaurea benedicta)	Blessed Thistle	Blessed thistle herb	Lack of appetite, dyspeptic symptoms	Positive
Cola nitida/ aquinata	Kola Nut	Kola nut (seed)	Psychological and physical exhaustion	Positive; HMPC
Colchicum autumnale	Autumn Crocus	Autumn crocus flowers, seeds, root tubers	Acute gout attacks	Positive
Convallaria majalis	Lily-of-the-Valley	Lily-of-the-valley herb	Aging heart, pulmonary heart disease (Cor pulmonare), mild congestive heart failure (CHF, NYHA I-II)	Positive
Coriandrum sativum	Coriander (cilantro)	Coriander seeds (Coriandri fructus)	Dyspeptic symptoms, lack of appetite, meteorism, Roemheld syndrome, carminative	Positive
Hintonia latiflora, syn. Coutarea latifolia ()	Copalchi	Copalchi bark	Diabetes mellitus	None
Crataegus laevigata	English Hawthorn	Hawthorn flowers, leaves, fruit (berries)	Aging heart, congestive heart failure (CHF) NYHA II (III), chronic pulmonary heart disease (Cor pulmonare)	Positive; ESCOP
Crataegus monogyna	Common Hawthorn			
Crocus sativus	Saffron	Saffron stigma (Croci stigma)	Calming nerves, spasms, asthma	Negative; WHO
Cucurbita pepo	Pumpkin	Pumpkin seeds	Irritable bladder, micturition problems due to benign prostatic hyperplasia (BPH, stages I–II)	Positive; HMPC
Curcuma longa/ domestica	Turmeric	Turmeric rootstock	Dyspeptic symptoms, stimulation of fat digestion	Positive; HMPC, WHO
Cyamopsis tetragonoloba	Guar Gum Bean	Guar Gum (Guaran)	Dietary supplement for overweight diabetics	None
Cynara cardunculus/ scolymus	Artichoke	Artichoke leaves	Dyspeptic symptoms, stimulation of fat digestion, lipid lowering	Positive
Cytisus scoparius	Scotch Broom	Scotch broom flowers, herb	Heart arrhythmia	Negative
Datura stramonium	Jimsonweed	Jimsonweed leaves and jimsonweed seeds	Many types of tremors, e.g., Parkinson's disease	Negative

(Continued)

Table 16.1 (Continued)

Botanical Name	English Name	Drug	Indication(s)	Monograph
Digitalis lanata Digitalis purpurea	Woolly Foxglove Purple Foxglove	Digitalis tincture	Treatment of torpid and chronic wounds of all types, also chronic ulcerations; as digitalis preparation, treatment of heart disorders	None
Drimia maritima	Squill (Sea Onion)	Squill bulb	Milder types of chronic heart failure, also for impaired kidney function	Positive
Drosera rotundifolia	Roundleaf Sundew	Roundleaf sundew herb	Spasmodic and irritable cough	Positive
Echinacea angustifolia	Echinacea Angustifolia, Narrow-Leafed Echinacea	Echinacea root	Colds, immune system support, inflammatory and purulent trauma, abscesses, boils, venous leg ulcers (Ulcus cruris)	Positive; ESCOP, HMPC, WHO
Echinacea pallida	Echinacea pallida, Pale-flowered Echinacea			
Echinacea purpurea	Purple Echinacea			
Eleutherococcus senticosus	Eleuthero	Eleuthero root	Fatigue, weakness, decreased stamina and ability to concentrate, during convalescence	Positive; HMPC
Elymus repens	Couch Grass	Couch grass rootstock	Flushing therapy for inflammatory disorders of the efferent urinary tract	Positive; HMPC
Ephedra sinica/shennungiana	Ephedra	Ephedra herb	Respiratory tract disorders with mild bronchial spasms	Positive; WHO
Chamaenerion angustifolium (Epilobium angustifolium)	Fireweed	Fireweed root and herb (Epilobii radix et herba)	Benign prostatic hyperplasia (BPH)	HMPC draft monograph
Equisetum arvense	Horsetail (Common)	Horsetail herb	Posttraumatic and static edema, flushing therapy with bacterial and inflammatory disorders of the efferent urinary tract and kidney gravel, poorly healing wounds	Positive; HMPC
Erodium cicutarium	Common Storksbill	Common storksbill herb	Uterine bleeding	None
Eryngium planum	Blue Eryngo	Blue eryngo herb	Folk remedy for whooping cough	None

(Continued)

Table 16.1 (Continued)

Botanical Name	English Name	Drug	Indication(s)	Monograph
Eschscholtzia californica	California Poppy	California poppy herb	Restlessness, sleep disorders, bed-wetting	Negative; HMPC
Eucalyptus globulus	Eucalyptus	Eucalyptus leaves	Colds	Positive; ESCOP, HMPC
Eupatorium perfoliatum	Boneset	Boneset herb	Colds	None
Euphorbia cyparissias	Cypress Spurge Sap (Wolf's Milk)	Cypress spurge sap	Chronic eczema, warts	None
Euphrasia officinalis	Eyebright	Eyebright herb (Euphrasiae herba)	Conjunctivitis, blepharitis, fresh eye injuries	HMPC assessment report
Fagopyrum esculentum	Buckwheat	Buckwheat herb (Fagopyri herba)	Venous system disorders	None
Fagus sylvatica	Beech	Beech tar	Dry, chronic eczema	None
Ferula assa-foetida	Asafetida	Asafetida resin (Ferulae resina)	Anxiety, restlessness	None
Filipendula ulmaria	Meadowsweet	Meadowsweet herb, flowers (also known as Spireae)	Supportive treatment for colds	Positive; HMPC
Foeniculum vulgare	Fennel	Fennel seeds (fruit)	Dyspeptic symptoms such as mild gastrointestinal spasms, bloating, flatulence, respiratory tract catarrh	Positive; ESCOP, HMPC
Frangula purshiana (Rhamnus purshiana)	Cascara sagrada	Cascara sagrada bark	Constipation, facilitating defecation with anal fissures, hemorrhoids, and after anorectal procedures	Positive; ESCOP, HMPC
Fraxinus excelsior	Common Ash	Ash bark	Analgesic, rheumatic disorders (as a component of the combination remedy Phytodolor)	HMPC
Fumaria officinalis	Fumitory	Fumitory herb	Gallbladder, biliary tract, and gastrointestinal spasms	Positive; HMPC assessment report
Galega officinalis	Goat's Rue	Goat's rue herb (Galegae herba)	Diabetes mellitus	Negative
Galeopsis ochroleuca	Hempnettle	Hempnettle herb (Galeopsidis herba)	Respiratory tract catarrh, lung tuberculosis (as a component of Kobert's Lung Tea)	Positive
Gelsemium sempervirens	Yellow Jessamine	Yellow Jessamine rootstock	Functional heart disorders	Negative

(Continued)

Table 16.1 (Continued)

Botanical Name	English Name	Drug	Indication(s)	Monograph
Gentiana lutea	Gentian	Gentian root	Digestive disorders such as lack of appetite, bloating, flatulence	Positive; ESCOP, HMPC
Geum urbanum	Avens	Avens root (Radix Caryophyllatae)	Anxiety	None
Ginkgo biloba	Ginkgo	Ginkgo leaves	Arterial peripheral circulation disorders, brain disorders, concentration and memory problems	Positive; HMPC, WHO
Glycyrrhiza glabra	Licorice	Licorice root	Ventricular/duodenal ulcers, respiratory tract catarrh	Positive; HMPC, WHO
Gratiola officinalis	Hedge Hyssop	Hedge hyssop herb	Emmenagogue	None
Hamamelis virginiana	Witch Hazel (Common, American)	Witch hazel leaves	Hemorrhoids, varicose vein symptoms, minor skin injuries, localized skin, and mucous membrane inflammation	Positive; ESCOP, HMPC
Harpagophytum procumbens	Devil's Claw	Devil's claw root	Lack of appetite, dyspeptic symptoms, supportive with generative locomotor system disorders	Positive; ESCOP; HMPC
Harungana madagascariensis	Haronga	Haronga leaves, bark	Dyspeptic symptoms, mild exocrine pancreas insufficiency	Positive
Hedera helix	Ivy	Ivy leaves	Upper respiratory tract catarrh, chronic inflammatory bronchial disorders	Positive; HMPC
Helianthus tuberosus	Jerusalem Artichoke	Jerusalem artichoke juice	Substitute for artificial sweeteners for diabetics	None
Helichrysum arenarium	Sandy Everlasting	Sandy everlasting flowers (Stoechados citrinae flos, Helichrysi flos)	Dyspeptic symptoms, diuretic, choleretic, hepatoprotective	Positive, WHO
Helleborus niger	Black Hellebore	Black Hellebore rootstock (Hellebori rhizoma)	Avolition	None
Herniaria glabra and Herniaria hirsuta	Rupturewort	Rupturewort herb	Flushing therapy, mild efferent urinary tract spasms	Negative
Hippophae rhamnoides	Sea Buckthorn	Sea buckthorn fruit (berries)	Supportive treatment for colds	None

(Continued)

Table 16.1 (Continued)

Botanical Name	English Name	Drug	Indication(s)	Monograph
Humulus lupulus	Hops	Hops strobiles	Sleep disorders, restlessness and anxiety	Positive; ESCOP; HMPC
Hypoxis rooperi	South African Star Grass	South African Star Grassroot (Hypoxis rooperi radix)	Benign prostatic hyperplasia (BPH)	None
Hyoscyamus niger	Henbane	Henbane leaves	Gastrointestinal spasms	Positive
Hypericum perforatum	St.-John's-wort	St.-John's-wort herb	Depressive mood disorders, fear, nervous restlessness, external use for trauma and myalgia	Positive; ESCOP, HMPC
Iberis amara	Bitter Candytuft	Bitter candytuft seeds, herb (Iberidis semen, Iberidis herba)	Bitter, functional dyspepsia, irritable colon (as a component of Iberogast Liquid)	None
Ilex paraguariensis	Yerba Mate	Yerba mate leaves	Psychological and physical exhaustion	Positive; HMPC
Illicum verum	Star Anise	Star anise fruit	Respiratory tract catarrh, dyspeptic symptoms	Positive
Iris florentina	Orris root	Orris root (Iris × germanica [Iridaceae])	Analgesic for teething children	Negative
Inula helenium	Elecampane	Elecampane root	Chronic cough, protracted bronchial catarrh, chronic obstructive pulmonary disease (COPD)	Negative
Jacobaea maritima (Cineraria maritima, Senecio cineraria)	Silver Ragwort	Cineraria mother tincture (plant juice)	Conjunctivitis, early stages of cataracts, asthenopia	None
Juglans regia	English Walnut	English walnut leaves	Superficial skin inflammation, excessive perspiration	Positive; HMPC
Juniperus communis	Juniper	Juniper berries	Dyspeptic symptoms, inflammation of the efferent urinary tract	Positive; ESCOP, HMPC
Lamium album	White Dead Nettle	White dead nettle flowers	Inflammation of the mouth and pharynx, nonspecific leucorrhea (Fluor albus), respiratory tract catarrh	Positive
Larix decidua	European Larch	European larch resin (Terebinthina Laricina)	Rheumatic and neuralgia symptoms, respiratory tract catarrh, boils	Positive

(Continued)

Table 16.1 (*Continued*)

Botanical Name	English Name	Drug	Indication(s)	Monograph
Lavandula angustifolia	Lavender	Lavender flowers	Problems falling asleep, restlessness, circulatory system disorders	Positive; HMPC
Leonurus cardiaca	Motherwort	Motherwort herb	Nervous heart symptoms, hyperthyroidism	Positive
Levisticum officinale	Lovage	Lovage root	Flushing therapy for nonspecific inflammation of the efferent urinary tract, kidney gravel	Positive; HMPC
Linum usitatissimum	Flax	Flax seeds	Habitual constipation, irritable colon, diverticulitis, as a cataplasm for localized inflammation	Positive; ESCOP, HMPC
Lithospermum officinale	European Stoneseed	European stoneseed seeds (Lithospermi semen, Semen Millii solis), leaves (Lithospermi folium)	Gallstones and urinary calculi, gout, antigonadotropic and antithyreotropic effect	None
Lycopus europaeus	Bugleweed (European)	Bugleweed herb	Mild hyperthyroidism, mastodynia	Positive
Lycopus virginicus	Bugleweed (American)			
Malva neglecta	Common Mallow (Cheeseweed)	Common mallow leaves, flowers	Exudative dermatitis	None
Malva sylvestris	Mallow	Mallow flowers, leaves	Mucous membrane irritations of the mouth and pharynx, dry, irritating cough	Positive
Marsdenia condurango	Condurango	Condurango bark	Lack of appetite	Positive
Matricaria matricarioides	Pineapple Weed	Chamomile flowers	Gastrointestinal spasms and inflammation; skin, gum, and mucous membrane inflammation	None
Matricaria recutita/ chamomilla	German Chamomile			Positive; ESCOP, WHO
Melilotus officinalis	Sweet Clover	Sweet clover herb	Chronic venous insufficiency symptoms such as leg pain and heaviness, nocturnal systremma (charley horse), itching, swelling, thrombophlebitis	Positive; ESCOP, HMPC
Melissa officinalis	Lemon Balm	Lemon balm leaves	Functional gastrointestinal symptoms, nervous sleep disorders (problems falling asleep)	Positive; ESCOP, HMPC

(Continued)

Table 16.1 (*Continued*)

Botanical Name	English Name	Drug	Indication(s)	Monograph
Mentha arvensis var. piperascens	Japanese Mint	Japanese mint essential oil (Menthae arvensis aetheroleum)	Internal use: meteorism, functional gastrointestinal and gallbladder symptoms, upper respiratory tract catarrh; External use: myalgia and neuralgia symptoms, upper respiratory tract catarrh	Positive
Mentha crispa	Spearmint	Spearmint leaves	Gastrointestinal, gallbladder and biliary tract spasms, tension headache, irritable colon	None
Mentha piperita	Peppermint	Peppermint leaves, oil		Positive; ESCOP, HMPC
Mentha pulegium	European Pennyroyal	European pennyroyal essential oil (Menthae pulegii aetheroleum)	Cultivated for menthol production	None
Mentha sylvestris (Mentha longifolia)	Horsemint	Horsemint herb (Herba Menthae sylvestris)	Colds (balneology)	None
Menyanthes trifoliata	Bogbean	Bogbean leaves	Lack of appetite, dyspeptic symptoms	Positive
Myroxylon balsamum	Peruvian Balsam	Peruvian balsam (Balsamum peruvianum)	Contusions, hematoma, sprains, prosthesis pressure points (external use)	Positive; HMPC draft monograph
Nelumbo nucifera	Lotus	Lotus seeds (Nelumbinis semen), leaves (Nelumbinis folium)	Tranquilizer, antiemetic	None
Nymphaea alba	European White Water Lily	European white water lily flowers (Nymphaeae albae flos)	Tranquilizer, antiemetic	None
Nymphaea lotus	White Egyptian Lotus	White Egyptian lotus leaves (Nymphaeae folium)	Tranquilizer, antiemetic	None
Oenothera biennis	Evening Primrose	Evening primrose oil	Atopic eczema	None; HMPC
Olea europaea	Olive	Olive leaves	Mild blood pressure-lowering effect	Negative; HMPC
Ononis spinosa	Spiny Restharrow	Spiny restharrow root	Flushing therapy for inflammatory efferent urinary tract disorders and kidney gravel	Positive; ESCOP, HMPC

(Continued)

Table 16.1 (*Continued*)

Botanical Name	English Name	Drug	Indication(s)	Monograph
Orthosiphon spicatus/stamineus/aristatus	Java Tea	Java tea leaves	Flushing therapy for inflammatory efferent urinary tract disorders and kidney gravel	Positive; ESCOP, HMPC
Panax ginseng	Ginseng	Ginseng root	Fatigue and weakness, declining performance and ability to concentrate	Positive; HMPC, WHO
Papaver somniferum	Poppy (Opium)	Opium tincture	Severe, acute diarrhea with painful spasms	None
Passiflora incarnata	Passionflower	Passionflower herb	Nervous restlessness (anxiety)	Positive; ESCOP; HMPC
Pelargonium sidoides DC.	African Geranium	African geranium root	Acute or acute exacerbating chronic bronchitis, sinusitis and nonpyogenic tonsillitis	None; HMPC
Petasites hybridus	Butterbur	Butterbur rootstock	Supportive for acute spastic pain of the efferent urinary tract, especially urolithiasis	Positive
Petroselinum crispum	Parsley	Parsley herb, root	Flushing therapy with efferent urinary tract disorders and with kidney gravel	Positive
Peumus boldus	Boldo	Boldo leaves	Mild spastic gastrointestinal symptoms, dyspeptic symptoms	Positive; ESCOP, HMPC
Phaseolus vulgaris	Kidney Bean (white)	Kidney bean pods	Supportive treatment for dysuria symptoms	Positive; HMPC
Picea abies	Spruce (Norway)	Spruce needle oil, Spruce bark oil	Rheumatic disorders, neuralgia, vasomotor headache	Positive
Pilocarpus pennatifolius	Jaborandi	Jaborandi leaves	Diaphoretic with colds	None
Pimpinella anisum	Anise	Anise fruit (seeds)	Respiratory tract catarrh, dyspeptic symptoms	Positive; ESCOP, HMPC
Pimpinella saxifraga/magna/nigra	Pimpinella	Pimpinella root	Respiratory tract catarrh	Positive
Pinguicula vulgaris	Common Butterwort	Common butterwort herb (Pinguiculae herba)	Spasmolytic for whooping cough	None
Pinus sylvestris	Pine (Scots)	Pine needle tar, wood tar	Dry chronic eczema	Positive
Piper methysticum	Kava	Kava rootstock	Nervous anxiety, tension, and restlessness	Positive

(Continued)

Table 16.1 (Continued)

Botanical Name	English Name	Drug	Indication(s)	Monograph
Plantago lanceolata	Narrowleaf Plantain	Narrowleaf plantain herb	Respiratory tract catarrh, mucous membrane inflammation of the mouth and pharynx	Positive; HMPC
Plantago ovata	Psyllium Seed (blond)	Psyllium seed husks	Habitual constipation, irritable colon, supportive for diarrhea	Positive; ESCOP, HMPC
Plantago psyllium	Psyllium Seed (black)	Psyllium seed	Habitual constipation, irritable colon	Positive; ESCOP, WHO
Podophyllum peltatum	Mayapple	Mayapple rootstock, resin	External use for removal of condyloma acuminatum (pointed genital warts)	Positive
Polygonum aviculare	Knotweed	Knotweed herb (Polygoni avicularis herba)	Mouth and pharynx inflammation, respiratory tract catarrh, lung tuberculosis (as a component in Kobert's Lung Tea)	Positive, WHO
Polygonum hydropiper	Water Pepper	Water pepper herb (Polygoni hydropiperis herba)	Hemorrhoids, uterine bleeding	None
Populus tremula	Quaking Aspen	Quaking aspen buds	Superficial skin injuries, hemorrhoids, chilblains, sunburn	Positive
Potentilla anserina	Potentilla	Potentilla herb	Mild mucous membrane inflammation of the mouth, supportive nonspecific diarrhea, mild dysmenorrhea symptoms	Positive
Potentilla aurea	Golden Cinquefoil	Golden cinquefoil herb (Potentillae aureae herba)	Diabetes mellitus	None
Poterium spinosum	Sarcopoterium (Prickly Burnet)	Sarcopoterium root (Poterii radix)	Diabetes mellitus	None
Potentilla tormentilla/erecta	Tormentil (Bloodroot)	Tormentil rootstock	Mild, nonspecific acute diarrhea, mild mucous membrane inflammation of the mouth and pharynx	Positive; HMPC assessment report
Primula elatior	Oxlip Primrose	Primrose flower, root	Respiratory tract catarrh	Positive; ESCOP, HMPC
Primula veris	Cowslip Primrose			
Pulsatilla vulgaris (Pulsatilla pratensis)	Pasque Flower	Pasque flower herb	Internal use for irititis, scleritis, retina disorders, cataracts and glaucoma	Negative

(Continued)

Table 16.1 (*Continued*)

Botanical Name	English Name	Drug	Indication(s)	Monograph
Quercus petraea Quercus robur	Sessile Oak Common Oak	Oak bark	Inflammatory skin disorders, mild inflammation of the mouth and pharynx as well as genital and anal areas	Positive; HMPC
Raphanus sativus	Radish	Radish root	Dyspeptic symptoms, respiratory tract catarrh	Positive
Rauwolfia serpentina	Indian Snakeroot	Indian snakeroot root	Mild essential hypertension with anxiety and tension, psychomotor agitation	Positive; WHO
Rhamnus cathartica	Buckthorn (Common)	Buckthorn berries	Constipation, facilitating defecation with anal fissures, hemorrhoids, and after anorectal procedures	Positive
Rhamnus frangula	Alder Buckthorn	Alder buckthorn bark	Constipation, facilitating defecation with anal fissures, hemorrhoids, and after anorectal procedures	Positive; HMPC
Rheum rhaponticum	Siberian Rhubarb	Sibirian rhubarb root (Rhei rhapontici radix)	Hormone disorders	None
Rheum palmatum/ officinale	Rhubarb	Rhubarb root	Constipation, facilitating defecation with anal fissures, hemorrhoids, and after anorectal procedures	Positive; ESCOP, HMPC, WHO
Rhus aromatica	Fragrant Sumac	Fragrant sumac bark	Enuresis	None
Ribes nigrum	Black Currant	Black currant berries, leaves	Mild, nonspecific diarrhea, colds	None; ESCOP
Ricinus communis	Castor Bean	Castor (bean) oil	Constipation	HMPC draft monograph
Rosa canina	Dog Rose	Dog rosehips	Colds	Negative
Rosmarinus officinalis	Rosemary	Rosemary leaves	Dyspeptic symptoms, hypotonic circulatory weakness (as a bath additive), supportive for rheumatic disorders	Positive; ESCOP, HMPC
Rubus fruticosus	Blackberry	Blackberry leaves	Nonspecific acute diarrhea, mild mucous membrane inflammation of the mouth and pharynx	Positive
Ruscus aculeatus	Butcher's-Broom	Butcher's-broom rootstock	Symptomatical for chronic venous insufficiency, hemorrhoids (itching, burning)	Positive; HMPC
Ruta graveolens	Rue	Rue leaves, herb (Rutae folium, Rutae herba)	Calming, sedative, emmenagogue	Negative

(Continued)

Table 16.1 (Continued)

Botanical Name	English Name	Drug	Indication(s)	Monograph
Salix purpurea/ daphnoides	Willow	Willow bark	Feverish disorders, rheumatic symptoms, headaches	Positive; ESCOP, HMPC
Salvia officinalis	Sage	Sage leaves	Mucous membrane inflammations of the mouth and pharynx, dyspeptic symptoms, increased perspiration	Positive; ESCOP, HMPC
Sambucus nigra	European Elderberry	European elderberry flowers	Colds	Positive; HMPC
Saponaria officinalis	Soapwort	Red soapwort root	Respiratory tract catarrh	Negative
Sarothamnus scoparius (see Cytisus scoparius)				
Smilax aristolochiifolia	Sarsaparilla Root	Sarsaparilla root (Sarsaparillae radix)	Psoriasis	Negative
Scilla maritima (see Drimia maritima)				
Senecio fuchsii	Senecio Herb	Senecio herb (Herba Senecionis fuchsii)	Uterine bleeding	Negative
Senna alexandrina (Cassia acutifolia/ angustifolia)	Senna	Senna leaves, fruit	Constipation	Positive; ESCOP, HMPC, WHO
Serenoa repens (Sabal serrulata)	Saw Palmetto	Saw palmetto fruit	Micturition disorders due to irritable bladder and benign prostatic hyperplasia (stages I–II)	Positive; HMPC draft monograph
Silybum marianum (Carduus marianus)	Milk Thistle	Milk thistle fruit (seeds)	Dyspeptic symptoms, toxic liver disorders; supportive for chronic inflammatory liver disorders, including cirrhosis of the liver	Positive; HMPC draft monograph
Solanum dulcamara	Woody Nightshade	Woody night-shade stems	Supportive treatment of chronic eczema	Positive; HMPC
Solidago canadensis Solidago gigantea (Solidago serotina)	Canadian Goldenrod Giant Goldenrod, Early Goldenrod	Goldenrod herb	Flushing therapy for inflammatory disorders of the efferent urinary tract, urinary calculi, and kidney gravel	Positive; ESCOP
Solidago virgaurea	European Goldenrod			HMPC

(Continued)

Table 16.1 (*Continued*)

Botanical Name	English Name	Drug	Indication(s)	Monograph
Strophanthus kombe/gratus	Strophanthus	Strophantus seeds	Congestive heart failure (cardiac insufficiency)	None
Strychnos nux vomica	Nux Vomica	Nux Vomica seeds	Bitter agent, avolition, tonic for older people, nervous stomach disorders	Negative
Symphytum officinale	Comfrey	Comfrey root, herb, leaves	External use for contusions, strains, sprains	Positive; HMPC
Swertia perennis	Star Gentian	Star gentian root (Radix swertiae)	Chronic gastritis, lack of appetite	None
Tabebuia impetiginosa	Pau d'arco (Lapacho)	Pau d'arco bark (Tabebuiae cortex)	Oncological disorders	None
Taraxacum officinale	Dandelion	Dandelion root, herb	Lack of appetite, dyspeptic symptoms such as bloating and flatulence, bile flow disorders	Positive; ESCOP, HMPC
Thuja occidentalis	Thuja	Thuja branch tips (Thujae summitates)	Colds, warts, oncological disorders	None
Thymus serpyllum	Wild Thyme	Wild thyme herb	External use for irritating cough	None
Thymus vulgaris	Thyme	Thyme herb	Spastic cough due to bronchitis and whooping cough, respiratory tract catarrh	Positive; ESCOP, HMPC, WHO
Tilia cordata	Littleleaf Linden	Linden flowers	Colds	Positive; HMPC
Tilia platyphyllos	Bigleaf Linden			
Triticum aestivum	Wheat	Wheat bran (Furfur tritici)	Atopic or dry eczema	Positive
Tropaeolum majus	Nasturtium	Nasturtium herb	Supportive treatment for urinary tract infections, respiratory tract catarrh	Positive pharmacological properties
Tussilago farfara	Coltsfoot	Coltsfoot leaves	Respiratory tract catarrh with coughing, hoarseness, mild mucous membrane inflammation of the mouth and pharynx	Positive
Urginea maritima see Scilla maritima				
Urtica dioica	Stinging Nettle	Nettle herb, leaves	Supportive for rheumatic symptoms, flushing therapy for inflammatory disorders of the efferent urinary tract, kidney gravel	Positive; ESCOP, HMPC

(Continued)

Table 16.1 (*Continued*)

Botanical Name	English Name	Drug	Indication(s)	Monograph
Urtica urens	Dwarf Nettle	Nettle root	Micturition disorders due to irritable bladder and benign prostatic hyperplasia (stages I–II)	Positive; ESCOP
Usnea barbata	Usnea	Usnea lichen	Mild mucous membrane inflammation of the mouth and pharynx	Positive
Vaccinium macrocarpon	Cranberry	Cranberries (fruit)	Chronic urinary tract infections, oral cavity infections	None
Vaccinium myrtillus	Bilberry (European Blueberry)	Bilberries (fruit)	Nonspecific acute diarrhea, mucous membrane inflammation of the mouth and pharynx	Positive
Valeriana officinalis	Valerian	Valerian root	Restlessness (anxiety), problems falling asleep due to nervous anxiety	Positive; ESCOP, HMPC, WHO
Verbascum densiflorum	Mullein	Mullein flowers	Respiratory tract catarrh	Positive; HMPC
Vinca minor	Periwinkle	Periwinkle herb	Peripheral and cerebral vascular disorders	Negative
Viola odorata	Sweet Violet	Sweet violet root	Mild, nonspecific cough	Positive pharmacological properties
Viola tricolor	Heart's Ease	Heart's ease herb	Mild seborrheic dermatitis, cradle cap in children	Positive; HMPC
Viscum album	Mistletoe	Mistletoe herb	Segmental therapy for inflammatory joint disorders, palliative treatment of malignant tumors	Positive; HMPC assessment report
Vitex agnus castus	Chaste Tree	Chaste tree fruit	Menstrual cycle disorders, premenstrual syndrome (PMS), mastodynia	Positive; HMPC
Vitis vinifera	Common Grape Vine	Red common grape vine leaves	Chronic venous insufficiency with symptoms of leg heaviness, swelling (edema), pain and tension	Positive; HMPC
Xysmalobium undulatum	Uzara	Uzara root	Nonspecific acute diarrhea	Positive
Zingiber officinalis	Ginger	Ginger rootstock	Dyspeptic symptoms, motion sickness	Positive; ESCOP, HMPC, WHO

17 Answer Key

Chapter 3.1, **see** Questions (p. 41)
1. Demulcents
2. Acute, painful inflammation
3. Tannins
4. Lemon balm (Melissa officinalis)

Answers

Chapter 3.2.1, **see** Questions (p. 50)
1. Chamomile, peppermint, lemon balm
2. Antiphlogistic, spasmolytic, carminative
3. See Chamomile Tea Regimen (p. 45)
4. Lamiaceae
5. Spasmolytic
6. Acidosis

Answers

Chapter 3.2.3, **see** Questions (p. 65)
1. Bitter, demulcent
2. Tonic bitter, aromatic bitter, acrid bitter
3. 1:20,000
4. Beta-asaron
5. Ginger, galangal
6. Flax, Iceland moss
7. See Tea for Chronic Gastritis (p. 64)

Answers

Chapter 3.2.4, **see** Questions (p. 71)
1. Licorice
2. Atropine

Answers

Chapter 3.3, **see** Questions (p. 102)
1. Remedy for meteorism
2. Caraway, fennel, anise
3. See "Four Winds Tea (p. 78)"
4. Yes, frankincense and wormwood
5. Tormentil, bilberry
6. Senna, Cascara sagrada/buckthorn, rhubarb
7. See Laxative Tea (p. 95)

Answers

Chapter 3.4, **see** Questions (p. 120)
1. RNA stimulation, stabilization of lipid structures, free radical scavenger, antifibrotic
2. Cynara cardunculus L. ssp. flavescens Wiklund
3. Asteraceae
4. Choleretic, cholekinetic, lipid regulating
5. Refers to a spastic, psychosomatically defined biliary tract syndrome
6. See Cholagogue Teas (p. 116)

Answers

Chapter 3.5, **see** Questions (p. 128)
1. See Functional Dyspepsia (p. 121)
2. See definition of Functional Dyspepsia (p. 121)
3. Turmeric rootstock, artichoke leaves, wormwood herb
4. Nine components
5. Bitter candytuft, Iberis amara

Answers

Chapter 3.6, see Questions (p. 135)
1. No
2. Yes, artichoke and garlic
3. Bugleweed, Lycopus virginicus/europaeus

Answers

Chapter 4, see Questions (p. 180)
1. See Hawthorn (p. 137)
2. Protects heart muscle against free radicals
3. 900–1800 mg
4. No
5. Tincture
6. Yes, lily-of-the-valley, squill, and oleander
7. Garlic, ginkgo
8. Rosemary, camphor

Answers

Chapter 5, see Questions (p. 212)
1. Demulcents, expectorants, antitussives
2. Marshmallow, mallow, coltsfoot
3. Saponins
4. Roundleaf sundew, Drosera rotundifolia
5. See Tea for Acute Urge to Cough (Acute Tracheobronchitis) (p. 199)
6. European elderberry, linden

Answers

Chapter 6, see Questions (p. 233)
1. Plant drugs that promote water diuresis
2. Horseradish, nasturtium, cranberry
3. Pure juniper berry oil
4. Silicic acid
5. See Bladder-Kidney Teas (p. 341)x
6. Pumpkin seeds, saw palmetto fruit, stinging nettle root
7. Fireweed

Answers

Chapter 7, see Questions (p. 250)
1. Plant drugs that promote excretion of substances
2. Dandelion
3. Leaves
4. Devil's claw
5. Willow bark
6. See Antirheumatic Teas (p. 244)
7. Colchicine

Answers

Chapter 8, see Questions (p. 285)
1. Valerian root, hops strobiles, lemon balm leaves, etc.
2. Valerian and hops
3. Passionflower
4. See "Sleep Teas" (p. 261)
5. Not at all
6. Cyclosporine, virostatics for treatment of HIV/AIDS, oral contraceptives
7. Yes, ginseng, kola nut, and yerba mate
8. Ginkgo biloba
9. Peppermint oil

Answers

Chapter 9, see Questions (p. 302)
1. Tannins
2. Evening primrose
3. Comfrey
4. See Foxglove (digitalis) Tincture (p. 300)
5. Calendula

Answers

Chapter 10, see Questions (p. 314)
1. Chaste tree, black cohosh
2. White dead nettle
3. Antispastic
4. Yes

Answers

Chapter 11, see Questions (p. 329)
1. Their comprehensive therapeutic range and tolerability
2. Hawthorn
3. See Stomachic Teas (Species stomachicae) (p. 323)
4. Valerian root with hops strobiles
5. Ginseng

Answers

Chapter 12, see Questions (p. 344)
1. Yes
2. Their therapeutic range
3. German chamomile flowers
4. Calamus
5. Coltsfoot
6. Lemon balm leaves, passionflower herb

Answers

Chapter 13, see Questions (p. 349)
1. No
2. For example, colchicine, vinca alkaloids, Taxol
3. Mistletoe

18 Photo Credits

Prof. Dr. Volker Fintelmann, Hamburg, Germany:
Fig. 3.14b, Fig. 3.28, Fig. 3.35, Fig. 4.10, Fig. 8.4, Fig. 8.5, Fig. 9.5

Naturfoto Franke Heckler, Panten-Hammer, Germany:
Fig. 3.26, Fig. 4.2, Fig. 5.12

Thieme, Stuttgart, Germany:
Fig. 3.27, Fig. 4.8a, Fig. 5.1, Fig. 8.1, Fig. 9.4

All other photographs: Dr. Roland Spohn, Engen, Germany

Index

Note: Page numbers set **bold** or *italic* indicate headings or figures, respectively.

Index

Index